Ultrasonography in Gynecology

Ultrasonography in Gynecology

Edited by

Botros R. M. B. Rizk, MD, FRCOG, FACOG, HCLD, FACS, FRCS(C)
Professor of Obstetrics and Gynecology and Director of the Division of Reproductive Endocrinology and Infertility, University of South Alabama College of Medicine, Mobile, AL, USA; President Elect, Middle East Fertility Society

Elizabeth E. Puscheck, MD, MS, FACOG
Professor and Chair of the Department of Obstetrics and Gynecology, Director of Gynecologic Ultrasound, Wayne State University Medical School, Detroit, MI, USA

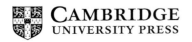

CAMBRIDGE
UNIVERSITY PRESS

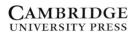

University Printing House, Cambridge CB2 8BS, United Kingdom

Cambridge University Press is part of the University of Cambridge.

It furthers the University's mission by disseminating knowledge in the pursuit of
education, learning and research at the highest international levels of excellence.

www.cambridge.org
Information on this title: www.cambridge.org/9781107029743

First published 2015

Printed in Spain by Grafos SA, Arte sobre papel

A catalogue record for this publication is available from the British Library

Library of Congress Cataloguing in Publication data
Ultrasonography in gynecology / [edited by] Botros R. M. B. Rizk,
Elizabeth E. Puscheck.
    p. ; cm.
Includes bibliographical references and index.
ISBN 978-1-107-02974-3 (hardback)
I. Rizk, Botros, editor.   II. Puscheck, Elizabeth E., editor.
[DNLM: 1. Genital Diseases, Female–ultrasonography.   2. Genitalia, Female–
ultrasonography.   3. Gynecologic Surgical Procedures–methods. WP 141]
RG527.5.U48
618.1'07543–dc23
2014032219

ISBN 978-1-107-02974-3 Hardback

I would like to dedicate this book
to my sisters Dr Sohair Mitry Rizk (1951–1994) and
Dr Mary Mitry Rizk
for their extraordinary love and support
Botros Rizk

Contents

About the editors

Botros Rizk

Dr. Botros R. M. B. Rizk is Professor of Obstetrics and Gynecology, Head of the Division of Reproductive Endocrinology and Infertility and Medical and Scientific Director of USA ART program at the University of South Alabama College of Medicine, Alabama, USA.

Dr. Rizk is the president elect of the Middle East Fertility Society, and past chair of the ASRM international membership committee. He is scientific advisory board member of the Mediterranean Society for Reproductive Medicine. Dr. Rizk chaired and lectured in many of the ASRM post-graduate courses over the last 20 years and the AIUM/ASRM post-graduate ultrasound course.

His main research interests are ovarian stimulation, ovarian hyperstimulation syndrome, and endoscopic surgery. Dr. Rizk has edited and authored 16 medical textbooks on infertility and assisted reproduction, ovarian stimulation, endometriosis, ultrasonography in reproductive medicine, ovarian hyperstimulation syndrome, and the future of ART. He has authored more than 400 peer-reviewed original and review papers, abstracts and book chapters.

Elizabeth Puscheck

Elizabeth Puscheck, MD is professor and chair of obstetrics and gynecology at Wayne State Medical School, Michigan, USA. Dr. Puscheck is an authority in ultrasound in gynecology and Director of Gynecologic Ultrasound unit at Wayne State Medical School. She chaired and lectured many of the AIUM/ASRM post-graduate courses.

Preface

This book of ultrasonography in gynecology represents the state-of-the-art in this ever-advancing field in medicine. The authors of every chapter of this book are world-renowned in their respective fields. The book layout and chapters allow the authors to present one of the largest collections of cases in benign and malignant gynecological disease as well as infertility. They take the reader step by step from the basic to the most complicated cases, and the text is rich in ultrasonographic figures rather than a theoretical text of limited value. Ultrasonograhy in gynecology is recommended reading for every gynecologist, ultrasonographer, radiologist, and infertility specialist.

The book is composed of five sections. The first section describes the techniques of ultrasonography such as three-dimensional ultrasonography, and compares the findings to other imaging techniques such as hysteroscopy and hysterosalpingography. The consents and patient counseling for ultrasonography are clearly described.

The second section covers benign gynecological diseases in great elegance. Polycystic ovarian syndrome, endometriosis and uterine septum are gracefully presented in clearly visualized cases. Pelvic floor ultrasound has become an area of interest that aids the gynecological surgeon in achieving a high precision and success of pelvic floor surgery. Uterine anomalies are presented case by case, comparing hysterosalpingography with hysteroscopy and 2D and 3D ultrasonography. The authors demonstrate that routine hysterosalpingography is inadequate to demonstrate the subtle anomalies, such as small uterine septae, for which hysteroscopy is recommended. The uterine fibroids are covered in three different chapters, one of which is dedicated to uterine artery embolization.

The third section is dedicated to ectopic pregnancy in six different chapters. The first chapter discusses the evaluation and management of ectopic pregnancy, providing tremendous clinical information that enables the ultrasonographer and clinician to evaluate and treat ectopic pregnancy. Interstitial and cesarean scar pregnancies are increasing in frequency. A good array of images helps the clinician to diagnose and manage these cases. Abdominal pregnancies are rare but clearly demonstrated. Heterotopic pregnancies are increasing as a result of assisted reproduction and multiple embryo transfer.

The fourth section is gynecological malignancies. Gestational trophoblastic neoplasia is elegantly presented. Ovarian and endometrial cancer affects a different demographic population, and ultrasound is very valuable in the preoperative assessment of these patients. Ovarian masses are very common in everyday clinical practice and are clearly presented to help make a spot diagnosis.

The fifth section deals with ultrasonography in infertility. The use of ultrasound imaging in onestop fertility diagnosis is of great convenience to infertile couples. Detailed ultrasound assessment before the IVF cycles ensures successful outcome. Assessment of ovarian reserve could be accomplished by hormonal evaluation such as anti-mullerian hormone; however, ultrasonographic assessment of antral follicle count is most predictive of the patient's response to gonadotropins. Ultrasound monitoring of ovulation induction and transvaginal ultrasonography for oocyte retrieval and embryo transfer is the cornerstone of successful in vitro fertilization cycle. Prediction, prevention and management of hyperstimulation syndrome could be safely accomplished by the expert ultrasonographic evaluation of patients undergoing assisted reproduction. It is possible that in the future self-operated vaginal ultrasound monitoring of follicular growth in assisted reproduction using the Internet could allow the monitoring of patients who do not have daily access to the ART program. Ultrasound-guided fallopian tube catheterization is of tremendous value in the management of tubal factor infertility. The application of ultrasonography to detect multiple pregnancies after ART and congenital anomalies is the basis for successful and safe outcome of pregnancies after ART. Finally, we put in your hands, our dear readers, a clinical text that we hope will be a great addition to your gynecological practice.

The editors would like to thank the authors and ultrasonographers for their most outstanding work. We would also like to thank the staff of Cambridge University Press for their skill and effort in the production of this valuable book.

Botros Rizk
Elizabeth Puscheck

Contributors

Amr Abbasy, MD
Lecturer in Obstetrics and Gynecology, National Research Centre, Cairo, Egypt

Mostafa I. Abuzeid, MD, FACOG, FRCOG
Director of Reproductive Endocrinology and Infertility, Division of Reproductive Endocrinology and Infertility, Department of Obstetrics and Gynecology, Hurley Medical Center, Flint, MI, USA; IVF Michigan, Rochester Hills, MI, USA; Professor of Obstetrics and Gynecology, Michigan State University College of Human Medicine, East Lansing (Flint Campus), MI, USA

Omar M. Abuzeid, BA
Research Assistant, IVF Michigan, Rochester Hills, MI, USA; Alfaisal University Medical School, Riyadh, Saudi Arabia

Gautam N. Allahbadia, MD, DNB, FNAMS
Medical Director, Rotunda – The Center for Human Reproduction, Rotunda Blue Fertility Clinic and Keyhole Surgery Center, Mumbai, India

Sarika Arora, MD
Chief Resident, Department of Obstetrics and Gynecology, Mount Sinai Hospital, Chicago, IL, USA

Norman Assad, MD
Associate Professor, Quillen Fertility and Women's Services, East Tennessee State University, Johnson City, TN, USA

Awoniyi O. Awonuga, MD, FACOG, FRCOG
Associate Professor, Residency Program Research Director, Division of Reproductive Endocrinology and Infertility, Department of Obstetrics and Gynecology, Wayne State University School of Medicine, Detroit, MI, USA

Osama M. Azmy, FRCOG, MD, DFFP
Professor of Obstetrics and Gynecology, National Research Centre, Cairo, Egypt

Shawky Z. A. Badawy, MD
Professor, Department of Obstetrics and Gynecology; Director, Division of Reproductive Endocrinology and Infertility, Upstate Medical University, Syracuse, NY, USA

Haitham Badran, MD
Lecturer in Obstetrics and Gynecology, Fayoum University, Egypt

Jashoman Banerjee, MD
Clinical Fellow, Reproductive Endocrinology and Infertility, Department of Obstetrics and Gynecology, Wayne State University School of Medicine, Detroit, MI, USA

M. N. Baumgarten, MD, MSc
Clinical Research Fellow, Nottingham University Research and Treatment Unit in Reproduction (NURTURE), Division of Obstetrics and Gynaecology, School of Clinical Sciences, University of Nottingham, UK

Donna C. Bennett, MD, FACOG
Assistant Professor, Division of Reproductive Endocrinology, Department of Obstetrics and Gynecology, University of South Alabama, AL, USA

Josef Blankstein, MD, ARDMS
Professor and Chairman, Department of Obstetrics and Gynecology, Rosalind Franklin University of Medicine and Science, The Chicago Medical School; Program Director, Mount Sinai Hospital, Chicago, IL, USA

Joel Brasch, MD
Assistant Professor, Department of Obstetrics and Gynecology, Rosalind Franklin University of Medicine and Science, The Chicago Medical School; Director, Chicago IVF, Chicago, IL, USA

Spyridon Chouliaras
Department of Reproductive Medicine, St. Mary's Hospital, CMFT University Hospitals, Manchester, UK

Kathryn H. Clarke, BS
Liberty University, Lynchburg, VA, USA; Life Interrupted Infertility Support Group Facilitator, Division of Reproductive Endocrinology and Infertility, Department of Obstetrics and Gynecology University of South Alabama, Mobile, AL, USA

Hans Peter Dietz, MD, PhD, FRANZCOG, DDU, CU

Professor, Department of Obstetrics and Gynaecology, Sydney Medical School Nepean, Penrith, NSW, Australia

Jan Gerris, MD, PhD

Professor, Centre for Reproductive Medicine, University Hospital Ghent, Ghent, Belgium

Harold Henning, MD

Clinical Assistant Professor, Department of Obstetrics and Gynecology, SUNY Upstate Medical University, Syracuse, NY

Candice P. Holliday, JD

Research Assistant, Division of Reproductive Endocrinology and Infertility, Department of Obstetrics and Gynecology, University of South Alabama, Mobile, AL, USA

Nicolette Holliday, MD

Assistant Professor, Co-Clerkship Director, Division of Reproductive Endocrinology and Infertility, Department of Obstetrics and Gynecology, University of South Alabama, Mobile, AL, USA

Sadie Hutson, PhD, RN, WHNP, BC

Associate Professor, College of Nursing, University of Tennessee-Knoxville, Knoxville, TN, USA

Kannamannadiar Jayaprakasan, MBBS, MD, MRCOG, PhD

Associate Professor in Reproductive Medicine and Surgery/ Consultant Gynaecologist, Division of Obstetrics and Gynaecology, School of Clinical Sciences, University of Nottingham, UK

Samuel Johnson, MD

Department of Radiology, Wayne State University School of Medicine, Detroit, MI, USA

Salem K. Joseph, BS

Research Assistant, IVF Michigan, Rochester Hills, MI, USA; University of Michigan, Ann Arbor, MI, USA

Asim Kurjak, MD, PhD

Professor, Department of Obstetrics and Gynecology, Medical School University of Zagreb, Zagreb, Croatia

John LaFleur, MD

Assistant Professor, Division of Reproductive Endocrinology and Infertility, Department of Obstetrics and Gynecology, University of South Alabama, Mobile, AL, USA

David F. Lewis, MD

Professor and Chair, Department of Obstetrics and Gynecology, University of South Alabama, Mobile, AL, USA

Kazuo Maeda

Department of Obstetrics and Gynecology (Emeritus), Tottori University Medical School, Yonago, Japan

Rizwan Malik, MD, FACOG

Clinical Assistant Professor, University of Indianapolis, Indianapolis, IN, USA

Ehab Abu Marar, MD

Fertility Specialist, Jeddah, Saudi Arabia and Fellow of UKS-H, Campus Luebeck, Germany

Rubina Merchant, PhD

Embryologist, Rotunda – Center for Human Reproduction, Mumbai, India

Luciano G. Nardo, MD, MRCOG

Clinical Director, Consultant Gynaecologist and Subspecialist in Reproductive Medicine Reproductive Health Group, Centre for Reproductive Health, Daresbury Park, Daresbury, UK

Geeta Nargund, MBBS, FRCOG

Head of Reproductive Medicine, St. George's Hospital, London; Medical Director, Centre for Reproduction and Advanced Technology (CREATE), London, UK

Sheri A. Owens, MD

Assistant Professor, Division of Reproductive Endocrinology and Infertility, Department of Obstetrics and Gynecology, University of South Alabama, Mobile, AL, USA

Sree Durga Patchava, MD, MRCOG

Department of Reproductive Medicine, St. Mary's Hospital, CMFT University Hospitals, Manchester, UK

L. T. Polanski, MBBS

Clinical Research Fellow, Nottingham University Research and Treatment Unit in Reproduction (NURTURE), Division of Obstetrics and Gynaecology, School of Clinical Sciences, University of Nottingham, UK

Misty M. Blanchette Porter, MD

Associate Professor and IVF/ART Medical Director, Department of Obstetrics and Gynecology, Dartmouth-Hitchcock Medical Center, Lebanon, NH, USA

Elizabeth E. Puscheck, MD, MS

Professor and Chair, Department of Obstetrics and Gynecology, Director of Gynecologic Ultrasound, Wayne State University Medical School, Detroit, MI, USA

Nicholas J. Raine-Fenning, MRCOG, MBChB, PhD

Reader in Reproductive Medicine and Surgery/Consultant Gynaecologist, Division of Obstetrics and Gynaecology, School of Clinical Sciences, University of Nottingham; Director of Research/Senior Consultant, Nottingham University Research and Treatment Unit in Reproduction (NURTURE), Nottingham, UK

Botros R. M. B. Rizk, MD, FRCOG, FACOG
Professor of Obstetrics and Gynecology and Director
of the Division of Reproductive Endocrinology and
Infertility, University of South Alabama College of
Medicine, Mobile, AL, USA; President Elect Middle East
Fertility Society

Valerie Shavell, MD
Department of Obstetrics and Gynecology, Wayne State
University Medical School, Detroit, MI, USA

Osama Shawki, MSc, MD
Professor, Department of Obstetrics and Gynecology,
Faculty of Medicine, Cairo University, Cairo, Egypt; Director,
Ebtesama Center for Advanced Endoscopic Surgery,
Al Ebtesama Hospital, Cairo, Egypt

James Shwayder, MD, JD
Professor and Chair, Department of Obstetrics and
Gynecology, University of Mississippi Medical Center,
Jackson, MS, USA

Bruce Singer, MD
Department of Radiology, Crouse Hospital, Syracuse,
NY, USA

Manvinder Singh, MD
Division of Reproductive Endocrinology and Infertility,
Department of Obstetrics and Gynecology, Wayne State
University School of Medicine, Detroit, MI, USA

Beverly A. Spirt, MD, FACR
Clinical Professor, Department of Radiology, Upstate Medical
University, Syracuse, NY, USA

Julie Sroga, MD
Clinical Instructor, Division of Reproductive Endocrinology,
University of Cincinnati, Cincinnati, OH, USA

Bradley J. Van Voorhis, MD
Vice Chair for Gynecology, Department of Obstetrics and
Gynecology, University of Iowa Hospitals, Iowa City, IA, USA

Amr Hassan Wahba, MD
Lecturer, Department of Obstetrics and Gynecology,
Faculty of Medicine, Cairo University, Cairo, Egypt;
Fellow of Cologne University Hospital, Cologne, Germany;
Department of Obstetrics and Gynecology,
Nottingham University Hospital, UK

Carrie Warshak, MD
Assistant Professor and Director of Ultrasound, Division of
Maternal Fetal Medicine, University of Cincinnati, Cincinnati,
OH, USA

Terri L. Woodard, MD
Clinical Fellow, Reproductive Endocrinology and Infertility,
Department of Obstetrics and Gynecology, Wayne State
University School of Medicine, Detroit, MI, USA

Three-dimensional ultrasonography in gynecology

Norman A. Assad and Sadie Hutson

3D ultrasound in gynecology

Three-dimensional ultrasound (3D US) was first developed by Olaf von Ramm and Stephen Smith at Duke University, Durham, NC in 1987. 3D US imaging extends the diagnostic acumen of the practitioner by providing an additional and very unique tool for the assessment and interpretation of both normal and abnormal pelvic anatomy. The images that are acquired and analyzed enable the operator to gain a perspective that goes beyond the physical examination and images produced by conventional two-dimensional US. The addition of power Doppler in 3D offers an additional clinical assessment of the vasculature of an organ, and may be an important research tool in the ongoing quest to diagnose pathology such as ovarian cancer at a much earlier and potentially treatable stage.

In general, current 3D US imaging systems are based on commercially available, one-dimensional, or annular transducer arrays whose position is known accurately or monitored by a position-sensing device. Position data may be obtained from stepping motors in the scan head, a translation or rotation device, or a position sensor that may be electromagnetic, acoustic, or mechanical. During acquisition, 2D US images and position data are stored in a computer for subsequent reconstruction into 3D US data. Depending on the type of acquisition utilized, the serial slices may be the pattern of a wedge, a series of parallel slices, a rotation around a central axis (i.e. from an endocavitary probe), or arbitrary orientations.

In 2005, the American Institute of Ultrasound in Medicine held a consensus conference on Three- and Four-Dimensional Ultrasound in Obstetrics and Gynecology [1]. The summary stated that 3D US is becoming an important part of state-of-the art sonographic imaging in obstetrics and gynecology. It is a problem-solving tool in selected circumstances. It has the potential to improve practice efficiency and patient throughput without jeopardizing diagnostic capabilities. To become widely accepted, however, work must be done by several groups, including manufacturers, to make the 3D US systems faster and more user-friendly. Additionally, standards must be established for transmission and storage of volume data; educational efforts must be expanded for teaching practitioners how to use and interpret these results. Further, medical societies and the industry need to reach a consensus about how to standardize imaging protocols and display. The panel proposed several recommendations to encourage the use of 3D US for clinical care, teaching, and research in obstetric and gynecologic ultrasound.

Acquisition of volume datasets

With the author's equipment (General Electric [GE] Voluson i) [2], the acquisition of volume datasets is performed by 2D scans with special transducers designed for 2D scans (Fig. 1.1). The 3D sweep and the real-time 4D scans are visualizations of the 3D images in real time. The volume acquisition is started using a 2D image with superimposed VOL-Box or using a 2D+Color image. In the case of a 2D+Color image, the Color-Box is at the same time as the VOL-Box. The 2D start image represents the central 2D scan of the volume. The volume scan itself sweeps from one margin to the other margin of the volume to be acquired. The VOL-Box frames the region of interest (ROI), which will be stored during the volume sweep. The display shows the actual 2D scan.

The sweep time varies and depends on the VOL-Box size (depth, range, and angle) and the quality (six positions). The probe must be held steady and in place during the 3D volume scan. The real-time display of the swept B frames allows continuous observation of the scan quality. During the real-time 4D scan, it is not necessary to hold the probe steady because of the continuous volume acquisition.

The volume scan is automatically performed by a tilt movement of the 2D scan head. The scanned volume is similar to a section of a torus (Fig. 1.2).

3D image rendering

The 3D image rendering is a calculation process to visualize certain 3D structures of a scanned volume via a 2D image. The gray value for each pixel of the 2D image is calculated from

Transducer type:

Fig. 1.1 Transducer types.

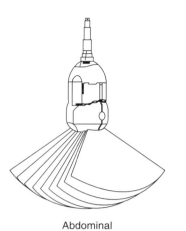 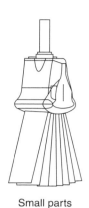 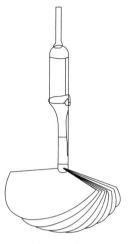

Abdominal   Small parts   Transvaginal

the voxels along the corresponding projection path (analyzing beam) through the volume. The render (calculation) algorithm surface or transparent mode decides which 3D structures are visualized.

All 3D imaging techniques using a transvaginal probe require that a planar beam of US be swept over the anatomy by use of a 1D transducer array, which is usually mechanical. With 3D ultrasonography, a volume of a target anatomic region, which contains an infinite number of planes, can be acquired. Such volume can then be displayed in three orthogonal 2D planes, representing the sagittal, transverse, and coronal planes of a reference 2D image within the volume. Using various rotations along the X, Y, and Z anatomic axes, the operator has the ability to display any reconstructed 2D plane within the volume. Despite the significant advances offered by 3D US, the acquisition, display, and manipulation of 3D volumes is a technique that requires a substantial learning curve. The ability to automate the retrieval of 2D diagnostic planes out of a 3D volume has significant advantages in clinical practice. This application, which is made available through the advances in 3D ultrasonography, has the potential to allow for an automated display out of a volume of all the 2D planes that are required for a complete anatomic evaluation of the targeted organ within the acquired volume (Fig. 1.3).

In some settings, the manner in which this can be accomplished is by holding a transvaginal probe stationary while the 3D volume is acquired with the push of a button. It is necessary for the patient to remain still during the acquisition of the volume in order to prevent artifacts and distortion. This is particularly important when acquiring power Doppler measurements. The original sweep is done by keeping the acquisition "box" as close to the scanned organ as possible, then on the rendered image any extraneous background can be removed with the Magicut feature (akin to cropping a photograph).

After the 2D US images have been acquired, the 3D US data can be reconstructed. The author's facility uses the GE Voluson

Central 20-gcan

Start 20-gcan

Range of VOL-sweed

Fig. 1.2 VOL-box: acquisition of the voxel for manipulation on the 3D software.

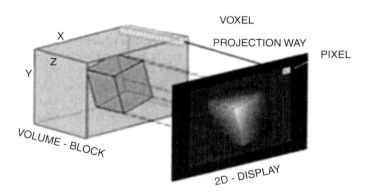

VOXEL

PROJECTION WAY

PIXEL

X

Z

Y

VOLUME - BLOCK

2D - DISPLAY

Fig. 1.3 "Voxel box": 3D sweep captures the entire organ being scanned.

i with E8 and 4D view software (4D view) provided by GE and designed by the Kretztechnik Company (Zipf, Austria). One challenge is that the software is only operative with Windows XP. Current modifications will make it compatible for use with Windows 7 software. Most manufacturers of 3D equipment offer their comparable version of software, which is compatible with their specific equipment.

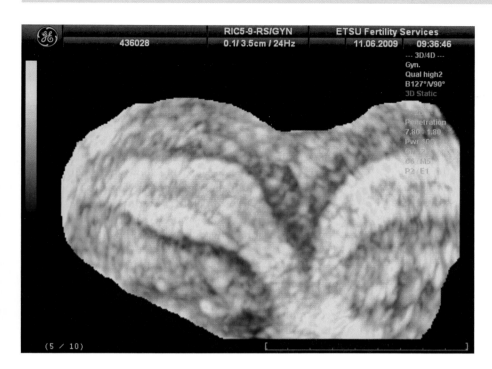

Fig. 1.4 Bicornuate uterus.

Volume data display modes

Volume data can be displayed in three ways: (1) color information alone, (2) grayscale information alone, or (3) a combination of both referred to as "glass body" mode.

Once the images have been rendered on the software, a vast array of features can be determined, including morphologic changes and assessments of color and power Doppler parameters. In addition, the Tomographic Ultrasound Imaging (TUI) feature will allow serial sectioning of the images similar to obtaining tissue slices of an organ in a pathology lab. The slice measurements can be varied. It is also possible to study both uterine and ovarian images using the Inversion Modalities on the software. These include surface rendering of the image – allowing for a more detailed look at the surface contours of a lesion. Image settings include six color settings. Some practitioners prefer to utilize the "candlelight" or "sepia" modalities as this seems to offer optimal visualization. Each individual provider, however, may prefer any of the color settings available with their particular software for optimal visualization of the organ being assessed. Utilizing Virtual Organ Computer-aided AnaLysis (VOCAL), it is possible to accurately determine the volume of an ovary or other pelvic structure. The software allows measurements from 6 degrees to 30 degrees; however, most of the author's assessments utilize the 15-degree parameter. VOCAL 2 software also has a "sphere" modality where power vascular parameters can be measured within a given area. The "Niche" features enable a cutaway of the central portion of an organ. It is also possible to utilize the "Magicut" feature to cut away extraneous images and areas around the focal area of the organ being studied and enables the organ to be "highlighted" for further study. It is then possible to rotate the images between 30 and 60 degrees at 15-degree increments. The axis can be rotated in either the X or Y plane. This is particularly useful to look into the contours of the uterus on study of a coronal plane of the uterus, to examine the details of the vasculature of an ovary, or to study the anatomic details of a fallopian tube.

Using the VOCAL software in 4D endometrial and ovarian volume datasets, Raine-Fenning et al. [3] tested the interobserver reliability of the results and determined an inter-class correlation coefficient of 0.9 in both organs. The authors concluded that 3D US can reliably be used to acquire, analyze, and define ovarian endometrial volumes.

Specific displays in 3D US

1. *Multiplanar navigation.* The image acquired during the 3D sweep is manipulated on the software to give a coronal view of the uterus. It is then possible to visualize congenital anomalies of the uterus, as well as any pathology, such as uterine fibroids, polyps, intrauterine synechiae, or in the case of a pregnant patient the location of the fetus within the uterine cavity including those pregnancies in an anomalous or abnormal uterus (Fig. 1.4).
2. *Thick slice VCI.* Thick slice VCI allows enhancement of picture quality and the ability to visualize abnormal contours or pathology within the uterus.
3. *Surface rendering.* Surface rendering allows visualization of the organ with varying degrees of contrast and light.
4. *Angiography.* Angiography allows visualization of vessel morphology in both color and power Doppler mode. It is possible to examine vessel aberrations including strictures,

dilatations, "lakes" (pools of color in the image), or orderly versus chaotic vascular patterns.

5. *Inversion.* Inversion mode rendering is a more recently introduced display mode, which starts from the minimum mode rendering and inverts merely the color of the information (similar to negative/positive film), thus presenting the hypoechoic structures as echogenic solids. It blackens most of the surrounding tissue information. By changing certain settings such as increasing the "threshold" and decreasing the transparency, the image can be improved. Choosing either the "gradient light" or the "light" rendering assists in getting the most from the image. This allows some unique views of uterine anomalies and also allows one to visualize antral follicles in the ovary. Two articles published in 2005, Timor-Tritsch et al. and Lee et al. [4,5], describe 3D inversion rendering in gynecology.

6. *X-ray mode.* X-ray mode also allows for visualization of denser structures within the scanned organ; however, the author has found little application for this modality in gynecologic US.

Pelvic organ scanning

It is essential when scanning patients to have a comprehensive medical history regarding their complaints, including the date of the last normal menstrual period. This is required in order to interpret the findings in relation to the day of the menstrual cycle. It is important to be able to distinguish normal anatomic changes from pathologic changes. Frequently, the word "cyst" is utilized instead of "follicle." This can engender much anxiety on the part of patients, who may misinterpret normal findings as "pathologic." It is important for the operator to interpret both uterine and ovarian findings in relation to the day of the cycle in order avoid confusion of normal findings as pathologic. It is also important to know the gynecologic history, obstetrical history, and any other pertinent symptom or history information that could assist in an accurate diagnosis.

Both the uterus and cervix can be rendered in 3D US. More frequently, the addition of the saline sonohysterogram (SIS) enhances uterine findings as it allows for more contrast imaging when interpreting findings. The author routinely uses either a Sonde rigid catheter (Laboratoire C.C.D. Paris, France) or a Gynecath Catheter (Cooper Surgical, Trumbull, CT) for the performance of this test. If possible, the author also prefers to avoid the catheter with a balloon as it is more likely to produce distortion artifact when interpreting 3D US images. Visualizing the coronal plane of the uterus on rendered US images allows for interpretation of a variety of conditions. In 2D studies, SIS is shown to improve the sensitivity, specificity, and positive predictive value in myomas. Further, SIS proved to have both a higher sensitivity than simple transvaginal sonography examination for diffuse lesions and a better specificity for focal lesions. SIS is superior to transvaginal sonography (TVS)

in the identification of endometrial polyps in the assessment of hysteroscopic operability of submucosal myomas [6]. SIS can reduce the number of unnecessary diagnostic hysteroscopies and permits a better surgical strategy in selected patients [7,8].

The entire uterus should be scanned in the 3D modality. It is important to keep the rendering box as close to the uterus as possible to exclude any other external artifacts. The angle of scan for a uterus is usually set to 90 degrees.

1. *Congenital anomalies.* The internal contours of the uterus are accurately imaged and allow for visualization of any uterine anomalies, including an arcuate, septate, bicornuate, or uterus didelphys. Uterine anomalies can result in impaired vascularization of a pregnancy and limited space for a fetus due to distortion of the uterine cavity.

    Inversion mode can be utilized with 3D US to give unique imaging in the instance of both unicornuate and bicornuate uteri. Approximately 12–15% of women with recurrent abortion have a uterine malformation. Of all of the possible uterine malformations, complete or partially septate uterus is the most common major anomaly, occurring about one-third of the time; it is associated with the poorest pregnancy outcomes. This anomaly is the most receptive to treatment and successful treatment results in a term delivery rate of 75% and a live birth rate of 85% [9]. The accuracy of diagnosing a septate uterus with 3D US is almost 98% [10].

2. *Uterine pathology.* Polyps and submucosal fibroids can be plainly visualized in relationship to the endometrial surface. In addition to the size and relationship of these pathologic processes to the endometrium, the consistency of the lesion can also be imaged. It is also possible to distinguish between type 0, type 1, and type 2 submucosal fibroids. Submucosal fibroids are by US typically hypoechoic and displace the basalis layer of the endometrium. The amount of extension into the myometrial layer is important in determining the intramural component and in determining the type of surgical procedure to be recommended. Superficial submucosal fibroids with a thin stalk may be removed by a wire loop or alligator forceps, whereas those that extend beyond the endometrial–myometrial interface may be better treated with vaporization or wire loop resection. Fibroids compared with polyps show more heterogeneous echogenicity and more often have a sessile attachment. Polyps tend to have homogeneous echogenicity and have a pedunculated attachment to the uterine wall without interruption of the endometrial lining. Color or power Doppler modes are useful to distinguish myomas from polyps or uterine malignancies. Myomas have a typical vascularization pattern of the capsule, which forms a circle, whereas polyps have a vascular pedicle. Malignancies have an abundant irregular vessel distribution [11] (Fig. 1.5).

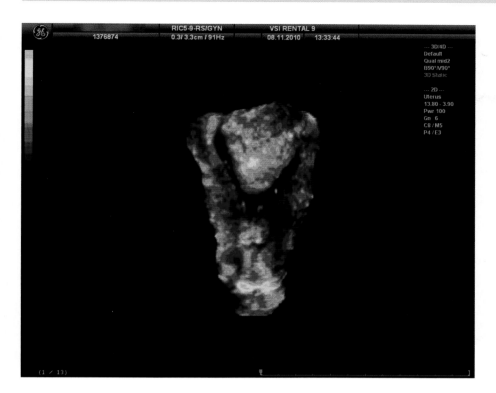

Fig. 1.5 Submucosal fibroid. Type 2.

- 3D US allows for postoperative evaluation of the endometrium to evaluate the results of surgery.
- 3D US also allows for complete visualization of an intrauterine contraceptive device (IUCD) by visualizing the device in the coronal plane.
- 3D US delineates intrauterine synechiae and these images assist the surgeon in preoperative planning when done prior to the surgery. Hysteroscopic treatment of synechiae can markedly improve both menstrual irregularity and reproductive outcome [12].
- 3D US utilizing SIS will also allow for coronal views of the uterus in patients with recurrent miscarriage to insure that there is no other intrauterine pathology or "funneling of the cervix," which may be associated with incompetent cervix.
- 3D SIS can be utilized to evaluate the endometrial changes seen with tamoxifen therapy and give greater detail of the anatomic changes present.
- 3D US can be used to diagnose complications in early pregnancy. These include early diagnosis of ectopic pregnancy, evaluation of the relationship between the gestational sac and uterine septum, and the location of an ectopic pregnancy. It can detect both the presence and volume of a subchorionic hemorrhage, and identify decreased gestational sac volume.

Analysis of the vascular pattern of the endometrium during the menstrual cycle has been described by Raine-Fenning et al. [13]. The study demonstrated that both endometrial and subendometrial vascular flow increased to a maximum 3 days prior to ovulation, then decreased until post-ovulatory day 5, and finally began a gradual increase during the remainder of the luteal phase. The proliferative phase increment was related to estradiol levels and its vasodilating effects, while the luteal phase increase was related to serum progesterone. The flow indices continued to increase during menstruation, regardless of the drastic fall in progesterone levels. This might be explained by the high endometrial vascular density due to progressive compaction of the spiral arteries. The reduction in the post-ovulatory vascular indices is explained by vasodilatation of the subepithelial capillary plexus, which induces the required stromal edema to allow embryo implantation. Therefore, 3D US is a reliable technique for investigating cyclic, physiologic changes in the endometrial vascularization. 3D US allows prompt, integrated evaluation of all known receptivity markers by measuring endometrial thickness, texture, pattern, volume, and global perfusion. While there is currently no reliable ultrasonographic predictor of endometrial receptivity for patients undergoing assisted reproductive technology (ART) (except to predict patients who will have little chance of conception), further comparative studies are needed to establish cut-off values in order to counsel patients about their prognosis regarding endometrial receptivity [14].

3. *Cervical pathology.* Visualization of nabothian follicles, cervical polyps, and endocervical cancer can be made with this modality. 3D US can also be useful in determining the features of a cervical pregnancy. By displaying the "thick

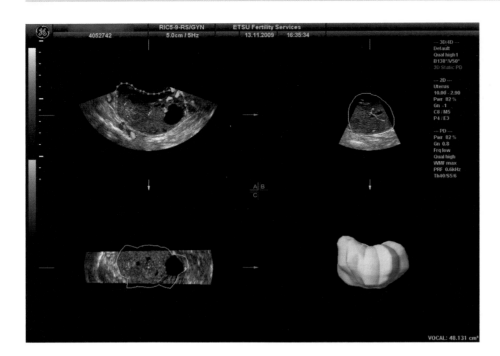

Fig. 1.6 Rendering "power Doppler" scan of ovary to give an accurate volume of that structure.

slice" mode, 3D can enhance the distinct features of the anatomy as well as the chorionic ring. The total separation between the cavity and the ectopic sac becomes more distinct, helping to make the diagnosis. Similar features are useful in diagnosing a cornual or interstitial pregnancy.

4. *Fallopian tube.* 3D scanning allows critical differentiation of the fallopian tube if pathology is involved. Hydrosalpinx has a definitive appearance on 3D ultrasound. After the volume of the tube is obtained, rendering of the images allows the best plane to determine the true nature of the pathology. Demonstration of incomplete septa helps to ascertain that a hydrosalpinx is the appropriate diagnosis. Tubo-ovarian masses can also be more accurately diagnosed using this modality. Using color and power Doppler assists in the diagnosis of tubal torsion; however, this subject will be covered more completely when discussing vascular changes on 3D scanning of the ovary.

5. *Ovary.* 3D evaluation of the ovary brings a unique perspective to the interpretation of pathology. Several modalities can be studied in order to gain information regarding pathologic or growth parameters within the ovary. While scanning the ovary it is necessary to keep the rendering box as close to the ovary as possible to rule out any extraneous artifacts. Most 3D sweeps through the ovary are done at the 60-degree setting on the ultrasound machine.

The first modality that is evaluated is the morphology of the ovary. Morphologic assessment by 3D US yields additional information over that of 2D scans. While endometriomas, benign cystic teratomas, and theca lutein cysts have a specific appearance on 2D scans, the unique features of malignancy are visualized in more detail utilizing 3D modality. The latter allows the ability to look inside the cyst and study the surface changes in more detail (Figs 1.6 and 1.7).

Features to be evaluated in an ovary to distinguish malignancy include the thickness of wall structures. Goldstein and Timor-Tritsch [15] use an arbitrary cut-off of 4 mm to distinguish lesions that are more likely to be malignant. Septation and loculation is also another finding that can raise the suspicion for malignancy. Multilocularity is more common in tumors of low malignant potential and malignant neoplasms. Papillations are also significant in assessing the morphology of the ovary and are more suspicious for malignant neoplasms. Papillae that contain blood vessels with detectable flow are more suspicious for malignancy. Exacoustos et al. [16] found that papillae as large as 15 mm in height and 10 mm in width were present in 48% of borderline tumors, but in only 4% of benign and 4% of malignant tumors. However, when papillations were larger, the lesions were present in 48% of invasive ovarian tumors, 18% of borderline tumors, and 7% of benign masses. Internal echo structure can indicate the present of particulate matter such as blood, cellular matter, or even mucoid material. A mass with mixed echogenicity can been found in either teratomas or malignancy. Shadowing, if present, may suggest the presence of an extremely dense tissue such as bone or calcification, indicating the probability of a benign teratoma. Malignant masses very rarely display frank shadowing.

In general, the larger the lesion, the more suspicious it is for malignancy. Malignant tumors usually have a complex appearance with thick walls greater than 4 mm, as well as a heterogeneous texture, multilocularity, solid

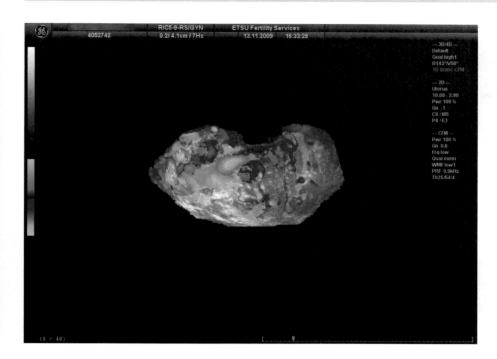

Fig. 1.7 Color Doppler acquisition of ovary showing "beach ball structures, strictures, and loss of tree-like vascularity" [32]. This lesion was a granulosa cell tumor of the ovary.

components, and papillary excrescences, particularly those demonstrating a lush blood supply. Timmerman and colleagues [17] published a report that illustrated five simple rules to predict malignancy: (1) irregular solid tumor, (2) ascites, (3) at least four papillary structures, (4) irregular multilocular-solid tumor with a largest diameter of at least 100 mm, and (5) very high color content on color Doppler examination. Five simple rules suggested a benign tumor: (1) unilocular cyst, (2) presence of solid components, where the largest solid component is less than 7 mm in largest diameter, (3) acoustic shadows, (4) smooth multilocular tumor less than 100 mm in largest diameter, and (5) no detectable blood flow on Doppler examination.

According to a technology assessment from the Agency for Healthcare Research and Quality (AHRQ), "conventional gray-scale ultrasonography is the most common imaging modality used to differentiate benign from malignant adnexal masses." Hopefully, 3D US using some of the study material displayed below will help to assist in the differentiation of benign from malignant lesions.

An opinion from the International Ovarian Tumor Analysis (IOTA) group regarding the terms, definitions, and measurements to describe the sonographic features of adnexal tumors [18] is described in this article.

Sensitivity and specificity of multimodal and ultrasound screening for ovarian cancer and stage distribution of detected cancers were published in the UK Collaborative Trial of Ovarian Cancer Screening (UKCTOCS) [19] and the results were encouraging as the sensitivity of the multimodal screening (MMS) was greater than the ultrasound screening (USS) group, resulting in lower rates of repeat testing and surgery. This in part reflects the high prevalence of benign adnexal abnormalities and the more frequent detection of borderline tumors in the USS group.

Amor et al. [20] described a Gynecologic Imaging Reporting and Data System that showed good diagnostic performance. The system is simple and could facilitate communication between sonographers/sonologists and clinicians.

3D power Doppler angiography

3D power Doppler angiography is a sonographic angiogram created by power Doppler-based identification of the blood flow of the vascular tree, where the vessel diameter is about 0.5–1 mm and blood velocity exceeds 2–3 mm per second [21].

For power Doppler scans, the author sets the Quality at high, the wall motion filter (WMF) at low, and the pulse repetition frequency (PRF) at 0.9. The scanning angle for ovaries is generally set at 60 degrees. These settings are used for scanning a known lesion. However, for screening, it has been suggested that the WMF is set to maximum. Unfortunately, the literature is confounded by the lack of standardization of settings, which can differ even within the 3D equipment of one manufacturer, much less the variation that occurs between different vendors and operators. Further research is urgently required in order to determine power Doppler parameters for the "normal" population. After the image is acquired, the render mode is then utilized to visualize the vessels in the entire volume after the color option is selected. Programs such as VOCAL software can be used to outline the contour of the ovary. Next, press the "Manual" button, followed by the degree tracing (6, 9, 15 or 30 degrees). Customarily, 15 degrees is utilized followed

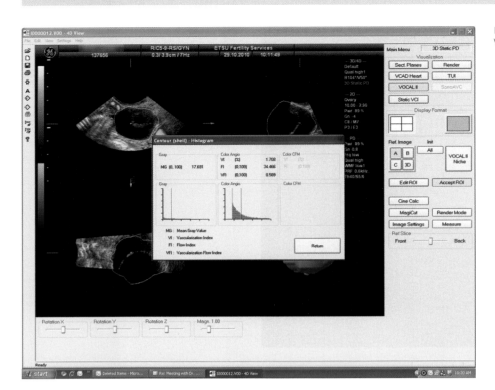

Fig. 1.8 . Histogram of the ovary documenting VI, FI, and VFI.

by employing the trace feature on the software to outline the ovary at each rotation. When the process is complete a volume shell of the ovary is displayed along with the volumetric assessment and size of the organ. From there it is possible to render the structure by the aforementioned "glass body" appearance, which then allows the user to visualize the vasculature within the ovary, display the vessels in the structure, or activate the histogram button on the software to give the various vascularization indices of the ovary. These are expressed as the vascularization index (VI), the flow index (FI), or the vascularization flow index (VFI) as a percentage between 1% and 100% (Fig. 1.8).

- The VI [22] represents the vessels in the tissue and is important in diagnosing high and low vascularization.
- The FI, a mean amplitude value, is important to characterize high-flow intensities that are seen more often in malignant tumors.
- The VFI is a combination of VI and FI, and identifies the extremes between low vascularization and low blood flow versus high vascularization and high blood flow.

Although VI and FI showed excellent reproducibility, VFI did not achieve accurate estimation between two observers, which might lead to unreliable measurements. In the future with further research there may be better evidence as to whether the VI and FI will become good predictors for neovascularization. This could then replace qualitative or semi-quantitative 3D power Doppler evaluations. Technologic developments, application of new indices for quantification of vascularization and

blood flow using the cube method, and simultaneous Doppler shift spectrum analysis will hopefully increase the usefulness of these new modalities.

Combining power Doppler and 3D tissue vascularization can be studied. Once the organ volume has been determined then the histogram produces various indices such as the VI, the FI, and the VFI.

A non-malignant source of morbidity involving the ovary is adnexal torsion. There is some suggestion that the diagnosis might be enhanced with power Doppler studies. Fleischer [23] has described changes consistent with adnexal torsion. These include detection of central flow, which is associated with still viable adnexa, and flow which is not present in the mass but in the capsular area around the mass. The "pedicle" sign [24,25] has been described and consists of color or power Doppler imaging of a spiral arrangement or coiling of the blood vessels that is highly suggestive of torsion of the fallopian tube or ovary. While not always present, when seen it is highly diagnostic for torsion.

Traditionally in 2D US scans, transvaginal color Doppler imaging allows tumor vascularization assessment. With publication of the study by Kurjak et al. in 1991 [26] there was hope that a resistance index (RI) of less than 0.4 would differentiate between benign and malignant masses. Fleischer et al. [27], in a group of ovarian masses using pulsatility index (PI) of less than 1 as the cut-off, found a sensitivity of 100% and a specificity of 83% with a positive predictive value of 73%. However, subsequent papers have failed to validate the predictive values of color flow assessment in ovarian tumors. There is no good published evidence that color or power

Doppler can be used to detect ovarian cancer in either pre-menopausal or postmenopausal women with normal-sized ovaries. Morphologic assessment of the ovaries with both 2D and 3D modalities continues to be scrutinized in an attempt to increase the likelihood of early detection and/or screening of ovarian cancer [28].

Various authors have endeavored to increase the sensitivity and specificity of diagnosis of ovarian carcinoma. Some major contributors include, but are not limited to, the following:

- In a study by Kurjak et al. [29], morphologic analysis by 3D US alone detected 74% of cancers ($N = 90$). Adding Doppler evaluation of tumor vascularity predicted 41 cases of stage 1 ovarian cancer, a 95.4% detection rate. Combined morphologic and 3D Doppler findings achieved a diagnostic accuracy of 97.7% [30].
- Chase et al. [31] published results of their study of preoperative diagnosis of ovarian malignancies using 3D vascular US. In this preliminary and observational study, chaotic vascular architecture correlated with malignancy in this group of high-risk patients.
- Crade [32] used a "Tissue Block" of data to analyze a variety of vascular features. These included loss of "treelike" branching of vessels, sacculation of arteries and veins, focal narrowing of arteries, internal shifts in velocity within arterial lumen, and the "Beach Ball" finding of abnormally increased and disorganized peripheral flow. Also noted was increased flow to the center of a solid region, crowding of vascularity and "start" and "stop" arteries found within a mass in a disjointed fashion losing the "tree-like" branching.
- Cohen et al. [33] concluded that 3D power Doppler evaluation defined the morphologic and vascular characteristics of ovarian lesions significantly better than 2D US alone. Specificity was significantly improved by the additional of 3D power Doppler analysis.
- Sladkevicius et al. [34] investigated the contribution of morphologic assessment of the vessel tree by 3D US to a correct diagnosis of malignancy in ovarian masses. The study concluded that subjective evaluation of the morphology of the vessel tree as depicted by 3D power Doppler US can be used to discriminate between benign and malignant tumors, but adds little to grayscale imaging in an ordinary population of tumors.
- Alcazar et al. [35] in an article entitled, "Three-dimensional sonographic morphologic assessment of adnexal masses: a reproducibility study" concluded that 3D sonography is a reproducible technique for morphologic assessment of adnexal masses.
- Other authors [36,37] have used "micro-bubble" (e.g. using harmonics or phase inverse imaging on grayscale or transient responses) enhanced sonography to depict microvessel perfusion. These techniques may allow assessment of tumor blood flow and changes that occur with treatment.

- Fleischer et al. [38] in an article entitled, "Contrast-enhanced transvaginal sonography of benign versus malignant ovarian masses," concluded that there was a significant difference in the contrast enhancement kinetic parameters between benign and malignant ovarian masses using "micro-bubble" technology.
- Prior to that, Marret et al. [39] showed that contrast-enhanced power Doppler imaging may easily and precisely discriminate benign from malignant adnexal lesions. Levomist was used in these studies.
- Several authors [40–42] have also used logistic regression analysis to further define the probability of malignancy in women with pelvic masses. Several prognostic variables were used in these articles to assess whether accuracy is better with a combination of variables than with the morphological Doppler criterion alone. This analysis shows promise and further studies are ongoing.
- Alcazar and Castillo [43] concluded that 3D power Doppler imaging did not have a better diagnostic performance than 2D power Doppler imaging for the discrimination of benign from malignant complex adnexal masses. However, another group of authors [44] concluded that evaluation by 3D US did improve the diagnosis of ovarian tumors.
- Kudla et al. [45] and Alcazar et al. [46,47] have utilized virtual spherical tissue sampling using 3D US power Doppler angiography to enhance differentiation between normal and pathologic ovaries. All three studies concluded that spherical sampling is a sensitive and promising approach to differentiate between ovarian tumors and normal ovaries. The most recent study from Alcazar depicted that 3D power Doppler vascular indices could be helpful for reducing the false-positive rate in cystic-solid and solid, vascularized adnexal masses [47].

The absolute critical values for these parameters (VI, VFI, and FI) remain to be determined; however, the higher the indices when interpreted in tandem with the morphologic changes in the ovaries, the greater the suspicion for ovarian carcinoma.

The utility of 3D US in the diagnosis of ovarian carcinoma is controversial and lacking in universal agreement. It has been established, however, that the morphology of both the ovaries and vasculature can be enhanced with this technology. When combined with an increase in the vascular parameters measured on the "histogram," the index of suspicion is enhanced with an increase in the vascularity of the lesion.

The morphologic structure of the blood vessels might also yield some valuable insight into the presence of a malignant lesion, particularly where a disordered pattern is noted. With the development of new and more sensitive probes such as matrix volume probes, it may be possible to study the micro-vasculature of the ovary in greater detail.

Undoubtedly, 3D US enhances the number of ways an ovary can be studied and each modality studied can yield another layer of information when attempting a diagnosis. Traditional ways of discriminating benign from malignant lesions as described in 2D US cannot be discounted, but merely enhanced by the further information gleaned from 3D assessment of the various parameters. Hopefully, ongoing research with this valuable tool will yield novel ways of studying the ovary in greater detail and subsequently inform more accurate and earlier diagnosis of serious pathology.

One of the most important steps is to determine the normal power Doppler parameters in both the pre- and postmenopausal population. The data are further confused by the different equipment and different machine parameters even within the equipment of the same manufacturer. Research is currently underway to determine the key settings to obtain the maximal information regarding the microvascularity of an organ, with particular reference to the ovary.

Conclusion

3D US of the pelvic organs provides an invaluable tool for enhancing diagnosis and, it is to be hoped, will result in more favorable outcomes for patients.

The findings of uterine anomalies as well as cervical and tubal pathology are greatly enhanced with this modality at a fraction of the cost, time, and inconvenience of an MRI. The scan times for the patients are quick and subsequent analysis can be done by the physician at a later time. The same holds true for cervical and tubal pathology. Most of the time, the patient can be informed of her results on the day of the scan, resulting in less patient anxiety and reduced wait-times for results.

While this tool is valuable for assessing vascular abnormalities, there is still untapped potential regarding the enhanced accuracy of diagnosing ovarian pathology. Hopefully, with technologic advances in equipment and software in the coming years, we will see major breakthroughs in the early diagnosis of ovarian cancer. Future research is required in order to provide a standardized protocol that can be developed for the advanced imaging of the ovaries.

Although the learning curve with this technology is long, the returns in the accuracy of the imaging obtained are well worth the effort.

Acknowledgments

The authors would like to express gratitude to Dr. Ilan Timor-Tritsch for his generous contribution of time in enhancing the skills of Dr. Norman Assad with the 3D US techniques described herein. Thanks also go to Sadie Hutson PhD for the many contributions to this chapter.

References

1. Benacerraf M, Benson CB, Abuhamad AZ, et al. Three and 4-dimensional ultrasound in obstetrics and gynecology: proceedings of the American Institute of Ultrasound in Medicine Consensus Conference. *J Ultrasound Med* 2005; **24**: 1587–1597.

2. GE Healthcare: Basic User Manual. Voluson i. Revision 2. KTI 106029–100.:10.1.1–10.1.2.

3. Raine-Fenning NJ, Campbell BK, Clews JS, et al. The interobserver reliability of three-dimensional power Doppler data acquisition within the female pelvis. *Ultrasound Rev Obstet Gynecol* 2004; **23**: 501–508.

4. Timor-Tritsch IE, Monteagudo A, Tsymbal T, Strok I. Three-dimensional inversion rendering. A new sonographic technique and its use in gynecology. *J Ultrasound Med* 2005; **24**: 681–688.

5. Lee W, Gonçalves LF, Espinoza J, Romero R. Inversion mode: a new volume analysis tool for 3-dimensional ultrasonography. *J Ultrasound Med* 2005; **24**: 201–207.

6. Cohen LS, Valle RF. Role of vaginal sonography and hysterosonography in the endoscopic treatment of uterine myomas. *Fertil Steril* 2000; **73**(2): 197–203.

7. Goldstein S. Saline infusion sonohysterography. *Clin Obstet Gynecol* 1996; **39**: 248–258.

8. Widrich T, Bradley LD, Mitchenson AR, Collins RL. Comparison of saline infusion sonography with office hysteroscopy for the evaluation of endometrium. *Am J Obstet Gynecol* 1996; **174**: 1327–1334.

9. Grimbizis GF, Camus M. Tarlatzis BC, et al. Clinical implications of uterine malformations and hysteroscopic treatment results. *Hum Reprod Update* 2001; **7**(2): 161–174.

10. Kupesic S. Three-dimensional ultrasound in reproductive medicine. *Ultrasound Rev Obstet Gynecol* 2005; **5**: 304–315.

11. Diagnosing the submucosal fibroids (SIS). Beyond Hysterectomy: The Contemporary Management of Uterine Fibroids – An International Conference; April 11–13, 2003.

12. Valle RF, Sciarra JJ. Intrauterine adhesions: hysteroscopic diagnosis, classification, treatment, and reproductive outcome. *Am J Obstet Gynecol* 1988; **158** (6 Pt 1): 1459–1470.

13. Raine-Fenning NJ, Campbell BK, Kendall NR, et al. Quantifying the changes in endometrial vascularity throughout the normal menstrual cycle with three-dimensional power Doppler angiography. *Hum Reprod* 2004; **19**: 330–338.

14. Alcazar JL. Three dimensional ultrasound assessment of endometrial receptivity: a review. *Reprod Biol Endocrinol* 2006; 456.

15. Timor-Tritsch IE, Goldstein SR. Skilled US imaging of the adnexae Part 2: the non-neoplastic mass. *Obg Management* 2010; **22**(10): 2–8.

16. Exacoustos C, Romanini ME, Rinaldo D, et al. Preoperative sonographic features of borderline ovarian tumors. *Ultrasound Obstet Gynecol* 2004; **25**(1): 50–59.

17. Timmerman D, Testa AC, Bourne T, et al. Simple ultrasound-based rules for the diagnosis of ovarian cancer. *Ultrasound Obstet Gynecol* 2008; **31**: 681–690.

18. Timmerman D, Valentin L, Bourne TH, et al. Terms, definitions and measurements to describe the sonographic features of adnexal tumors: a consensus opinion from the International Ovarian Tumor Analysis (IOTA) Group. *Ultrasound Obstet Gynecol* 2000; **16**: 500–505.

19. Menon U, Gentry-Maharaj A, Hallett R, et al. Sensitivity and specificity of multimodal and ultrasound screening for ovarian cancer, and stage distribution of detected cancers: results of

the prevalence screen of the UK Collaborative Trial of Ovarian Cancer Screening (UKCTOCS). *Lancet Oncol* 2009; **10**: 327–340.

20. Amor F, Vaccaro H, Alcázar JL, León M, Craig JM, Martinez J. Gynecologic Imaging Reporting and Data System: a new proposal for classifying adnexal masses on the basis of sonographic findings. *J Ultrasound* 2009; **28**: 285–291.

21. Timor-Tritsch IE, Goldstein SR. *Three Dimensional Ultrasound in Gynecology. Ultrasound in Gynecology*, 2nd edn. Philadelphia, PA: Churchill Livingstone; 2007: 282.

22. Kupesic S. Early ovarian cancer: 3D Power doppler. *Abdom Imaging* 2006; **31**: 613–619.

23. Fleischer A. Color Doppler sonography of adnexal torsion. 39th Annual Convention of AIUM; March 26–29, 1995.

24. Auslander R, Lavie O, Kaurman Y. Coiling of the ovarian vessels: a color Doppler sign for adnexal torsion without strangulation. *Ultrasound Obstet Gynecol* 2002; **20**: 96–97.

25. Lee EJ, Kwon HC, Joo HJ. Diagnosis of ovarian torsion with color Doppler sonography: depiction of twisted vascular pedicle. *J Ultrasound Med* 1998; **17**: 83–89.

26. Kurjak A, Zalud I, Aldfirevic Z. Evaluation of adnexal masses with transvaginal color ultrasound. *J Ultrasound Med* 1991; **10**: 295–297.

27. Fleischer A, Rodgers W, Rao B, et al. Assessment of ovarian tumor vascularity with transvaginal color Doppler sonography. *J Ultrasound Med* 1991; **10**: 563–568.

28. Timor-Tritsch IE, Goldstein SR. *Transvaginal Sonography and Ovarian Cancer*, 2nd edn. Philadelphia, PA: Churchill Livingstone; 2007: 260.

29. Kurjac A, Kupesic S, Sparac V, Kosuta D. Three dimensional ultrasonographic and power Doppler characterization of ovarian lesions. *Ultrasound Obstet Gynecol* 2000; **16**: 365–371.

30. Kurjak A, Kupesic S, Sparac V, et al. The detection of stage 1 ovarian cancer by three-dimensional sonography and power Doppler. *Gynecol Oncol* 2003; **90**: 258–264.

31. Chase DM, Crade M, Basu T, Saffari B, Berman ML. Preoperative diagnosis of ovarian malignancy: preliminary results of the use of 3-dimensional vascular ultrasound. *Intl J Gynecol Cancer* 2009; **19**(3): 354–360.

32. Crade M. Tissue block ultrasound and ovarian cancer – a pictorial presentation of findings. *Donald School J Ultrasound Obstet Gynecol* 2009; **3**(1): 40–46.

33. Cohen LS, Escobar PF, Scharm C, Glimco B, Fishman DA. Three-dimensional power Doppler ultrasound improves the diagnostic accuracy for ovarian cancer prediction. *Gynecol Oncol* 2001; **82**: 40–48.

34. Sladkevicius P, Jokubkiene L, Valentin L. Contribution of morphological assessment of the vessel tree by three-dimensional ultrasound to a correct diagnosis of malignancy in ovarian masses. *Ultrasound Obstet Gynecol* 2007; **30**: 874–882.

35. Alcazar JL, Garcia-Manero M, Galvan R. Three-dimensional sonographic morphologic assessment of adnexal masses: a reproducibility study. *J Ultrasound Med* 2007; **26**: 1007–1011.

36. Fleischer A, Niermann KJ, Donnelly EF, et al. Sonographic depiction of microvessel perfusion: principles and potential. *J Ultrasound Med* 2004; **23**: 1499–1506.

37. Cosgrove D. Microbubble enhancement of tumor neovascularity. *Eur Radiol* 1999; **9** (Suppl 3): 413–414.

38. Fleischer AC, Lyshchik A, Jones HW Jr, et al. Contrast-enhanced transvaginal sonography of benign versus malignant ovarian masses. *J Ultrasound Med* 2008; **27**: 1011–1018.

39. Marret H, Sauget S, Giraudeau B, et al. Contrast-enhanced sonography helps in discrimination of benign from malignant adnexal masses. *J Ultrasound Med* 2004; **23**: 1629–1639.

40. Tailor A, Jurkovic D, Bourne TH, et al. Sonographic prediction of malignancy in adnexal masses using multivariate logistic regression analysis. *Ultrasound Obstet Gynecol* 1997; **10**: 41–47.

41. Mousavi AS, Borna S, Moeinoddini S. Estimation of probability of malignancy using a logistic model combining color Doppler ultrasonography, serum CA125 level in women with a pelvic mass. *Int J Gynecol Cancer* 2006; **16** (Suppl 1):92–98.

42. Timmerman D, Testa AC, Bourne T, et al. Logistic regression model to distinguish between the benign and malignant adnexal mass before surgery: a multicenter study by the International Ovarian Tumor Analysis Group. *J Clin Oncol* 2005; **23**(24): 8794–8801.

43. Alcazar JS, Castillo G. Comparison of 2-dimensional and 3-dimensional power-Doppler imaging in complex adnexal masses for the prediction of ovarian cancer. *Am J Obstet Gynecol* 2005; **192**: 807–812.

44. Laban M, Metawee H, Elyan A, Kamal M, Kamel M, Mansour G. Three-dimensional ultrasound and three dimensional power Doppler in the assessment of ovarian tumors. *Intl J Gynecol Obstet* 2007; **99**: 201–205.

45. Kudla MJ, Timor-Tritsch IE, Hope JM, et al. Spherical tissue sampling 3-dimensional power Doppler angiography. *J Ultrasound Med* 2008; **27**: 425–433.

46. Alcazar JL, Merce LT, Garcia-Manero M. Three-dimensional power Doppler vascular sampling. *J Ultrasound Med* 2005; **24**: 689–696.

47. Alcazar JL, Rodriguez D. Three-dimensional power Doppler vascular sonographic sampling for predicting ovarian cancer in cystic-solid and solid vascularized masses. *J Ultrasound Med* 2009; **28**: 275–281.

Hysterosalpingography

Shawky Z. A. Badawy

Introduction

During ancient history, human reproduction was the subject of much research and study in order to diagnose the cause of infertility or to help people prevent pregnancy. Herbal formulas were used for the diagnosis as well as management of infertility. This was documented in ancient Egypt, ancient Greece, and also ancient Rome [1].

In the early part of the sixteenth century, Gabriel Fallopio, an Italian anatomist and physician, described the fallopian tube in a poetic sense as resembling a trumpet and it has carried his name up to the present time. The fallopian tube facilitates the passage of the oocyte from the ovary towards the uterus. It also facilitates the passage of sperm from the uterus for the process of fertilization [2].

Pathology of the fallopian tube leading to various kinds of distortion and obstruction is a very significant cause of infertility. Tubal disease is responsible for almost half of the patients presenting for evaluation because of failure to achieve pregnancy [3,4]. Hence, tubal testing to check for patency is an important part of the workup of the infertile woman.

In the early part of the twentieth century, Dr. Isidor Rubin introduced the testing for patency of the fallopian tube by a procedure called insufflation [5]. An insufflation cannula is introduced into the cervical canal and held tight. The insufflation medium was oxygen and that was modified to the use of carbon dioxide. It was found that carbon dioxide is easily absorbable from the peritoneal cavity and less likely than oxygen to produce an air embolism. The diagnosis of a patent tube was accomplished by listening with a stethoscope placed at the lower part of the abdomen to hear any wheezing sound indicating the passage of carbon dioxide through the tube and this would make the diagnosis of at least patency of one fallopian tube. Later on, a kymograph was attached to the device to register the pressure and oscillation [6]. Usually the pressure rises up to 60 or 80 mm of mercury and then plateaus and decreases if the tube is patent, or remains as it is if the tube is obstructed.

The introduction of the X-ray diagnostic methods by Dr. Roentgen [7] facilitated the use of radiopaque contrast media to inject into the uterine cavity to help the diagnosis of tubal pathology. The introduction of the radiographic evaluation of the uterine cavity and fallopian tube using contrast media has revolutionized our knowledge of the pathophysiology and various anatomical variations of the uterus and fallopian tubes. Hysterosalpingography is the name of this procedure and it is performed as an outpatient procedure [8].

Indications for hysterosalpingography

Infertility

This procedure is a basic evaluation of the uterine cavity and fallopian tubes in infertile women. It is a noninvasive procedure and usually many congenital and acquired pathological findings will be easily diagnosed and prepare the patient for management [9].

Uterine anomalies

Hysterosalpingography has been very valuable in defining many of the uterine anomalies, including the septate uterus, bicornuate uterus, arcuate uterus, and the didelphys. The diagnosis is usually supported by MRI evaluation of the pelvis. Both hysterosalpingography and MRI will give a definitive diagnosis of the uterine anomaly [10].

Uterine cavity abnormalities

Hysterosalpingography has been very valuable in the diagnosis of submucous fibroids, polyps, as well as intrauterine adhesions [11].

Recurrent pregnancy losses

Hysterosalpingography is one of the basic evaluation procedures for patients with recurrent miscarriages and premature

---

Ultrasonography in Gynecology, ed. Botros R. M. B. Rizk and Elizabeth E. Puscheck. Published by Cambridge University Press. © Cambridge University Press 2015.

labor. This might be due to a submucous lesion, or in many cases, due to incompetent cervix [12].

Recently, sonohysterography became a standard procedure to evaluate the uterine cavity. It is quick and carried out as an office procedure with the insertion of saline into the uterine cavity through the hysterosalpingogram catheter. The uterine cavity is distended and any lesion can be easily diagnosed using the vaginal probe ultrasound technology [13].

Patient preparation and procedure of hysterosalpingography

The patient is instructed that the procedure will be performed during the proliferative phase of the cycle within 2–7 days after completion of her menstrual flow. The patient is given instructions to administer 600–800 mg of ibuprofen 2 hours before the procedure. This has been found to be very helpful in prevention and alleviation of any uterine contractions due to the prostaglandin effect from the endometrium during the procedure [14]. The patient is then taken to the fluoroscopy room. She is placed in the dorsal lithotomy position. She is covered with sterile towels. The speculum is then inserted in the vagina with the aid of a suitable lighting system. The cervix and vagina are cleaned with Betadine solution. The anterior lip of the cervix is then grasped with a tenaculum.

There are two systems used for delivery of the contrast material to the uterine cavity. One system is in the form of a thin hysterogram catheter with an inflatable balloon at the end. This catheter is introduced through the cervix into the lower uterine segment and then the balloon is distended with air, thus preventing any reflux of the contrast material through the cervical canal.

The second system uses the Rubin cannula with a plastic tip that fits into the cervical canal and then the contrast material is delivered through it into the lower uterine segment. After the insertion of the delivery cannula, the speculum is taken out. A syringe is attached to the end of the cannula or the catheter. The patient is then centralized on the fluoroscopy table, and fluoroscopy is activated while the injection of the contrast medium is taking place. As such, we follow the contrast medium into the uterine cavity and then into the fallopian tubes. During the fluoroscopic evaluation, pictures can be taken electronically and reviewed later on with the radiologist. At the end of the procedure, the cannula or catheter is removed. A speculum is used again in order to inspect the cervix to be sure that there is no bleeding.

The patient is usually instructed that she will have some drainage from the vagina for a few hours. This is due to the reflux of the dye outside the uterus into the vagina. She is given the necessary pads to help her during this period of time. She is also instructed to take ibuprofen as needed on that day. Usually the patients do very well and go home right after the procedure. Many patients will be able to drive themselves home. However, we advise them to have their husband or friend with them in case they are needed to drive the patient home.

Contrast medium for hysterosalpingography

There are two types of contrast media that have been used over the years for hysterosalpingography: oil-based and water-based [15].

Hysterosalpingography started with the use of the oil-based contrast medium. The picture is well-defined. However, in order to know whether the tubes are patent, the patient has to come to the office 24 hours later for another flat plate of the pelvis. If there is contrast material in the pelvic cavity, then it suggests tubal patency. Otherwise, the tubes are not patent. This has been the standard in the past and patients are used to it. However, one of the side effects is development of oil granulomas in the pelvis and this could be detected for many years following the hysterosalpingogram [16].

The water-based contrast medium is now the standard used in this procedure. It is less thick than the oil-based medium. Usually the diagnosis of tubal patency is done immediately during the injection of the contrast medium. Therefore, the patient should know the results and the exact diagnosis straight away.

Diagnostic and therapeutic values

Hysterosalpingography has two goals. One is the diagnosis of uterine and tubal pathology and the second is its therapeutic value. It has been found that approximately one-third of the women who undergo this procedure for infertility achieve pregnancy spontaneously within a few months after the procedure. Various authors have compared the oil-based and water-based therapeutic values after hysterosalpingography. All these authors agreed that there is a success rate with regard to pregnancy following the procedure. However, some investigators found that the oil-based procedure is associated with a higher pregnancy rate and the pregnancies occur sooner after the procedure as compared with the water-based procedure. Other investigators found no difference between the two contrast media in pregnancy rates [17–20].

Complications of hysterosalpingogram include infection, pain, intravasation of the contrast medium into the vascular plexus in the pelvis, embolization of the dye into distant locations, and vasovagal attacks [21,22].

In order to prevent pelvic infection after hysterosalpingography, it is essential that patients undergoing this procedure have no history of recent pelvic infections. If the patient had an infection that was treated in the past and at the present time she is 2–3 months past the incident with a normal white count and normal temperature, then the procedure can be performed to check the effect of the past infection on the tubes.

In order to prevent pain, women are given ibuprofen prior to the procedure, as we stated. In addition, the injection of the contrast medium into the uterus should be slow and the medium should be previously warmed to body temperature. If these precautions are followed, then pain is very rare. If they are not followed, then the patient could get severe pain, which predisposes her to vasovagal attack. The patient in these circumstances will feel dizzy, hypotensive, and tachycardic. The

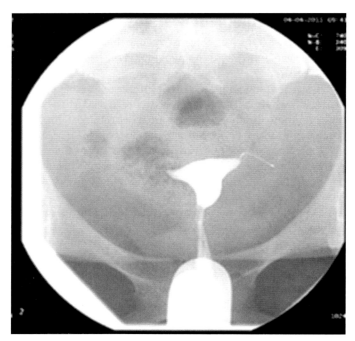

Fig. 2.1 Hysterosalpingogram showing normal uterine cavity and Essure device in isthmus of left fallopian tube. The right fallopian tube is absent.

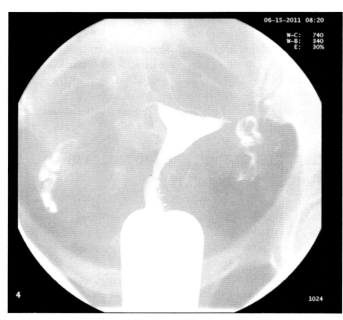

Fig. 2.3 Hysterosalpingogram showing normal uterine cavity and both fallopian tubes with spillage, suggesting patency.

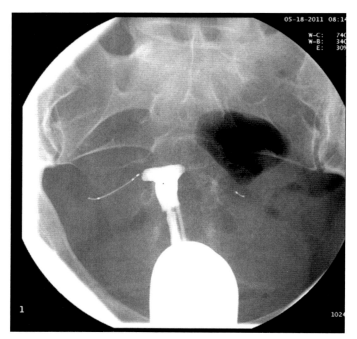

Fig. 2.2 Hysterosalpingogram showing Essure device in isthmus of right and left fallopian tubes.

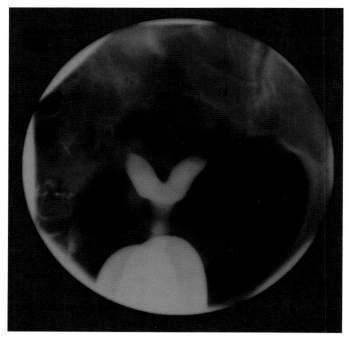

Fig. 2.4 Hysterosalpingogram showing a bicornuate or septate uterus. MRI is needed to confirm diagnosis.

patient should be immediately started on intravenous (IV) fluid therapy, given IV sedation, and watched for several hours in the Recovery Room.

Intravasation of the contrast medium will occur if undue pressure is used during the injection of the contrast medium and especially if there is cornual obstruction of the fallopian tube. This is why fluoroscopy is of great value in these patients because you will see the contrast medium traveling up the uterus and tubes; and you can stop at any time if there is obstruction.

Findings at hysterosalpingography

Figs 2.1–2.5 represent the various abnormalities that may be encountered during this procedure and suggest that its use is

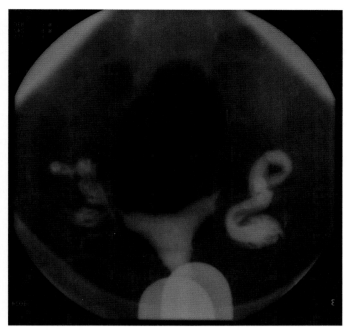

Fig. 2.5 Hysterosalpingogram showing normal uterine cavity, left hydrosalpinx. Right tube shows marked convolutions suggesting adhesions.

very beneficial as the first step in evaluation of the infertile patient. One of the most recent indications for hysterosalpingography is to diagnose the condition of the tubes following the insertion of transuterine implants in the tubes. Patients are instructed to continue the use of contraception until 3 months after the procedure and a hysterosalpingogram is done. In these cases, you will see the implant in the tubes, the tubes are blocked, and there is no dye beyond the isthmus of the tube.

References

1. DeCherney AH, Harris TC. The barren woman through history. In: DeCherney AH (Ed.) *Reproductive Failure*. Churchill Livingstone; 1986: 1–5.

2. Speert H. *Obstetric and Gynecologic Milestones: Essays in Eponymy*. New York: Macmillan; 1958.

3. Eschenbach DA. Acute pelvic inflammatory disease: etiology, risk factors and pathogenesis. *Clin Obstet Gynecol* 1976; **19**: 147.

4. Holmes KK, Eschenbach DA, Knapp JD. Salpingitis: overview of etiology and epidemiology. *Am J Obstet Gynecol* 1980; **138**: 893.

5. Rubin IC. Non-operative determination of patency in fallopian tubes in sterility: intrauterine insufflation with oxygen and production of pneumoperitoneum, preliminary report. *JAMA* 1920; **74**: 1017.

6. Rubin IC. Rhythmic contractions and peristaltic movements in the human fallopian tube as determined by peri-uterine gas insufflation and the kymograph, experimental and clinical study. *Am J Obstet Gynecol* 1927; **14**: 557.

7. Navelline R. *Squire's Fundamentals of Radiology*, 5th edn. Harvard University Press; 1997.

8. Siegler AM. Hysterosalpingography. *Fertil Steril* 1983; **40**: 139.

9. Geary WL, Holland JB, Weed JC, Weed, Jr JC. Ultrasonography. *Am J Obstet Gynecol* 1969; **104**(5): 687–692.

10. Braun P, Gray FV, Pons RM, Enguix DP. Is hysterosalpingography able to diagnose all uterine malformations correctly? A retrospective study. *Eur J Radiol* 2005; **53**(2): 274–279.

11. Steinkeler JA, Woodfield CA, Lazarus E, Hillstrom MM. Female infertility: a systematic approach to radiologic imaging and diagnosis. *Radiographics* 2009; **29**: 1353–1370.

12. Filho HAG, Mattar R, Pires CR, et al. Comparison of hysterosalpingography, hysterosonography, and hysteroscopy in evaluation of the uterine cavity in patients with recurrent pregnancy losses. *Arch Gynecol Obstet* 2006; **274**(5): 284–288.

13. Goldbert JM, Falcone T, Attaran M. Sonohysterographic evaluation of uterine anomalies noted on hysterosalpingography. *Hum Reprod* 1997; **12**(10): 1251–2153.

14. Anserilia P. Strategies to minimize discomfort during diagnostic hysterosalpingography with disposable balloon catheters: a randomized placebo-controlled study with oral nonsteroidal pain medication. *Fertil Steril* 2008; **90**: 846.

15. Deboer AD, Vemer HM, Willemsen WNP, Sanders FBM. Oil or aqueous contrast media for hysterosalpingography: a perspective, randomized, clinical study. *Eur J Obstet Gynecol and Reprod Biol* 1988; **28**(1): 65–68.

16. Aaron JD, Levine W. Endometrial oil granuloma following hysterosalpingography. *Am J Obstet Gynecol* 1954; **68**(6): 1594–1597.

17. Decherney AH, Kort H, Barney JB, et al. Increased pregnancy rate with oil soluble hysterosalpingography dyes. *Fertil Steril* 1989; **33**: 407.

18. Schawabe MG, Shapiro SS, Haning RV Jr. Hysterosalpingography with oil contrast medium enhances infertility in patients with infertility of unknown etiology. *Fertil Steril* 1983; **40**: 604.

19. Steiner AZ, Meyer WR, Clark RL, Hartman KE. Oil-soluble contrast during hysterosalpingography in women with proven tubal patency. *Obstet Gynecol* 2003; **101**(1): 109–113.

20. Barqawi R, Bani-Irshaid I, Bdor AN. The effects of contrast media in patients undergoing salpingography on pregnancy rates. *J Bahrain Med Soc* 2007; **19**(4): 133–136.

21. Williams ER. Venous intravasation during hysterosalpingography. *Br J Radiol* 1944; **17**: 13.

22. Karshmer N, Stein W. Oil embolism complicating hysterosalpingography. *J Med Soc New Jersey* 1951; **48**: 496.

3

Ultrasonography and hysteroscopy in gynecologic evaluation: are they competitive or complementary to each other?

Amr Hassan Wahba and Osama Shawki

Introduction

Ultrasonography and hysteroscopy have established themselves as invaluable and essential tools in the modern practice of gynecology, allowing for the proper evaluation of most gynecologic complaints.

Imaging of the female reproductive tract using ultrasonography was first reported by Kratochwil et al. in 1972 [1] and currently represents one of the most common procedures performed by gynecologists. It is very well tolerated by patients, besides being noninvasive and cost effective. On the other hand, although hysteroscopy was described in 1869 by Pantaleoni to treat abnormal bleeding from an endometrial polyp [2], its clinical importance was only realized a few decades ago.

The introduction of more advanced scopes in 1990, with smaller diameters ranging between 1.2 and 3 mm, as well as the use of small operative sheaths with an outer diameter not exceeding 5 mm, has not only made the diagnosis of uterine lesions possible but has also allowed for eye-guided biopsies and treatment of most endo-uterine pathologies during the same procedure introducing the attractive concept of "*see* and *treat.*"

Ultrasonography is privileged over hysteroscopy in visualizing the ovaries, adnexa, the pouch of Douglas, and the uterine wall, while hysteroscopy is privileged over ultrasonography in visualizing the vagina (acting as a vaginoscop) and ectocervix (acting as a colposcope). However, both ultrasonography and hysteroscopy compete together in the visualization of the uterine cavity; the former achieves this indirectly and the latter directly. Which procedure is superior over the other has been a source of debate and continuous research, especially with the unremitting development of both tools.

This chapter will explore the role of ultrasonography and hysteroscopy in the evaluation of common gynecologic complaints, aiming to highlight the value and limits of each diagnostic tool.

Intrauterine abnormalities; the culprit behind most gynecologic presentations

Intrauterine abnormalities may include the presence of polyps, endometrial hyperplasia, submucous myomas, and adhesions. Such lesions contribute to most gynecologic presentations, including abnormal uterine bleeding (AUB), infertility, amenorrhea, and recurrent miscarriage.

Intrauterine abnormalities have been reported in more than 40% of affected women with AUB [3], in 19–62% of infertile women [4], and in as many as 50% of women with recurrent implantation failure [4]. Thus, the proper assessment of the uterine cavity can provide a clue to unravel the majority of gynecologic complaints.

Evaluation of uterine cavity

The methods available for evaluation of the uterine cavity have developed considerably over the last few decades. Hysterosalpingography (HSG) has traditionally, been the most commonly used technique. However, it has been associated with high false-positive and false-negative results, besides other disadvantages inherent to the technique [4].

Being noninvasive, transvaginal sonography (TVS) has been used as a screening test for the assessment of the uterine cavity. The diagnosis of specific disorders is directly dependent on the phase of the menstrual cycle. For example, endometrial polyps are best seen during the proliferative phase, while submucous myomas, uterine anomalies, and adhesions are best observed during the secretory phase. Consequently, the changes in the echogenicity of the endometrium may result in missing the diagnosis and accurate location of the lesions.

Instillation of saline into the uterine cavity during ultrasound examination, known as saline infusion sonography (SIS), distends the uterine cavity and serves as a negative contrast agent, thus improving the delineation of the uterine cavity and showing structural abnormalities of the endometrium with high sensitivity and specificity [4,5]. Unlike TVS, the intracavitary infusion of saline during SIS makes it possible to reliably examine the uterine cavity at any stage of the menstrual cycle.

Hysteroscopy is considered the definitive diagnostic tool to evaluate any intrauterine abnormality suspected on HSG, TVS, or SIS during routine investigation of common gynecologic complaints. Given its high diagnostic accuracy, it has become a diagnostic gold standard against which other methods are assessed.

Ultrasonography in Gynecology, ed. Botros R. M. B. Rizk and Elizabeth E. Puscheck. Published by Cambridge University Press. © Cambridge University Press 2015.

When TVS and SIS were compared with hysteroscopy in the assessment of uterine cavity prior to in vitro fertilization (IVF), the overall sensitivity of TVS increased after SIS (from 84.5% to 87.5%), as did the specificity (from 98.7% to 100%) [5]. Similar findings were observed when TVS, SIS, and diagnostic hysteroscopy were evaluated in patients with AUB. The overall sensitivity of TVS improved after SIS (from 67% to 87%), as did the specificity (from 89% to 91%) [6].

Thus, abnormal findings on a baseline scan with TVS can be further evaluated with SIS or hysteroscopy. Interestingly, when women were given the choice between SIS and office hysteroscopy for further evaluation of the uterine cavity, the majority preferred to undergo office hysteroscopy [7], even though more pain was experienced during hysteroscopy compared with SIS [8]. This preference was explained by the completeness of diagnosis and therapy in one visit with hysteroscopy.

Evaluation of endometrial pathology

The evaluation of endometrium has historically been conducted through dilation and curettage (D&C) especially when malignancy is of concern, despite being an invasive inpatient procedure with inherent diagnostic limitations [9]. D&C relies on blindly sampling endometrial specimens; in most cases, it samples less than half of the uterine cavity [10].

Thick endometrial echo on ultrasonography may result from endometrial polyp, hyperplasia, endometrial carcinoma, or endometritis [11]. TVS can measure endometrial thickness accurately, but it cannot distinguish between a hyperplastic endometrium and an endometrial polyp [12,13].

Endometrial polyp

Diagnosis of endometrial polyp can be inconclusive with TVS, but using SIS, an intracavitary polyp will be clearly surrounded by anechoic fluid [14]. Moreover, SIS can provide realistic information about the location and size of the endometrial polyps (Figs 3.1 and 3.2) [12]. When compared with hysteroscopy, SIS showed a 7% false-positive rate in patients with polyps [12]. Figs 3.3 and 3.4 show hysteroscopic views of endometrial polyp and polypoid endometrium, respectively.

In a retrospective study of a mixed population of 300 women with polyps, 24.3% of whom were asymptomatic, the underlying rate of malignancy and complex hyperplasia with atypia was 1.6%. All of the cancer cases were in peri- or postmenopausal patients symptomatic with AUB [15]. Malignant changes within polyps can rarely be detected with ultrasound including Doppler flow or hysteroscopic visualization alone. Accordingly, histological evaluation is mandatory, which entails resection of such lesions [15]. Fig. 3.5 shows a hysteroscopic view of a malignant polyp.

Endometrial hyperplasia and endometrial carcinoma

Endometrial carcinoma is the overriding concern that needs to be reliably excluded, especially in postmenopausal and

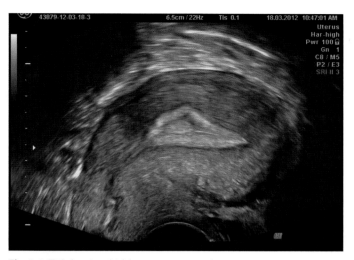

Fig. 3.1 TVS showing thick heterogeneous endometrium.

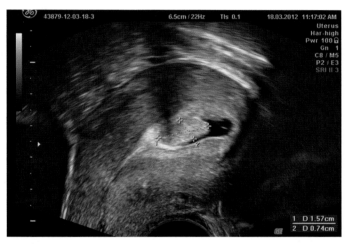

Fig. 3.2 SIS (same case) showing endometrial polyp arising from the anterior endometrial lining.

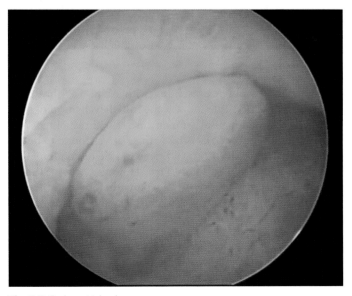

Fig. 3.3 Endometrial polyp.

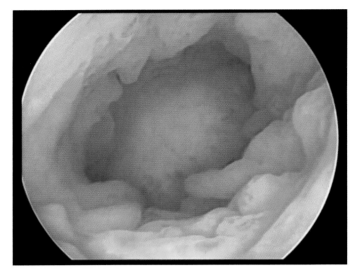

Fig. 3.4 Polypoid endometrium.

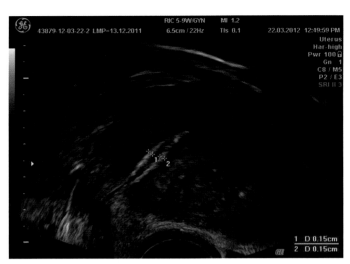

Fig. 3.6 SIS showing symmetrical endometrial thickness in a postmenopausal woman.

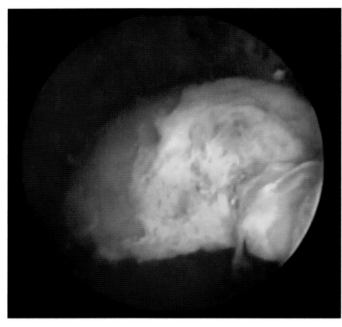

Fig. 3.5 Malignant polyp.

premenopausal women presenting with AUB. TVS has been proposed as the first-line tool for the initial evaluation of such cases. In postmenopausal women, using a threshold of less than 5 mm for endometrial echo with TVS was found to be the most cost-effective diagnostic strategy to rule out endometrial pathology with good certainty [16]. However, when SIS was used to evaluate postmenopausal women before the initiation of hormone replacement therapy, intracavitary abnormalities were found in 37% of patients with an endometrial thickness of less than or equal to 5 mm. Consequently, endometrial thickness of less than or equal to 5 mm can exclude hyperplasia, but does not eliminate other intrauterine abnormalities, e.g. polyps and submucous myomas [17].

Distinguishing endometrial cancer or hyperplasia from other conditions is not possible based solely on unenhanced measurements of the endometrial echo. Distension of the uterine cavity during SIS separates the endometrial layers, allowing for proper examination of the whole endometrial lining as shown in Fig. 3.6. In such a case, demonstration of asymmetric thickening of the endometrium can be suggestive of endometrial hyperplasia or carcinoma [14]. The inability to distend the endometrial cavity during attempted SIS has been reported as a finding consistent with endometrial carcinoma [11].

For the assessment of endometrial carcinoma, TVS and hysteroscopy revealed sensitivity of 77.8% and 98.3% and specificity of 93.3% and 98.3%, respectively. The combined use of both methods revealed sensitivity of 100% and specificity of 91.7% [18].

Hysteroscopy is a superior diagnostic procedure in postmenopausal women and should be performed whenever there is endometrial thickness greater than 4 mm, ill-defined endometrial lining, recurrent bleeding, or risk factors for endometrial carcinoma [18]. Hence, a clinician should seriously consider hysteroscopy with directed biopsy if there is persistent postmenopausal bleeding, even if TVS and endometrial biopsy are normal [19]. Figs 3.7 and 3.8 show hysteroscopic views of endometrial hyperplasia and endometrial cancer, respectively.

Unlike cases with postmenopausal bleeding, cut-off values for endometrial thickness are not recommended in the workup of premenopausal patients with AUB since the endometrial thickness varies throughout the menstrual cycle and a thickened stripe might merely be secondary to secretory endometrium [20]. Also, polyps and fibroids may be found even in women with endometrial stripe thicknesses less than 5 mm [21].

Evaluation of submucous myomas

Myomas can originate anywhere in the myometrium; however, those projecting into the uterine cavity are more problematic.

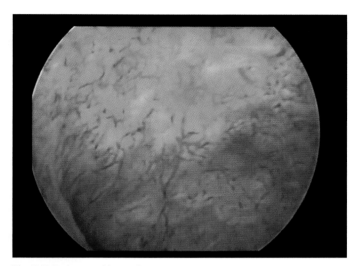

Fig. 3.7 Endometrial hyperplasia.

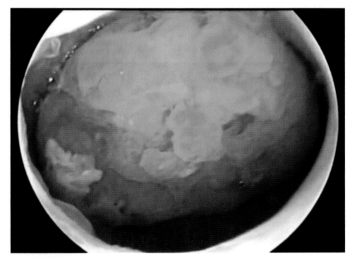

Fig. 3.8 Endometrial cancer.

Traditionally, symptomatic submucous myomas were treated surgically by either hysterectomy or abdominal myomectomy, depending on whether pregnancy is desired or not. However, the latter approach requires the opening of the uterine cavity, which may compromise any future parturition as it requires cesarean delivery; moreover, it may lead to the development of pelvic postoperative adhesions, which may further reduce rather than enhance fertility [22]. Operative hysteroscopy has recently provided a better alternative for resection of these submucous myomas transcervically, thus avoiding the drawbacks of laparotomy and uterine incision.

It is essential not only to establish the diagnosis of submucous myomas, but also to properly evaluate such lesions to determine the best route through which they can be managed as well as the level of hysteroscopic skills needed (to ensure successful complete resection and to reduce the occurrence of possible complications such as perforation and hemorrhage).

A proper preoperative evaluation should include precise assessment of the *number, size, location, degree of intramural extension of the submucous myomas,* as well as *the distance between the myoma and the serosa.* According to the degree of intramural growth, submucous myomas have been classified into three categories: type 0 (no intramural extension), type 1 (intramural part <50%), and type 2 (intramural part ≥50%) [23].

Submucous myomas can be easily diagnosed by TVS as well-defined hypoechoic structures clearly distinguishable from the endometrium. Fedele et al. reported that TVS was as sensitive and specific as hysteroscopy in the diagnosis of submucous myomas [24]; however, in the study by Cicinelli et al., TVS was found to be less sensitive (since it missed the diagnosis of a myoma prolapsing through the cervix) and less specific (identifying an endometrial polyp as myoma) [25]. Both studies agreed that TVS was more precise than hysteroscopy in estimating the size of the myomas and in mapping them, but less accurate in estimating the percentage of intracavitary growth and in diagnosing the location of the tumor. Failure of TVS to accurately distinguish the wall to which the myoma is attached may be explained by the inability to visualize the endometrial echoes in correspondence with the myoma, especially with large intracavitary tumors, particularly when TVS is performed during the follicular phase when the endometrium is thin [25].

SIS can distinguish myomas from polyps based on the complete endoluminal location of the polyp, its motility during fluid injection, the less echogenic nature of myoma, and the possibility of recognizing continuity between the myoma and the myometrium. It was reported to be as sensitive and specific as hysteroscopy [25]. More importantly, it can accurately estimate the percentage of intracavitary growth, which is related to the failure rate of transcervical resection and the subsequent recurrence rate [23]. Moreover, SIS can precisely define the tumor location, a crucial piece of information to counter the increased risk of uterine perforation or hemorrhagic complications when the myoma is located in the cornual region or near the cervix [26].

Hysteroscopy provides a definitive diagnosis of a submucous myoma and can distinguish it from an endometrial polyp (Figs 3.9 and 3.10). Preoperative diagnostic hysteroscopy will accurately confirm the number of submucous myomas, their precise location, and the feasibility of hysteroscopic resection, but it does not offer a precise evaluation of the size, intramyometrial extension, or the distance between the myoma and the serosa, which can be determined by TVS and SIS.

Consequently, the combination of ultrasonography and hysteroscopy is now considered the most effective diagnostic approach for selecting the best method and strategy for excising submucous myomas [27].

Evaluation of congenital uterine anomalies

Establishing a definite diagnosis of a suspected uterine anomaly with duplication of the uterine cavity is important, since a

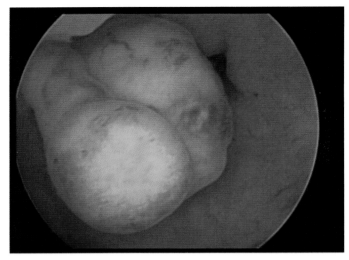

Fig. 3.9 Submucous fibroid polyp (superficial blood vessels are easily visible through overlying stretched pale endometrium).

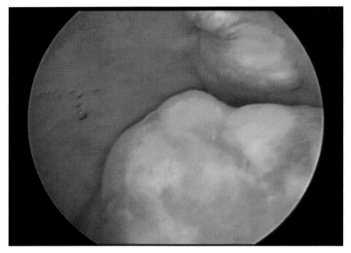

Fig. 3.10 Multiple myomas.

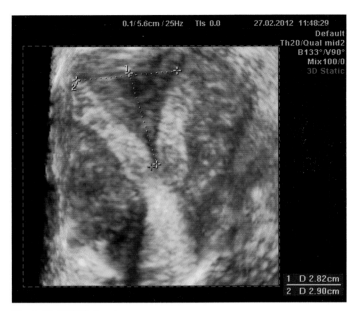

Fig. 3.11 3D TVS showing a septate uterus.

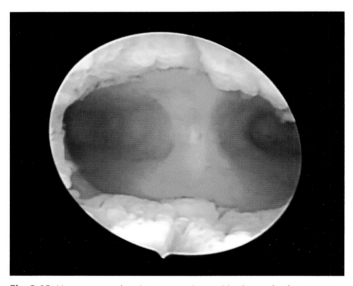

Fig. 3.12 Hysteroscopy showing two uterine cavities (proved to be a septate uterus by laparoscopy) .

septate uterus can be treated by resection of the septum while reunification of a bicornuate uterus is no longer performed. In one study, TVS, SIS, and diagnostic hysteroscopy were found to have a sensitivity of 44%, 44%, and 77% with a specificity of 96%, 100%, and 100%, respectively, in the diagnosis of uterine malformations [13].

The laparoscopic visualization of a single uterine fundus has been the gold standard for differentiating a septate uterus from a bicornuate uterus. TVS allows visualization of the fundal contour and can, thus, diagnose such anomalies with an accuracy of 90–92% [28]. The addition of three-dimensional (3D) sonography allows for coronal imaging, making the differentiation between bicornuate and wide septa more accurate with a sensitivity of 93% and a specificity of 100% [29]. For diagnosed septa, it can also measure its depth and width (Fig. 3.11).

Hysteroscopy allows direct visualization of the uterine cavity, identifying a number of cavities (Fig. 3.12). Nevertheless, similar to HSG, it does not allow visualization of the uterine fundus, which is necessary to differentiate a septate uterus from a bicornuate uterus. Despite this limitation of hysteroscopy, Bettocchi et al. have suggested three "diagnostic criteria" that can differentiate between septate uteri and bicornuate uteri during office hysteroscopic metroplasty, namely *the presence of vascularized tissue, sensitive innervation*, and *appearance of the tissue at the incision of a supposed septum* allowing both confirmation of diagnosis as well as treatment in an office setting [30].

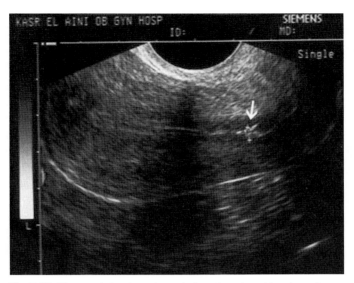

Fig. 3.13 Ultrasound showing echogenic focus in endometrium (arrow) denoting IUAs (confirmed by hysteroscopy).

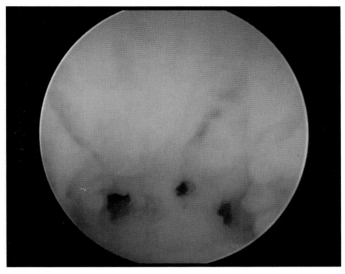

Fig. 3.14 Central fibrotic IUAs.

Evaluation of intrauterine adhesions

Intrauterine adhesions (IUAs), known as Asherman's syndrome, occur as a result of the destruction of the basalis layer of the endometrium, usually by the over-enthusiastic curettage of the endometrial cavity, especially in the postpartal or postabortal period, resulting in infertility, amenorrhea, or recurrent spontaneous abortion.

HSG has been reported to be the most accurate screening method in the diagnosis of IUAs [31] with a sensitivity, specificity, positive predictive value (PPV), and negative predictive value (NPV) of 75%, 95%, 50%, and 98%, respectively [13]. HSG may show a small, fragmented, and distorted uterine cavity as a result of IUAs.

The occurrence of IUAs can be suspected during TVS by the presence of small echogenic foci related to the endometrial cavity or asymmetric thickness of endometrium (Fig. 3.13). [32] TVS was found to be highly specific (95%), but insensitive (0%), with a PPV of 50% and an NPV of 95% [13]. Although some have reported a significantly better sensitivity and PPV, such results can be difficult to achieve by most ultrasonographers [13]. Thus, generally, TVS is not a reliable diagnostic test for detection of IUAs [13]; however, it may be of prognostic value by being helpful in planning hysteroscopic adhesiolysis. Patients with an endometrium thinner than 2 mm in the luteal phase were found not to benefit from hysteroscopic adhesiolysis [33].

Uterine distension during SIS permits detection of IUAs, which usually appear as mobile, thin, echogenic bands that bridge a normally distensible endometrial cavity. Occasionally, thicker, broad-based bands or complete obliteration of the endometrial cavity may be observed [34] with inability to distend the uterine cavity [14]. SIS has been reported to have a diagnostic accuracy comparable to HSG for identification of IUAs with a sensitivity, specificity, PPV, and NPV of 75%, 93%,

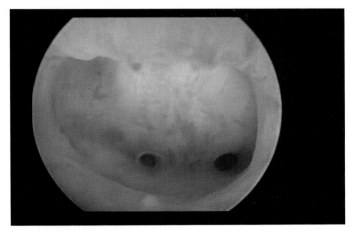

Fig. 3.15 Central fibromuscular IUAs.

43%, and 98%, respectively. The relatively low PPV of both SIS and HSG may relate to artifacts produced by the inadvertent injection of air bubbles or the presence of cervical mucus [13].

The introduction of 3D sonography now allows interactive visualization of the endometrial cavity through multiplanar reformatting and provides an improved depiction of adhesions and extent of cavity damage compared with 2D sonography [35].

In view of the relatively low sensitivity of both HSG and SIS, a direct hysteroscopic examination of the uterine cavity is clearly a superior method, representing the gold standard for the diagnosis of IUAs against which other methods must be compared [13]. It does not only establish the diagnosis, but also permits precise assessment of the *tissue type* of the adhesions (endometrial, fibromuscular, or connective tissue), *location* (central or marginal), and *extent* of the adhesions (mild, moderate, or severe); all are important factors in determining therapy and prognosis [31]. Figs 3.14–3.17 show hysteroscopic views of IUAs.

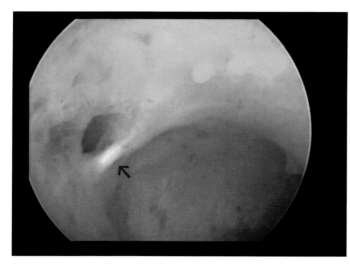

Fig. 3.16 Marginal adhesions at the cornu (arrow).

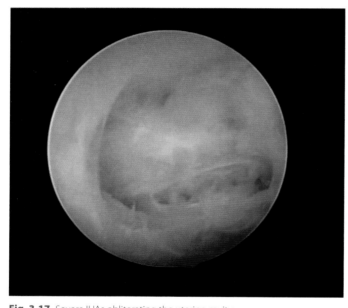

Fig. 3.17 Severe IUAs obliterating the uterine cavity.

Evaluation of other challenging conditions

Adenomyosis

TVS can provide a clue to the diagnosis of adenomyosis through some sonographic features suggestive of the lesion. Although hysteroscopy cannot provide a reliable diagnosis for this condition, some authors suspect it when the endometrium shows irregularity with endometrial defects, altered vascularization, and a cystic hemorrhagic lesion, as seen in Fig. 3.18(A and B). Hysteroscopy also may offer the possibility of obtaining endometrial-myometrial biopsies under visual control [36], allowing for histopathological examination, which remains the definitive diagnosis of such pathology.

Problems associated with intrauterine contraceptive devices (IUDs)

Abnormal bleeding and pain caused by IUDs may result from malposition or displacement of the IUD or can be premonitory of an organic lesion that otherwise would have been asymptomatic, prompting a thorough investigation of the uterine cavity. Although sonographic evaluation may be helpful to exclude translocation of the device, malposition could be easily missed and proper evaluation of the endometrium may be limited by the shadowing caused by the IUD. Performance of hysteroscopy in such cases would be more useful not only to detect malposition (Fig. 3.19), but also to correct the position of the device or safely remove it, instead of the blind extraction which can be traumatic. Moreover, it can be valuable in identifying a coexisting pathology.

Summary

Enthusiasts of hysteroscopy and those of ultrasonography often appear to be in an endless fierce competition, each group trying to prove the superiority of its diagnostic modality. Yet, in fact, both are integral parts of the gynecologist's armamentar-

A

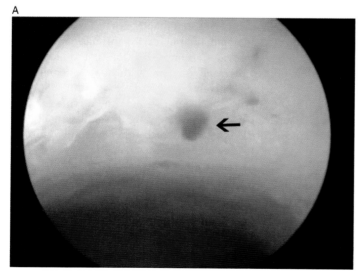

B

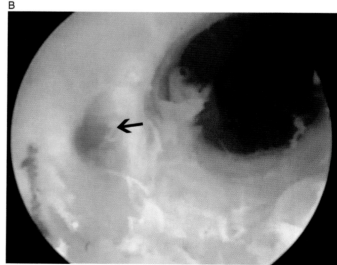

Fig. 3.18 (A and B) Cystic hemorrhagic lesions (arrow) suggestive of adenomyosis.

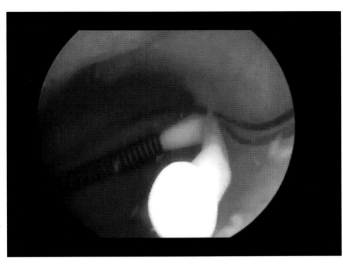

Fig. 3.19 Malposition of IUD (turned upside down).

ium and are actually complementary to each other, rather than being exclusive to one another.

The simplicity of the ultrasound examination has led gynecologists to consider it as the "first step" procedure in the evaluation of the uterine cavity. However, the accuracy provided by hysteroscopic examination, with its ability to provide histological examination, has led gynecologists to consider hysteroscopy as the "gold standard" in the evaluation of the uterine cavity. Nevertheless, the decision about the roles of ultrasonography and hysteroscopy should be based primarily upon the available evidence regarding feasibility, accuracy, and cost-effectiveness.

References

1. Kratochwil A, Urban GU, Friedrich F. Ultrasonic tomography of the ovaries. *Ann Chir Gynecol* 1972; **61**: 211.

2. Pantaleoni DC. On endoscopic examination of the cavity of the womb. *Med Press Circ* 1869; **8**: 26.

3. de Kroon CD, Jansen FW. Saline infusion sonography in women with abnormal uterine bleeding: an update of recent findings. *Curr Opin Obstet Gynecol* 2006; **18**: 653–657.

4. Brown SE, Coddington CC, Schnorr J, et al. Evaluation of outpatient hysteroscopy, saline infusion hysterosonography, and hysterosalpingography in infertile women: a prospective, randomized study. *Fertil Steril* 2000; **74**: 1029–1034.

5. Ayida G, Chamberlain P, Barlow D, Kennedy S. Uterine cavity assessment prior to *in vitro* fertilization: comparison of transvaginal scanning, saline contrast hysterosonography and hysteroscopy. *Ultrasound Obstet Gynecol* 1997; **10**(1): 59–62.

6. Schwärzler P, Concin H, Bösch H, et al. An evaluation of sonohysterography and diagnostic hysteroscopy for the assessment of intrauterine pathology. *Ultrasound Obstet Gynecol* 1998; **11**: 337–342.

7. van Dongen H, Timmermans A, Jacobi CE, et al. Diagnostic hysteroscopy and saline infusion sonography in the diagnosis of intrauterine abnormalities: an assessment of patient preference. *Gynecol Surg* 2011; **8**(1): 65–70.

8. van Dongen H, de Kroon CD, van den Tillaart S, et al. A randomized comparison of office vaginoscopic hysteroscopy with saline infusion sonography: a patient compliance study. *BJOG* 2008; **115**: 1232–1237.

9. Büyük E, Durmusoglu F, Erenus M, Karakoç B. Endometrial disease diagnosed by transvaginal ultrasound and dilatation and curettage. *Acta Obstet Gynecol Scand* 1999; **78**: 419–422.

10. de Wit AC, Vleugels MP, de Kruif JH. Diagnostic hysteroscopy: a valuable diagnostic tool in the diagnosis of structural intra-cavital pathology and endometrial hyperplasia or carcinoma? Six years of experience with non-clinical diagnostic hysteroscopy. *Eur J Obstet Gynecol Reprod Biol* 2003; **110**: 79–82.

11. Laing FC, Brown DL, DiSalvo DN. Gynecologic ultrasound. *Radiol Clin North Am* 2001; **39**: 523–540.

12. Bingol B, Gunenc Z, Gedikbasi A, et al. Comparison of diagnostic accuracy of saline infusion sonohysterography, transvaginal sonography and hysteroscopy. *J Obstet Gynaecol* 2011; **31**(1): 54–58.

13. Soares SR, Barbosa dos Reis MM, Camargos AF. Diagnostic accuracy of sonohysterography, transvaginal sonography, and hysterosalpingography in patients with uterine cavity diseases. *Fertil Steril* 2000; **73**: 406–411.

14. Cullinan JA, Fleischer AC, Kepple DM, Arnold AL. Sonohysterography: a technique for endometrial evaluation. *Radiographics* 1995; **15**(3): 501–514; discussion 515–516.

15. Shushan A, Revel A, Rojansky N. How often are endometrial polyps malignant? *Gynecol Obstet Invest* 2004; **58**(4): 212–215.

16. Gupta JK, Chien PFW, Voit D, Clark TJ, et al. Ultrasonographic endometrial thickness for diagnosing endometrial pathology in women with postmenopausal bleeding: a meta-analysis. *Acta Obstetricia et Gynecologica Scandinavica* 2002; **81**: 799–816.

17. Cohen MA, Sauer MV, Keltz M, Lindheim SR. Utilizing routine sonohysterography to detect intrauterine pathology before initiating hormone replacement therapy. *Menopause* 1999; **6**: 68–70

18. Sousa R, Silvestre M, Almeida e Sousa L, et al. Transvaginal ultrasonography and hysteroscopy in postmenopausal bleeding: a prospective study. *Acta Obstet Gynecol Scand* 2001; **80**(9): 856–862.

19. Runowicz CD. Can radiological procedures replace histologic examination in the evaluation of abnormal vaginal bleeding? *Obstet Gynecol* 2002; **99**: 529–530.

20. Goldstein SR, Zeltser I, Horan CK. Ultrasonography-based triage for perimenopausal patients with abnormal uterine bleeding. *Am J Obstet Gynecol* 1997; **177**: 102–108.

21. Breitkopf DM, Frederickson RA, Snyder RR. Detection of benign endometrial masses by endometrial stripe measurement in premenopausal women. *Obstet Gynecol* 2004; **104**: 120–125.

22. Ubaldi F, Tournaye H, Camus M, et al. Fertility after hysteroscopic myomectomy. *Hum Reprod Update* 1995; **1**: 81–90.

23. Wamsteker K, Emanuel MH, de Kruif JH. Transcervical hysteroscopic resection of submucous fibroids for abnormal uterine bleeding: results regarding the degree of intramural extension. *Obstet Gynecol* 1993; **82**: 736–740.

24. Fedele L, Bianchi S, Dorta M, et al. Transvaginal ultrasonography versus hysteroscopy in the diagnosis of uterine submucous myoma. *Obstet Gynecol* 1991; **77**: 745–748.

25. Cicinelli E, Romano F, Anastasio PS, et al. Transabdominal sonohysterography, transvaginal sonography, and hysteroscopy in the evaluation of submucous myomas. *Obstet Gynecol* 1995; **85**(1): 42–47.

26. Friedman AJ. Use of gonadotropin-releasing hormone agonists before myomectomy. *Clin Obstet Gynecol* 1993; **36**: 650–659.

27. Jamieson WM. Hysteroscopic excision of symptomatic submucosal leiomyomas using the Nd: YAG laser. In: Corfman RS, Diamond MP, DeCherney A (Eds.) *Complications of Laparoscopy and Hysteroscopy*. Cambridge, MA: Blackwell Scientific Publications; 1993: 203–209.

28. Troiano RN, McCarthy SM. Müllerian duct anomalies: Imaging and clinical issues. *Radiology* 2004; **233**: 19–34.

29. Raga F, Bonilla-Musoles F, Blanes J, Osborne NG. Congenital müllerian anomalies: diagnostic accuracy of three-dimensional ultrasound. *Fertil Steril* 1996; **65**: 523–528.

30. Bettocchi S, Ceci O, Nappi L, et al. Office hysteroscopic metroplasty: three "diagnostic criteria" to differentiate between septate and bicornuate uteri. *J Minim Invasive Gynecol* 2007; **14**(3): 324–328.

31. Donnez J, Nisolle M. Operative laser hysteroscopy in Müllerian fusion defects and uterine adhesions. In: Donnez J (Ed.) *Operative Laser Laparoscopy and Hysteroscopy*. Leuven, Belgium: Nauwelaerts Printing; 1989: 249–261.

32. Confino E, Friberg J, Giglia RV, Fleicher N. Sonographic imaging of intrauterine adhesions. *Obstet Gynecol* 1985; **66**: 596–598.

33. Schlaff WD, Hurst BS. Preoperative sonographic measurement of endometrial pattern predicts outcome of surgical repair in patients with severe Asherman's syndrome. *Fertil Steril* 1995; **63**: 410.

34. Davis PC, O'Neill MJ, Yoder IC, et al. Sonohysterographic findings of endometrial and subendometrial conditions. *Radiographics* 2002; **22**: 803–816.

35. Sylvestre C, Child T, Tulandi T, Tan SL. A prospective study to evaluate the efficacy of two- and three-dimensional sonohysterography in women with intrauterine lesions. *Fertil Steril* 2003; **79**: 1222–1225.

36. Molinas CR, Campo R. Office hysteroscopy and adenomyosis. *Best Pract Res Clin Obstet Gynaecol* 2006; **20**(4): 557–567.

Chapter

4

Consent and legal counseling for gynecologic ultrasound examinations

James Shwayder

Consent

The legal precedent for informed consent began with a 1914 court case in which a patient underwent surgical removal of a tumor to which he had not agreed. Justice Cardozo, then of the New York Supreme Court, opined that "Every human being of adult years and sound mind has a right to determine what shall be done with his own body" [1]. This remains the basis for patient autonomy in making decisions related to their medical care and treatment. The phrase "informed consent" was introduced in a 1957 California medical negligence case, *Salgo v. Stanford University* [2]. A patient's legs became paralyzed following an aortogram. The treating physician allegedly failed to advise the patient of this inherent risk of the procedure. The court held that "a physician violates his duty to his patient and subjects himself to liability if he withholds any facts which are necessary to form the basis of an intelligent consent by the patient to the proposed treatment" [2].

The ethical concept of "informed consent" involves comprehension, or understanding, and free consent, or voluntary choice [3]. There are two standards of consent: (a) the reasonable person (patient) and (b) the reasonable physician, which may vary with each jurisdiction. The *reasonable patient standard* holds that the communication to the patient is adequate and sufficient enough that a reasonable person could make a reasonable decision based on the provided information. The *reasonable physician standard* holds that the information communicated to the patient is that which a reasonable physician would have discussed with the patient. In actuality, most informed consent discussions encompass both standards. It is recognized that informed consent is an interactive process between the physician and the patient [3]. The "informed consent" form merely memorializes the discussions [3]

The elements of consent require a description or discussion of the following: (a) the diagnosis or nature of the condition; (b) the planned procedure; (c) the alternatives to the procedure, including doing nothing; and (d) the substantial risks of the procedure (Table 4.1). Further, a discussion of the anticipated success or benefit of the procedure and the risks if

Table 4.1 Elements of informed consent

1. The diagnosis or nature of condition
2. The planned procedure or treatment
3. The alternatives to the procedure or treatment, including doing nothing
4. The substantial risks of the procedure or treatment

the procedure is not done are inherent to adequate informed consent [4].

Consent for ultrasound is the process by which someone agrees to the performance of an ultrasound study. Most gynecologic ultrasound includes some combination of vaginal and abdominal ultrasound. Many patients are familiar and comfortable with abdominal ultrasound. This may not be true with vaginal ultrasound. A discussion of the vaginal procedure should include a brief description of its performance and the relative merits of vaginal sonography. This discussion should also include the diagnostic limitations of ultrasound; whether the sonologist is acting as a consultant; and, if so, that the patient's primary provider is responsible for clinical care decisions.

Vaginal studies may not be feasible in some elderly patients or patients who have never used tampons or been sexually active. In these instances, informed consent should include the limitations that may exist in relying on findings from the abdominal study only. Alternatives to a vaginal ultrasound include transperineal or transrectal ultrasound. These warrant further discussion as they are not a part of a typical gynecologic ultrasound. Whether a formal written consent is required for the various ultrasound approaches is highly dependent on local and regional norms, as well as institutional policy.

The request for a pelvic ultrasound should originate from an appropriately licensed health care provider and should include sufficient information for appropriate performance and interpretation of the ultrasound study [5]. Some institutions require a specific order or requisition for the transvaginal component of a pelvic ultrasound examination [6]. AIUM guidelines state

Ultrasonography in Gynecology, ed. Botros R. M. B. Rizk and Elizabeth E. Puscheck. Published by Cambridge University Press. © Cambridge University Press 2015.

that "All relevant structures should be identified by a transabdominal and/or transvaginal approach. In some cases, both will be needed" [5]. It is recognized that the transabdominal approach is beneficial with an enlarged or midplane uterus or a large pelvic/abdominal mass. Vaginal ultrasound enhances the morphologic and dynamic assessment of the pelvis and cul-de-sac. Thus, it is the author's opinion that a pelvic ultrasound inherently encompasses both abdominal and transvaginal approaches. Therefore, a request for a pelvic ultrasound infers the use of either or both approaches.

3D pelvic ultrasound and Doppler require additional comment. 3D multiplanar reconstruction and rendering offer unique capabilities in visualizing and diagnosing many uterine, tubal, and adnexal/ovarian abnormalities. Doppler evaluation may enhance the further differentiation of malignant versus benign masses or the possibility of torsion. Thus, if clinically indicated, a request for a pelvic ultrasound inherently includes 3D and Doppler studies as well. However, prudent use dictates the use of these modalities for appropriate clinical indications, not financial gain.

The performance of sonohysterography, sonosalpingography, and ultrasound-guided puncture procedures resides outside the normal pelvic ultrasound examination. As such, these procedures are not considered integral to a request for a pelvic ultrasound. Each procedure should be performed with an appropriate provider request. There are no express standards regarding the use of written informed consent for these procedures [7]. Each institution or practice should establish standard policies and procedures regarding written consent, pre-procedure pregnancy testing, and antibiotic prophylaxis. However, the basis of appropriate informed consent is the discussion with the patient, not just a signed consent form.

Types of consent

Consent may either be implied or express. Implied consent is consent that is inferred from signs, actions, or facts, or by inaction or silence [8]. Implied consent exists when a patient presents for a diagnostic study. Her presence implies that she consents to the performance of necessary procedures.

Express consent comprises the discussion or communication of the elements of informed consent with the patient's express consent either verbally or in writing that requires no inference or implication to supply its meaning [8]. Often, a patient's written consent to sonographic procedures is obtained at the registration area. This may be sufficient for standard procedures, such as abdominal and vaginal ultrasound. An informal survey of gynecologic experts in vaginal sonography revealed that none obtained specific consent for vaginal sonography. However, the addition of sonohysterography, sonosalpingography, or an associated biopsy procedure may warrant specific informed consent, often in writing.

Whether consent is implied or expressed, written or verbal, providers should recognize that patients can retract their consent at any time. This injects the concept of informed refusal

where the sonologist must inform the patient of the potential for adverse outcomes if a recommended diagnostic or therapeutic procedure is refused. This counseling should be documented in the patient's chart; and, in critical situations, a written refusal signed by the patient should be obtained.

The use of chaperones during vaginal ultrasound presents a unique situation. Chaperones are generally recommended for either female or male providers during any pelvic exam. Logically, this should apply to vaginal ultrasound as well. However, the routine, habit, and custom of most diagnostic units is that female and, occasionally, male sonographers do not routinely have chaperones during sonographic studies. It is recommended that chaperones be present when males perform vaginal, transperineal, or rectal studies. Patients should have the option for the presence of a chaperone and should consent, either verbally or in writing, to the lack of a chaperone in all instances.

Recommendations (Table 4.2)

As noted, regional and institutional differences exist regarding the specific consent requirements for performing pelvic ultrasound and the related procedures. Not all institutions require a requisition for transvaginal ultrasound when performing pelvic sonography. However, most require specific requisitions for sonohysterography, sonosalpingography, and ultrasound-guided puncture procedures.

Differences also exist regarding the use of written consent for ultrasound. Providers of ultrasound services should check with their malpractice carrier and institution to determine whether written consent to any specific procedure is required. If so, such written consent should include a description of the procedure, its alternatives, and any significant risks or benefits. Policies regarding specific consent forms for sonohysterography, sonosalpingography, and ultrasound-guided puncture procedures should be established by each institution and practice. Ideally, written consent should also incorporate a disclaimer regarding the limitations of ultrasound procedures and clearly state that clinical management decisions rest with the patient's primary provider.

Informed refusal forms should be available in unique, critical clinical circumstances (Table 4.3).

One should document whether there is a chance of pregnancy at the time of the pelvic ultrasound. This can include

Table 4.2 Informed consent recommendations

1. Determine requisition requirements for ultrasound procedures
2. Determine norms for written consent for pelvic ultrasound
3. Establish policies regarding written consent for ultrasound procedures
4. Incorporate disclaimers into consent forms
5. Develop a generic "informed refusal" form for use when clinically indicated
6. Develop a policy regarding the use of chaperones
7. Document the possibility of pregnancy prior to ultrasound study

Table 4.3 Informed consent recommended for the following*

1. Sonohysterography
2. Sonosalpingography
3. Ultrasound-guided puncture procedures
4. Use of non-FDA-approved contrast agents
5. Use of intravenous contrast agents

*1 and 2 based on regional or institutional policy.

documenting a patient's last menstrual period, contraceptive use, the patient's voluntary declaration, or a documented pregnancy test. If vaginal ultrasound is anticipated, the registration form or consent form should include the unit's policy on the presence of chaperones during the procedure. If a chaperone is not used, the patient's consent can be obtained at this time.

Legal counseling

Counseling patients with respect to ultrasound-related liability requires an understanding of what underlies most ultrasound-related cases. Although the specialties affected by ultrasound-related liability have changed over the past 30 years, obstetrics and gynecology remain the focus of most litigation (Fig. 4.1). Ultrasound-related liability generally falls under several categories [9]:

1. Missed diagnosis
2. Misinterpreted sonograms
3. Invented lesions
4. Delay (or failure) in communication
5. Failure to perform ultrasound
6. Fraud cases
7. Procedure-related cases
8. Sonographer-related cases.

Missed diagnosis is also known as an error in perception and occurs when the abnormality is seen in retrospect, but it was missed when interpreting the initial study [10]. An example would be an ectopic pregnancy visualized on the ultrasound study, but not identified by the interpreting sonologist.

Patients should be counseled regarding the limitations of the study, the potential errors in diagnosis, and the importance of immediate communication with their primary provider if their clinical condition deteriorates. Although the error rate in radiology may be as high as 30% [11], the critical question is, "Was it below the standard of care for the physician not to have seen the abnormality?" [12]. It is difficult to defend such an error as the plaintiff's expert usually identifies the abnormality on the radiologic study and allows the jury or judge to draw their own conclusion. It is estimated that 80% of cases are lost if they go to jury verdict [12]. Thus, many suits regarding an error in perception or a missed diagnosis are settled.

Misinterpreted ultrasounds, so-called errors in interpretation, occur when an abnormality is perceived, but is incorrectly described [10]. This most often occurs when a malignant

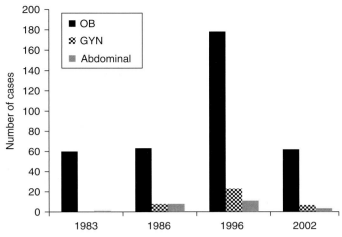

Fig. 4.1 Litigation cases related to ultrasound by specialty area, in the United States [9].

lesion is called benign or a benign lesion is called malignant. A common example is a hemorrhagic corpus luteum that is called a cancer, which leads to unnecessary surgery, particularly if complications occur during the surgical procedure. As before, counseling a patient regarding the findings, concerns, and need for follow-up is critical to patient compliance. Also, direct communication with the requesting provider allows further discussion of diagnostic and treatment options. The best defense in such cases is an appropriate differential diagnosis, preferably including the correct diagnosis [12]. By including such differential diagnoses, most cases are won if they go to jury verdict.

An example of an invented lesion is when an early intrauterine pregnancy with a corpus luteum is called an ectopic pregnancy. This error is compounded when methotrexate is given with an adverse outcome. Unfortunately, this error is increasing in frequency [13]. A discussion of preventing such errors is beyond this chapter. However, methotrexate use should be withheld until a definitive diagnosis of ectopic pregnancy is made or serial quantitative hCG levels and ultrasounds fail to demonstrate the pregnancy's location, the so-called "pregnancy of unknown location" [14].

A delay, or failure, to communicate significant findings in a timely and clinically appropriate manner may result in litigation, particularly when immediate or urgent intervention is required [10]. Although the final written report is considered the definitive means of communicating the results of an imaging study or procedure, direct or personal communication must occur in certain situations. Examples would be an ectopic pregnancy with hemoperitoneum; a torsed, or twisted, ovary; or an obvious malignancy. Direct communication to the ordering provider, or in their absence the responsible party, is recommended. The type of communication and the person receiving the communication should be documented in the report. It is preferable to include the date and time of the communication as well. In other cases, one should establish standard

Table 4.4 Legal issues in ultrasound

1. Perform studies in accordance with established standards
2. Counsel patients regarding the limitations of ultrasound diagnosis
3. Communicate directly with the ordering provider in critical situations
4. Avoid inappropriate diagnosis codes to allow insurance coverage
5. Counsel patients as to the anticipated adverse reactions to ultrasound-related procedures
6. Obtain appropriate informed consent when performing procedures or utilizing agents outside their approved use

reporting routines, such as required by AIUM accreditation [15]. However, email and text messaging provide alternatives to standard communication. It may be beneficial to adopt such methods of communication with frequent referrers.

In the final report, the prudent sonologist should suggest the next appropriate study or procedure based upon the findings and clinical information [10]. Communicating this recommendation to the patient enhances their understanding and compliance. The additional studies should add meaningful information to clarify or confirm the initial impression, and not for the sole purpose of enhancing referral income.

Failure to perform an ultrasound in the recommended fashion, visualizing all of the pelvic anatomy, can subject one to litigation for missed diagnosis and incomplete studies (Table 4.4). One should follow AIUM or ACOG guidelines for appropriate exam performance and content [5,7]. If a limited study is performed, the patient should be counseled as to the limited nature of the study and the need for a complete pelvic ultrasound for diagnostic purposes.

Health care fraud in ultrasound is an important concern. In the context of patient counseling, the prime issue is advising the patient that diagnoses cannot be altered to justify insurance coverage for a procedure. A classic example is a patient undergoing ovulation induction for fertility who requests that the diagnosis be entered as polycystic ovarian disease for ovulation monitoring. If the patient lacks infertility coverage this would constitute fraud on the part of the sonologist. Ethically, one is obligated to advise the patient that such accommodations are not possible as it subjects the sonologist and their practice or institution to litigation and punitive action.

Procedure-related litigation is an area in which patient counseling and informed consent are critical. The risks of sonohysterography and sonosalpingography are minimal. In general, patients should be counseled as to the risks of cramping, vasovagal reactions, infection, allergic reactions to cleansing solutions, and possible vaginal drainage and bleeding following the procedure. It is preferable to avoid latex probe covers and catheters due to the increasing incidence of latex-related adverse reactions.

Contrast agents require special counseling and consent. Efforts to enhance visualization of the fallopian tubes and the uterine cavity have led to the development of contrast agents such as specialized foams or gels. Although available in other countries, these are currently not Food and Drug

Administration (FDA)-approved for use in the United States. As such, their current use should be restricted to research protocols. This requires appropriate counseling and written consent. Similarly, intravenous contrast agents for assessment of ovarian malignancy are under study. Although many of the agents are approved for use in cardiac evaluation, for example, gynecologic use is investigational. These research protocols clearly require written consent.

Ultrasound-guided puncture procedures, such as follicular aspiration or ultrasound-guided injection of ectopic pregnancies should incorporate written consent for the procedure, incorporating the required elements for informed consent. This should include any additional risks germane to the procedure, such as vascular or intestinal injury.

Conclusion

Gynecologic ultrasound is critical to the evaluation and treatment of patients. Innovative applications are rapidly evolving. Written informed consent for routine pelvic ultrasound is highly dependent on the region and institution where one practices. However, non-traditional uses, such as intravenous contrast agents and various puncture procedures, warrant focused counseling and appropriate written informed consent.

References

1. *Schloendorff* v. *Society of New York Hospital*. 105 NE 92 (NY 1914).
2. *Salgo* v. *Leland Stanford, Jr. University Board of Trustees*. 317 P2d. 170 (Ca. App 1957).
3. American College of Obstetricians and Gynecologists. Informed Consent. Washington, DC. ACOG August 2009, Number 439.
4. American Medical Association. Informed Consent. Chicago: AMA. http://www.ama-assn.org//ama/pub/physician-resources/medical-ethics/code-medical-ethics/opinion808.page (accessed April 26, 2014).
5. AIUM (American Institute of Ultrasound in Medicine). *AIUM Practice Guideline for the Performance of Pelvic Ultrasound Examinations*. Laurel, MD: AIUM; 2009.
6. Daftary. *Requisition Needed for Transvaginal Ultrasound Component?* Laurel, MD: AIUM; 2010. http://www.aiumcommunities.org/group/gynecologic/forum/topics/requisition-needed-for (accessed May 16, 2011).
7. AIUM. *AIUM Practice Guideline for the Performance of Saline Infusion Sonohysterography*. Laurel, MD: American Institute of Ultrasound in Medicine; 2011. http://www.aium.org/resources/guidelines/sonohysterography.pdf (accessed May 16, 2011).
8. *Black's Law Dictionary*, 7th edn. St. Paul, MN: West Group; 1999.
9. Sanders RC. Changing patterns in ultrasound-related litigation. *J Ultrasound Med* 2003; **22**: 1009–1015.
10. Raskin MM. Why radiologists get sued. *Appl Radiol* 2001; **30**: 9–13.
11. Berlin L, Hendrix R. Perceptual errors and negligence. *Am J Roentgenol* 1998; **170**(4): 863–867.
12. Berlin L. Malpractice issues in radiology: defending the "missed" radiographic diagnosis. *Am J Roentgenol* 2001; **176**: 317–332.

13. Shwayder JM. Waiting for the tide to change: reducing risk in the turbulent sea of liability. *Obstet Gynecol* 2010; **116**(1): 8–15.

14. Barnhart K, van Mello NM, Bourne T, et al. Pregnancy of unknown location: a consensus statement of nomenclature, definitions, and outcome. *Fertil Steril* 2011; **95**(3): 857–866.

15. AIUM. *Standards and Guidelines for the Accreditation of Ultrasound Practices*. Laurel, MD: AIUM; 2010 (updated December 17, 2010). Available from www.aium.org/officialStatements/26 (accessed April 18, 2014).

5

Ultrasound imaging in polycystic ovary syndrome

Misty M. Blanchette Porter

Introduction

Polycystic ovary syndrome (PCOS) is the single most common endocrine disorder of women of reproductive age. The major clinical features are menstrual irregularity (anovulation or infrequent ovulation), clinical or biochemical evidence of hyperandrogenism (HA), and/or the presence of polycystic ovaries (PCO), as defined by transvaginal ultrasound (US). The prevalence of the disorder is 6–8% of women worldwide and 12% in women with increasing body mass index (BMI) [1], when the National Institutes of Health (NIH) 1990 criteria are applied [2]. This triad of symptoms is also frequently accompanied by infertility, obesity, insulin resistance, and the resultant compensatory hyperinsulinemia.

Definition

There has been little international consensus on the definition of PCOS. Until recently, two definitions were accepted: (a) the more conservative 1990 NIH conference criteria [3] and (b) one suggested by the European Society of Human Reproduction and Embryology (ESHRE)/American Society for Reproductive Medicine (ASRM) [2]. The Androgen Excess and PCOS (AE-PCOS) Society has proposed a third definition [4]. The AE-PCOS Society suggests that there should be acceptance of the original NIH criteria, but with modification. It acknowledged the opinions expressed during the 2003 Rotterdam ESHRE/ASRM consensus conference that a cardinal feature of PCOS is the PCO, also referred to as the polycystic ovarian morphology (PCOM) (Fig. 5.1). However, a principal conclusion of the AE-PCOS report is that PCOS should first be considered a disorder of androgen excess or HA [4]. The three definitions are summarized in Table 5.1.

The establishment of the diagnosis of PCOS imparts substantial psychological, social, and economic consequences in the care of these women. The diagnosis implies an increased risk for type 2 diabetes mellitus, dyslipidemia, hypertension, endometrial adenocarcinoma, dysfunctional uterine bleeding, metabolic syndrome, and possibly cardiovascular disease for these patients [4]. Furthermore, the diagnosis may have important familial implications for the patient's sisters, brothers, father, mother, and her children [5]. Family members of women with PCOS have been found to have a higher risk of exhibiting the hyperandrogenic or metabolic traits of the disorder [5]. Careful selection of patients with PCOS would allow for the appropriate screening and treatment of women who are at significant risk for life-long sequelae, and the appropriate identification of women with PCOS would provide a guide for current and future research.

The 2003 ESHRE/ASRM-sponsored PCOS consensus group re-emphasized the importance of PCOM by US in the diagnostic criteria. However, the inclusion of the use of US to diagnose PCOS sparked an international controversy. Application of these criteria allowed for the inclusion of two phenotypes of PCOS: (a) patients with hirsutism and/or HA with PCOM, but who ovulate normally, and (b) patients with PCOM and irregular ovulation, but no signs of androgen excess. Further adding to the controversy is the observation that while PCOM is found consistently in women with PCOS [6], similar ovarian findings are often seen in up to 25% of normal controls [7]. Nonetheless, debate continues about the utilization of ovarian morphology in the diagnosis of PCOS.

Clinical presentation

The characteristic clinical features used to establish the diagnosis of PCOS include: (a) ovulatory or menstrual dysfunction, (b) hyperandrogenism, and/or (c) PCOM. The menstrual dysfunction associated with PCOS is generally characterized by infrequent or absent menstrual bleeding and affects 75–85% of women with the disorder [4]. Menstrual irregularity may begin at menarche, or may follow an initial duration of regular periods, and is often hallmarked by oligomenorrhea or amenorrhea. Although menstrual dysfunction is a common presenting symptom of patients with PCOS, 20–30% of women with PCOS will present with eumenorrhea [4]. Patients who present with clinical evidence of HA, but give a history of regular menses, should have their ovulatory function further evaluated. Between 20% and 50% of these women may ultimately be diagnosed with menstrual dysfunction and be considered to be affected by PCOS [4].

Ultrasonography in Gynecology, ed. Botros R. M. B. Rizk and Elizabeth E. Puscheck. Published by Cambridge University Press. © Cambridge University Press 2015.

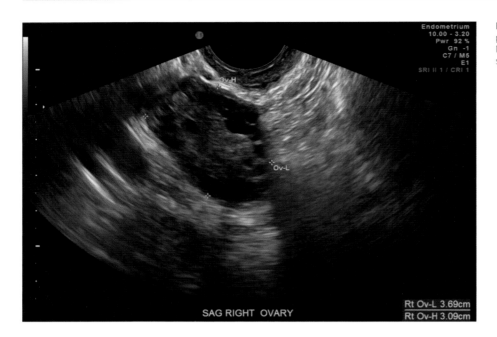

Fig. 5.1 Transvaginal ultrasound in the sagittal plane showing polycystic ovarian morphology. Numerous small follicles surround a dense central stroma.

Table 5.1 Criteria for PCOS

	NIH 1990	Rotterdam 2003	AE-PCOS 2009
Diagnostic criteria	Requires simultaneous presence of: 1. Clinical and/or biochemical hyperandrogenism 2. Menstrual dysfunction	Requires the presence of at least two criteria: 1. Clinical and/or biochemical hyperandrogenism 2. Ovulatory dysfunction 3. PCOM	Requires the presence of: 1. Hyperandrogenism and/or hyperandrogenemia 2. Ovarian dysfunction: oligo-anovulation, and/or polycystic ovaries
Exclusion criteria	Congenital adrenal hyperplasia, androgen-secreting tumors, Cushing's syndrome, and hyperprolactinemia	Congenital adrenal hyperplasia, androgen-secreting tumors, and Cushing's syndrome	21-hydroxylase-deficient nonclassic adrenal hyperplasia, androgen-secreting neoplasms, androgenic/anabolic drug use or abuse, the hyperandrogenic–insulin resistance–acanthosis nigricans syndrome, thyroid dysfunction, and hyperprolactinemia
Clinical traits	Hirsutism, acne, and alopecia	Hirsutism, acne, and androgenic alopecia	Hirsutism
Biochemical traits	1. Total testosterone 2. Free testosterone 3. Androstenedione 4. DHEAS	1. Free androgen index and free testosterone 2. Total testosterone 3. DHEAS	1. Free androgen index or free testosterone 2. Total testosterone 3. DHEAS
PCOM	Not included	At least one ovary showing either: 1. Twelve or more follicles of 2–9 mm in diameter 2. Ovarian volume – 10 mL	At least one ovary showing either: 1. Twelve or more follicles of 2–9 mm in diameter 2. Ovarian volume – 10 mL

AE-PCOS, Androgen Excess and PCOS Society; DHEAS, dehydroepiandrosterone sulfate; NIH, National Institutes of Health; PCOM, polycystic morphology by US.

HA is the most constant and prominent diagnostic component of PCOS. It is assessed by clinical features and/or biochemical indices. The degree to which patients exhibit evidence of HA can vary substantially based on ethnic origin, body weight, and age. HA is clinically diagnosed by the subjective assessment of hirsutism (~70%), acne (12–40%), and androgenic alopecia (~10–40%) [4]. The most commonly used assessment tool to visually score hirsutism is a modification of the method originally reported by Ferriman and Gallwey [8]. Nine body areas, including upper lip, chin, chest, upper and lower back, upper and lower abdomen, upper arm, and the thigh are visually scored for the density of terminal hairs. A cut-off value between 6 and 8 has been used to define hirsutism.

Biochemically, HA is most commonly assessed by measurement of serum testosterone (T) levels, total and unbound or free. Serum T and sex hormone-binding globulin (SHBG) values are utilized to calculate the free or bioavailable fraction of the free androgen index (T/SHBG × 100). The concentrations of other serum androgens, such as androstenedione and dihydroepiandrostenedione sulfate (DHEAS), are often high in women with PCOS, but their measurement is thought to add little to the diagnosis of the syndrome in most clinical settings. Other conditions known to mimic the features of PCOS must be excluded. These conditions include nonclassic congenital adrenal hyperplasia, androgen-secreting tumors, androgenic or anabolic drug use or abuse, the hyperandrogenic–insulin–resistance–acanthosis nigricans (HAIR-AN) syndrome, thyroid dysfunction, and hyperprolactinemia. Although obesity and metabolic syndrome are frequently present in women with PCOS, they are not regarded as intrinsic disturbances of the disorder. Overall, 50–70% of women with PCOS have demonstrable insulin resistance [4].

The diagnosis of polycystic ovary syndrome in adolescents

The application of the Rotterdam criteria to make the diagnosis of PCOS in the adolescent may prove problematic. In the adolescent, some clinical features consistent with PCOS may be in evolution or, in fact, transitory [9]. Prematurely assigning a label of PCOS to an adolescent may result in unnecessary treatments and impose psychological distress [9]. During pubertal transition, adolescents have relative androgenemia, insulin resistance, cystic ovaries, and anovulatory cycles, which transition into an estrogenic state later in puberty [10]. However, while there is no agreement concerning how to diagnose PCOS in the adolescent, the potential benefits of early intervention have led to growing attention to identifying those individuals with the highest probability of having the disorder.

In a recent clinical opinion, Carmina et al. suggested more stringent criteria for establishing the diagnosis of PCOS in the adolescent than would be allowed by both the Rotterdam and NIH guidelines [9]. These authors suggest that, during adolescence, all three elements of the Rotterdam criteria should be met and that HA be defined as hyperandrogenemia, using ultrasensitive serum androgen assays with the exception of well-documented progressive hirsutism [9]. By this definition, patients should be considered only if they are at least 2 years post-menarche, have oligoamenorrhea present for at least 2 years, and demonstrate the diagnosis of PCOM by abdominal US (increased ovarian size >10 cm³) (Fig. 5.2). For other patients who may not demonstrate all three criteria, but have features suggestive of PCOS, these authors suggest careful follow-up into adulthood to be certain that those with the disorder are not missed [9].

Table 5.2 Table demonstrating a large ovarian volume associated with polycystic ovary. Ovarian volume can be auto-calculated from three orthogonal measurements of the ovary by most ultrasound machines

GYN	
General GYN	
Uterus	
Uterus volume	72.80 ml
Uterus length	8.65 cm
Uterus height	3.93 cm
Uterus width	4.09 cm
Right ovary	
R ov volume	18.32 ml
R ov length	3.84 cm
R ov height	2.43 cm
R ov width	3.75 cm
Left ovary	
L ov volume	12.81 ml

ESHRE/ASRM consensus definition

The ESHRE/ASRM consensus workshop definition for the PCOM is one that contains 12 or more follicles in each ovary of 2–9 mm in diameter and/or increased ovarian volume (OV) (>10 cm³) [11] (Fig. 5.3). To establish the follicular number (FN), each ovary is scanned in a longitudinal plane from the inner to outer margin with the total number of follicles noted. Follicular number is estimated in two planes of the ovary, noting their size and number. The diameter of the follicles is measured as the mean of three diameters (longitudinal, transverse, and anteroposterior) [11]. If there is evidence of a dominant follicle (>10 mm) or a corpus luteum, the scan should be repeated in the next cycle. The finding of only one ovary fitting this definition, or an occurrence of one of the above criteria (i.e. FN or follicular volume only), is considered sufficient to define the PCOM. This definition does not apply to women taking the oral contraceptive pill, as ovarian size is reduced, even though the "polycystic" appearance may persist. The scan should be performed with "state of the art" equipment, by a transvaginal approach when possible, and in the follicular phase or 3–5 days following a progestin-induced bleed or at random within the cycle.

The FN per ovary and size of those follicles accepted to meet the criteria for the PCOM was established primarily based on the work of Jonard et al. [12]. In a study comparing 214 women with PCOS (oligo-/amenorrhea, elevated serum luteinizing hormone and/or T, and/or ovarian area (OA) >5.5 cm²) to 112 controls, these authors utilized 2D transvaginal US to determine total FN, and to classify follicular size into three different

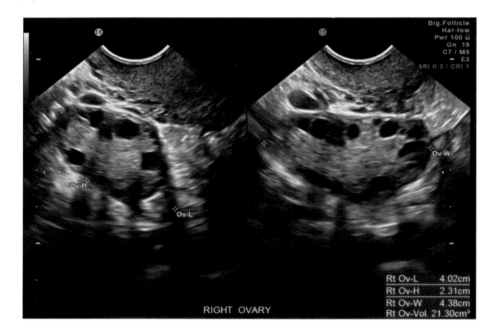

Fig. 5.2 Transvaginal ultrasound of an ovary in both sagittal and longitudinal planes demonstrating a large ovarian volume.

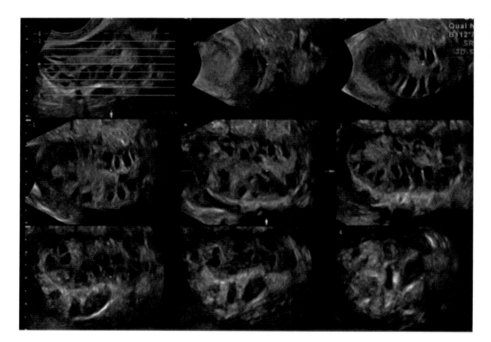

Fig. 5.3 Transvaginal ultrasound with topographic assessment of an ovary demonstrating multiple small follicles from one lateral margin to the opposite margin.

categories (2–5 mm, 6–9 mm, and 2–9 mm). Their study demonstrated that, with a threshold set at ≥12 follicles of 2–9 mm size, the best compromise was reached with regard to sensitivity (75%) and specificity (99%) [12]. Furthermore, in evaluating the subcategories of follicles, this group demonstrated that the mean FN was similar between normal and PCOS in the 6–9 mm range, but significantly higher in PCOS in the 2–5 mm and 2–9 mm ranges [12] (Fig. 5.4). In subsequent work, the size of the 2–5 mm follicular pool has been shown to be strongly associated with the severity of the menstrual disorder (Table 5.2) [13].

Multicystic (multifollicular) versus polycystic ovarian morphology

A multifollicular ovary (MFO) has been described as one in which the ovaries are normal in size or slightly enlarged, have multiple (≥6) follicles (usually 4–10 mm in diameter), and have normal stromal size (Figs 5.5 and 5.6) [14]. An increase in number of 2–9 mm follicles from 10 to 12 was proposed to help discriminate the PCO from the multifollicular ovary (MFO), or "multicystic" ovary [14]. In these patients, the uterus is often small, consistent with estrogen deficiency. In

Table 5.3 Median values with the 5–95th percentiles (in parentheses) of the tested variables in PCOS and control groups

	PCOS Amenorrhea (*n* = 63)	PCOS Oligoamenorrhea (*n* = 284)	PCOS Regular cycles (*n* = 110)	Controls (*n* = 188)
Age (years)	26.0 (17.2–36.2)[a,b]	28 (20.0–35.5)	28.0 (21.4–35.2)	29.0 (22.4–36.0)
BMI (kg/m^2)	28.2 (19.4–42.5)	25.2 (18.8–41.9)	24.6 (18.4–39.9)	22.9 (18.1–35.0)
Waist circumference (cm)	90.0 (64.0–123.0)[b]	82.0 (64.3–117.7)	80.0 (62.5–113.5)	73.0 (60.0–102.2)
Testosterone (ng/mL)	0.58 (0.28–1.16)[a,b]	0.46 (0.13–.92)[c]	0.38 (0.16–.75)	0.25 (0.08–0.54)
Insulin (mIU/L)	7.8 (1.2–34.4)[a,b]	5.2 (1.0–20.3)	4.4 (0.9–15.3)	3.4 (0.9–10.1)
2–5 mm FN	17.5 (6.6–40.2)[a,b]	13.5 (4.0–28.4)[c]	11.5 (3.7–24.6)	4.5 (2.2–9.5)
6–9 mm FN	1.5 (0–10.0)[a,b]	3.5 (0–12.0)	4.0 (0–12.2)	2.3 (0–5.5)
Ovarian area (cm^2)	6.68 (3.9–9.3)[a,b]	5.9 (3.8–8.6)[c]	5.47 (3.7–7.4)	3.9 (2.8–5.1)

BMI, body mass index; FN, follicular number
[a]Amenorrhea subgroup significantly different from oligoamenorrhea subgroup (ANOVA with post hoc analysis, $P < 0.05$).
[b]Amenorrhea subgroup significantly different from regular cycle subgroup (ANOVA with post hoc analysis, $P < 0.05$).
[c]Oligoamenorrhea subgroup significantly different from regular cycle subgroup (ANOVA with post hoc analysis, $P < 0.05$).
Source: Adapted from Dewailly D, Catteau-Jonard S, Reyss AC, et al. *Hum Reprod* 2007; **22**(6): 1562.

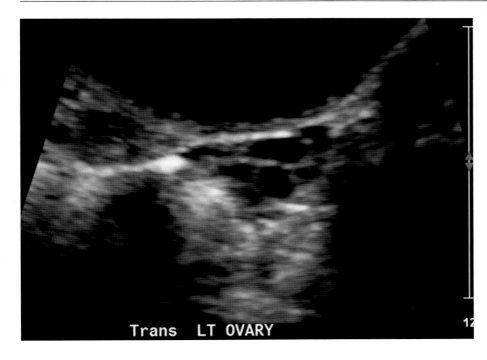

Trans LT OVARY

Fig. 5.4 Transabdominal ultrasound of a multifollicular ovary (transverse view). Note the multiple follicles with little intervening stroma.

contrast to the PCO, the MFO is characteristically seen in normal puberty, central precocious puberty, hyperprolactinemia, and in women with hypothalamic amenorrhea, such as those patients with eating disorders. These clinical situations are often associated with follicular growth without the consistent recruitment of a dominant follicle. Although the clinical picture of hypothalamic amenorrhea is different, the combination of amenorrhea and presence of an MFO could lead to the erroneous diagnosis of PCOS. As the finding of an MFO is relatively common, careful consideration of the association of these US findings with the patient's clinical and endocrinologic profile is imperative before the diagnosis of PCOS is established.

Ovarian volume and ovarian area

The ESHRE/ASRM consensus definition for PCOM includes an OV of >10 cm^3. OV is calculated by utilizing a simplified formula for a prolate ellipse. It is recognized that any calculation of the volume of a sphere or prolate ellipse (0.5 × length × width × thickness) based on 2D measurements assumes a degree of regularity of the ovary, and yet ovaries with PCOM are generally less regular. The selected threshold of OV of 10 cm^3 was based on an evaluation of results of many studies in which the upper normal threshold of OV was either defined as the maximal value of control subjects, or the 95th percentile of the control subject range. While this criterion

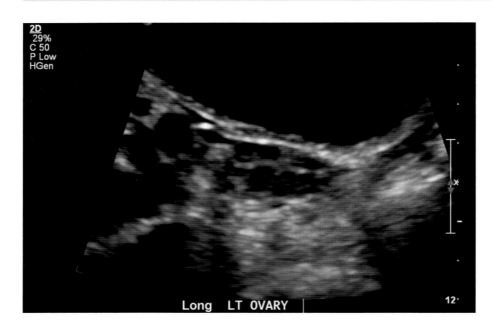

Fig. 5.5 Same ovary as in Fig. 5.5 (longitudinal view).

Table 5.4 ROC curve data

	Area under the ROC curve	Threshold	Sensitivity (%)	Specificity (%)
OA (cm²)	0.941	4	95.9	55.4
		4.5	90	75
		5.0	77.6	94.7
		5.5	67	100
		5	53.1	100
OV (cm³)	0.905	6	89.8	77.2
		7	67.5	91.2
		8	63.3	94.7
		9	53.1	98.2
		10	45.9	98.2
2–9 mm FN	0.956	10	91.5	85
		11	89.4	90.2
		12	79	97
		13	76.3	100
		14	68.9	100
		15	65	100

OA, ovarian area; OV, ovarian volume; FN, follicular number.

Source: Adapted from Jonard S, Robert Y, Dewailly D. *Hum Reprod* 2005; 20(10): 2893.

guarantees a specificity of 98%, it does not offer the best sensitivity [15].

In a study completed to define the optimal values for OV, OA, and FN in the PCOM, Jonard et al. utilized receiver operator characteristic (ROC) analysis comparing 154 patients with PCOS to 57 age-matched control women (Table 5.3) [15]. In this study, the Rotterdam ESHRE/ARSM guidelines were carefully applied with imaging completed in the follicular phase of cycling women. These authors suggested lowering the OV threshold to 7 cm³, which allowed for a sensitivity of 67.5% and a specificity of 91.2% [15]. They suggested that while there is considerable controversy in the literature with regard to normative data for the upper limit of OV, when the imaging studies are restricted to the very early follicular phase of natural cycles, the mean normal OV is observed to be 4.5 cm³ [15].

In 2D US, OA is calculated by one of three methods: (a) utilizing the formula for an ellipse (length × width × π/4); (b) fitting an ellipse to the ovary with the area calculated by the US machine; and (c) outlining by hand the ovary with the

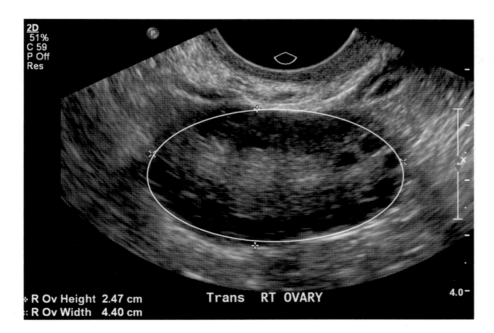

Fig. 5.6 Transvaginal ultrasound in a patient with polycystic ovarian syndrome demonstrating the calculation of the ovarian area by fitting an ellipse to the ovary.

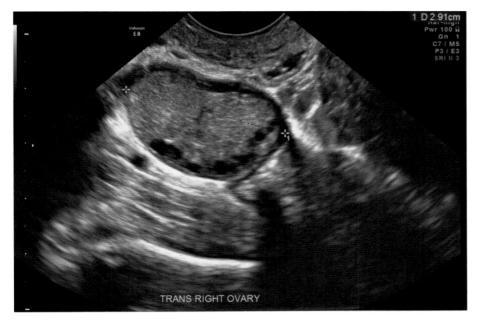

Fig. 5.7 Transvaginal ultrasound in a patient with polycystic ovarian morphology demonstrating stromal hypertrophy.

automatic calculation of the outlined area by the US machine (Fig. 5.7). Although OA is less frequently utilized in research protocols, it has better diagnostic power than OV (Table 5.3) [15]. A threshold for OA of 5.0 cm², a sensitivity of 77.6%, and a specificity of 94.7% have been observed [15]. Recognizing the substantial intra- and inter-observer variability in determining OV, these authors also noted that OA is less operator dependent and allows for good reproducibility [15].

Ovarian stromal area and total ovarian area

Improvements in US technology have increased the ability to differentiate between the ovarian stromal and follicular compartments, and thereby quantify ovarian stromal area. Stromal hypertrophy was recognized as a frequent and specific feature in ovarian androgenic dysfunction [16] (Fig. 5.8). Assessment of the stromal area, specifically the stromal to total OA ratio (S/A ratio), was suggested to help differentiate between PCOM, control, and MFOs [16]. In a study evaluating 80 consecutive amenorrheic or oligoamenorrheic patients aged 18–38 years, Fulghesu et al. correlated ovarian morphologic findings with serum androgen levels [16]. OA was evaluated by outlining with a US caliper the external limits of the ovary in the maximum longitudinal plane. The stromal area was determined by outlining with the caliper the outer peripheral profile

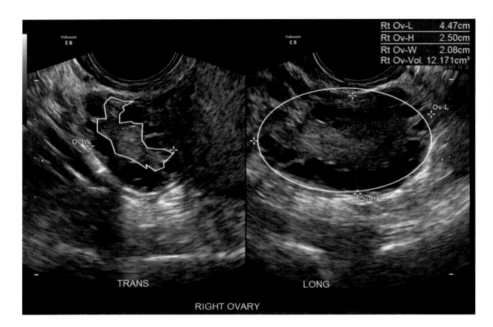

Fig. 5.8 Transvaginal ultrasound demonstrating assessment of the ovarian stromal area to the total ovarian area and calculation of the ratio in the maximal longitudinal plane of the ovary. The stromal area is determined by outlining the outer peripheral profile of the stroma (central hyperechoic area devoid of follicles). The ovarian area is determined by outlining the periphery of the ovary.

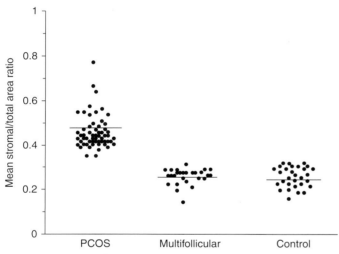

Fig. 5.9 Ovarian stromal/total area ratio in PCOS. (From Fulghesu AM, Ciampelli M, Belosi C, et al. *Fertil Steril* 2001; **76**(2): 326.)

of the stroma, identified as a hyperechoic area center devoid of follicles, and the S/A ratio noted (Fig. 5.9). A mean OV, area, stromal area, and S/A ratio for each individual patient was determined by adding the measurements of each component for both ovaries and then dividing by two.

In this study, patients with PCOS showed significantly higher OV, total area, and stromal area when compared to both controls and patients with MFOs [16]. Androstenedione (A), T, 17 alpha-hydroxyprogesterone (17-OHP), and the free androgen index (FAI) were found to be higher in the PCOS group compared with the other groups [16]. Based on the mean value +2 standard deviations (SD) in the control group, a cut-off value for an S/A ratio of 0.34 showed a sensitivity of 100% and specificity of 100% for PCOS diagnosis [16]. All of the patients with MFO were below the upper limit of the S/A ratio without overlap with the PCOS group [16] (Fig. 5.10). Despite criticism that this measure might be difficult to apply in clinical practice, a subsequent multicentric study demonstrated reproducibility of this scanning technique and further refined the criteria to an S/A ratio of 0.32 as the best cut-off [17].

Three-dimensional ultrasound

The innovation of 3D US may provide a tool to further refine the criteria for the PCO and further differentiate this finding from the MFO. Technical advances in the acquisition, storage, and analysis of ovarian imaging data have facilitated the quantitative measurement of the individual ovarian compartments. The advantage of 3D systems is their ability to obtain more accurate and reproducible OV. Once the total OV is obtained, the stromal volume is measured by subtraction of the total follicular volume. As compared with the "full planar" method of 3D volume data analysis, the use of the virtual organ computer-aided analysis imaging program (VOCAL) allows for a highly reliable assessment of OVs [18]. Several studies utilizing initial 3D technology confirmed the presence of more antral follicles, and a larger OV in the PCO, although by 3D technique a higher threshold of antral follicles has been suggested to meet the criteria of PCOM [19] (Fig. 5.11).

Magnetic resonance imaging in PCOS

The use of magnetic resonance imaging (MRI) to evaluate the morphology of the ovary has been reported [20]. In a pilot study comparing MRI and transabdominal US in obese adolescents, Yoo et al. demonstrated that MRI provided clarity in the assessment of FN and distribution, as well as better definition in the distinction between the ovarian capsule, follicle, and stroma [20]. With MRI, follicular borders were easily discernible separate from the ovarian stroma, whereas with approximately half

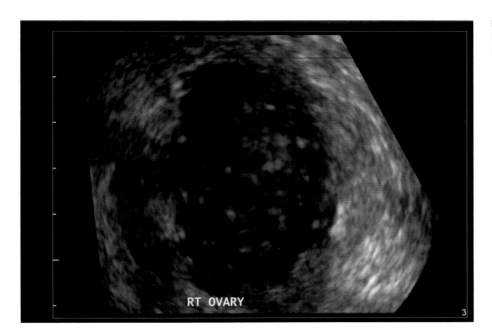

Fig. 5.10 Three-dimensional transvaginal ultrasound of an ovary with polycystic ovarian morphology in a rendered reconstructed view.

of the patients, delineation and detail of these compartments was not achievable by images obtained on transabdominal US. Given the precision with which MRI revealed the structural components of the ovary, the use of MRI was suggested to provide an excellent investigational tool for studies that involve young women with PCOS and increased central obesity. However, the cost and lack of easy accessibility may limit the use of this imaging modality. In those patients for whom the transvaginal approach is less favorable, transrectal imaging has been suggested as an alternative to evaluate the pelvis.

The phenotypes of PCOS

The Androgen Excess Society recently reported the results of an evidence-based review of the phenotypes for PCOS [21]. These authors concluded that PCOS should first be considered a disorder of androgen biosynthesis, utilization, and/or metabolism in women [4]. In terms of the phenotypes of PCOS, ovulatory women with HA and PCOM may have a milder form of the disorder, but for women with PCOM in the absence of anovulation or hyperandrogenism, the diagnosis is less certain [4].

To clarify the whole phenotypic spectrum of PCOS, Diamanti-Kandarakis and Panidis reported their results of a large prospective study [22]. Women in this study comprised 634 Greek women (18–35 years) diagnosed with PCOS by ESHRE/ASRM criteria and 108 healthy controls with comparable BMI. The PCOS group was then subdivided into two main phenotypes: (a) "classic (NIH) PCOS" and (b) "nonclassic (ESHRE/ASRM) PCOS." These phenotypic groups were then further divided into sub-phenotypes based on their androgen and ovulatory status and the presence or absence of PCOM [22]. In addition to the epidemiologic data obtained, an evaluation was completed between the hormonal and metabolic abnormalities of each sub-phenotype. The classic phenotype

for PCOS was the most frequent (85.96%) as compared with the nonclassic phenotype (14.04%) [22]. In this study, subjects with classic PCOS and biochemical HA (74.76%) were more insulin resistant than controls. In women with classic PCOS, FN was positively related to insulin resistance and biochemical HA. Forty-three (6.78%) of the patients were defined as having PCOS without evidence of HA, but met the diagnostic criteria based on a history of chronic anovulation and PCOM [22].

Alternatives to imaging in the diagnosis of the PCOM

In adolescents, a clear diagnosis of PCOS may be clinically challenging. Irregular menstrual patterns may be similar in both adolescent girls with PCOS and normal post-menarchal girls. The ability to perform transvaginal US may be limited in girls, and details of the ovarian morphology are often difficult to discern on transabdominal US in obese adolescents. Anti-müllerian hormone (AMH) is a member of the transforming growth factor (TGF)β family and is a peptide with exclusive production of the granulosa cells of early growing pre-antral and small-antral follicles. With the development of a second-generation AMH ultrasensitive assay, interest arose in determining whether AMH could be used as a surrogate marker for the FN in the diagnosis of the PCO and aid in diagnosis of PCOS.

In an initial study, Pigny et al. compared serum follicular phase AMH levels from 73 patients with a diagnosis of PCOS by the Rotterdam criteria to those of 96 control women [23]. The mean serum AMH level was three fold higher in the PCOS patients than in controls, and the mean 2- to 9-mm FN per ovary was three fold higher in PCOS patients than in controls [23]. Because of the improvement in US technology, the currently established FN (i.e. 12 follicles per ovary) has led to an

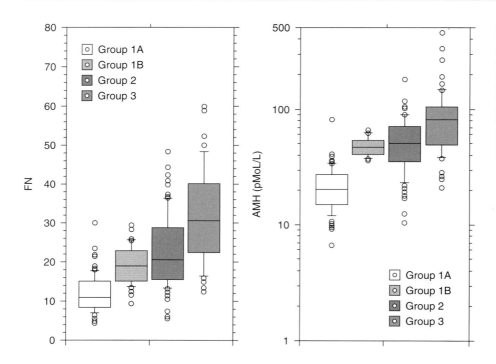

Fig. 5.11 Box-and-whisker plot showing the values of the follicle count (left) and AMH level (right, logarithmic scale) in four subgroups of patients. Group 1A: control; group 1B: asymptomatic women with PCOM; group 2: presumption of PCOS with only HA or only oligo-anovulation; group 3: PCOS with HA and oligo-anovulation. Horizontal small bars represent the 5–95th percentile range, and the boxes indicate the 25–75th percentile range. The horizontal line in each box corresponds to the median. From Dewailly et al. [24] with permission.

Table 5.5 Adaptation of the previous classifications for the diagnosis of PCOS, proposing an excessive FN of >19 or serum AMH concentration of >35 pmol/L or >5 ng/mL as a surrogate when either oligo-anovulation or hyperandrogenism is missing

Oligo-anovulation	Clinical and/or biochemical HA	FN >19 and/or serum AMH[a] >35 pmol/L (5 ng/mL)	Diagnosis
+	+	(+/−)[b]	PCOS
+	−	+	PCOS
−	+	+	PCOS[c]
−	−	+	Normal women with PCOM
+	−	−	Idiopathic anovulation
−	+	−	Idiopathic hyperandrogenism

FN, follicular number; AMH, anti-müllerian hormone; PCOS, polycystic ovary syndrome; PCOM, polycystic ovarian morphology
[a]To be used preferentially.
[b]Not necessary for the diagnosis.
[c]Consider the risk for ovarian hyperstimulation syndrome.

From Dewailly D, Gronier H, Poncelet, et al. Diagnosis of polycystic ovary syndrome (PCOS): revisiting the threshold values of follicle count on ultrasound and of the serum AMH level for the definition of polycystic ovaries. *Hum Reprod* 2011; **26**(11): 3123–3129.

artificial increase in the prevalence of PCOM in normal populations (especially in women aged <30 years) [24].

In a recent study published by Dewailly et al. [24], the threshold for FN and AMH levels consistent with the diagnosis of PCOS was further refined. Clinical, hormonal, and US data were compared in 240 patients with HA, menstrual disorders, and/or infertility. The subjects were grouped only according to their symptoms. Group 1A consisted of control subjects. Group 1B subjects had PCOM but were asymptomatic. Group 2 subjects had presumed PCOS, but with only HA or oligo-anovulation. Group 3 subjects had PCOS, as defined by the presence of HA and oligo-anovulation [24]. In this study, FN per ovary was determined using the highest possible magnification in 2D and the total number of visible follicles smaller than 10 mm was counted. Group 1B differed from group 1A by a significantly higher mean rank of FN and AMH (Fig. 5.12). Groups 1B and 2 had similar FN and AMH, but group 1B had lower mean ranks of total T and serum A levels [24]. Compared with group 3, group 1B subjects had significantly lower mean ranks of FN, AMH, total T and A levels [24].

When ROC analysis was applied, the best compromise to distinguish the control patients from those with PCOS with HA and oligo-anovulation, the best compromise between sensitivity (81% and 92%) and specificity (92% and 97%) was obtained with threshold values of 19 follicles and an AMH level of 35 pmol/L [24]. These authors concluded that with newer US technology and the increase in the resolution of US images, the FN threshold retained at the Rotterdam conference in 2003 is now obsolete [24]. Acknowledging the negative effect of age on FN and AMH levels, these authors emphasized that the criteria proposed here should not be applied to women <35 years old. In their conclusion, these authors suggested that an international consortium validate the threshold value for AMH and suggested a simplified algorithm for the diagnosis of PCOS [24] (Table 5.4).

Conclusion

The definition for PCOS is a topic of intense international debate. The 1990 NIH criteria require the presence of chronic anovulation plus clinical and/or biochemical signs of hyperandrogenemia, whereas the 2003 Rotterdam criteria require the presence of two or more of the following: chronic anovulation, clinical and/or biochemical signs of hyperandrogenism, and PCOM. A third definition proposed by AE-PCOS suggests that there should be acceptance of the original NIH criteria, but with modification. The principal conclusion of its report is that PCOS should first be considered a disorder of androgen excess or HA.

The US findings for establishing the diagnosis of the PCO, or PCOM, require strict criteria and should not be based solely on a multicystic appearance of the ovary. By 2D US the FN and size of the 2–5 mm follicular pool have been associated with the severity of the menstrual disorder. Utilizing the ESHRE/ASRM criteria of OV on 2D US lacks sensitivity, but has a reasonable specificity in making the diagnosis of PCOM. Calculation of the ovarian stromal/total area ratio may provide a more sensitive and specific test and allow for the appropriate identification of those patients who are at risk for long-term sequelae associated with PCOS. While still a research tool, 3D US may provide a more effective method in quantifying ovarian compartmental volumes and calculating an S/A ratio. In recognition of the emerging evidence that serum AMH levels correlate with the FN in patients with PCOS, this biologic surrogate may be useful in establishing the diagnosis in patients for whom FN cannot be determined by US, and/or be a useful biomarker for the presence of the disorder.

References

1. Yildiz BO, Knochenhauer ES, Azziz R. Impact of obesity on the risk for polycystic ovary syndrome. *J Clin Endocrinol Metab* 2008; **93**: 162–168.

2. Rotterdam ESHRE/ASRM-Sponsored PCOS consensus workshop group. Revised 2003 consensus on diagnostic criteria and long-term health risks related to polycystic ovary syndrome (PCOS). *Hum Reprod* 2004; **19**: 41–47.

3. Zawadski JK, Dunaif A. Diagnostic criteria for polycystic ovary syndrome: towards a rational approach. In: Dunaif A, Givens JR, Haseltine FP, Merriam GE (Eds.) *Polycystic Ovary Syndrome (Current Issues in Endocrinology and Metabolism)*. Boston: Blackwell Scientific Inc.; 1992: 377.

4. Azziz R, Carmina E, Dewailly D, et al. The Androgen Excess and PCOS Society criteria for the polycystic ovary syndrome: the complete task force report. *Fertil Steril* 2009; **91**: 456–488.

5. Azziz R. Polycystic ovary syndrome is a family affair. *J Clin Endocrinol Metab* 2008; **93**: 1579–1581.

6. Legro RS, Chiu P, Kunselman AR, et al. Polycystic ovaries are common in women with hyperandrogenic chronic anovulation but do not predict metabolic or reproductive phenotype. *J Clin Endocrinol Metab* 2005; **90**: 2571–2579.

7. Polson DW, Adams J, Wadsworth J, Franks S. Polycystic ovaries – a common finding in normal women. *Lancet* 1988; **1**: 870–872.

8. Ferriman D, Gallwey JD. Clinical assessment of body hair growth in women. *J Clin Endocrinol Metab* 1961; **21**: 1440–1447.

9. Carmina E, Oberfield SE, Lobo RA. The diagnosis of polycystic ovary syndrome in adolescents. *Am J Obstet Gynecol* 2010; **203**: 201 e1–5.

10. Pfeifer SM, Kives S. Polycystic ovary syndrome in the adolescent. *Obstet Gynecol Clin North Am* 2009; **36**: 129–152.

11. Balen AH, Laven JS, Tan SL, Dewailly D. Ultrasound assessment of the polycystic ovary: international consensus definitions. *Hum Reprod Update* 2003; **9**: 505–514.

12. Jonard S, Robert Y, Cortet-Rudelli C, et al. Ultrasound examination of polycystic ovaries: is it worth counting the follicles? *Hum Reprod* 2003; **18**: 598–603.

13. Dewailly D, Catteau-Jonard S, Reyss AC, et al. The excess in 2–5 mm follicles seen at ovarian ultrasonography is tightly associated to the follicular arrest of the polycystic ovary syndrome. *Hum Reprod* 2007; **22**: 1562–1566.

14. Adams J, Franks S, Polson DW, et al. Multifollicular ovaries: clinical and endocrine features and response to pulsatile gonadotropin releasing hormone. *Lancet* 1985; **2**: 1375–1379.

15. Jonard S, Robert Y, Dewailly D. Revisiting the ovarian volume as a diagnostic criterion for polycystic ovaries. *Hum Reprod* 2005; **20**: 2893–1898.

16. Fulghesu AM, Ciampelli M, Belosi C, et al. A new ultrasound criterion for the diagnosis of polycystic ovary syndrome: the ovarian stroma/total area ratio. *Fertil Steril* 2001; **76**: 326–331.

17. Fulghesu AM, Angioni S, Frau E, et al. Ultrasound in polycystic ovary syndrome – the measuring of ovarian stroma and relationship with circulating androgens: results of a multicentric study. *Hum Reprod* 2007; **22**: 2501–2508.

18. Raine-Fenning NJ, Campbell BK, Clewes JS, Johnson IR. The interobserver reliability of ovarian volume measurement is improved with three-dimensional ultrasound, but dependent upon technique. *Ultrasound Med Biol* 2003; **29**: 1685–1690.

19. Lam PM, Raine-Fenning N. The role of three-dimensional ultrasonography in polycystic ovary syndrome. *Hum Reprod* 2006; **21**: 2209–2215.

20. Yoo RY, Sirlin CB, Gottschalk M, Chang RJ. Ovarian imaging by magnetic resonance in obese adolescent girls with polycystic ovary syndrome: a pilot study. *Fertil Steril* 2005; **84**: 985–995.

21. Azziz R, Carmina E, Dewailly D, et al. Positions statement: criteria for defining polycystic ovary syndrome as a predominantly hyperandrogenic syndrome: an Androgen Excess Society guideline. *J Clin Endocrinol Metab* 2006; **91**: 4237–4245.

22. Diamanti-Kandarakis E, Panidis D. Unravelling the phenotypic map of polycystic ovary syndrome (PCOS): a prospective study of 634 women with PCOS. *Clin Endocrinol (Oxf)* 2007; **67**: 735–742.

23. Pigny P, Jonard S, Robert Y, Dewailly D. Serum anti-Mullerian hormone as a surrogate for antral follicle count for definition of the polycystic ovary syndrome. *J Clin Endocrinol Metab* 2006; **91**: 941–945.

24. Dewailly D, Gronier H, Poncelet E, et al. Diagnosis of polycystic ovary syndrome (PCOS): revisiting the threshold values of follicle count on ultrasound and of the serum AMH level for the definition of polycystic ovaries. *Hum Reprod* 2011; **26**(11): 3123–3129.

Müllerian anomaly and ultrasonographic diagnosis

Awoniyi O. Awonuga, Samuel Johnson, Manvinder Singh and Elizabeth E. Puscheck

Introduction

The combination of radiologic imaging techniques, hysteroscopy, and laparoscopy has traditionally been the cornerstone for making the diagnosis of müllerian duct anomalies (MDA). Patients with MDA may present with symptoms of acute abdominal pain, cyclic pelvic pain, recurrent pregnancy loss (early or late), or infertility. However, several patients with these types of anomalies do not have any symptoms at all and go undetected. This chapter will focus on the embryologic development and the reproductive consequences of MDA, the criteria for making a diagnosis of MDA, and comparison of the different imaging modalities (hysterosalpingogram [HSG], two- and three-dimensional ultrasound (2D US and 3D US), and magnetic resonance imaging [MRI])[1] used to make an accurate diagnosis of an MDA.

MDA development

Embryologically, the uterus and the upper vagina form from two müllerian ducts (MDs), which become developed by 5–6 weeks of gestation from infolding of the coelomic epithelium lateral to mesonephric ducts or wolffian ducts. This process occurs when there is an absence of anti-müllerian hormone (AMH), which is typically produced in the developing testis. The MDs come together and fuse to form a single uterine corpus and the lower third of the MD elongates caudally to the urogenital sinus to form the upper third of the vagina, while the urogenital sinus forms the lower two-thirds of the vagina. Two theories have been evoked to explain the fusion of the two MDs to create one uterus and subsequent recanalization of the inner upper part of the MDs to form the uterine cavity. The conventional or unidirectional theory suggests that fusion and subsequent recanalization commences caudally and proceeds in cephalad fashion. The bi-directional theory suggests that fusion and resorption begin at the isthmus and proceed simultaneously in both cranial and caudal directions. Whilst there are proponents of each theory, recent reports of patients with a single uterus (consistent with fusion), complete uterine septum (indicating resorption), cervical duplication (indicating

incomplete fusion), and complete longitudinal vaginal septum (indicating incomplete fusion of both the MD and urogenital sinus) favor the bi-directional mechanism [2].

Although a detailed description of the uterovaginal embryology is beyond the scope of this chapter, a brief description is necessary for the imaging diagnosis of MDAs. Suffice it to mention here that faulty development of the MD system results in various uterine, vaginal, and renal abnormalities. Complete or partial absence of MD fusion and/or canalization results in didelphic (double), bicornuate, septate, or subseptate uterus, and the specific anomaly depends upon the degree of fusion and recanalization. In the majority of cases, the etiology is unknown; while some have multifactorial inheritance, others have a clear genetic cause that gives rise to MDAs: (a) the presence of B-cell leukemia/lymphoma 2 protein (anti-reabsorption protein) [3]; (b) alteration of HOX genes (Hox-9, 10, 11, 13 are expressed along the length of MDs) and their transcription factors [4]; and (c) the loss of function mutation in Wingless-related MMTV (mouse tumor virus) integration site 4 (WNT4) – critical for successful nephrogenesis, normal ovarian differentiation, and initial differentiation of the MDs [5]. In addition, teratogens such as diethylstilbestrol, thalidomide, and radiation exposure of the fetus in utero may account for MDAs seen in fetuses of exposed women [6–8].

Incidence

The incidence of congenital anomaly of the female reproductive system is estimated at 0.001–10% in the general population [1,8], with uterine malformation from müllerian defect being the most common. The wide range quoted above depends on the study population and the modality used for diagnosis. In one study in which 3D ultrasound (US) was used, the incidence was as high as 13% in patients undergoing assisted reproductive technology (ART) [9]. Saravelos and colleagues [10] performed a critical analysis of published studies and found that the prevalence of congenital uterine anomalies is approximately 6.7% in the general population, 7.3% in the infertile population, and 16.7% in the recurrent miscarriage population. These studies are all estimates since all rely on the study population having an

Ultrasonography in Gynecology, ed. Botros R. M. B. Rizk and Elizabeth E. Puscheck. Published by Cambridge University Press. © Cambridge University Press 2015.

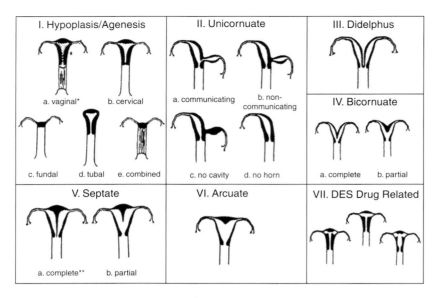

Fig 6.1 American Fertility Society classification of müllerian duct anomalies

DES, diethylstilbestrol. *Uterus may be normal or take a variety of abnormal forms. **May have two distinct cervices.

indication to have the imaging test; the true incidence would require scanning the entire population. Although various modifications [11] of the original American Fertility Society (now called the American Society for Reproductive Medicine) classification for uterine anomalies (Fig. 6.1) [12,13] exist in the literature, this classification still remains the cornerstone for the description of uterine anomalies.

Why is accurate diagnosis of the nature of uterine anomaly essential?

Use of 2D ultrasound to screen for MDAs

An effective diagnostic modality should be simple, reproducible, and inexpensive. In addition, it should have high sensitivity and specificity since diagnostic accuracy is important for treatment. Such a modality should be able to define the precise nature of each uterine anomaly so that the findings can help with patient selection and aid in determining the feasibility, type of surgical approach, and safety of surgical correction. The ideal investigational tool should also be able to demonstrate the fundal contour of the uterus and the zonal anatomy of the corpus, cervix, and vagina. Hysterosalpingography (HSG) is a radiologic procedure where radiopaque contrast material is injected into the uterus under fluoroscopy and X-rays are taken to evaluate the uterine cavity and the fallopian tubes. The contrast material outlines the inner contour of the uterine cavity and fallopian tubes to confirm patency. For an accurate diagnosis of an MDA, one needs to have information not only about the inner cavity of the uterus but also about the outer surface. Consequently, the HSG has a low accuracy rate for making the diagnosis. Two-dimensional (2D) transvaginal sonography is able to show the uterus with the endometrium of a different echogenicity than the myometrium. However, 2D US has a

relatively low sensitivity because of its inability to effectively demonstrate the contour of the uterine fundus and reconstruct the uterine coronal axis (Fig. 6.2). Imaging of this axis has major significance in the diagnosis of uterine fundus malformation. However, ultrasonographers and reproductive endocrinologists have become more experienced in the use of US in gynecology, since the declaration by McArdle and Berezin [14] in 1980 that US examination detected uterus subseptus only during the second trimester of pregnancy. The conclusion at the time was that US was not sufficiently sensitive to supplant hysterography in the detection of MDAs [15].

Association with significant morbidity and pregnancy complications

Congenital uterine anomaly is associated with significant morbidity and pregnancy complications. Such complications include dysmenorrhea from obstructed outflow tract or non-communicating, but functional uterine horn [16,17], and chronic pelvic pain from endometriosis because of increased retrograde menstruation and intraperitoneal implanting of endometrial fragments because of obstruction to menstrual flow [7]. In addition, there is associated increased risk of miscarriages [9], preterm labor/delivery, and malpresentation/abnormal lie with increased cesarean delivery rate [8,18–20]. Timely surgical correction after a correct diagnosis but before pregnancy is contemplated by women with MDAs may avert some of these complications, as well as rare cases of reported fetal deformities in women with bicornuate uterus [21]. Some MDAs (such as müllerian agenesis) result in infertility.

Due to the intimate association of the development of the mesonephric ducts and MDs, the renal organs may be affected when an MDA occurs. The renal anomalies range from agenesis

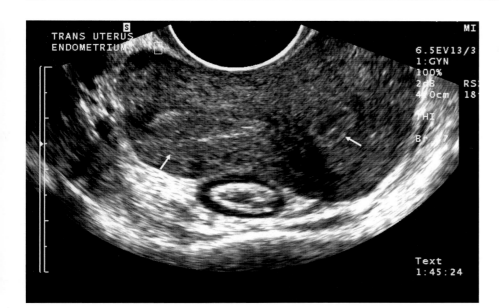

Fig. 6.2 Bicornuate uterus. Transverse transvaginal ultrasound shows widened transverse uterine diameter with subdivision of the endometrium into right and left components (arrows).

to malformations (e.g. horseshoe kidney) to abnormal or duplication of the collecting duct systems. Upon diagnosing an MDA, one should evaluate the kidneys, ureters, and the bladder [7,22,23], given the high association of prenatal dysplastic and postnatal absent kidneys [16] and abnormal ureteric insertions [24,25]. The renal system may be evaluated by US, intravenous pyelogram, computed tomography (CT) scan, or MRI. Müllerian defects are also associated with a higher incidence of other congenital malformations in other organ systems, such as gastrointestinal tract [26], musculoskeletal system [27], cardiac [28,29], and facio-auriculo [30] anomalies.

Role of ultrasonography in the differential diagnosis of uterine anomaly

3D ultrasound versus MRI

Depending on the MDA, the anomaly may be suggested at the time of physical exam (i.e. müllerian agenesis) whereas most other MDAs are first diagnosed during surgical procedures (i.e. laparotomy or laparoscopy/hysteroscopy), either as an incidental finding or in relation to symptoms such as pain from an outflow track obstruction or sequelae of the anomaly (e.g. chronic pain associated with endometriosis). Invasive methods such as laparoscopy/hysteroscopy have been called the gold standard with which to compare all other imaging techniques to diagnose MDAs. Noninvasive 2D US, 3D US [31], and MRI [13] and slightly more invasive imaging techniques such as HSG, saline infusion sonography (SIS) [32,33], or a combination of these investigative modalities, have been used for the assessment of uterine morphology.

If a couple presents with infertility then an HSG [34] may be the first imaging technique to indicate that an MDA exists;

however, as mentioned above, it does not give information about the outer surface of the uterus, hence its low accuracy for making the diagnosis of MDAs. Although 2D US can show more information, such as the myometrium of the uterus and the presence of ovaries, it also has limitations. Similar to HSG, 2D US alone is not adequate to image the uterine fundal serosal surface. Many sonographers will note on a transverse US image of the uterus that there is a separation of the endometrium (Fig. 6.2). Some will call this a bicornuate uterus erroneously. This finding is consistent with multiple diagnoses (arcuate uterus, septate uterus, subseptate uterus, and bicornuate uterus). The treatments for these various MDAs are different, so diagnostic accuracy is important.

In recent years further advances in ultrasonography have led to 3D US. In this method the structure of interest is placed within an artificial box by the sonographer and a volume acquisition is performed. It takes less than 10 seconds to obtain this volume. This data is represented in three orthogonal planes on the screen and, typically, there is a dot on the image noting the same spot in each of the three planes. The method utilizes plane interrogation with 3D software to generate a coronal plane. The coronal view can be visualized no matter what the anatomic orientation. These volumes can be stored for later processing or the sonographer can manipulate the images at the time of the US. Abuhamad and colleagues [35] described the Z technique, which allows for easy manipulation of the image within seconds to identify the best orientation to see the mid-fundal region of the uterus, both internally and externally. This technique enables uterine anomalies to be quickly and accurately identified. Indeed, several authors have reported a sensitivity of 93–100% and a specificity of 94–100% when 3D US was used for the diagnosis of MDAs [36–39]. Salim and colleagues [40] evaluated 35 cases of congenital uterine anomalies as assessed by two observers who measured the width of the uterine cavity (W), fundal distortion (F), and the length of unaffected uterine cavity (C) using 3D US volumes. The intra-observer variability for each of the three measurements (W, F, and C) was satisfactory with limits of agreement ranging from ±1.43 to ±2.51 mm. The examination of the inter-observer variability showed no significant differences between the two observers ($F = 0.484$, $P > 0.05$). These authors concluded that 3D US is a reproducible method for the diagnosis of congenital uterine anomalies and for the measurement of uterine cavity dimensions. Caliskan and collaborators [36] compared 3D US performed in the follicular phase with that performed in the luteal phase in the same patients, taking advantage of the increased thickness and echogenicity of the endometrium associated with the later phase of the cycle, and reported a higher sensitivity and specificity in the diagnosis of MDAs and suggested that 3D US examinations be performed in the luteal phase of the menstrual cycle. Similar sensitivity and specificity to 3D US have been reported when MRI was used as a diagnostic modality for MDAs [13,15,41]. We believe that a careful examination of the lower genital tract together with use of speculum can delineate the nature of associated lower genital tract anomaly when combined with 3D US.

As with coronal and transverse T2-weighted MRI (Figs 6.2 and 6.3), visualization of fundal convex exterior and internal indentation, and partial or complete duplication of the endometrial cavity by real-time 3D US enables the differentiation between a bicornuate uterus (Fig. 6.5A–D) and a septate uterus (Fig. 6.6A and B) [36,42,43]. Differentiation between these two anomalies can be based on the presence or absence of a characteristic fundal notch and bilateral cornual separation. The presence of a 1 cm or greater fundal indentation was the criterion for the differentiation of a septate uterus (Fig. 6.6A) from a bicornuate uterus (Fig. 6.3) [37,44]. In addition, the elongated wide cervical canal which contributes to the Y-shaped appearance of the uterus can be visualized on 3D US when performed along with SIS (Fig. 6.7). Therefore, the concomitant use of SIS with 3D US imaging will further increase the accuracy of diagnosis of MDAs and may obviate the need to perform HSG. Thus, similar to MRI, 3D US can differentiate between a bicornuate and a septate uterus. Distinguishing between these two entities is important since hysteroscopic surgery improves pregnancy outcomes in patients with a septate uterus [1].

Given that, like MRI, the echogenicity of endometrium, myometrium, and fibrous tissue can be delineated on US, 3D US can differentiate a bicornuate uterus from a uterus didelphys. Uterus didelphys appears on MRI (Fig. 6.8A) and 3D US (Fig. 6.9A) as separate divergent horns with a large fundal cleft and two cervices [45]. However, distinguishing uterus didelphys from uterus bicornis bicollis may be a challenge and both can be associated with obstructed hemivagina [46]. The vaginal septum is more apparent (Figs 6.7B–D, 6.8B and C) when it causes obstruction with associated severe dysmenorrhea and chronic pelvic pain.

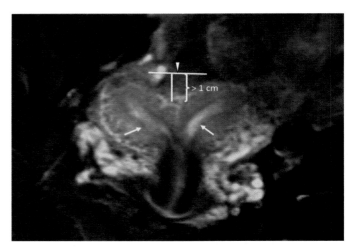

Fig. 6.3 Bicornuate uterus. Coronal reformatted T2 MRI of uterus demonstrates adjacent right and left uterine horns (arrows) with concavity of uterine fundus (arrowhead). The presence of a 1 cm or greater fundal indentation was the criterion for the differentiation of a bicornuate uterus from a septate uterus.

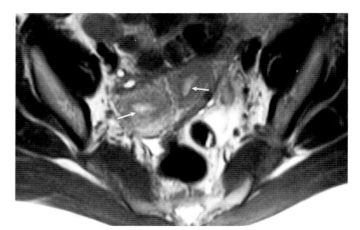

Fig. 6.4 Bicornuate uterus. Transverse T2 MRI demonstrates adjacent right and left uterine horns (arrows).

The volume of the unicornuate uterus is decreased, with ellipsoidal and asymmetric configuration when viewed on MRI and US. Both 3D US (Fig. 6.10A–E) and MRI (Fig. 6.11A and B) will identify one uterine horn of a unicornuate uterus, which is associated with lack of widening of the endometrial canal toward the fundus. Although a unicornuate uterus can be confused with a normal uterus on 2D US, 3D US will reveal the diagnosis. An HSG may be required to confirm the presence of a single fallopian tube. Similar to MRI, careful US scanning will identify the presence of a communicating or non-communicating rudimentary second horn, especially if it contains a functional endometrium.

Finally, the arcuate uterus is characterized by a mild indentation of the endometrium at the uterine fundus. This results from a near complete resorption of the uterovaginal septum

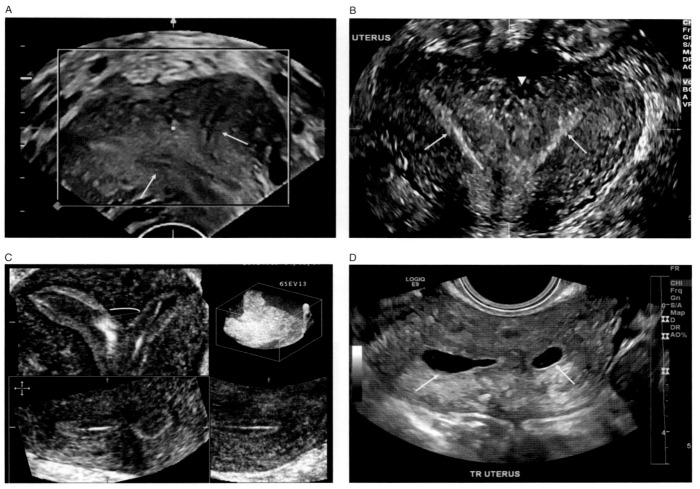

Fig. 6.5 Bicornuate uterus. (A) Coronal 3D reconstructed ultrasound image of the uterus showing subtle subdivision of right and left uterine horns (arrows). (B) Coronal 3D reconstructed ultrasound image of the uterus showing the right and left uterine horns at an obtuse angle (arrows). Concavity along the fundal contour of the uterus (arrowhead) is characteristic of a bicornuate uterus. (C) Multiplanar 3D reconstructed ultrasound images of the uterus show an obtuse angle between the uterine horns (white arc). (D) Transverse transvaginal of uterus following saline infusion sonohysterogram clearly shows subdivision of the uterine cavity into right and left horns (arrows).

and it gives a myometrial signal to the subdividing echo of < 1 cm on pelvic US. It is debatable whether this uterine variant should be classified as a true anomaly or as an anatomic variant of normal. US can distinguish arcuate (Fig. 6.12A and B) from a bicornuate (presence of fundal indentation) (Fig. 6.5C) and septate uterus (Fig. 6.6A).

To date, no randomized controlled trials exist in the literature comparing the accuracy of 3D US and MRI for the diagnosis of MDAs. Given that 3D US is cheaper, quicker, and widely available, it should be the initial investigation tool of choice in screening for and confirming the nature and type of MDAs. The caveat for 3D US must be acknowledged. The limitations of 3D US are mainly anything that obscures the path of sound waves such as the presence of fibroids or adenomyoma in the area of interest. Shadowing from fibroids or calcifications can obscure valuable information if in the wrong location. In patients with imperforate hymen, atretic vagina, or transverse vaginal septum, transvaginal 3D US is not technically possible. In such

cases, 3D US can be done abdominally with a full bladder. However, US becomes less informative in the obese patient, and MRI will be a better choice despite cost. Concomitant use of SIS with 3D US can help in the diagnosis when the patient presents in the early follicular time period or in situations where intracavitary abnormalities, such as polyps, submucosal myomas, or synechiae, are suspected.

Classification

Although multiple classifications of congenital uterine anomalies have been proposed, the American Fertility Society system (Fig. 6.1) is the most widely accepted and will be utilized below to illustrate the various anomalies. It should be noted that the true incidence of MDA in the general population is not known, with widely disparate prevalence quoted in the literature [1,13,47–50]. These variations have depended on the population studied and the diagnostic method or methods used to evaluate

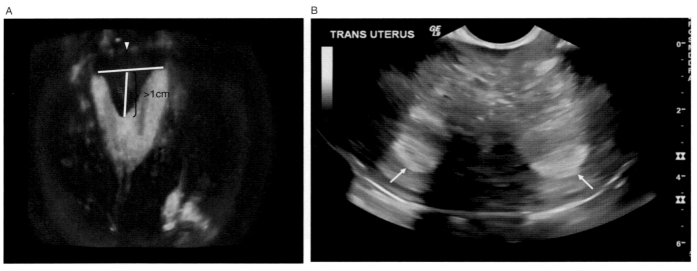

Fig. 6.6 Septate uterus. (A) Coronal 3D reconstructed ultrasound image of the uterus showing a partial uterine septum(s) subdividing the endometrial echo. Arrowhead shows convex fundal contour. Subdividing echo >1 cm separates an arcuate from a septate uterus. (B) Transverse transvaginal ultrasound through the proximal uterus showing a duplicated endometrial echo (arrows).

patients. In addition, an unknown number of MDAs remain undiagnosed, especially in those who are asymptomatic.

American Fertility Society classification of uterine anomalies: distribution

Class I – uterine agenesis or hypoplasia (4–10%) [13,47]

Class II – unicornuate uterus (10–20%) [1,13]

    A. Cavity with endometrium and communicating (10%)

    B. Cavity with endometrium but non-communicating with endometrium of the contralateral horn (22%)

    C. No cavity and no endometrium (35%)

    D. No rudimentary horn (33%)

Class III – uterus didelphys (5–11%) [1,13,47]

Class IV – bicornuate uterus (10–25%) [1,13]

Class V – septate and subseptate uterus (35–55%) [1,13,48–50]

Class VI – arcuate uterus (15–20%) [1,47]

Class VII – DES-exposed uterus

Class I – uterine agenesis or hypoplasia

Müllerian agenesis (Mayer–Rokitansky–Küster–Hauser syndrome) or uterine and vaginal hypoplasia results from early failure of MD development. Agenesis or hypoplasia of the vagina commonly occurs in association with uterine agenesis, but rarely may be seen in isolation. The ovaries are usually normal. Patients usually present with normal secondary sexual characteristics and primary amenorrhea given the absence of a uterus. In most cases the vagina can be created by progressive dilatation over time. Patience and support are helpful and this approach has the least risk. If not successful, then a surgical approach can be done when the patient is mentally and physically mature.

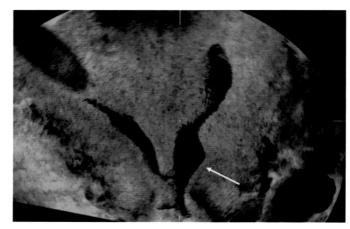

Fig. 6.7 Bicornuate uterus. Coronal 3D reconstructed ultrasound image of the uterus following saline infusion sonohysterogram demonstrating an obtuse angle between the uterine horns and Y-shaped appearance of the uterus (arrow).

Occasionally, there is a uterine remnant or rudimentary tubes; rarely, the anlagen may have functioning endometrium which can cause a hematometra with pelvic pain, requiring removal. From the reproductive perspective, patients with müllerian agenesis do not have a functional uterus and will not be able to conceive. However, their ovaries have normal function and advanced reproductive technology can be used to stimulate the ovaries and undertake a US-guided oocyte retrieval with subsequent insemination to create embryos, which would need to be transferred into a gestational carrier.

The diagnosis of these individuals is typically made with a physical exam and transabdominal US. HSG cannot be performed on these individuals since the uterus, cervix, and vagina are not present. Ultrasound, whether 2D or 3D, will show no

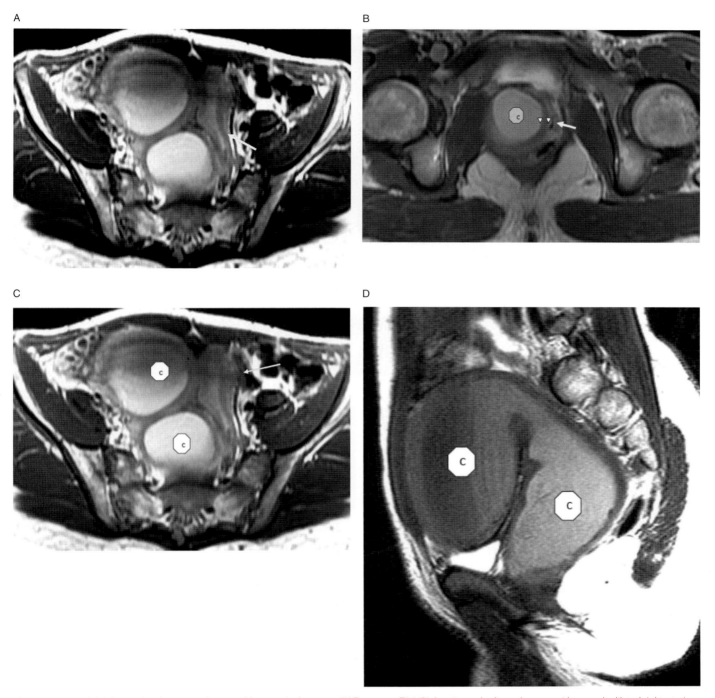

Fig. 6.8 Uterus didelphys with right uterus obstructed by a vaginal septum. (A) Transverse T2 MRI showing a duplicated uterus with severely dilated right uterine cavity. The normal left uterus (arrow) is displaced laterally. (B) Transverse T2 MRI through the lower pelvis showing a severely dilated right vaginal canal (c) that displaces the left vaginal canal laterally (arrow). A thick longitudinal septum (arrowheads) is present between the right and left vaginal canals. (C) Transverse T2 MRI showing a duplicated uterus with severely dilated right uterine cavity (c). The normal left uterus (arrow) is displaced laterally. (D) Sagittal T2 MRI demonstrates a severe right hematometrocolpos (c).

uterus, but ovaries will be present. Ultrasound may be limited in identifying or characterizing a hypoplastic uterus, and may falsely identify a possible uterine remnant. One French study stated that the US diagnosis of müllerian agenesis was accurate in 32% of cases, but wrong in 68% where a uterine remnant was identified [51]. When there is uncertainty in the diagnosis,

MRI can be helpful as the next noninvasive step to characterize this condition. On MRI, T2-weighted images note abnormally low signal myometrium with poor definition of zonal anatomy in uterine hypoplasia. Normal ovaries are identified by both US and MRI. Once a vagina has been created, transvaginal US can be used to visualize the ovaries.

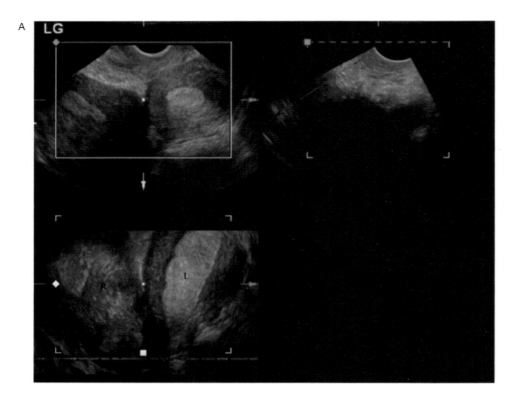

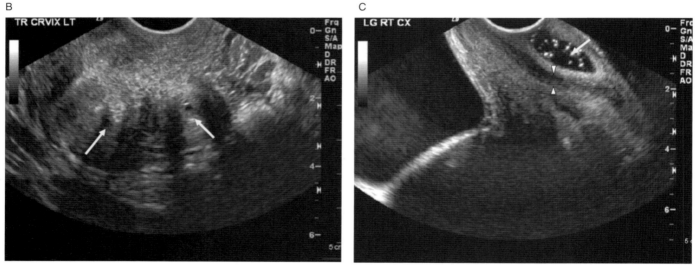

Fig. 6.9 Uterus didelphys with right uterus obstructed by a vaginal septum. (A) Multiplanar 3D reconstructed ultrasound images of the uterus showing the right (R) and left (L) uteri in the coronal plane. (B) Transverse transvaginal ultrasound displays the adjacent right and left cervices (arrows). (C) Sagittal transvaginal ultrasound performed after distension of left vaginal canal (arrow) with saline. A thick longitudinal vaginal septum is evident (arrowheads).

Class II – unicornuate uterus

A unicornuate uterus results from the normal development of only one MD with contralateral agenesis (Figs. 6.10A–D) (rudimentary horn is absent in approximately one-third of cases) or hypoplasia (rudimentary horn present, approximately two-thirds of cases). The majority of rudimentary horns either have no endometrial tissue or have endometrial tissue that does not communicate with the contralateral side (Fig. 6.10C and D). In a minority of cases, there is communication of the endometrial cavities between the normal side and rudimentary horn. Renal anomalies are frequently seen in association with a unicornuate uterus and the most common side for renal agenesis is contralateral to the normal uterine horn. Complications of a unicornuate uterus include endometriosis due to retrograde menstruation from a non-communicating rudimentary horn with functioning endometrial tissue.

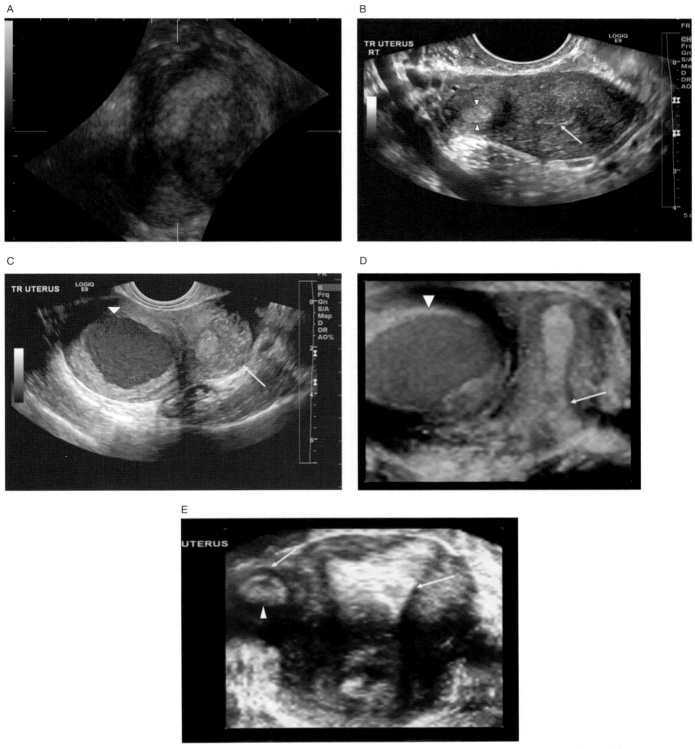

Fig. 6.10 (A) 3D ultrasound with unicornuate uterus. Notice that the rendered image is angled to the side it is located on. In this case, this is a left unicornuate uterus. (B) Unicornuate uterus with rudimentary horn. Transverse transvaginal ultrasound of uterus showing a normal left side of the uterus with a thin endometrium (arrow). The right side of the uterus (short arrowheads) is small with a mildly dilated central cavity containing hyperechoic endometrium and debris. (C) Unicornuate uterus with obstructed non-communicating rudimentary horn. Transverse transvaginal ultrasound of uterus showing a normal left side of the uterus with hyperechoic endometrium (arrow). The right side of the uterus is enlarged, non-separated, and with a dilated cavity (arrowhead) filled with echogenic fluid. (D) Unicornuate uterus with obstructed non-communicating rudimentary horn. Three-dimensional coronal reconstructed image of the uterus demonstrates absence of communication between the obstructed right rudimentary horn (arrowhead) and the normal left endometrium and cervical canal (arrow). (E) Unicornuate uterus with rudimentary horn. 3D coronal reconstructed image of the uterus demonstrates a small right rudimentary horn protruding from the left uterus (arrowhead). Note the thin hypoechoic layer of inner myometrium surrounding each uterine cavity (arrows).

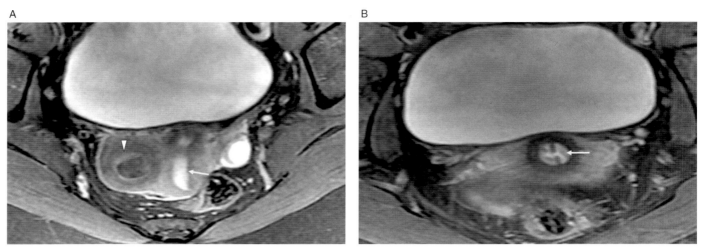

Fig. 6.11 Unicornuate uterus with obstructed non-communicating rudimentary horn. (A) Axial T2 fat saturation MRI image showing similar features of dilated right rudimentary horn (arrowhead) and normal left uterine cavity (arrow). (B) Axial T2 fat saturation MRI image showing the additional finding of a longitudinal vaginal septum (arrow).

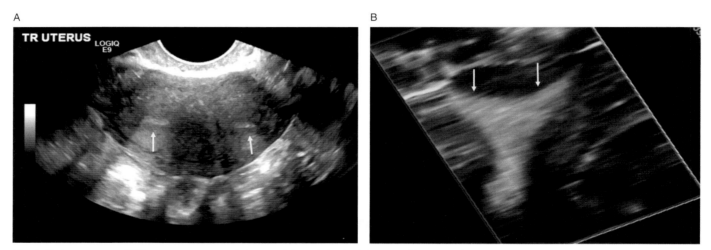

Fig. 6.12 Arcuate uterus. (A) Transverse transvaginal ultrasound through the fundal aspect of the uterus showing a duplicated endometrial echo (arrows). (B) Coronal 3D reconstructed ultrasound image of the uterus demonstrating a shallow curvilinear impression upon the fundal aspect of the endometrial echo (arrows).

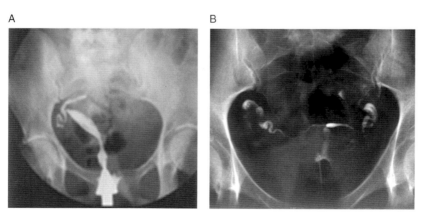

Fig. 6.13 (A) Unicornuate uterus. HSG showing the endometrial cavity is fusiform-shaped, tapering at the apex and draining into a solitary fallopian tube. The uterus is generally shifted off the midline. (B) HSG of a patient with in utero DES exposure showing a narrowed irregular endocervical canal, an endometrial cavity that is small, and a shortened upper uterine segment resulting in the characteristic T configuration.

Most patients with a unicornuate uterus have no difficulty achieving pregnancy. Common complications of pregnancy include preterm labor and abnormal lie. Poor fetal survival has been reported in patients with a unicornuate uterus due to preterm delivery, poor uteroplacental blood supply, and dystocia at delivery. Treatment is usually expectant. If a non-communicating rudimentary horn is present, it can be removed to prevent endometriosis, pain, or the possibility of ectopic pregnancy in that horn. Cerclage can be considered for patients who have incompetent cervix.

HSG demonstrates a small fusiform uterine cavity that is deviated to one side and drains into a single fallopian tube (Fig. 6.13A). An HSG cannot distinguish a unicornuate from didelphic uterus if the second vagina and cervix are not cannulated when the latter MDA exists. An HSG can demonstrate a communicating rudimentary horn, if there is one. But an HSG cannot distinguish the absence of a rudimentary horn, a rudimentary horn with a non-communicating cavity, or a rudimentary horn with no cavity. Two-dimensional transvaginal US images show a uterus off of midline, but the diagnosis is difficult to make. However, 3D US with rendering can make the diagnosis easily (Fig. 6.10A). US can also detect a rudimentary horn and the sonographer will need to identify that the mass is contiguous with the uterus. Occasionally, the rudimentary horn may be confused with an adnexal mass. MRI and 3D transvaginal US demonstrate an elongated, narrowed uterus that is deviated to one side, with preserved zonal anatomy.

Class III – uterus didelphys

Uterus didelphys results from near complete failure of MD fusion and the subsequent formation of two separate uterine horns and cervices. Therefore, the uterine horns are usually widely divergent. A longitudinal vaginal septum is present in the majority of these cases. Patients are usually asymptomatic. On occasion, a hemi-obstructed vagina due to an obstructing longitudinal or transverse vaginal septum associated with a uterus didelphys could present with hematocolpos, hematometra, dysmenorrhea, and endometriosis. Ultrasound reveals two separate endometrial and endocervical cavities with widely divergent uterine horns, separated by a large fundal cleft. MRI demonstrates two usually widely separate uterine horns and two cervices with normal zonal anatomy (Fig. 6.8A–D). A longitudinal vaginal septum is often identified on physical exam. Typically, one is dominant and can be overlooked during an examination.

HSG can only make this diagnosis when both cervices are identified and injected, demonstrating that each cavity opens into a single fallopian tube. The second vagina or cervix may be difficult to identify and, therefore, the HSG would only have one side injected with contrast and a misdiagnosis of a unicornuate uterus would be made. The role of MRI and 3D US (Fig. 6.9A–C) [45] in the diagnosis was discussed earlier in this chapter, although distinguishing uterine didelphys from uterus bicornis bicollis may be a challenge [46]. A 3D transvaginal US of the cervix with rendering can help make the correct diagnosis.

The live birth rate in patients with uterine didelphys has been reported to be 57–71% [52–55], similar to that for a unicornuate uterus. Treatment is usually expectant. Rarely, a Strassman metroplasty [56] or Tomkins metroplasty [57] is needed for treatment of recurrent pregnancy loss and these procedures surgically fuse the two horns. Surgical treatment is reserved for a patient without other identifiable causes of infertility and multiple pregnancy losses.

Class IV – bicornuate uterus

Bicornuate uterus results from incomplete fusion of the MDs, resulting in a concave fundal contour with two divergent uterine horns and concave fundal indentation. Both indentations need to be more than 1 cm to make the diagnosis. Incomplete fusion may extend to the external cervical os (bicornuate bicollis), the internal cervical os (bicornuate unicollis), or to lesser degrees within the uterus. Except for bicornuate bicollis, there is communication of the uterine cavities. A vaginal septum is occasionally present. Women with a bicornuate uterus have a small increased incidence of premature childbirth, spontaneous abortion, and dystocia. Surgical treatment with fusion of the uterine horns is rarely needed and is reserved for patients with repeated fetal loss in whom other potential causes have been excluded.

On HSG, identifying two endometrial cavities with an intercornual angle of greater than 105 degrees is suggestive of a bicornuate uterus. However, the intercornual angle is often less than 105 degrees and, therefore, HSG cannot reliably distinguish a bicornuate from a septate uterus. An intercornual distance of greater than 4 cm is also suggestive of a bicornuate uterus, but again, this is suggestive only. The definition relies on both the serosal surface and the fundal endometrial surface indenting (concavely) by more than 1 cm. On transvaginal 2D US the serosal surface cannot be seen (Figs 6.1 and 6.5B). The longitudinal or sagittal view is normal and the transverse view shows separation of the endometrium. This is an unreliable finding upon which to make the diagnosis.

The differential diagnosis with this finding is arcuate, bicornuate, or subseptate uterus. It requires 3D US with either a multiplanar approach or rendering to evaluate the coronal view, which shows the serosal surface (Fig. 6.5A and B). It is recommended that this US be done in the luteal time frame so that the endometrium is thickened and homogeneously hyperechoic, giving the sonographer an endogenous contrast material without being invasive. It is easy to see both the serosal and fundal indentations to make the diagnosis of a bicornuate uterus (Fig. 6.5A and B). MRI needs to be done using a gynecology protocol so that the MRI axis aligns with the uterus, then it is easy to make this diagnosis as well (Figs 6.2 and 6.3).

Class V – septate and subseptate uterus

The subseptate uterus is the most common congenital uterine anomaly (Fig. 6.6B). A complete septate uterus results from failure of resorption of the septum after fusion of the two MDs and a subseptate uterus results from partial resorption. The septum may contain muscle, fibrous tissue, or elements of both; hence, the signal intensity of the septum cannot be used to reliably distinguish a septate from a bicornuate uterus. On HSG, an intercornual angle of less than 75 degrees or an intercornual distance of less than 4 cm is suggestive of a septate uterus; however, a septate uterus cannot be reliably distinguished from a bicornuate uterus on an HSG because the serosal surface is not imaged. The diagnosis of a subseptate uterus relies on a normal serosal surface (convex, flat, or slightly concave <1 cm) and an indentation in the mid-fundal endometrial surface by >1 cm [45,53].

On US, the septum is typically of similar echogenicity as the myometrium. 3D US with either the multiplanar or rendering mode enables one to see the coronal view so the serosal surface can be seen and the differentiation between a bicornuate uterus (Figs 6.5A and 6.6) and a septate uterus can easily be made (Figs 6.7 and 6.8) [36,42,43]. Again, it is best to perform the 3D US during the luteal phase as this is a time when the endometrium is homogeneously thickened and hyperechoic, providing a natural contrast material without being invasive. Early in the follicular phase, the endometrium is thin and not useful in identifying the endometrial cavity. Consequently, combining a 3D US with an SIS during the early follicular phase demonstrates the endometrial cavity with a hypoechoic echo that differentiates the inner cavity from the myometrium, and the fundal indentation can easily be measured and, if greater than 1 cm with the convex serosal surface, the diagnosis is made of a subseptate or complete septate uterus. A vaginal septum may be present in some cases.

This entity is associated with poor reproductive and obstetric outcomes, with rates of spontaneous abortion ranging from 26% to 94% [49,55,58–63] and premature birth rates ranging from 9% to 33% [59,62–65]. Treatment involves hysteroscopic resection of the septum, ideally leaving a remnant of less than 1 cm. Correction of the subseptum or septum leads to a marked improvement in pregnancy outcome.

Class VI – arcuate uterus

The arcuate uterus has a mild, broad depression on the fundal portion of the endometrium (less than 1 cm) and a normal serosal surface (convex, flat, or less than 1 cm indentation) secondary to near complete resorption of the uterovaginal septum. The diagnosis is made by drawing a horizontal line between the two cornua and then measuring the distance of a vertical drop at the mid-fundal portion to the endometrium. If this distance is less than 1 cm, then it qualifies as an arcuate uterus. Most consider the arcuate uterus as a normal variant that has no definite association with infertility or recurrent pregnancy loss.

However, recently there does appear to be a higher incidence of late second or third trimester obstetric complications. More data are being collected (Fig. 6.12A and B).

Class VII – uterine anomaly related to in utero diethylstilbestrol (DES) exposure

Diethylstilbestrol is a synthetic estrogen that was used extensively in the 1940s and 1950s to prevent pregnancy loss in women. It was discontinued in the 1970s. There is a 69% incidence of congenital uterine anomalies detected on HSG in females exposed to DES in utero [66]. Anomalies related to DES exposure include a T-shaped uterus. Hypoplasia, constrictions, synechiae, polypoid defects, a widened lower uterine segment, and irregular margins of endometrial cavity are well depicted on HSG (Fig. 6.13B). These anomalies are associated with increased rates of ectopic pregnancy, preterm delivery, and spontaneous abortion. Ultrasound findings are often nonspecific. Saline infusion sonohysterography can assist in showing this disorder either visually or with the increased resistance and rapid effusion of fluid. MRI may demonstrate local junctional-zone thickening at sites of constriction on T2-weighted imaging. The T-shaped configuration and irregularity of the endometrium can also be demonstrated on MRI and 3D US, especially with SIS.

Misdiagnosis of müllerian anomalies

Misdiagnosis of the exact nature of uterine anomalies is common. For example, complete uterine and vaginal septum can be easily confused with uterus didelphys and management of these two MDAs is different [17]. In addition, misdiagnoses with inappropriate abdominal surgeries leading to infertility attributable to contralateral isthmic stenosis after a hysterectomy of the obstructed hemiuterus have been reported [16]. Several reports in the literature also allude to misdiagnosis leading to increased morbidity such as severe dysmenorrhea, dyspareunia [67,68], infertility [8,69], and pregnancy complications as mentioned previously, including ruptured rudimentary uterine horn [70–72]. To that end, it is now widely accepted that surgical treatment should be performed by the vaginal approach to avoid infertility, especially in patients with obstructive utero vaginal duplication [16], while the presence of uterine anomaly can be a cause of failure of sterilization if undetected [73].

Prior detection of a uterine anomaly may alert the obstetrician to the possibility of cervical incompetence, which may prompt serial US surveillance with a view to determining whether prophylactic cerclage is appropriate. Recently, a new variety of MDA termed accessory and cavitated uterine masses (ACUM) with functional endometrium, often erroneously diagnosed as juvenile cystic adenomyoma (JCA), has been described. This entity is also a cause of severe dysmenorrhea and chronic pelvic pain, may be multiple, and, rarely, can be associated with an adjacent accessory rudimentary tube [74]. The diagnosis ACUM is problematic because of a broad differential diagnosis, including rudimentary and cavitated uterine horns; however, with a high index of suspicion, diagnosis can be made with transvaginal US and MRI.

In all cases of suspected uterine anomaly, timely and accurate diagnosis is essential to identify the underlying problem and formulate an appropriate therapeutic plan in order to avoid complications and prevent further sequelae. The role of imaging, therefore, is not only to detect and diagnose MDAs, but also to help distinguish surgically correctable forms of these anomalies from nonsurgical forms. Thus, correct classification of an anomaly can spare the patient unnecessary laparoscopy or surgery. In addition, coincidental leiomyomas, adenomyosis, and ovarian masses may also be detected and classified by appropriate imaging and can influence treatment modality.

Conclusion

Müllerian anomalies include a constellation of congenital malformations. There is significant diversity in their respective long-term sexual and reproductive outcomes. Some of these malformations can be surgically corrected; hence, presurgical pelvic imaging has a diagnostic and therapeutic value. Three-D US enables multiplanar 3D reconstruction of the uterus, which can be evaluated at the time of the US imaging or the 3D acquisition can be saved for post-procedure processing and not be technician dependent. If done in the follicular phase, then SIS combined with 3D US may be helpful. In either case, 3D US provides a rapid (within minutes), low-cost investigational modality to diagnose MDAs.

In most instances, 3D US and MRI are comparable methods to diagnose MDAs. Given that 3D US is cheaper, quicker, and more accessible, it should be the first line of investigation. If the diagnosis cannot be made with 3D US, or there is some uncertainty, then MRI with a gynecologic protocol should be utilized. There are circumstances where MRI images are more useful since MRI can penetrate easily through fibroids and calcifications so that the images are not obscured and an accurate diagnosis can be made. This accuracy depends on the alignment of the MRI image with the alignment of the uterus, which does not always occur with the sagittal orientation that is required in a gynecologic protocol.

Most hospitals need to be aware of the need to apply the gynecologic protocol when performing MRI as some do not follow this protocol. In addition, the MRI can be extended beyond the pelvis to evaluate the kidneys and collecting ducts. However, MRIs are more expensive and take more time to perform. Both procedures are noninvasive so one of these modalities should be performed to confirm the diagnosis prior to surgery.

References

1. Grimbizis GF, Camus M, Tarlatzis BC, Bontis JN, Devroey P. Clinical implications of uterine malformations and hysteroscopic treatment results. *Hum Reprod Update* 2001; **7**(2): 161–174.

2. Chang AS, Siegel CL, Moley KH, Ratts VS, Odem RR. Septate uterus with cervical duplication and longitudinal vaginal septum: a report of five new cases. *Fertil Steril* 2004; **81**(4): 1133–1136.

3. Lee DM, Osathanondh R, Yeh J. Localization of Bcl-2 in the human fetal mullerian tract. *Fertil Steril* 1998; **70**(1): 135–140.

4. Miller C, Pavlova A, Sassoon DA. Differential expression patterns of Wnt genes in the murine female reproductive tract during development and the estrous cycle. *Mech Dev* 1998; **76**(1–2): 91–99.

5. Vainio S, Heikkila M, Kispert A, Chin N, McMahon AP. Female development in mammals is regulated by Wnt-4 signalling. *Nature* 1999; **397**(6718): 405–409.

6. Rennell CL: T-shaped uterus in diethylstilbestrol (DES) exposure. *AJR Am J Roentgenol* 1979; **132**(6): 979–980.

7. Golan A, Langer R, Bukovsky I, Caspi E. Congenital anomalies of the mullerian system. *Fertil Steril* 1989; **51**(5): 747–755.

8. Sharara FI. Complete uterine septum with cervical duplication, longitudinal vaginal septum and duplication of a renal collecting system. A case report. *J Reprod Med* 1998; **43**(12): 1055–1059.

9. Jayaprakasan K, Chan YY, Sur S, Deb S, Clewes JS, Raine-Fenning NJ. Prevalence of uterine anomalies and their impact on early pregnancy in women conceiving after assisted reproduction treatment. *Ultrasound Obstet Gynecol* 2011; **37**(6): 727–732.

10. Saravelos SH, Cocksedge KA, Li TC. Prevalence and diagnosis of congenital uterine anomalies in women with reproductive failure: a critical appraisal. *Hum Reprod Update* 2008; **14**(5): 415–429.

11. Gubbini G, Di Spiezio Sardo A, Nascetti D, Marra E, Spinelli M, Greco E, Casadio P, Nappi C. New outpatient subclassification system for American Fertility Society Classes V and VI uterine anomalies. *J Minim Invasive Gynecol* 2009; **16**(5): 554–561.

12. The American Fertility Society classifications of adnexal adhesions, distal tubal occlusion, tubal occlusion secondary to tubal ligation, tubal pregnancies, mullerian anomalies and intrauterine adhesions. *Fertil Steril* 1988; **49**(6): 944–955.

13. Troiano RN, McCarthy SM. Mullerian duct anomalies: imaging and clinical issues. *Radiology* 2004; **233**(1): 19–34.

14. McArdle CR, Berezin AF. Ultrasound demonstration of uterus subseptus. *J Clin Ultrasound* 1980; **8**(2): 139–141.

15. Carrington BM, Hricak H, Nuruddin RN, Secaf E, Laros RK, Jr., Hill EC. Mullerian duct anomalies: MR imaging evaluation. *Radiology* 1990; **176**(3): 715–720.

16. Capito C, Echaieb A, Lortat-Jacob S, Thibaud E, Sarnacki S, Nihoul-Fekete C. Pitfalls in the diagnosis and management of obstructive uterovaginal duplication: a series of 32 cases. *Pediatrics* 2008; **122**(4): e891–897.

17. Patton PE, Novy MJ, Lee DM, Hickok LR. The diagnosis and reproductive outcome after surgical treatment of the complete septate uterus, duplicated cervix and vaginal septum. *Am J Obstet Gynecol* 2004; **190**(6): 1669–1675; discussion 1675–1668.

18. Stein AL, March CM. Pregnancy outcome in women with mullerian duct anomalies. *J Reprod Med* 1990; **35**(4): 411–414.

19. Hua M, Odibo AO, Longman RE, Macones GA, Roehl KA, Cahill AG. Congenital uterine anomalies and adverse pregnancy outcomes. *Am J Obstet Gynecol* 2011; **205**(6): 558 e551–555.

20. Devi Wold AS, Pham N, Arici A. Anatomic factors in recurrent pregnancy loss. *Semin Reprod Med* 2006; **24**(1): 25–32.

21. Crabtree GS, Machin GA, Martin JM, Nicholson SF, Nimrod CA. Fetal deformation caused by uterine malformation. *Pediatr Pathol* 1984; **2**(3): 305–312.

22. Li S, Qayyum A, Coakley FV, Hricak H. Association of renal agenesis and mullerian duct anomalies. *J Comput Assist Tomogr* 2000; **24**(6): 829–834.

23. Tanaka YO, Kurosaki Y, Kobayashi T, Eguchi N, Mori K, Satoh Y, Nishida M, Kubo T, Itai Y. Uterus didelphys associated with obstructed hemivagina and ipsilateral renal agenesis: MR findings in seven cases. *Abdom Imaging* 1998; **23**(4): 437–441.

24. Li YW, Sheih CP, Chen WJ. Unilateral occlusion of duplicated uterus with ipsilateral renal anomaly in young girls: a study with MRI. *Pediatr Radiol* 1995; **25**(Suppl 1): S54–59.

25. Kiechl-Kohlendorfer U, Geley T, Maurer K, Gassner I. Uterus didelphys with unilateral vaginal atresia: multicystic dysplastic kidney is the precursor of "renal agenesis" and the key to early diagnosis of this genital anomaly. *Pediatr Radiol* 2011; **41**(9): 1112–1116.

26. Kanamori Y, Iwanaka T, Nakahara S, Kawashima H, Komura M, Sugiyama M, et al. Survival in a neonate with complete urorectal septum malformation sequence after fetal vesico-amniotic shunting for a prominently dilated cloaca. *Fetal Diagn Ther* 2008; **24**(4): 458–461.

27. Pittock ST, Babovic-Vuksanovic D, Lteif A. Mayer-Rokitansky-Kuster-Hauser anomaly and its associated malformations. *Am J Med Genet A* 200; **135**(3): 314–316.

28. Ganie MA, Laway BA, Ahmed S, Alai MS, Lone GN. Mayer-Rokintansky-Kuster-Hauser syndrome associated with atrial septal defect, partial anomalous pulmonary venous connection and unilateral kidney – an unusual triad of anomalies. *J Pediatr Endocrinol Metab* 2010; **23**(10): 1087–1091.

29. Calaluce RD, Huang TH, Quesenberry JT, Evans ML, Luger AM, O'Connor TA. Hypoplastic left heart syndrome with male pseudohermaphroditism and bicornuate uterus bicollis. *Pediatr Cardiol* 1995; **16**(5): 239–241.

30. David A, Mercier J, Verloes A. Child with manifestations of Nager acrofacial dysostosis, and the MURCS, VACTERL, and pulmonary agenesis associations: complex defect of blastogenesis? *Am J Med Genet* 1996; **62**(1): 1–5.

31. Jurkovic D, Geipel A, Gruboeck K, Jauniaux E, Natucci M, Campbell S. Three-dimensional ultrasound for the assessment of uterine anatomy and detection of congenital anomalies: a comparison with hysterosalpingography and two-dimensional sonography. *Ultrasound Obstet Gynecol* 1995; **5**(4): 233–237.

32. Fayez JA, Mutie G, Schneider PJ. The diagnostic value of hysterosalpingography and hysteroscopy in infertility investigation. *Am J Obstet Gynecol* 1987; **156**(3): 558–560.

33. Pellerito JS, McCarthy SM, Doyle MB, Glickman MG, DeCherney AH. Diagnosis of uterine anomalies: relative accuracy of MR imaging, endovaginal sonography, and hysterosalpingography. *Radiology* 1992; **183**(3): 795–800.

34. Braun P, Grau FV, Pons RM, Enguix DP. Is hysterosalpingography able to diagnose all uterine malformations correctly? A retrospective study. *Eur J Radiol* 2005; **53**(2): 274–279.

35. Abuhamad AZ, Singleton S, Zhao Y, Bocca S. The Z technique: an easy approach to the display of the mid-coronal plane of the uterus in volume sonography. *J Ultrasound Med* 2006; **25**(5): 607–612.

36. Caliskan E, Ozkan S, Cakiroglu Y, Sarisoy HT, Corakci A, Ozeren S. Diagnostic accuracy of real-time 3D sonography in the diagnosis of congenital Mullerian anomalies in high-risk patients with respect to the phase of the menstrual cycle. *J Clin Ultrasound* 2010; **38**(3): 123–127.

37. Wu MH, Hsu CC, Huang KE. Detection of congenital mullerian duct anomalies using three-dimensional ultrasound. *J Clin Ultrasound* 1997; **25**(9): 487–492.

38. Kupesic SKA: Ultrasound and Doppler assessment of uterine anomalies. In: Kupesic S, de Ziegler D, eds. *Ultrasound and Infertility*. Pearl River, NY: Parthenon; 2000.

39. Raga F, Bonilla-Musoles F, Blanes J, Osborne NG. Congenital Mullerian anomalies: diagnostic accuracy of three-dimensional ultrasound. *Fertil Steril* 1996; **65**(3): 523–528.

40. Salim R, Woelfer B, Backos M, Regan L, Jurkovic D. Reproducibility of three-dimensional ultrasound diagnosis of congenital uterine anomalies. *Ultrasound Obstet Gynecol* 2003; **21**(6): 578–582.

41. Deutch TD, Abuhamad AZ. The role of 3-dimensional ultrasonography and magnetic resonance imaging in the diagnosis of mullerian duct anomalies: a review of the literature. *J Ultrasound Med* 2008; **27**(3): 413–423.

42. Mazouni C, Girard G, Deter R, Haumonte JB, Blanc B, Bretelle F. Diagnosis of Mullerian anomalies in adults: evaluation of practice. *Fertil Steril* 2008; **89**(1): 219–222.

43. Ghi T, Casadio P, Kuleva M, Perrone AM, Savelli L, Giunchi S, et al. Accuracy of three-dimensional ultrasound in diagnosis and classification of congenital uterine anomalies. *Fertil Steril* 2009; **92**(2): 808–813.

44. Salim R, Jurkovic D. Assessing congenital uterine anomalies: the role of three-dimensional ultrasonography. *Best Pract Res Clin Obstet Gynaecol* 2004; **18**(1): 29–36.

45. Pui MH. Imaging diagnosis of congenital uterine malformation. *Comput Med Imaging Graph* 2004; **28**(7): 425–433.

46. Acien P, Acien M. Unilateral renal agenesis and female genital tract pathologies. *Acta Obstet Gynecol Scand* 2010; **89**(11): 1424–1431.

47. Acien P. Incidence of Mullerian defects in fertile and infertile women. *Hum Reprod* 1997; **12**(7): 1372–1376.

48. Homer HA, Li TC, Cooke ID. The septate uterus: a review of management and reproductive outcome. *Fertil Steril* 2000; **73**(1): 1–14.

49. Raga F, Bauset C, Remohi J, Bonilla-Musoles F, Simon C, Pellicer A. Reproductive impact of congenital Mullerian anomalies. *Hum Reprod* 1997; **12**(10): 2277–2281.

50. Fedele L, Bianchi S: Hysteroscopic metroplasty for septate uterus. *Obstet Gynecol Clin North Am* 1995; **22**(3): 473–489.

51. Paniel BJ, Haddad B, el Medjadji M, Vincent Y. [Value of ultrasonography in utero-vaginal aplasia]. *J Gynecol Obstet Biol Reprod (Paris)* 1996; **25**(2): 128–130.

52. Moutos DM, Damewood MD, Schlaff WD, Rock JA. A comparison of the reproductive outcome between women with a unicornuate uterus and women with a didelphic uterus. *Fertil Steril* 1992; **58**(1): 88–93.

53. Acien P: Reproductive performance of women with uterine malformations. *Hum Reprod* 1993; **8**(1): 122–126.

54. Ludmir J, Samuels P, Brooks S, Mennuti MT. Pregnancy outcome of patients with uncorrected uterine anomalies managed in a high-risk obstetric setting. *Obstet Gynecol* 1990; **75**(6): 906–910.

55. Heinonen PK, Saarikoski S, Pystynen P. Reproductive performance of women with uterine anomalies. An evaluation of 182 cases. *Acta Obstet Gynecol Scand* 1982; **61**(2): 157–162.

56. Mercer CA, Long WN, Thompson JD. Uterine unification: indications and technique. *Clin Obstet Gynecol* 1981; **24**(4): 1199–1216.

57. D'Addato F, Andreoli C, Repinto A, Malagnino F. [Comparison of metroplasty by Strassman's method and by Tomkins' method. Retrospective study of 30 years]. *Minerva Ginecol* 1991; **43**(5): 223–226.

58. Harger JH, Archer DF, Marchese SG, Muracca-Clemens M, Garver KL. Etiology of recurrent pregnancy losses and outcome of subsequent pregnancies. *Obstet Gynecol* 1983; **62**(5): 574–581.

59. Buttram VC, Jr. Mullerian anomalies and their management. *Fertil Steril* 1983; **40**(2): 159–163.

60. Raziel A, Arieli S, Bukovsky I, Caspi E, Golan A. Investigation of the uterine cavity in recurrent aborters. *Fertil Steril* 1994; **62**(5): 1080–1082.

61. Clifford K, Rai R, Watson H, Regan L. An informative protocol for the investigation of recurrent miscarriage: preliminary experience of 500 consecutive cases. *Hum Reprod* 1994; **9**(7): 1328–1332.

62. Maneschi F, Zupi E, Marconi D, Valli E, Romanini C, Mancuso S. Hysteroscopically detected asymptomatic mullerian anomalies. Prevalence and reproductive implications. *J Reprod Med* 1995; **40**(10): 684–688.

63. Propst AM, Hill JA, 3rd. Anatomic factors associated with recurrent pregnancy loss. *Semin Reprod Med* 2000; **18**(4): 341–350.

64. Fedele L, Bianchi S, Agnoli B, Tozzi L, Vignali M. Urinary tract anomalies associated with unicornuate uterus. *J Urol* 1996; **155**(3): 847–848.

65. Gray SE RD, Franklin RR. Fertility after metroplasty of the uterus. *J Reprod Med* 1984; **29**: 185–188.

66. Kaufman RH, Adam E, Binder GL, Gerthoffer E. Upper genital tract changes and pregnancy outcome in offspring exposed in utero to diethylstilbestrol. *Am J Obstet Gynecol* 1980; **137**(3): 299–308.

67. Ziebarth A, Eyster K, Hansen K. Delayed diagnosis of partially obstructed longitudinal vaginal septa. *Fertil Steril* 2007; **87**(3): 697 e617–620.

68. Paniel BJ, Truc JB, Poitout P. [110 cases of longitudinal septa of the vagina]. *J Gynecol Obstet Biol Reprod (Paris)* 1985; **14**(8): 1011–1024.

69. Taylor E, Gomel V. The uterus and fertility. *Fertil Steril* 2008; **89**(1): 1–16.

70. Samuels TA, Awonuga A. Second-trimester rudimentary uterine horn pregnancy: rupture after labor induction with misoprostol. *Obstet Gynecol* 2005; **106**(5 Pt 2): 1160–1162.

71. Abreu R, Barros S, Jardim O, Morais C. Failure of prostaglandin induction labor in a Mullerian abnormality. *Arch Gynecol Obstet* 2010; **282**(2): 143–147.

72. van der Veen NM, Brouns JF, Doornbos JP, van Wijngaarden WJ. Misoprostol and termination of pregnancy: is there a need for ultrasound screening in a general population to assess the risk for adverse outcome in cases of uterine anomaly? *Arch Gynecol Obstet* 2011; **283**(1): 1–5.

73. Ferreira CR, Magalhaes DR, Lippes J. Sonographic recognition of three cases of septate uteri diminishes failures of quinacrine sterilization. *Contraception* 2006; **73**(4): 433–436.

74. Acien P, Bataller A, Fernandez F, Acien MI, Rodriguez JM, Mayol MJ. New cases of accessory and cavitated uterine masses (ACUM): a significant cause of severe dysmenorrhea and recurrent pelvic pain in young women. *Hum Reprod* 2012; **27**(3): 683–694.

Ultrasound imaging in hydrosalpinges

Gautam N. Allahbadia and Rubina Merchant

Introduction

Tubal factor infertility, which accounts for 15–30% of infertility in all women, is common in developing countries with high rates of pelvic inflammatory disease (PID) but limited resources [1], with distal tubal disease accounting for 85% of such cases [2]. Distal tubal disease is caused by PID due to infection, adhesions from previous surgery, endometriosis, and hydrosalpinx. Fallopian tubes affected by PID, mostly caused by *Chlamydia trachomatis* and/or *Neisseria gonorrhoeae*, may have a spectrum of sequelae ranging from a patent, apparently unaffected tube to a thick-walled hydrosalpinx showing chronic inflammation with irreversibly destroyed mucosa [3]. Fig. 7.1 depicts normal fallopian tubes while Fig. 7.2 depicts an ultrasound image of hydrosalpinges. Distal tubal disease may be classified as mild, moderate, or severe based on the extent of adhesions, degree of fimbrial preservation, appearance of the endosalpinx on hysterosalpingography (HSG), and size of hydrosalpinx [2]. A hydrosalpinx essentially involves distal tubal occlusion and accumulation of fluid within the fallopian tube as a result of a range of inflammatory conditions. It adversely affects early pregnancy events by altering the uterine and tubal environment and interfering with tubal transport of gametes and embryos through mechanical and functional damage, resulting in infertility [2,4]. A higher incidence of pelvic pathology has been reported in patients with chronic pelvic pain (CPP) compared with those without CPP and only infertility (76.7% vs. 42.6% $P \leq 0.0001$), hydrosalpinges with pelvic adhesions being significantly more frequent in cases with CPP [5] Hence, an optimal initial infertility investigation protocol that is diagnostically accurate, expeditious, cost-effective, reliable, as minimally invasive as possible, and that provides the clinician with useful prognostic information regarding possible future treatment is mandatory.

Ultrasound for the diagnosis and treatment of infertility has progressed rapidly to become an integral part of the management of the infertile woman. It enables a non-invasive, refined, and detailed evaluation of the pelvic cavity, thus facilitating the diagnosis of uterine, tubal, and ovarian pathology [6].

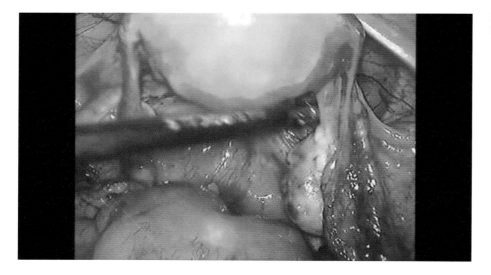

Fig. 7.1 Normal fallopian tubes. (Courtesy of Dr. Ameya Padmawar, Mumbai, India.)

Ultrasonography in Gynecology, ed. Botros R. M. B. Rizk and Elizabeth E. Puscheck. Published by Cambridge University Press. © Cambridge University Press 2015.

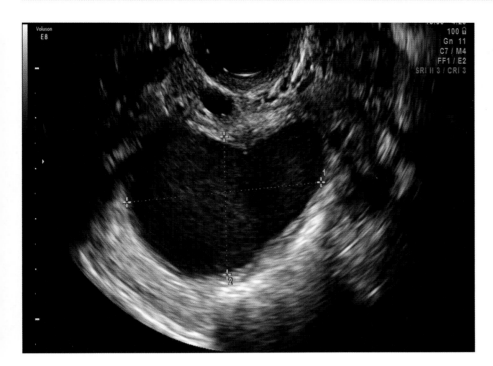

Fig. 7.2 Ultrasound image of hydrosalpinges. (Courtesy of Dr. Umesh Athavale, Athavale Imaging Centre, Mumbai, India.)

Pathophysiology

Hydrosalpinx is a common cause of female infertility that has a detrimental effect on the outcome of in vitro fertilization (IVF) [7,8]. Several authors have reported significantly reduced clinical pregnancy rates, ongoing pregnancy rates, and implantation rates after IVF in women with hydrosalpinges compared with women who had tubal disease, but no hydrosalpinges [9], and in the presence of an ultrasound-visible hydrosalpinx, but not in the presence of a hydrosalpinx not visible by ultrasound. The cumulative chance of achieving an ongoing pregnancy after one or more IVF cycles was also significantly reduced in the presence of an ultrasound-visible hydrosalpinx [10]. The mechanism of increased tubal ectopic pregnancy rates during IVF with hydrosalpinges remains unexplained; however, abnormal embryo migration due to the hydrosalpinx may be a contributing factor [11].

Though the adverse effects of hydrosalpinx on the outcome of IVF have been well documented, the mechanism by which hydrosalpinges exert their negative impact on fertility and assisted reproductive technology (ART) outcomes is poorly understood [8,12]. Several mechanisms have been proposed. Mechanical factors, toxicity of the hydrosalpingeal fluid, and receptivity dysfunction may explain the impaired IVF outcome in the presence of hydrosalpinx [8]. Genital *C. trachomatis* infection has been recognized as the single most common cause of PID, leading to severe tubal damage, ectopic pregnancy, infertility, and hydrosalpinx [13].

Ajonuma et al. [13] have suggested the involvement of fallopian tube epithelial transporters and ion channels, particularly the cystic fibrosis transmembrane conductance regulator (CFTR), as a possible mechanism underlying hydrosalpinx

formation following PID and possible links between *C. trachomatis* in PID and the subsequent CFTR-mediated events in hydrosalpinx formation that lead to infertility [12]. Using Western blot analysis, they demonstrated up-regulated expression of CFTR (a cAMP-activated chloride channel that regulates epithelial electrolyte and fluid secretion in hydrosalpinx fluid formation) in ultrasound-visible hydrosalpinx tissues of infertile patients with detectable serum levels of *C. trachomatis* antibody (immunoglobulin G), as further proof of the possible involvement of CFTR in the pathogenesis of hydrosalpinx fluid formation. However, further research on the mechanisms underlying the formation of hydrosalpinx induced by *C. trachomatis* infection is necessary to explain the causes for reduced implantation in hydrosalpinx patients and provide more avenues of treatment [12,14].

Clinical discussion

It is important to make an accurate diagnosis of hydrosalpinges prior to management, as bilateral megaureters may masquerade as hydrosalpinges on ultrasound [15]. The possibility of complications, such as ruptured tubo-ovarian abscess, owing to reactivation of latent pelvic infection due to previous PID after transvaginal ultrasound-directed follicle aspiration–transcervical embryo transfer despite aspiration of bilateral hydrosalpinges at the time of oocyte retrieval has been reported. This further emphasizes the significance of a proper diagnosis and management of pelvic infection prior to proceeding with ART [16]. Testing all patients for hydrosalpinges, as well as ovarian reserve and endometrial defects, is a common clinical practice identified among consistently high-performing IVF programs [17].

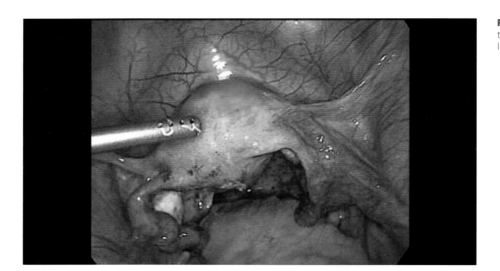

Fig. 7.3 "Beads on a string" view of the fallopian tube. (Courtesy of Dr. Ameya Padmawar, Mumbai, India.)

Diagnosis of hydrosalpinges

The role of ultrasound

Recent advances in gynecologic ultrasonography have shown that ultrasound can replace routine invasive investigative procedures, with the advantages of decreased cost, decreased time, and increased patient acceptability [1,18]. Most pathological conditions of the fallopian tubes have characteristic appearances on ultrasound and the diagnostic accuracy with transvaginal ultrasound, using high-frequency, high-resolution probes, is high. The routine use of ultrasound in this setting has also contributed to a better understanding of the natural history of conditions affecting the fallopian tubes and enables a triage of patients suitable for expectant or surgical management [4].

It is possible to outline the fallopian tubes by injecting isotonic saline transcervically during transvaginal ultrasound scanning of the pelvis, and both color flow Doppler and 3-dimensional (3D) scanning modes have been employed to improve visualization of the tubes with varying success [1]. Pelvic ultrasonography should be a part of the routine infertility investigation, followed, if necessary, by diagnostic laparoscopy, especially in symptomatic patients [15], for confirmation and further management. The major limitation of ultrasound, however, is the fact that it is not useful in air/gaseous containing media [5].

Normal fallopian tubes are rarely visible with transvaginal ultrasound unless they are pathologically altered and filled with fluid in cases such as hydro- or pyosalpinx [19]. The accumulation of fluid within the fallopian tube provides a sonographic contrast agent [4]. Ultrasonographically, the dilated fallopian tube presents as a thick- (>3 mm) or thin (<3 mm)-walled tubular and elongated structure, with a thin wall usually being seen in chronic tubal disease and longitudinal endosalpingeal folds seen in cross-section as small hyperechoic nodules when inflamed. The thickened, edematous folds give the appearance that is typically described as the "cogwheel" sign in acute infection, and as the "beads on a string" sign in chronic disease when the active inflammation has settled and the folds are less edematous, less congested, and therefore, smaller. Kinking of the tube gives the typical ultrasound appearance of an incomplete septation [20]. Fig. 7.3 depicts the "beads on a string" view of the fallopian tubes. The overall sensitivity and specificity of conventional B-mode transvaginal ultrasound in the diagnosis of a hydrosalpinx has been reported to be 93.3% and 99.6%, respectively [21]. Ultrasound additionally offers the ability to distinguish peritoneal pseudocysts, which have typical ultrasound features, and ovarian cysts from hydrosalpinges. In patients with ultrasound-visible hydrosalpinges, ultrasonography before embryo transfer is useful to detect newly developed hydrometra [22].

Patel et al. [23] attempted to describe the "waist" sign as a feature of hydrosalpinx and to calculate the likelihood ratio of sonographic findings for predicting that a cystic adnexal mass is a hydrosalpinx. They reported hydrosalpinges in 39% of the 67 cystic adnexal masses, with the waist sign occurring in combination with the tubular shape on the sonograms in 12 hydrosalpinges and no other masses (likelihood ratio of between 18.9 and infinity for the sonographic findings) and small round projections combined with tubular shape in 14 hydrosalpinges and one other mass (likelihood ratio of 22.1). They concluded that hydrosalpinx can be diagnosed with the highest likelihood when a tubular mass in combination with the waist sign or small round projections is encountered. Incomplete septations and short linear projections are less discriminating findings of hydrosalpinx [23].

Three-dimensional ultrasound evaluation

Volume sonography, or 3D ultrasound, is a major advance in ultrasound technology that essentially takes multiple 2D ultrasound slices and molds them into a composite volume, enabling the practitioner to evaluate an entire organ instead of just

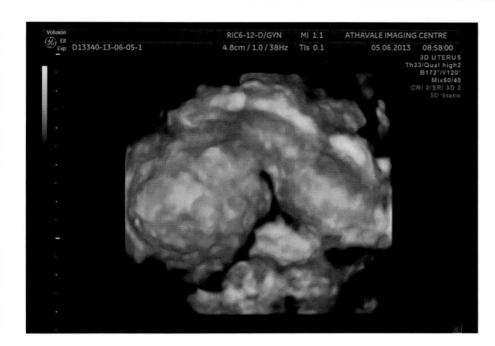

Fig. 7.4 3D image of a hydrosalpinx. (Courtesy of Dr. Umesh Athavale, Athavale Imaging Centre, Mumbai, India.)

one slice. Further, the composite volumes can be viewed from any angle and with a variety of different modes. Fig. 7.4 depicts a 3D image of a hydrosalpinx. With 2D ultrasound, it can often be difficult to differentiate between a hydrosalpinx and ovarian pathology, including multiple or complex cysts [24].

3D transvaginal ultrasound (TVUS) inversion technique

The 3D transvaginal ultrasound (TVUS) inversion technique is a simple and effective way to render fluid-filled spaces, which may be tortuous and follow various directions [3]. The 3D software inverts anechoic into echogenic voxels, which, against the black background of the monitor screen, displays the fluid-filled structure as a "cast" of it. A relatively short learning curve is required to master the inversion rendering technique and it may be used in selected gynecologic cases to offer a more accurate diagnosis somewhat faster than 2D sonography or even the 3D orthogonal planes [25] The rendered images increased the confidence in diagnosing hydrosalpinx. In a utility test of the 3D ultrasound inversion rendering technique in the evaluation of fluid-distended fallopian tubes, Timor-Tritsch et al. [26] demonstrated that 52/58 inversion renderings in patients with fluid-filled adnexal masses, suspected of being abnormal fallopian tubes, yielded acceptable images of hydrosalpinges. The acquired volumes on 3D TVUS were then "inverted" to display a cast-like appearance of the fluid-filled structures. The tubes in the patients with acute tubal disease ($n = 5$) were all successfully inverted. Only in four patients were the 2D images more informative than the 3D-rendered and inverted views [26]. While the technique may have marginal value over the 2D and 3D images in the diagnosis of uterine

disease, rendering the inverted fluid-filled adnexal structures provides an accurate diagnosis of tubal origin of pathology (chronic hydrosalpinges) [25].

Grayscale and Doppler ultrasonography

Subjective evaluation of grayscale and Doppler ultrasound findings enables an almost conclusive diagnosis of hydrosalpinx with a positive and negative likelihood ratio of pattern recognition of 38.9 and 0.15, respectively, with regard to hydrosalpinges and a specificity of 86%. Though other adnexal pathologies can be recognized, they cannot be confidently confirmed or excluded. In one study, a total of 1066 women were included, of whom 800 had benign masses and 266 had malignant masses [27]. Grayscale ultrasound morphology ("pattern recognition"), for the characterization of a pelvic mass, provides images with the same information as that obtained from postsurgical tissue histology [14].

The Sion procedure

The Sion procedure includes filling up the pouch of Douglas with approximately 300 mL of sterile normal saline, not only to elucidate the patency, but also to visualize the motility, the fimbriae, and peritubal adhesions, if present [28]. When surrounded by fluid, such as normal saline, a contrast is created and the normal tube appears as a 4 mm diameter tubular echogenic structure that usually courses from the lateral aspect of the uterine cornu posterolaterally into the adnexal regions and cul-de-sac. This procedure (negative contrast hydrogynecography) facilitates the visualization of minor tubal disorders, particularly thickened or abnormally dilated fallopian tubes, and is particularly helpful in distinguishing inflammatory disorders, such as tubo-ovarian masses, from simple hydrosalpinx [29].

Transvaginal hysterosalpingo-contrast-sonography (HyCoSy)

Transvaginal HyCoSy has been suggested as a simple, safe, and cheap method for the early assessment of the uterine cavity and fallopian tubes that can be employed as a routine, first-line infertility investigation, useful in the decision-making for future diagnostic and therapeutic procedures. It involves the instillation of an echogenic (hypo/hyperechogenic) contrast medium into the uterine cavity through a transcervical catheter (balloon catheter 5F or 7F in diameter), accompanied by transvaginal sonography with or without Doppler to assess tubal flow of contrast material and/or accumulation of contrast material in the pouch of Douglas. The hypoechogenic fluid is sterile normal saline and the hyperechogenic contrast fluid is usually Echovist-200 (a galactose-based echo-enhancing agent) [30].

Vaginal sonographic hydrotubation, using "agitated" saline during transvaginal sonography, has been shown to be more effective than HSG in detecting abnormalities of both interstitial and distal parts of the tube and has the advantage of being performed in an office setting [31]. When performed by experienced operators, it serves as a valuable, first-line screening test for the more invasive procedures of laparoscopy and hysteroscopy [32].

Alternatives to ultrasound

The effect of a hydrosalpinx on medically assisted reproduction requires an understanding of the complex pathophysiology of the hydrosalpinx and its clinical management, whether by functional surgery or IVF, preceded or not by salpingectomy [33]. Direct endoscopic evaluation of the tubal mucosa in hydrosalpinges offers the most advanced, office-based, and reliable technique to assess the quality of the tubal mucosa and to discriminate between a hydrosalpinx that should be treated with functional surgery or preventive salpingectomy [33,34]. Also, transvaginal ultrasound is not appropriate for selecting patients for further surgical management by salpingectomy or salpingostomy [34].

Magnetic resonance imaging (MRI) enables the diagnosis of hydrosalpinges with high confidence [35].

Management of hydrosalpinges

Hydrosalpinges have adverse effects on IVF outcomes. The accumulation of hydrosalpingeal fluid in the uterine cavity during an IVF-embryo transfer (IVF-ET) cycle is a rare complication of hydrosalpinges. The retrograde flow of tubal fluid may disturb intrauterine embryo development [36]. Surgical intervention such as salpingectomy, tubal occlusion, salpingostomy, or aspiration of the hydrosalpinx fluid, prior to the IVF procedure in women with hydrosalpinges, is thought to

improve the likelihood of a successful outcome [7]. Though salpingectomy is effective in improving outcomes, it is not always practical or safe [37].

Ultrasound-guided management

Randomized controlled trials comparing ultrasound-guided aspiration of hydrosalpingeal fluid prior to IVF-ET and no intervention prior to IVF-ET in patients with ultrasound-visible hydrosalpinges have reported significantly favorable pregnancy outcomes following aspiration of hydrosalpinges prior to IVF-ET [9,37,38].

Following computer-generated randomization and allocation concealment, Hammadieh et al. [37] reported biochemical pregnancy rates of 43.8% vs. 20.6%, $P = 0.04$, and clinical pregnancy rates of 31.3% vs. 17.6%, $P = 0.20$, in patients ≤39 years, following TVUS aspiration of hydrosalpinges at oocyte collection under antibiotic cover compared with controls, respectively. They observed no differences in the implantation rate, spontaneous abortion risk, ectopic pregnancy rates, or infection rates [37]. Van Voorhis et al. [9] reported higher clinical pregnancy rates (31 vs. 5%, $P = 0.07$), ongoing pregnancy rates (31 vs. 0%, $P = 0.015$), and implantation rates (14 vs. 1%, $P = 0.015$) following aspiration of hydrosalpinges at the time of oocyte retrieval compared with the no-aspiration group [9]. Hence, the presence of hydrosalpinges is associated with poor IVF outcomes and aspiration of hydrosalpingeal fluid at the time of oocyte retrieval in patients with ultrasound-visible hydrosalpinges is a simple, safe, and effective procedure that results in improved pregnancy outcomes [9,37], particularly for those without rapid reaccumulation of hydrosalpingeal fluid after aspiration or uterine fluid collection during the IVF-ET cycles [1]. Ultrasound-guided aspiration of hydrosalpinges at the time of oocyte retrieval may be an acceptable alternative to salpingectomy for the treatment of these patients [9].

However, according to certain authors, aspiration of the uterine fluid is unlikely to help because of rapid reaccumulation of hydrometra and failure to cure the underlying pathology. Cancellation of the treatment cycle and cryopreservation of oocytes in the pronucleate stage, or the embryos for future transfer, after surgical correction of the tubes is recommended [21,36].

Alternative management

Surgery

Surgical options for the management of hydrosalpinges apart from TVUS-guided drainage of hydrosalpinx before or during oocyte retrieval include laparoscopic salpingostomy, laparoscopic or hysteroscopic tubal occlusion, and laparoscopic salpingectomy. Laparoscopic surgery has a place in the diagnosis and management of hydrosalpinx, with a positive impact on fertility outcomes. Laparoscopic salpingectomy is a treatment option in women with bilateral disease or in patients with ultrasound-visible hydrosalpinges [8]. Salpingectomy in patients with ultrasound-visible hydrosalpinges has been suggested as a method to overcome the negative influence of the hydrosalpingeal fluid on implantation and embryo development, with significantly higher clinical pregnancy and birth rates following IVF [21,39,40]. Significantly higher implantation rates (30.3% vs. 17.1%, P = 0.003) and live birth rates (P = 0.004) have been reported in patients with ultrasound-visible hydrosalpinges who had undergone salpingectomy as compared with patients undergoing salpingectomy for other reasons [41]. The results of the cumulative cycles strengthen the recommendation for a laparoscopic salpingectomy prior to IVF in patients with ultrasound-visible hydrosalpinges [41].

In a review of five randomized controlled trials involving 646 patients, Johnson et al. [7] reported an increase in the odds of ongoing pregnancy and clinical pregnancy with laparoscopic salpingectomy for hydrosalpinges prior to IVF versus no intervention. However, laparoscopic occlusion of the fallopian tube did not increase the odds of ongoing pregnancy significantly but the odds of clinical pregnancy had sufficient power to show a significant increase versus no intervention. Comparison of tubal occlusion to salpingectomy did not show a significant advantage of either surgical procedure in terms of ongoing pregnancy or clinical pregnancy. The authors concluded that (i) surgical treatment should be considered for all women with hydrosalpinges prior to IVF treatment, (ii) laparoscopic tubal occlusion is an alternative to laparoscopic salpingectomy in improving IVF pregnancy rates in women with hydrosalpinges, and (iii) there were no significant differences in adverse effects of surgical treatments across the different comparisons. While laparoscopic tubal occlusion is an effective alternative to laparoscopic salpingectomy in improving IVF pregnancy rates in women with hydrosalpinges, further research is required to assess the value of aspiration of hydrosalpinges prior to or during IVF procedures and also the value of tubal restorative surgery as an alternative (or as a preliminary procedure) to IVF [7].

However, preserved tubal mucosa indicates a good prognosis for tubal surgery, therefore an appropriate mucosal assessment should be routine prior to deciding upon further management to avoid unnecessary salpingectomies. As salpingectomy is a definitive procedure, it is recommended that it should be performed prior to IVF in select patients with large ultrasound-visible hydrosalpinges beyond repair, with severely damaged tubal mucosa, in cases of IVF failure or re-occlusion of tubes to achieve improved pregnancy outcomes. Tubal surgery should be preferred to salpingectomy in patients with hydrosalpinges with preserved mucosa and in mild to moderate tubal disease [21,34]. Prophylactic salpingectomy prior to IVF and tubal surgery is not competing but complementary in the treatment of hydrosalpinges-related infertility [21]. A randomized controlled trial, analyzing the efficacy of salpingectomy prior to IVF in patients with ultrasound-visible hydrosalpinges and the cost-effectiveness of this strategy (intervention) compared with that of optional salpingectomy after a failed cycle (control), reported a higher live birth rate (60.8% vs. 40.9%)

following salpingectomy compared with controls and concluded that the incremental cost of the intervention strategy to achieve the higher birth rate was reasonable [42].

In patients requiring occlusion of unilateral or bilateral ultrasound-visible hydrosalpinges before IVF and with contraindications to abdominal surgery because of previous extensive abdominopelvic surgery, hysteroscopic placement of the Essure microinsert under general anesthesia may offer a safer, minimally invasive option. This may also be achieved by fluoroscopically-guided placement. Preoperative documentation of proximal tubal patency helps predict placement success. However, further research into this unique clinical scenario is required [43].

Conclusion

Hydrosalpinges have a detrimental impact on fertility as they interfere with the mechanical and functional roles of the fallopian tubes and uterus in achieving conception, thus necessitating an accurate diagnosis and management. Ultrasonography, enhanced by grayscale, Doppler and the 3D TVUS inversion technique serves as the cornerstone for the accurate diagnosis and therapeutic management of hydrosalpinges, and is often superior to both 2D and 3D orthogonal images in the diagnosis of hydrosalpinges. TVUS-guided aspiration of hydrosalpingeal fluid at oocyte retrieval in select patients with ultrasound-visible hydrosalpinges offers a non-invasive, office-based, and safe treatment option compared with surgical alternatives like laparoscopic tubal occlusion, salpingostomy, and salpingectomy, with improved pregnancy outcomes following IVF. However, it is not a widely accepted procedure yet, and may be accompanied with complications such as rapid reaccumulation of hydrometra, necessitating cycle cancellation, and embryo cryopreservation for future transfer. Though laparoscopic salpingectomy prior to IVF is a definite treatment option in the management of hydrosalpinges with improved pregnant outcomes, it is invasive and should ideally be reserved for patients with irreversibly damaged tubal mucosa, failure of tubal occlusion, or conception failure. Patients with healthy tubal mucosa following a failed attempt at ultrasound-guided hydrosalpinges aspiration should be referred for functional tubal surgery. Tubal endoscopy has a significant role in the evaluation of the quality of tubal mucosa to direct further surgical management because ultrasonography is inappropriate for this. Hence, management of hydrosalpinges should be directed by thorough patient evaluation, an accurate diagnosis of the severity of tubal disease, and the possibility of success with the treatment option considered in the given patient.

References

1. Hoffman L, Chan K, Smith B, Okolo S. The value of saline salpingosonography as a surrogate test of tubal patency in low-resource settings. *Int J Fertil Womens Med* 2005; **50**: 135–139.

2. Bhattacharya S, Logan S. Evidence-based management of tubal factor infertility. In: Allahbadia GN, Djahanbakhch O, Saridogan

E (Eds.) *The Fallopian Tube*. Tunbridge Wells, UK: Anshan Publishers; 2009: 215–223.

3. Puttemans PJ, De Bruyne F, Heylen SM. A decade of salpingoscopy. *Eur J Obstet Gynecol Reprod Biol* 1998; **81**: 197–206.

4. Salim R, Jurkovic D. The ultrasound of fallopian tubes In: Allahbadia GN, Djahanbakhch O, Saridogan E (Eds.) *The Fallopian Tube*. Tunbridge Wells, UK: Anshan Publishers; 2009: 191–197.

5. Milingos S, Protopapas A, Kallipolitis G, et al. Laparoscopic evaluation of infertile patients with chronic pelvic pain. *Reprod Biomed Online* 2006; **12**(3): 347–353.

6. Shapiro BS, DeCherney AH. Ultrasound and infertility. *J Reprod Med* 1989; **34**(2): 151–155.

7. Johnson N, van Voorst S, Sowter MC, et al. Surgical treatment for tubal disease in women due to undergo in vitro fertilisation. *Cochrane Database Syst Rev* 2010; (1): CD002125.

8. Bontis JN, Theodoridis TD. Laparoscopic management of hydrosalpinx. *Ann N Y Acad Sci* 2006; **1092**: 199–210.

9. Van Voorhis BJ, Sparks AE, Syrop CH, Stovall DW. Ultrasound-guided aspiration of hydrosalpinges is associated with improved pregnancy and implantation rates after in-vitro fertilization cycles. *Hum Reprod* 1998; **13**(3): 736–739.

10. de Wit W, Gowrising CJ, Kuik DJ, et al. Only hydrosalpinges visible on ultrasound are associated with reduced implantation and pregnancy rates after in-vitro fertilization. *Hum Reprod* 1998; **13**(6): 1696–1701.

11. Garde RV, Jovanovic VP, Couchman GM, et al. Ectopic pregnancy in a preexisting hydrosalpinx during a spontaneous pregnancy. *Fertil Steril* 2006; **86**(4): 1001.e11–13.

12. Ajonuma LC, Ng EH, Chan HC. New insights into the mechanisms underlying hydrosalpinx fluid formation and its adverse effect on IVF outcome. *Hum Reprod Update* 2002; **8**(3): 255–264.

13. Ajonuma LC, Chan PK, Ng EH, et al. Involvement of cystic fibrosis transmembrane conductance regulator (CFTR) in the pathogenesis of hydrosalpinx induced by *Chlamydia trachomatis* infection. *J Obstet Gynaecol Res* 2008; **34**(6): 923–930.

14. Valentin L. Use of morphology to characterize and manage common adnexal masses. *Best Pract Res Clin Obstet Gynaecol* 2004; **18**(1): 71–89.

15. Choi JM, Wang J, Guarnaccia MM, Sauer MV. Bilateral megaureters may masquerade as hydrosalpinges on ultrasound. *Reprod Biomed Online* 2009; **18**(6): 821–823.

16. Varras M, Polyzos D, Tsikini A, et al. Ruptured tubo-ovarian abscess as a complication of IVF treatment: clinical, ultrasonographic and histopathologic findings. A case report. *Clin Exp Obstet Gynecol* 2003; **30**(2–3): 164–168.

17. Van Voorhis BJ, Thomas M, Surrey ES, Sparks A. What do consistently high-performing in vitro fertilization programs in the U.S. do? *Fertil Steril* 2010; **94**(4): 1346–1349.

18. Ekerhovd E, Fried G, Granberg S. An ultrasound-based approach to the assessment of infertility, including the evaluation of tubal patency. *Best Pract Res Clin Obstet Gynaecol* 2004; **18**: 13–28.

19. Horrow MM. Ultrasound of pelvic inflammatory disease. *Ultrasound Q* 2004; **20**: 171–179.

20. Timor-Tritsch IE, Lerner JP, Monteagudo A, et al. Transvaginal sonographic markers of tubal inflammatory disease. *Ultrasound Obstet Gynecol* 1998; **12**: 56–66.

21. Sabatini L, Davis C. The management of hydrosalpinges: tubal surgery or salpingectomy? *Curr Opin Obstet Gynecol* 2005; **17**(4): 323–328.

22. Hinckley MD, Milki AA. Rapid reaccumulation of hydrometra after drainage at embryo transfer in patients with hydrosalpinx. *Fertil Steril* 2003; **80**(5): 1268–1271.

23. Patel MD, Acord DL, Young SW. Likelihood ratio of sonographic findings in discriminating hydrosalpinx from other adnexal masses. *AJR Am J Roentgenol* 2006; **186**(4): 1033–1038.

24. Deutch T, Stadtmauer L. The role of three-dimensional ultrasound in determining fallopian tube patency. In: Allahbadia GN, Djahanbakhch O, Saridogan E (Eds.) *The Fallopian Tube*. Tunbridge Wells, UK: Anshan Publishers; 2009: 173–179.

25. Timor-Tritsch IE, Monteagudo A, Tsymbal T, Strok I. Three-dimensional inversion rendering: a new sonographic technique and its use in gynecology. *J Ultrasound Med* 2005; **24**(5): 681–688.

26. Timor-Tritsch IE, Monteagudo A, Tsymbal T. Three-dimensional ultrasound inversion rendering technique facilitates the diagnosis of hydrosalpinx. *J Clin Ultrasound* 2010; **38**(7): 372–376.

27. Sokalska A, Timmerman D, Testa AC, et al. Diagnostic accuracy of transvaginal ultrasound examination for assigning a specific diagnosis to adnexal masses. *Ultrasound Obstet Gynecol* 2009; **34**(4): 462–470.

28. Allahbadia GN. Fallopian tubes and ultrasonography: the Sion experience. *Fertil Steril* 1992; **58**: 901–907.

29. Allahbadia GN. Negative contrast hydrogynecography. In: Allahbadia GN, Djahanbakhch O, Saridogan E (Eds.) *The Fallopian Tube*. Tunbridge Wells, UK: Anshan Publishers; 2009; 163–170.

30. Alborzi S, Dehbashi S, Khodaee R. Sonohysterosalpingographic screening for infertile patients. *Int J Gynaecol Obstet* 2003; **82**: 57–62.

31. Lupaşcu I, Vegheş S, Solomiţchi V, et al. [Sono-hysterosalpingography in the assessment of tubal infertility] [Article in Romanian] *Rev Med Chir Soc Med Nat Iasi* 2003; **107**: 841–845.

32. Radić V, Canić T, Valetić J, Duić Z. Advantages and disadvantages of hysterosonosalpingography in the assessment of the reproductive status of uterine cavity and fallopian tubes. *Eur J Radiol* 2005; **53**: 268–273.

33. Puttemans P, Campo R, Gordts S, Brosens I. Hydrosalpinx and ART: hydrosalpinx – functional surgery or salpingectomy? *Hum Reprod* 2000; **15**(7): 1427–1430.

34. Strandell A, Lindhard A. Hydrosalpinx and ART. Salpingectomy prior to IVF can be recommended to a well-defined subgroup of patients. *Hum Reprod* 2000; **15**(10): 2072–2074.

35. Rajkotia K, Veeramani M, Macura KJ. Magnetic resonance imaging of adnexal masses. *Top Magn Reson Imaging* 2006; **17**(6): 379–397.

36. Bloechle M, Schreiner T, Lisse K. Recurrence of hydrosalpinges after transvaginal aspiration of tubal fluid in an IVF cycle with development of a serometra. *Hum Reprod* 1997; **12**(4): 703–705.

37. Hammadieh N, Coomarasamy A, Ola B, et al. Ultrasound-guided hydrosalpinx aspiration during oocyte collection improves

pregnancy outcome in IVF: a randomized controlled trial. *Hum Reprod* 2008; **23**(5): 1113–1117.

38. Fouda UM, Sayed AM. Effect of ultrasound-guided aspiration of hydrosalpingeal fluid during oocyte retrieval on the outcomes of in vitro fertilisation-embryo transfer: a randomised controlled trial (NCT01040351). *Gynecol Endocrinol* 2011; **27**(8): 562–567.

39. Strandell A. How to treat hydrosalpinges: IVF as the treatment of choice. *Reprod Biomed Online* 2002; **4** Suppl 3: 37–39.

40. Johnson NP, Norris J. An Australasian survey of the management of hydrosalpinges in women due to undergo in vitro fertilisation. *Aust N Z J Obstet Gynaecol* 2002; **42**(3): 271–276.

41. Strandell A, Lindhard A, Waldenström U, Thorburn J. Hydrosalpinx and IVF outcome: cumulative results after salpingectomy in a randomized controlled trial. *Hum Reprod* 2001; **16**(11): 2403–2410.

42. Strandell A, Lindhard A, Eckerlund I. Cost-effectiveness analysis of salpingectomy prior to IVF, based on a randomized controlled trial. *Hum Reprod* 2005; **20**(12): 3284–3292.

43. Hitkari JA, Singh SS, Shapiro HM, Leyland N. Essure treatment of hydrosalpinges. *Fertil Steril* 2007; **88**(6): 1663–1666.

Chapter

8

Three-dimensional ultrasonography of subtle uterine anomalies: correlation with hysterosalpingogram, two-dimensional ultrasonography, and hysteroscopy

Mostafa I. Abuzeid and Omar M. Abuzeid

Introduction

A septate uterus has been shown to be associated with a very high pregnancy wastage rate of >70% [1]. More recently, a small uterine septum, or arcuate uterus, has been considered an important risk variable for preterm birth [2]. In addition, there is higher prevalence of a septate uterus in patients with repeated in vitro fertilization and embryo transfer (IVF-ET) failure (18.2%) [3]. Furthermore, some reports suggested higher prevalence of a septate uterus in patients with early pregnancy loss after IVF-ET (9.7%) [4].

The overall belief of experts in the area of ultrasonography of uterine cavity disorders is that transvaginal saline infusion hysterosonogram (SIH) with three-dimensional ultrasonography (3D US) and hysterosalpingogram (HSG) is highly sensitive in the diagnosis of major uterine malformations [5]. However, it is not sufficiently sensitive in the diagnosis of minor uterine abnormalities [5]. In our experience, transvaginal 2D US and SIH with 2D US are only useful in the presence of a complete uterine septum or significant incomplete uterine septum, but not helpful in the diagnosis of subtle cases of incomplete septum and arcuate uterus [6].

The gold standard for diagnosing a uterine septum and arcuate uterus is transvaginal SIH with 3D US and diagnostic hysteroscopy [6,7]. However, HSG is a test that is still being used during evaluation of infertility and in some cases of recurrent pregnancy loss (RPL). Fayez et al. reported high sensitivity of HSG in detecting significant uterine septum [8]. In addition, we observed high accuracy of HSG in detecting significant incomplete uterine septum [6,7]. Recent data from our unit suggested that the accuracy and sensitivity of HSG in detecting subtle uterine anomalies is poor [9]. Limited data in the literature suggested poor sensitivity of HSG in detecting endometrial cavity abnormalities in general [10,11].

The purpose of this chapter is to illustrate that when dealing with an arcuate uterus or a subtle incomplete septum there appear to be conflicting findings on various imaging studies. This may result in under-diagnosis of such anomalies. In turn, it is not unreasonable to think that such undiagnosed subtle uterine anomalies may account for some cases of unexplained infertility and RPL. In 50% of patients with RPL, the etiology is unexplained [12] and in 25–30% of infertile patients the etiology is unexplained [13,14]. The diagnosis and management of these subtle uterine anomalies may improve pregnancy rates and reproductive outcome in such patients. Specifically, we will focus on the two imaging studies that are now considered the gold standard for the diagnosis of uterine anomalies. These are transvaginal 3D US and SIH with 3D US. We will compare the findings of these tests with the findings on HSG, 2D US, and diagnostic hysteroscopy in the following eight cases.

Significant incomplete uterine septum diagnosed by all imaging studies (Case 1)

A 38-year-old white female presented with primary infertility of one year's duration. In this patient, the HSG (Fig. 8.1A and B) suggested the presence of an incomplete uterine septum versus incomplete bicornuate uterus and possible endometrial polyps. Both transvaginal 3D US (Fig. 8.2) and SIH with 3D US (Fig. 8.3) confirmed the presence of an incomplete uterine septum, and SIH with 3D US suggested the presence of possible endometrial polyps (Fig. 8.3). It is worthy of note that transvaginal 2D US and SIH with 2D US suggested the same diagnosis. The findings on hysteroscopy confirmed the presence of significant incomplete uterine septum and endometrial polyps (Fig. 8.4A–D). This case illustrates that when the uterine anomaly (in this case, an incomplete uterine septum) is relatively significant (15 mm in length in the mid-fundal region), it can be diagnosed easily by any of the imaging methods mentioned above. Two months after hysteroscopic division of an incomplete uterine septum and polypectomy, a postoperative SIH with 3D US was completely normal. The patient conceived spontaneously through IVF-ET treatment and delivered twins at 36 weeks gestation.

Ultrasonography in Gynecology, ed. Botros R. M. B. Rizk and Elizabeth E. Puscheck. Published by Cambridge University Press. © Cambridge University Press 2015.

A

B

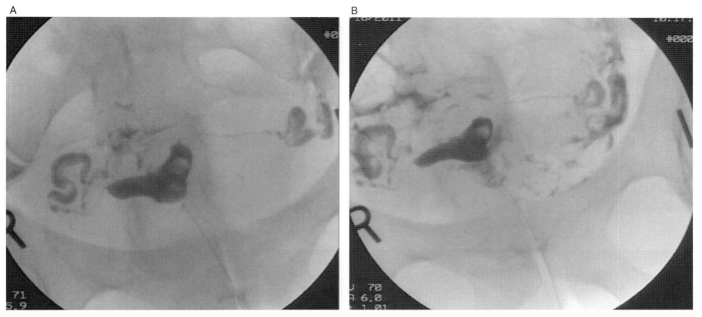

Fig. 8.1 (A) HSG film suggesting a slight arcuate uterus with two filling defects most probably as a result of endometrial polyps. (B) HSG film showing that as more dye is injected the fundal region appears normal but the two filling defects are still present.

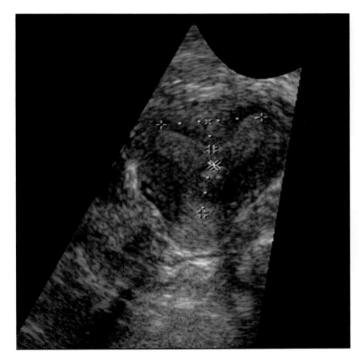

Fig. 8.2 Transvaginal 3D US picture showing an incomplete uterine septum (9.5 mm in length in the mid-fundal region).

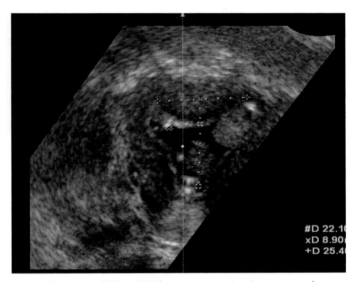

Fig. 8.3 Transvaginal SIH on 3D US picture suggesting the presence of an incomplete uterine septum (8.9 mm in length in the mid-fundal region) and SIH on 3D US and possible endometrial polyps.

Significant arcuate uterus: normal uterine fundus on 3D US and SIH with 3D US (Case 2)

A 31-year-old white female presented with primary infertility of one year's duration. In this patient, the HSG suggested a significant arcuate uterus (Fig. 8.5A and B) versus an incomplete

bicornuate uterus. Both transvaginal 3D US (Fig. 8.6) and SIH with 3D US (Fig. 8.7) revealed normal uterine fundus and possible small endometrial polyp in the right cornual region. Transvaginal 2D US with and without SIH were negative. The findings on hysteroscopy (Fig. 8.8) confirmed the presence of a significant arcuate uterus (15 mm length in the mid-fundal region). This case illustrates that the findings on transvaginal 3D US and SIH with 3D US can be misleading, even in the presence of a significant arcuate uterus. This patient had

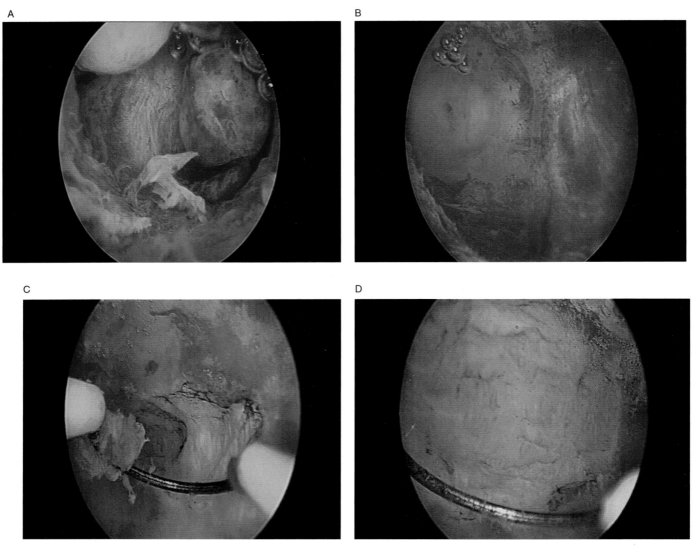

Fig. 8.4 Hysteroscopic pictures depicting (A) two large endometrial polyps masking the uterine fundus; (B) a significant incomplete uterine septum with the right side of the upper uterine segment seen; (C) the steps of septum division; and (D) the final appearance of the uterine fundus at the completion of the procedure. Notice the extent of divide septum (~15 mm in length in mid-fundal region).

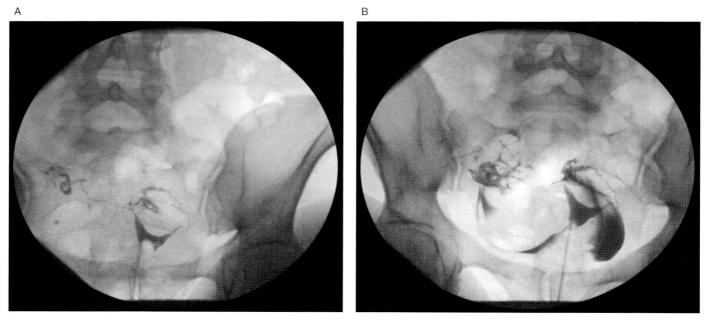

Fig. 8.5 (A) HSG film suggesting a significant arcuate uterus. (B) HSG film showing that as more dye is injected the fundal region appears almost normal.

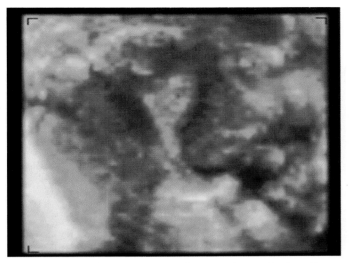

Fig. 8.6 Transvaginal 3D US picture revealing normal uterine fundus with no evidence of arcuate uterus and possible filling defect in the right corneal region, most probably representing an endometrial polyp.

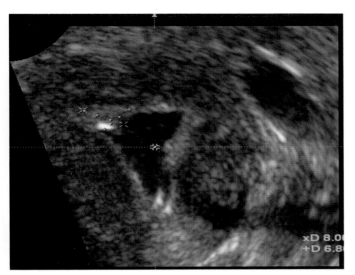

Fig. 8.7 Transvaginal SIH on 3D US picture revealing normal uterine fundus with no evidence of arcuate uterus and possible filling defect in the right corneal region, most probably representing an endometrial polyp.

A

B

C

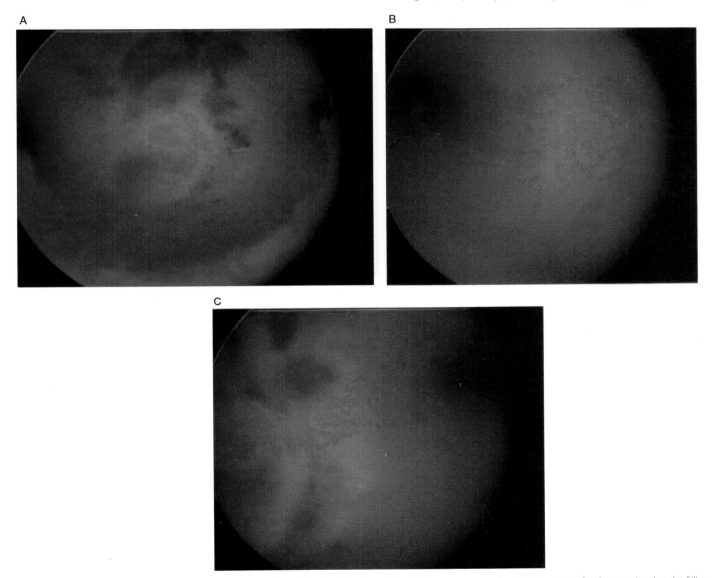

Fig. 8.8 Hysteroscopic pictures depicting (A) a panoramic view of the fundal region with a typical appearance of an arcuate uterine fundus – notice that the filling defect extends from one tubal ostium to the other and it has a wide base and rounded tip; (B) the right cornual region with tubal ostium and right portion of the arcuate fundus; and (C) the left cornual region with tubal ostium and the left portion of the arcuate fundus.

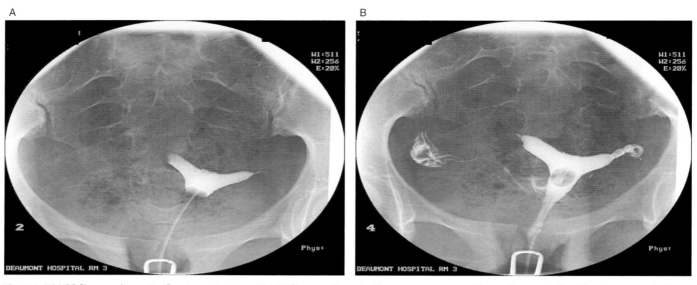

Fig. 8.9 (A) HSG film revealing a significant arcuate uterus. (B) HSG film revealing a significant arcuate uterus with no effect on the fundal region as a result of injecting more dye.

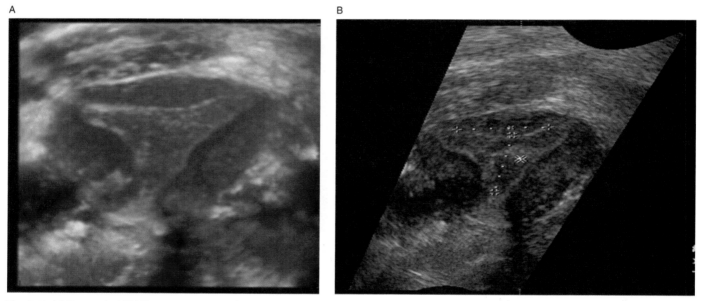

Fig. 8.10 (A) Transvaginal 3D US picture suggesting the presence of a very subtle arcuate uterus. (B) Transvaginal 3D US picture suggesting the presence of a very subtle arcuate uterus (mid-fundal length of 4.1 mm).

one failed IVF-ET cycle prior to her surgery. Following hysteroscopic division of the arcuate fundus, the patient conceived with intracytoplasmic sperm injection (ICSI)-ET and delivered a singleton at term.

Significant arcuate uterus: discrepancy between HSG and 3D US findings (Case 3)

A 28-year-old Asian female presented with primary infertility of 4 years' duration. In this patient, the HSG suggested a significant arcuate uterus versus incomplete bicornuate uterus (Fig. 8.9A and B), while transvaginal 3D US (Fig. 8.10A and B) suggested the presence of a very subtle arcuate uterus (mid-

fundal length of 4 mm). Transvaginal 2D US revealed slight endometrial separation in the fundal region in the transverse view. The findings on hysteroscopy confirmed the presence of a significant arcuate uterus (12 mm length in the mid-fundal region) (Fig. 8.11A–C). This case illustrates that the findings on transvaginal 3D US and SIH with 3D US can be misleading, even in the presence of a significant arcuate uterus. Two months after hysteroscopic division of a significant arcuate uterus, a postoperative SIH with 3D US was completely normal. One month later the patient underwent ICSI–ET for associated severe endometriosis and she conceived. The patient started with a twin pregnancy, which reduced spontaneously to a singleton. She delivered a singleton at term.

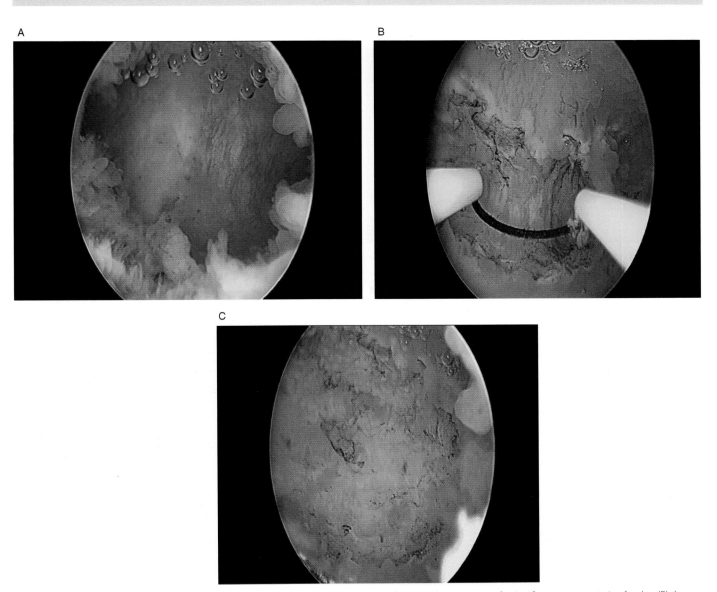

Fig. 8.11 Hysteroscopic pictures depicting (A) a panoramic view of the fundal region with a typical appearance of a significant arcuate uterine fundus; (B) the steps of septum division; and (C) the final appearance of the uterine fundus at the completion of the procedure. Notice the extent of divide septum (~12 mm in length in mid-fundal region).

Short incomplete uterine septum: normal uterine fundus on 3D US and SIH with 3D US (Case 4)

This is a 27-year-old white female who presented with primary infertility of 3 years' duration. In this patient, HSG suggested a subtle incomplete septum versus a subtle incomplete bicornuate uterus (Fig. 8.12A and B), while both transvaginal 3D US (Fig. 8.13) and SIS on 3D US were completely normal (Fig. 8.14). In addition, transvaginal 2D US with and without SIH was negative. The findings on hysteroscopy confirmed the presence of a short incomplete uterine septum (10 mm length in the mid-fundal region) (Fig. 8.15). This case illustrates that the findings on HSG and both transvaginal 3D US and SIH with 3D US can be misleading in the presence of a short incomplete

uterine septum. The patient underwent hysteroscopic division of the short uterine septum and conservative laparoscopic surgery for stage III endometriosis. She subsequently underwent IVF-ET, and she conceived and delivered a singleton at term.

Arcuate uterus: discrepancy between HSG and 3D US findings (Case 5)

A 30-year-old white female presented with primary infertility of one year's duration. In this patient, HSG film revealed an essentially normal appearance of the endometrial cavity (Fig. 8.16). Transvaginal 2D US with and without SIH were negative. Both transvaginal 3D US (Fig. 8.17) and SIH with 3D US (Fig. 8.18) suggested a slight arcuate uterus. The findings on hysteroscopy confirmed the presence of an arcuate uterus (Fig. 8.19A–C).

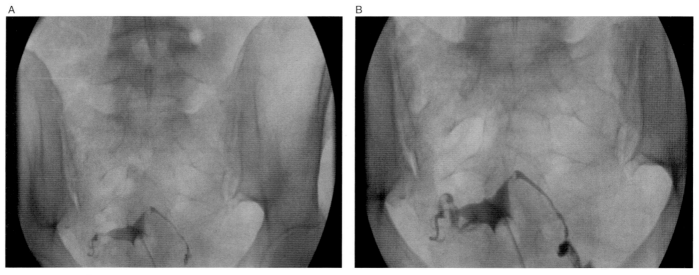

Fig. 8.12 (A) HSG film suggesting a subtle incomplete uterine septum. (B) HSG film showing that as more dye is injected the fundal region appears almost normal.

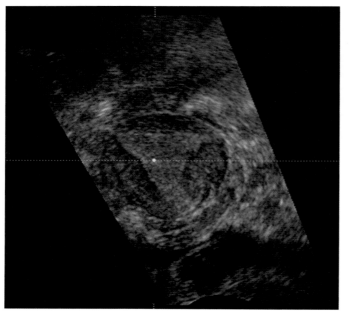

Fig. 8.13 Transvaginal 3D US picture showing a completely normal endometrial cavity.

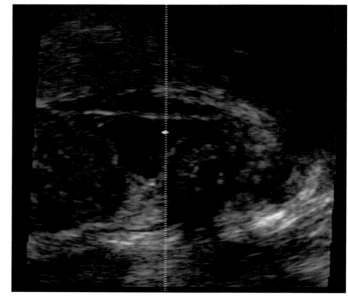

Fig. 8.14 Transvaginal SIH on 3D US picture showing a completely normal endometrial cavity.

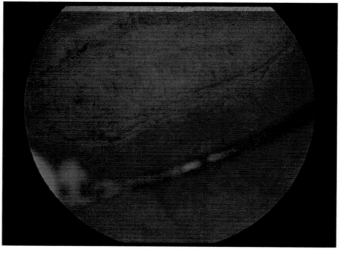

Fig. 8.15 Hysteroscopic picture showing the fundal region after dividing a short uterine septum (~10 mm length in the mid-fundal region).

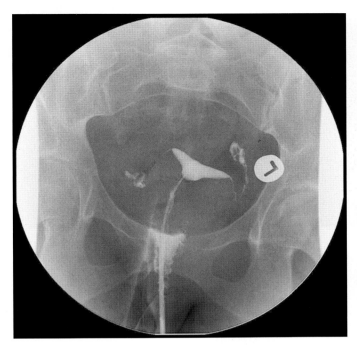

Fig. 8.16 HSG film revealing an essentially normal appearance of the endometrial cavity.

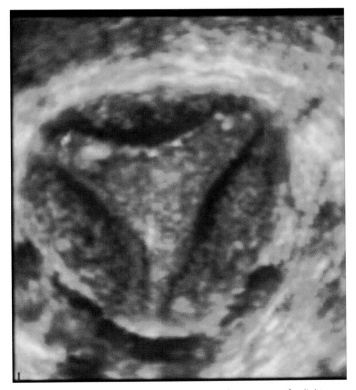

Fig. 8.17 Transvaginal 3D US picture suggesting the presence of a slight arcuate uterus.

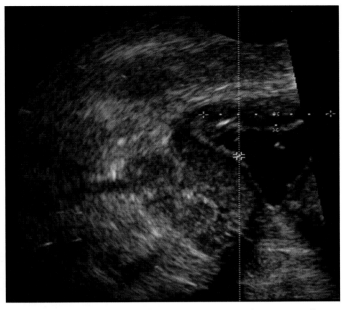

Fig. 8.18 Transvaginal SIH on 3D US picture suggesting the presence of a slight arcuate uterus (6.9 mm in length at the mid-fundal region).

This case illustrates that HSG and both transvaginal 3D US and SIH with 3D US can sometimes underestimate the extent of subtle uterine septum. In turn, the clinical significance of the presence of an arcuate uterus and its contribution to reproductive difficulty in this patient could have been overlooked if hysteroscopy had not been performed. The patient underwent IVF-ET treatment. Two blastocysts were transferred and she conceived with a triplet pregnancy, one embryo split resulting in a monochorionic diamniotic twins. She delivered by CS at 28 weeks of gestation. One of the identical twins died after 6 days and the other two babies survived and did well.

Significant arcuate uterus: discrepancy between HSG and 3D US findings (Case 6)

A 28-year-old white female presented with primary infertility of 2 years' duration. HSG suggested a normal endometrial cavity (Fig. 8.20), and transvaginal 2D US with and without SIH were negative. Both transvaginal 3D US (Fig. 8.21) and SIH with 3D US (Fig. 8.22) suggested the presence of a subtle arcuate uterus. This patient had a significant arcuate uterus on hysteroscopy (~14 mm in length at mid-fundal region) (Fig. 8.23A–C). The case illustrates that in the presence of normal findings on HSG, transvaginal 2D US with and without SIH, and what most clinicians and radiologists would accept as a variant of normal on transvaginal 3D US and SIH with 3D US, could be associated with a significant arcuate uterus. This patient delivered a singleton at term following ICSI–ET for associated male-factor infertility.

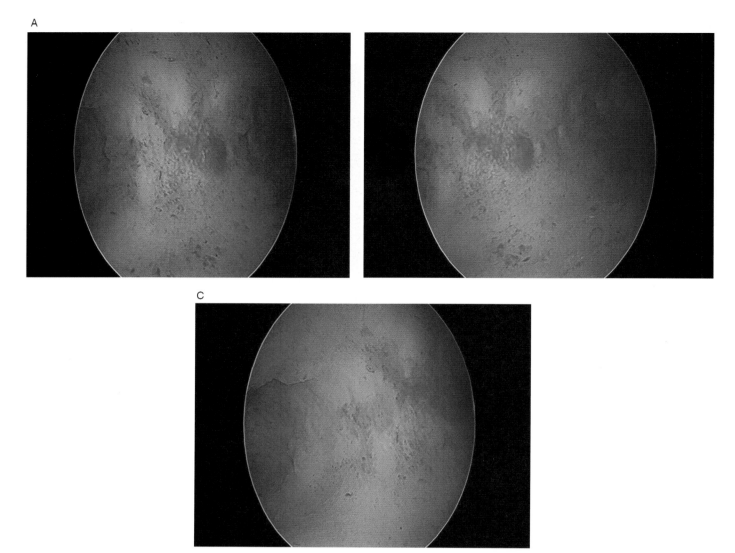

Fig. 8.19 Hysteroscopic pictures depicting (A) a panoramic view of the fundal region with a typical appearance of an arcuate uterine fundus; (B) the left cornual region with tubal ostium and the left portion of the arcuate fundus; and (C) the right cornual region with tubal ostium and the right portion of the arcuate fundus.

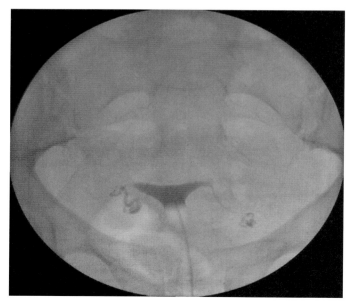

Fig. 8.20 HSG film revealing an essentially normal appearance of the endometrial cavity.

Significant arcuate uterus – unequal size of the cornual regions: discrepancy between HSG and 3D US findings (Case 7)

A 28-year-old Asian female presented with primary infertility of 2 years' duration. In this patient, an evaluation of HSG films suggested a normal endometrial cavity (Fig. 8.24) and transvaginal 2D US with and without SIH were negative. Transvaginal 3D US suggested a slight arcuate uterus (mid-fundal length of 5.1 mm) (Fig. 8.25), while transvaginal SIH with 3D US suggested a normal endometrial cavity (Fig. 8.26). The findings on hysteroscopy confirmed the presence of a significant arcuate uterus with unequal size of the cornual regions (right > left) (length is 12 mm in the mid-fundal region) (Fig. 8.27A–C). This case illustrates that the findings on HSG, transvaginal 2D US with and without SIH, and both transvaginal 3D US and SIH with 3D US can be misleading, even in the presence of a significant arcuate uterus. Following hysteroscopic division of the arcuate fundus, the patient conceived with ICSI–ET for associated stage II endometriosis and delivered a singleton at term.

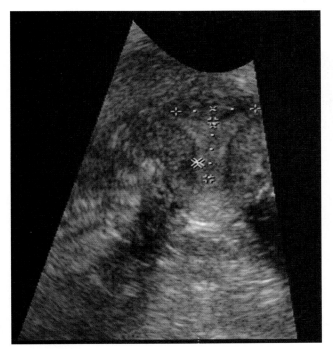

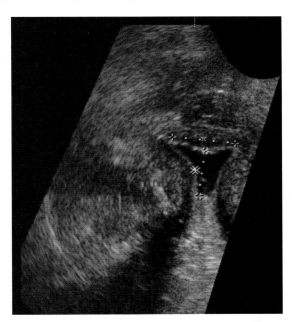

Fig. 8.22 Transvaginal SIH on 3D US picture suggesting the presence of a slight arcuate uterus (6.1 mm in length at the mid-fundal region).

Fig. 8.21 Transvaginal 3D US picture suggesting the presence of a slight arcuate uterus (6.4 mm in length at the mid-fundal region).

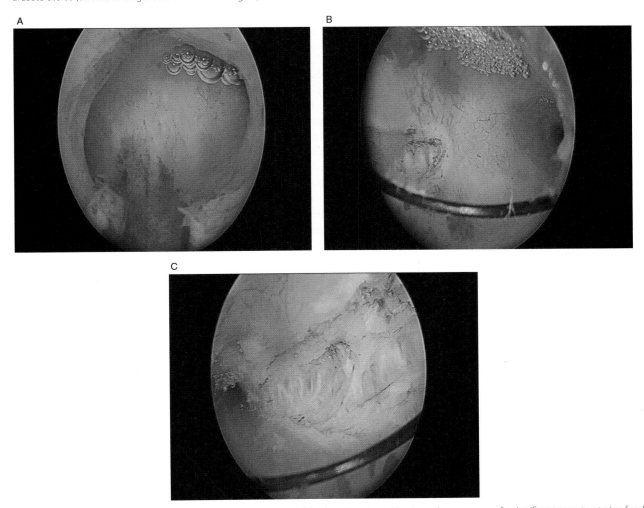

Fig. 8.23 Hysteroscopic pictures depicting (A) a panoramic view of the fundal region with a typical appearance of a significant arcuate uterine fundus; (B) the left cornual region with tubal ostium and the left portion of the arcuate fundus and a view of part the divided right portion of the septum; and (C) the fundal region after dividing an arcuate fundus (~10 mm length in the mid-fundal region).

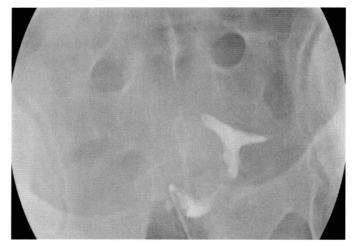

Fig. 8.24 HSG film reveals an essentially normal appearance of the endometrial cavity.

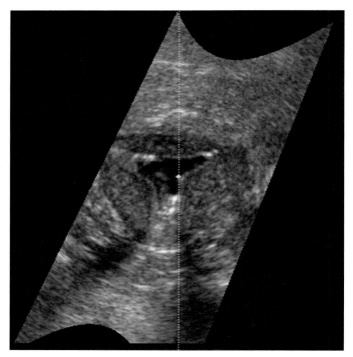

Fig. 8.26 Transvaginal SIH on 3D US picture suggesting normal endometrial cavity.

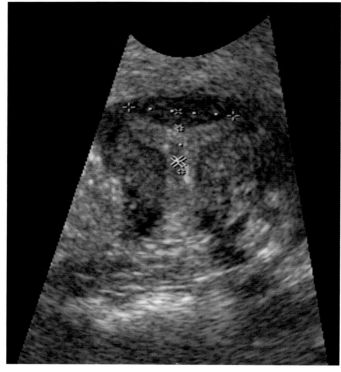

Fig. 8.25 Transvaginal 3D US picture suggesting a slight arcuate uterus (mid-fundal length of 5.1 mm).

Significant arcuate uterus: unequal size of the cornual regions (Case 8)

A 30-year-old white female presented with primary infertility of one year's duration. In this patient, transvaginal 2D US with and without SIH were normal; however, a slight arcuate uterus with unequal cornual regions (right more than left) was suggested on both HSG (Fig. 8.28A and B) and a transvaginal 3D US (Fig. 8.29). The findings on hysteroscopy confirmed

the above-mentioned findings (Fig. 8.30A–C). This case illustrates a rare type of arcuate uterus that was described previously by our group and others [6,7,15,16]. Most practitioners are not familiar with this type of arcuate uterus (which is rare) and therefore it is very unlikely to be diagnosed. We are hoping that this case will increase the awareness of practitioners regarding this rather rare type of arcuate uterus. Before this uterine anomaly was diagnosed, the patient conceived with twins after IVF-ET. Unfortunately, she lost them at 20 weeks gestation. Following hysteroscopic correction of the arcuate anomaly, the patient conceived with ICSI–ET and delivered twins at 34 weeks.

Discussion

Subtle uterine septum appears to be underdiagnosed. Therefore, the incidence of subtle uterine septum in patients presenting with reproductive failure may be much higher than previously reported. In the diagnosis of subtle congenital anomalies of the uterine cavity, the accuracy and sensitivity of HSG is poor (Cases 4–8). Transvaginal 2D US and 2D with SIH are poor diagnostic tools in screening for subtle uterine septum (Cases 2, 4–8). Transvaginal 3D US and 3D with SIH are excellent diagnostic tools in screening for subtle uterine septum. However, these imaging studies can still be misleading. They could be negative in some patients (Cases 2, 4). In other patients, the findings on transvaginal 3D US and 3D with SIH may underestimate the extent of the uterine anomalies (Cases 3, 5–8). This is especially the case if the uterus is retroverted, acutely anteflexed, or tilted in position (Cases 6, 7). Diagnostic hysteroscopy appears

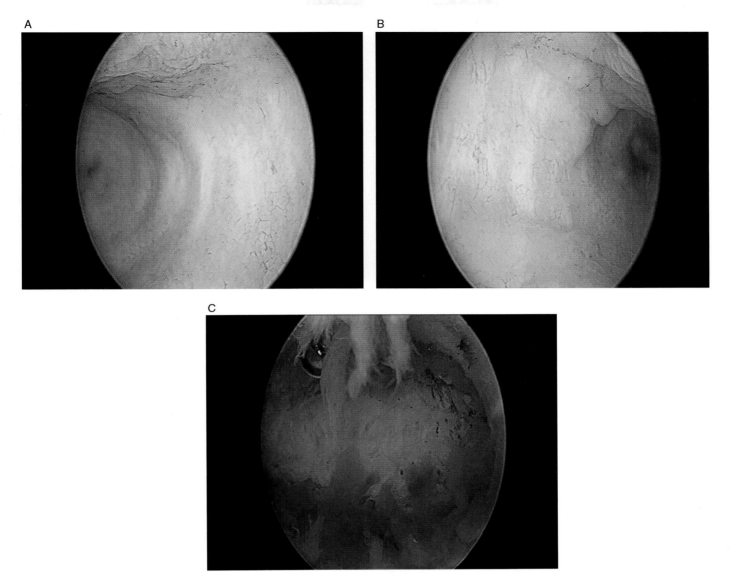

Fig. 8.27 Hysteroscopic pictures depicting a significant arcuate uterus with unequal size of the cornual regions (right > left) (length is 12 mm in the mid-fundal region). (A) The larger right cornual region and tubal ostium. (B) The smaller left cornual region and tubal ostium. (C) The fundal region after dividing an arcuate fundus (~12 mm length in the mid-fundal region).

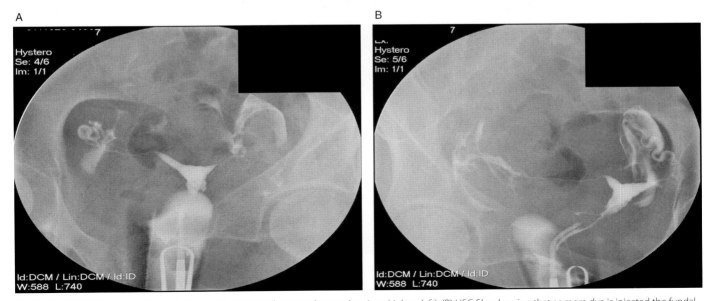

Fig. 8.28 (A) HSG film suggesting a slight arcuate uterus with unequal cornual regions (right > left). (B) HSG film showing that as more dye is injected the fundal region appears almost normal.

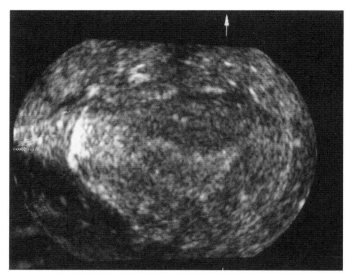

Fig. 8.29 Transvaginal 3D US picture revealing a slight arcuate uterus with unequal cornual regions (right > left).

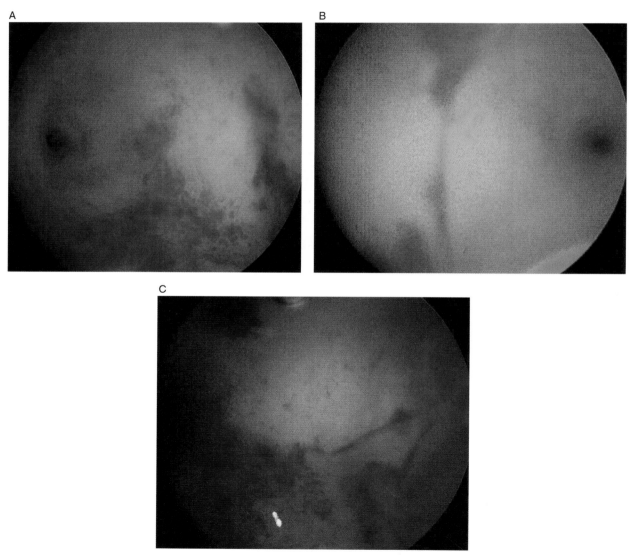

Fig. 8.30 Hysteroscopic pictures depicting a slight arcuate uterus with unequal size of the cornual regions (right > left) (length is ~10 mm in the mid-fundal region. (A) The larger right cornual region and tubal ostium. (B) The smaller left cornual region and tubal ostium. (C) A panoramic view of the fundal region showing a slight arcuate uterine fundus.

to be the gold standard for accurate diagnosis of subtle uterine septum. Diagnostic hysteroscopy should be performed by an experienced reproductive surgeon. Moreover, diagnostic hysteroscopy should be performed whenever there is a very subtle uterine septum on radiological studies, there is a discrepancy between various radiological studies, and when subtle uterine septum is suspected but not confirmed by imaging studies.

Conclusion

In the diagnosis of subtle congenital anomalies of the uterine cavity, the accuracy and sensitivity of HSG, transvaginal 2D US, and SIH with 2D US is poor. Although transvaginal 3D US and SIH with 3D US are the gold standard for imaging studies in the diagnosis of such anomalies, they can still be misleading. A negative imaging study is highly questionable in the presence of an abnormal uterine position. Diagnostic hysteroscopy by an experienced reproductive surgeon is the gold standard before ruling out subtle incomplete uterine septum or arcuate uterus in patients with unexplained infertility, unexplained repeated implantation failure after IVF-ET, unexplained RPL, and unexplained bad obstetric history.

References

1. Buttram VC, Gibbons WE. Muellerian anomalies: a proposed classification (an analysis of 144 cases). *Fertil Steril* 1979; **32**: 40–46.

2. Tomazevic T, Ban-Frangez H, Ribic-Pucelj M, et al. Small uterine septum is an important risk variable for preterm birth. *Eur J Obstet Gynecol Reprod Biol* 2007; **135**(2): 154–157.

3. Raga F, Bauset C, Remohi J, et al. Reproductive impact of congenital Müllerian anomalies. *Hum Reprod* 1997; **12**: 2277–2281.

4. Dicker D, Ashkenazi J, Dekel A, et al. The value of hysteroscopic evaluation in patients with preclinical in-vitro fertilization abortions. *Hum Reprod* 1996; **11**: 730–731.

5. Kupesic S. Clinical implications of sonographic detection of uterine anomalies for reproductive outcome. *US Obstet Gynecol* 2001; **18**: 387–400.

6. Mitwally MFM, Abuzeid M. Operative hysteroscopy for uterine septum. In: Rizk B, Garcia-Velasco JA, Sallam H, Makrigiannakis A. (Eds.) *Infertility and Assisted Reproduction*. Cambridge University Press; 2008: 115–131.

7. Mitwally MFM, Abuzeid M. Uterine septum. In: Rizk B (Ed.) *Ultrasonography in Reproductive Medicine and Infertility*. Cambridge University Press; 2010: 141–154.

8. Fayez JA, Mutie G, Schneider PJ. The diagnostic value of hysterosalpingography and hysteroscopy in infertility investigation. *Am J Obstet Gynecol* 1987; **156**: 558–560.

9. Kallia N, Abuzeid O, Ashraf M, Abuzeid M. Role of hysteroscopy in diagnosis of subtle uterine anomalies in patients with normal hysterosalpingography. *Fertil Steril* 2011; **96**(3; Suppl): S12.

10. Soares SR, Camargos AF, Barbosa do Reis MMB. Diagnostic accuracy of sonohysterography, transvaginal sonography, and hysterosalpingography in patients with uterine cavity diseases. *Fertil Steril* 2000; **73**: 406–411.

11. Filo GHA, Mattar R, Pires CR, et al. Comparison of hysterosalpingography, hysterosonography and hysteroscopy in evaluation of the uterine cavity in patients with recurrent pregnancy losses. *Arch Gynecol Obstet* 2006; **274**(5): 284–288.

12. Kiwi R. Recurrent pregnancy loss: evaluation and discussion of the causes and their management. *Cleveland Clinic J Med* 2006; **73**(10): 913–921.

13. Evers JLH. Female subfertility. *Lancet* 2002; **360**(9327): 151–159.

14. Templeton AA, Penney GC. The incidence, characteristics, and prognosis of patients whose infertility is unexplained. *Fertil Steril* 1982; **37**(2): 175–182.

15. Abuzeid OM, Sakhel K, Abuzeid MI. Diagnosis of various types of uterine septum in infertile patients. *J Min Inv Gynecol* 2005; **12**(5; Suppl): 117.

16. Hartman A. *Uterine Imaging – Malformations, Fibroids and Adenomyosis, Thirty-Ninth Annual Postgraduate Program, Course 17 Reproductive Imaging – How to Improve the Outcome of Assisted Reproductive Technology*, October 22, 2006, New Orleans, Louisiana, sponsored by ASRM; 2006.

Chapter 9

Transvaginal ultrasonography of uterine fibroids

Mostafa I. Abuzeid and Salem K. Joseph

Introduction

A uterine fibroid is a very common benign tumor of the uterus [1]. Submucous myomas are classified according to the European Society for Gynecological Endoscopy (ESGE) into three types: type 0 has no intramural extension, type I has less than 50% intramural extension, and type II has greater than 50% intramural extension [2]. A submucous fibroid is the only type that has been found to adversely affect reproductive function [3]. Some limited data suggests that an intramural fibroid may also have a negative impact on reproduction [4,5]. In addition, myomas may cause symptoms requiring treatment, such as menorrhagia, dysmenorrhea, dyspareunia, pelvic pain, and pressure symptoms [6,7]. Transabdominal and transvaginal two-dimensional (2D) ultrasonography (US) has played a significant role in the diagnosis of uterine fibroids for the past three decades. More recently, the introduction of saline infusion hysterosonogram (SIH) and 3D US has improved the diagnostic ability of US in determining the type, extent, and location of uterine fibroids [8].

The purpose of this chapter is to discuss a few challenging cases in which US helped not only in making the diagnosis, but also in selecting the appropriate treatment plan. The first two cases present the potential problem of missing the diagnosis of an associated subtle uterine septum (Case 1) or arcuate uterus (Case 2) in the presence of uterine fibroid. Case 3 presents the challenge of determining the best treatment choice for a patient with a large submucous, intramural, subserous fibroid who wishes to preserve her reproductive potential. In Case 4, we discuss a rare complication of myomectomy of a cervical fibroid and its management with a minimally invasive technique. The value of transvaginal US in establishing the diagnosis and follow-up during treatment is illustrated. Cases 5 and 6 present the challenge of managing large, broad ligament fibroids in patients who wish to preserve their reproductive potential. In these two latter cases, transvaginal US played a major role in the choice of the appropriate surgical procedure.

Coexisting fundal submucous fibroid and incomplete uterine septum in a patient presenting with recurrent pregnancy loss (Case 1)

A 30-year-old white female presented with recurrent pregnancy loss (RPL) secondary to concurrent uterine factors. The couple's workup for RPL was normal, except for a fundal type II submucosal fibroid on transvaginal 3D US with SIH (Fig. 9.1). Laparoscopic myomectomy and repair of the myometrial defect was performed (Figs 9.2–9.4). At the conclusion of the procedure, a diagnostic hysteroscopy suggested a possible concurrent, incomplete short uterine septum, which could not be corrected for fear of cutting the myomectomy sutures (Fig. 9.5). The patient did not come for follow-up, which led her to have three more miscarriages and one chemical pregnancy. The presence of a short uterine septum was confirmed on SIH with 3D US. The patient underwent hysteroscopic division of a short uterine septum. Postoperative SIH showed normal uterine cavity. The patient conceived twins through IVF-ET treatment and delivered at 36 weeks gestation.

The aim of presenting this case is to bring attention to the unique diagnostic and surgical dilemma of dealing with coexisting fundal submucous uterine leiomyoma and incomplete uterine septum in a patient with RPL. The real challenge in this case was to suspect a concurrent uterine pathology based on the hysteroscopic findings at the conclusion of laparoscopic myomectomy. Surgical management of such coexisting uterine pathology cannot be performed in a single session.

Coexisting multiple uterine fibroids and arcuate uterus in an infertile patient (Case 2)

The patient was a 34-year-old white female who presented with secondary infertility of 4 years' duration with a history of one early miscarriage 5 years previously. Infertility problems included moderate male factor, right distal tubal blockage,

Ultrasonography in Gynecology, ed. Botros R. M. B. Rizk and Elizabeth E. Puscheck. Published by Cambridge University Press.

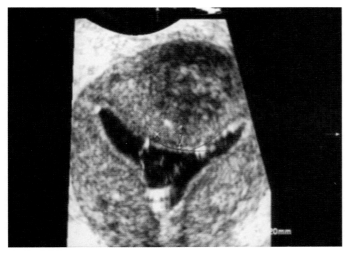

Fig. 9.1 Transvaginal 3D US with SIH showing a 3 × 2 cm submucosal-intramural-subserosal fundal fibroid (type II submucosal fibroid).

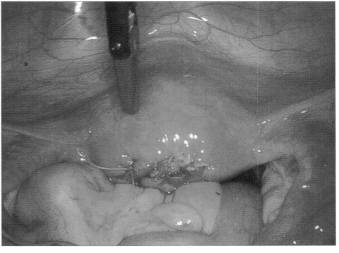

Fig. 9.4 Laparoscopic picture showing myometrial defect sutured in two layers.

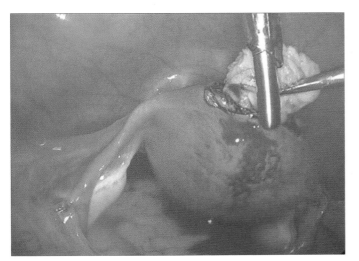

Fig. 9.2 Laparoscopic picture showing dissection of fundal uterine fibroid.

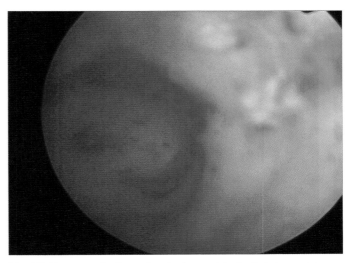

Fig. 9.5 Hysteroscopic picture showing incomplete short uterine septum.

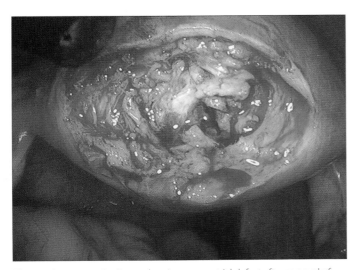

Fig. 9.3 Laparoscopic picture showing myometrial defect after removal of fundal uterine fibroid.

and multiple small intramural and subserous uterine fibroids. Her menstrual cycles were regular and ovulation was documented. In this patient, HSG suggested a normal endometrial cavity and right partial distal tubal occlusion (Fig. 9.6). The patient was treated with five cycles of Clomid and one cycle of in vitro fertilization and embryo transfer (IVF-ET) at another unit without any success. She was then referred to our unit for further management. Transvaginal 2D US revealed multiple intramural and subserous fibroids (Fig. 9.7), the largest of which measured 25 mm in diameter. Transvaginal 3D US with and without SIH suggested a subtle arcuate fundus with mid-fundal length of 6.8 mm (Figs 9.8, 9.9). Operative laparoscopy was performed during which right fimbrioplasty, coagulation of endometriosis using an argon beam coagulator, laparoscopic myomectomy, and mini-laparotomy for repair of the myometrial defect were performed (Figs 9.10–9.12). The findings on hysteroscopy confirmed the presence of a significant arcuate uterus (12 mm length in the mid-fundal region) (Fig. 9.13).

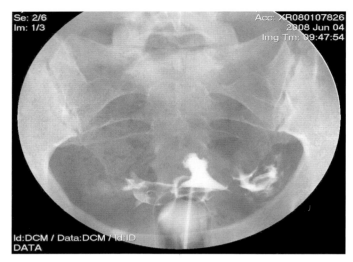

Fig. 9.6 HSG film revealing an essentially normal appearance of the endometrial cavity. The uterus is acutely anteflexed in position.

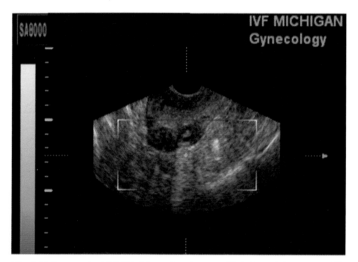

Fig. 9.7 Transvaginal 2D US picture showing a sagittal view of the uterus with two subserous uterine fibroids.

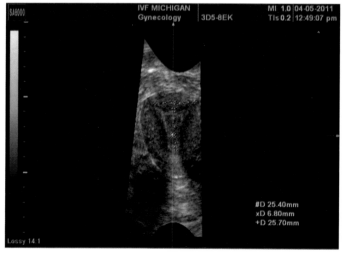

Fig. 9.8 Transvaginal 3D US picture suggesting the presence of a slight arcuate uterus (6.8 mm in length at the mid-fundal region).

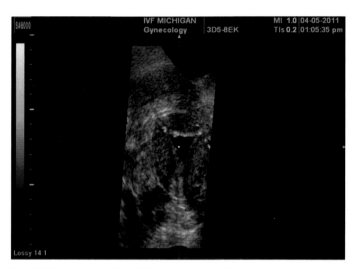

Fig. 9.9 Transvaginal SIH on 3D US picture suggesting the presence of a slight arcuate uterus.

Therefore, hysteroscopic metroplasty for the arcuate uterus was performed. The patient conceived on her own 3 months later and she delivered a singleton at term.

The aim of presenting this case is to demonstrate the value of transvaginal 3D US with and without SIH in detecting a subtle arcuate uterus in the presence of multiple uterine fibroids in a patient with a long history of infertility. Laparoscopy helped in determining that hysteroscopic metroplasty of the arcuate uterus could be done at the same time as myomectomy in a single session.

Management of a large type II submucous fibroid by minimally invasive procedure (Case 3)

The patient was a 36-year-old woman who presented with primary infertility of 2 years' duration. Her associated complaints were menorrhagia and a known uterine fibroid. She had undergone hysteroscopic myomectomy in the past without any improvement. HSG revealed that the uterine cavity was occupied by a single, large submucosal fibroid (Fig. 9.14). Transvaginal 2D US and SIH showed a large anterior type II submucous, intramural, subserous fibroid (Fig. 9.15). Diagnostic hysteroscopy and laparoscopy revealed a type II submucous fibroid occupying the entire anterior wall of the uterus. Laparoscopic myomectomy was performed and a fibroid measuring 8 cm was dissected (Fig. 9.16). During this procedure, the endometrial cavity was entered (Fig. 9.17) and mini-laparotomy through a transverse incision (5 cm in length) was performed to repair the endometrial cavity and overlying myometrium adequately and to remove the myoma (Fig. 9.18). Postoperative course was uneventful. Six weeks later, SIH revealed a uniform endometrial cavity with no filling defects or synechiae. Five months later, the patient conceived spontaneously. Unfortunately, the pregnancy was terminated at 20 weeks gestation because of trisomy 18.

The purpose of presenting this case is to describe a patient with a single, large type II submucous fibroid distorting and

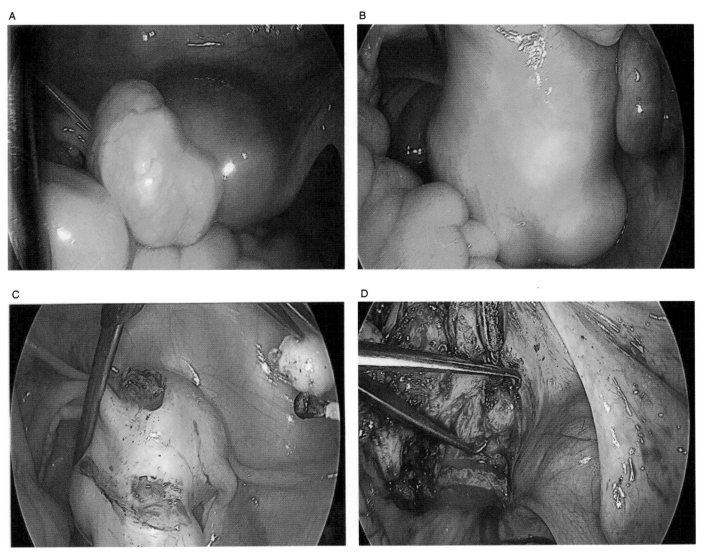

Fig. 9.10 Laparoscopic pictures showing (A) a pedunculated subserous fibroid in the fundal region; (B) a large pedunculated subserous fibroid in the posterior wall of the uterus; (C) the uterus after removal of the fundal and the posterior wall fibroids; and (D) laparoscopic dissection and removal of other posterior wall intramural fibroids.

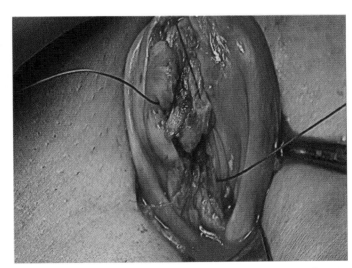

Fig. 9.11 Repair of the large myometrial defect in the posterior wall of the uterus via a mini-laparotomy.

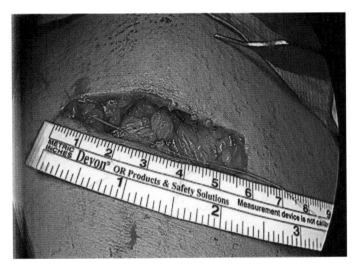

Fig. 9.12 A 5 cm transverse suprapubic mini-laparotomy incision through which the repair of the large myometrial defect in the posterior wall of the uterus was performed.

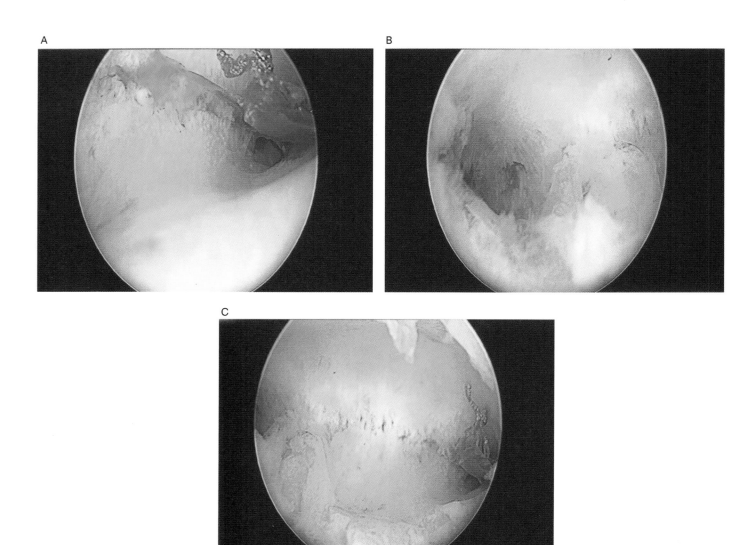

Fig. 9.13 Hysteroscopic pictures depicting (A) the left cornual region with tubal ostium and the left portion of the arcuate fundus; (B) the right cornual region with tubal ostium and the right portion of the arcuate fundus; and (C) a panoramic view of the fundal region with a typical appearance of a significant arcuate uterine fundus.

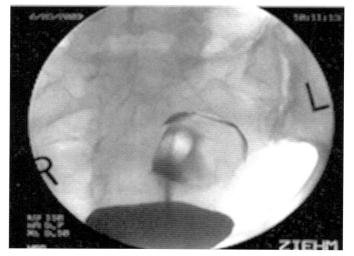

Fig. 9.14 HSG film showing the uterine cavity to be occupied and compromised by a large filling defect with smooth surface, most probably representing a submucous myoma.

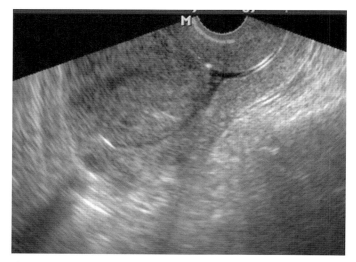

Fig. 9.15 Transvaginal 2D ultrasound with SIH picture showing an 8 cm anterior-fundal submucous intramural fibroid reaching and stretching the serosal layer (type II submucous fibroid).

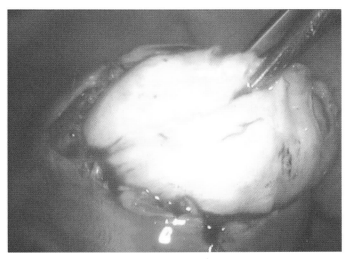

Fig. 9.16 Laparoscopic picture depicting the dissection of the myoma.

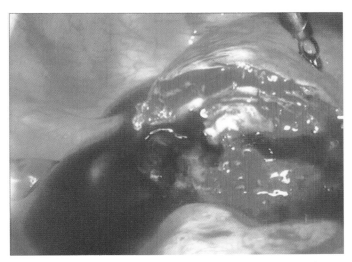

Fig. 9.17 Laparoscopic picture depicting the myoma bed; notice that the endometrial cavity was entered in a small area (about 1 cm) and a moderate amount of bleeding from the myometrium was observed.

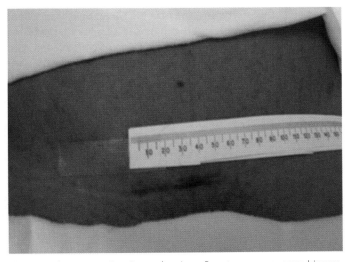

Fig. 9.18 A postoperative picture showing a 5 cm transverse suprapubic scar of mini-laparotomy.

occupying the entire endometrial cavity that was managed successfully with a minimally invasive approach. Laparoscopic myomectomy with mini-laparotomy is a safe and cost-effective minimally invasive approach for treatment of patients with a large type II submucous fibroid who want to preserve their reproductive potential. This procedure can be performed successfully by a gynecologist with adequate laparoscopic training, but limited laparoscopic suturing abilities. It also avoids the need for traditional laparotomy, in most cases of uterine fibroids without the expense associated with robotic assisted laparoscopic myomectomy.

Myometrial abscess: a complication of myomectomy of a large cervical myoma (Case 4)

A 39-year-old African American female gravida 3, para 1, with a history of two early miscarriages, presented with menorrhagia and recurrence of multiple fibroids. She had undergone laparotomy and myomectomy 9 years earlier. Transvaginal 2D US revealed an enlarged uterus with at least six uterine fibroids, the largest being 9 cm in diameter (Figs 9.19, 9.20). An attempt at robotic assisted laparoscopic myomectomy was abandoned as the largest fibroid was found to be arising from the lower uterine segment and because of the multiple fibroids. Laparotomy and myomectomy were performed.

The postoperative course was complicated by a drop in hemoglobin of 2 g/dL, requiring transfusion of 2 units of pre-donated blood from the patient. In addition, the patient had an element of paralytic ileus, which resolved by supportive measures in 2 days and, therefore, the patient was discharged home. Four weeks later, the patient presented with a complaint of pelvic pain, nausea, vomiting, constipation, and fever of one day's duration. On examination, her temperature was 102°F, pulse was 120/minute, blood pressure was 120/78, and respiration was 16/minute. Examination of the abdomen revealed left lower quadrant tenderness, rebound tenderness, and guarding, but no rigidity. Transvaginal 2D US revealed a slightly enlarged uterus due to possibly infected hematoma in the posterior wall of the lower uterine segment measuring 42–52 mm in diameter. The possible infected hematoma was located where the largest fibroid was removed (Fig. 9.21). The patient was admitted to hospital and she was started on intravenous antibiotics (Cefotetan and clindamycin) after a blood culture was obtained. The diagnosis of myometrial abscess was confirmed by CT scan of the abdomen and pelvis with and without contrast. No other pathology was detected. One day later, the patient underwent CT scan-guided placement of a pigtail catheter in the center of the myometrial abscess for continuous drainage (Fig. 9.22A and B) by an interventional radiologist.

The patient continued to have spiking of temperature for 2 days. The blood culture was negative. The result of the culture of the pus obtained from the abscess revealed Gram-negative rods, Gram-positive cocci, and *Staphylococcus aureus*. A consult was made for an infectious disease specialist to assist in the management. The infectious disease specialist added

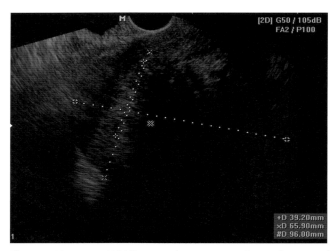

Fig. 9.19 Transvaginal 2D US picture showing a sagittal view of uterus with a large fibroid (96 × 66 cm) occupying the lower uterine segment and upper part of the cervical canal.

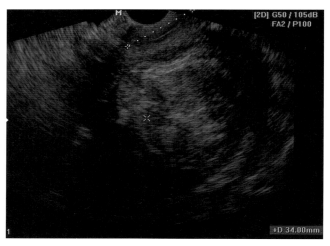

Fig. 9.20 Transvaginal 2D US picture showing a sagittal view of uterus with a part of the fibroid occupying the lower uterine segment and upper part of the cervical canal.

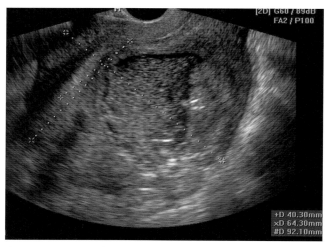

Fig. 9.21 Transvaginal 2D US picture showing a sagittal view of uterus with a well-circumscribed area of hyperechogenicity (5 cm in diameter) occupying the lower uterine segment and upper part of the cervical canal, most probably representing an infected hematoma in the myometrium (myometrial abscess).

gentamicin and replaced clindamycin with Flagyl as the patient experienced diarrhea. The patient received 2 units of packed red blood cells for low hemoglobin (8.0 g/dL). Her temperature came down and remained normal thereafter. The size of the myometrial abscess decreased with time (Fig. 9.22C and D). The pigtail catheter continued to drain more than 30 mL of fluid, therefore the decision was made to discharge the patient home with the pigtail catheter in place. She was discharged home 8 days after hospital admission with a PICC line in place to continue intravenous antibiotics (cefepime hydrochloride 1 g every 12 hours) and Flagyl orally 500 mg three times a day for an additional 14 days. Arrangements were made with Home Care to help with her care. The pigtail catheter was removed once there was no drainage 2 weeks after its initial insertion (Fig. 9.23). The PICC line was removed after she completed the antibiotic course. Two months after her discharge, a transvaginal US was essentially normal (Fig. 9.24).

The purpose of presenting this case is to illustrate the value of transvaginal US in the diagnosis of myometrial abscess, a very rare late complication of myomectomy. We believe that the best way to avoid this complication is to ensure complete obliteration of the dead space in the myometrial bed and to secure complete homeostasis after myomectomy. We also discussed a minimally invasive technique for management of myometrial abscess and the role of transvaginal US during follow-up.

A huge broad ligament uterine fibroid: successful myomectomy to preserve reproductive potential via laparotomy (Case 5)

A 31-year-old nulliparous Asian female, married for 2 years, was evaluated for infertility and a large abdominal mass, which was found to be rapidly growing for 3 months. Transvaginal 2D US suggested a large broad ligament fibroid on the right side, pushing the uterus to the left side and occupying most of the pelvic cavity (Fig. 9.25A–C). The diagnosis was also confirmed on transvaginal SIH on 2D US with and without Doppler flow study (Fig. 9.26A and B). There was an increase in the vascularity between the uterus and the fibroid. The patient underwent diagnostic laparoscopy and the diagnosis of a very large broad ligament fibroid was confirmed (Fig. 9.27). We proceeded with exploratory laparotomy after ureteric stents were placed bilaterally. Intraoperatively the mass was noticed to be in the right broad ligament, measuring approximately 20 cm in length. Myomectomy was performed with preservation of the uterus. The procedure was complicated by intraoperative bleeding, resulting from injury to the uterine vein, which was controlled by two figure-of-8 sutures. Diagnostic hysteroscopy, performed at the end of the procedure, revealed a normal endometrial cavity (Fig. 9.28). The pathology report confirmed the diagnosis of a uterine fibroid weighing 2191.4 g and measuring 19 × 19.5 cm with no evidence of malignancy. The patient had an uneventful recovery. Transvaginal 2D US 3 months postoperatively was essentially normal (Fig. 9.29). Two years later, the patient conceived spontaneously and delivered a singleton at term.

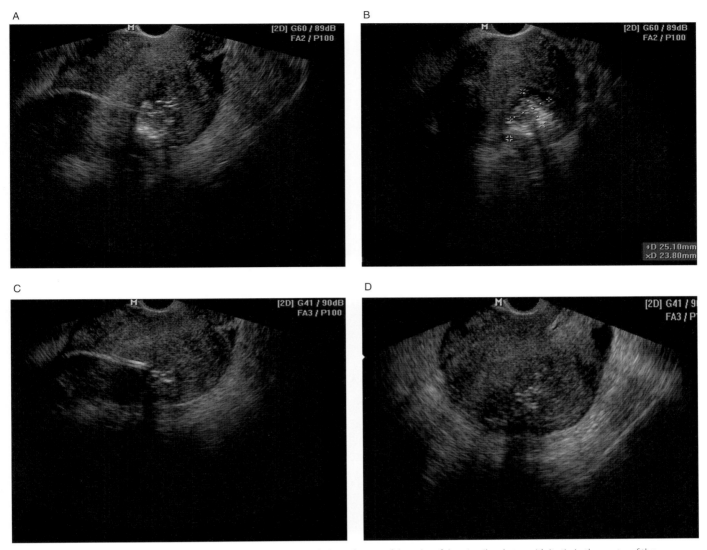

Fig. 9.22 Transvaginal 2D US: sagittal view of uterus showing (A) the radiologic feature of the tube of the pigtail catheter with its tip in the center of the myometrial abscess 7 days after its insertion; (B) the marked reduction in the size of the myometrial abscess (2.4–2.5 cm) 7 days after the insertion of the pigtail catheter; (C) the radiologic feature of the tube of the pigtail catheter with its tip in the center of the myometrial abscess 14 days after its insertion; and (D) the marked reduction in the size of the myometrial abscess 14 days after the insertion of the pigtail catheter.

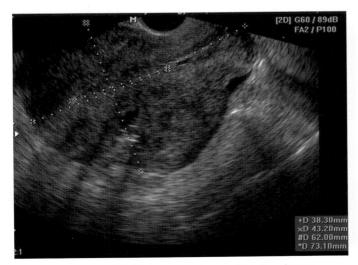

Fig. 9.23 Transvaginal 2D US picture showing a sagittal view of uterus revealing the uterine dimensions and disappearance of the myometrial abscess 10 days after the removal of the pigtail catheter.

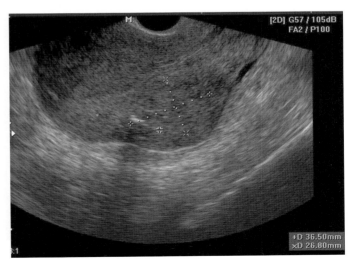

Fig. 9.24 Transvaginal 2D US picture showing a sagittal view of uterus 60 days after the removal of the pigtail catheter.

87

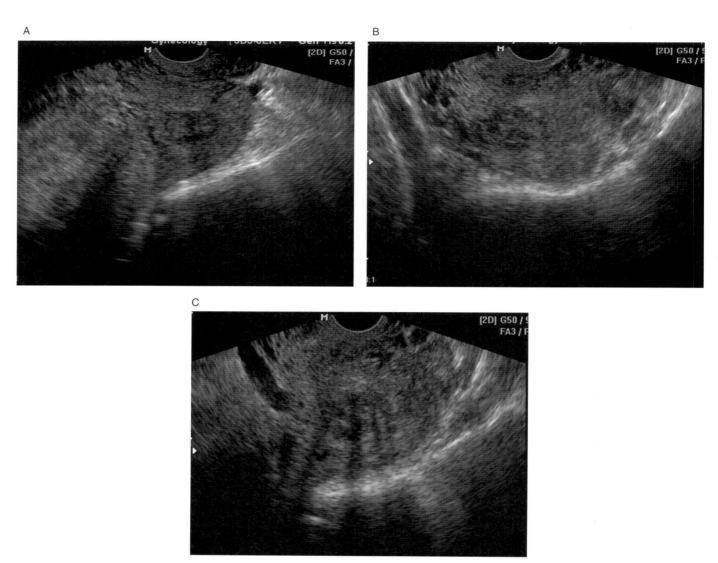

Fig. 9.25 Transvaginal 2D US pictures showing: (A) a transverse view of uterus pushed to the left by a large broad ligament fibroid (only a part of the fibroid is seen in this picture); (B) a transverse view of a large uterine fibroid that appears to occupy the whole pelvic cavity; (C) a transverse view of a large uterine fibroid that appears to occupy the whole pelvic cavity with a large blood vessel seen between the fibroid and pelvic sidewall.

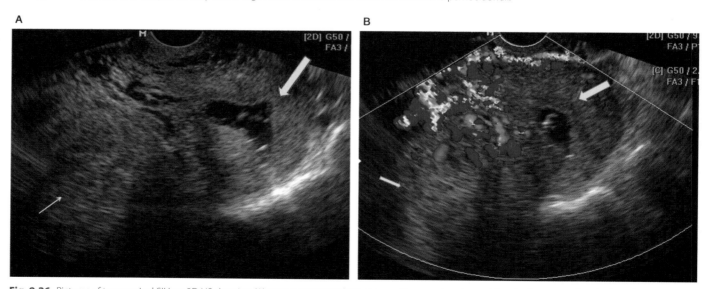

Fig. 9.26 Pictures of transvaginal SIH on 2D US showing (A) transverse view of the uterus with normal endometrial cavity (large arrow) and a large broad ligament fibroid (small arrow). Notice the marked increase in vascularity between the uterus and the fibroid; (B) transverse view of the uterus with Doppler flow study showing a normal endometrial cavity (large arrow) and a large broad ligament fibroid (small arrow). Notice the marked increase in vascularity between the uterus and the fibroid.

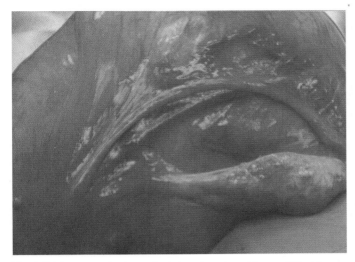

Fig. 9.27 Laparoscopic picture depicting a large broad ligament fibroid pushing the uterus to the left. Notice that the right fallopian tube is stretched over the large fibroid.

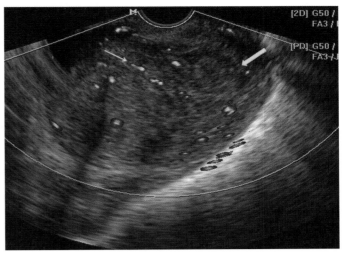

Fig. 9.30 Transvaginal 2D US with Doppler flow study showing transverse view of the uterus (thick arrow) and a large broad ligament fibroid (thin arrow). Notice that there is minimum vascularity between the uterus and the fibroid.

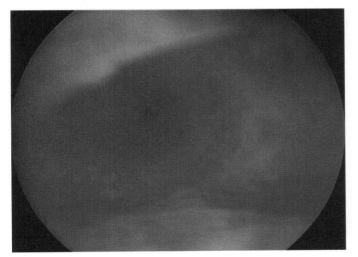

Fig. 9.28 Hysteroscopic picture showing a normal endometrial cavity.

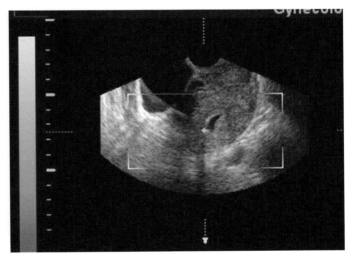

Fig. 9.31 Picture of a transvaginal SIH on 2D US showing a sagittal view of the uterus with normal endometrial cavity.

The aim of presenting this case is to demonstrate that in infertile patients with a huge broad ligament fibroid, myomectomy and preservation of the uterus is possible. However, preoperative planning and surgical expertise are mandatory to achieve this goal. Transvaginal US plays an important role in determining the extent of attachment and vascularity between the uterus and the broad ligament fibroid. Such findings may help in the choice of surgical procedure.

A large broad ligament uterine fibroid: successful myomectomy with robotic assisted laparoscopic myomectomy (Case 6)

A 40-year-old nulliparous white female presented with dysmenorrhea, menorrhagia, and an abdominal mass. Transvaginal 2D US revealed an enlarged uterus 9.6 × 6.1 × 7.9 cm in dimension.

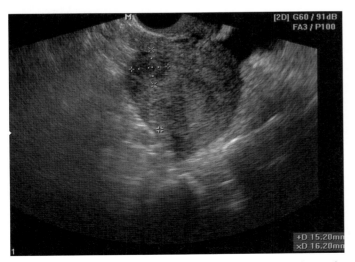

Fig. 9.29 Transvaginal 2D US picture showing postoperative sagittal view of the uterus, which appears normal.

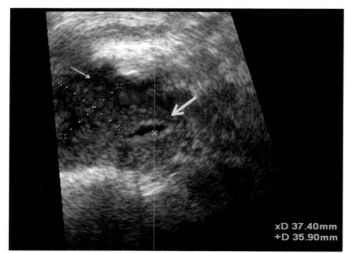

Fig. 9.32 Picture of a transvaginal 2D US with SIH showing a transverse view of the uterus with normal endometrial cavity (thick arrow) and part of a large broad ligament fibroid (thin arrow).

xD 37.40mm
+D 35.90mm

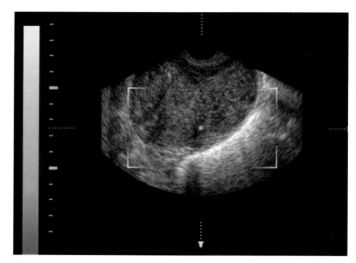

Fig. 9.33 Transvaginal 3D US picture of a large broad ligament fibroid.

A

B

C

D

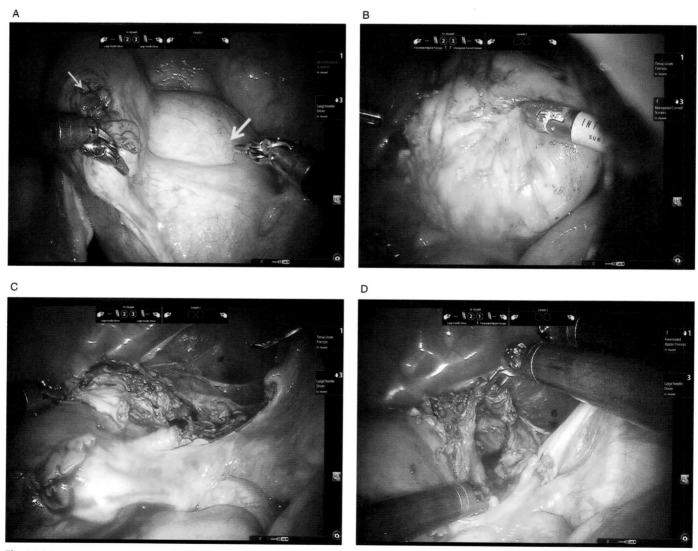

Fig. 9.34 Laparoscopic pictures using Da Vinci laparoscope and camera showing (A) a large broad ligament fibroid pushing the uterus to the left (large arrow). An area where a 5 cm fibroid was dissected and removed from the fundal region of the uterus is seen (small arrow); (B) the fibroid being dissected from the broad ligament; (C) a gap in the broad ligament after removal of the fibroid; (D) careful inspection of the gap in the broad ligament to insure homeostasis; (E) the posterior leaf of the broad ligament is seen intact; (F) the anterior leaf of the broad ligament is repaired; and (G) an apparently normal uterus and pelvic anatomy at the conclusion of the procedure.

E

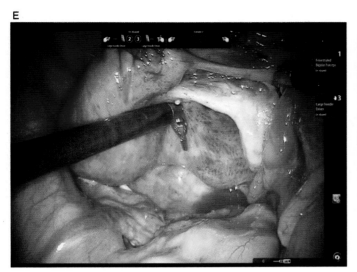

F

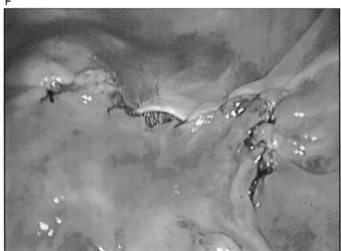

G

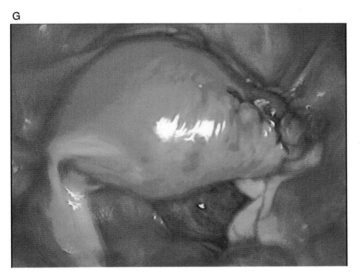

Fig. 9.34 (*cont.*)

Two uterine fibroids, intramural subserous in nature, were seen on transvaginal 2D US measuring 7.1 × 6.2 cm and 3.6 × 4.2 cm in diameter. A transvaginal US with Doppler flow study suggested that the larger fibroid was broad ligament in nature and that there was minimal vascularity in the area of attachment between the broad ligament fibroid and the uterus (Fig. 9.30). Transvaginal 2D US with SIH showed that the endometrial cavity was not affected (Fig. 9.31) and suggested a large broad ligament fibroid (Fig. 9.32). Transvaginal 3D US confirmed the presence of a large broad ligament fibroid (Fig. 9.33). The patient underwent robotic assisted laparoscopic myomectomy. First, a 4 cm intramural subserous fibroid was removed, then a large broad ligament fibroid (10 cm in diameter) was dissected from the uterus and the anterior leaf of the broad ligament was sutured (Fig. 9.34A–G). Care was taken to avoid injury to the right ureter and uterine vessels. Blood loss during the procedure was minimal. The fibroids were morcellated and removed from the peritoneal cavity. Diagnostic hysteroscopy, performed at the end of the procedure, revealed a normal endometrial cavity (Fig. 9.35). The pathology report confirmed the diagnosis of a uterine fibroid weighing 300 g and measuring 13 × 10 cm (aggregate of morcellated leiomyoma tissue). The postoperative course was uneventful and the patient was discharged home the next day. Three months later, an HSG was performed and it revealed a normal endometrial cavity and possible bilateral cornual blockage. Alternatively, the possibility of bilateral cornual spasm should be considered (Fig. 9.36). It is also possible that the reason for failure of filling of the fallopian tubes was leakage of radiopaque material in the cervical canal and upper vagina due to the anteverted position of the uterus.

The aim of presenting this case is to demonstrate that in infertile patients with a large broad ligament fibroid, who want to preserve their reproductive potential, robotic assisted laparoscopic myomectomy and preservation of the uterus is possible. However, preoperative planning and surgical expertise are mandatory to achieve this goal. Transvaginal US may play

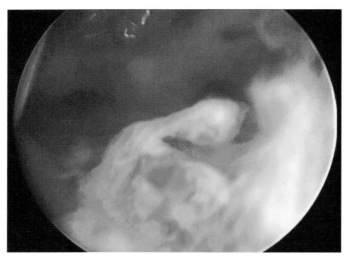

Fig. 9.35 A hysteroscopic picture revealing a normal endometrial cavity at the conclusion of the procedure.

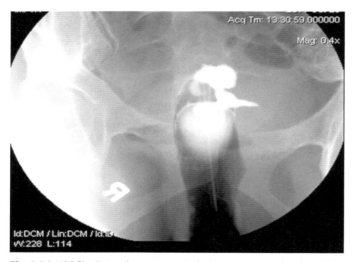

Fig. 9.36 HSG film 3 months postoperatively showing a normal endometrial cavity. The fallopian tubes did not fully visualize, most likely due to leakage of radio-opaque material in the cervical canal and upper vagina due to the anteverted position of the uterus.

an important role in determining the degree of attachment and vascularity between the uterus and the broad ligament fibroid, which helps in the choice of surgical procedure and technique.

Discussion

Removal of submucosal and intramural fibroids distorting the endometrial cavity has been shown to improve the fertility outcome [3,9]. Hysteroscopic division of a uterine septum has been shown to be safe and effective in improving reproductive outcome in patients with RPL [10,11]. The coexistence of a uterine septum and uterine fibroids in patients during their reproductive years (as in Cases 1 and 2) may present certain challenges. Coexistence of a submucous fibroid in the fundal region of the uterus and incomplete uterine septum (as in Case 1) is indeed not only a diagnostic but also a surgical challenge [12]. Removal of only the fibroid can still result in RPL.

Surgical management of such coexisting uterine pathology cannot be performed in a single session. We believe that the ideal approach to this challenge should take place in two separate sessions. First, myomectomy should be performed. Then hysteroscopic metroplasty to correct the incomplete uterine septum can be performed after at least 3–4 months to allow for myometrial healing [12]. Transvaginal 2D US is very helpful in detecting uterine fibroids, and 3D US with and without SIH can be helpful in detecting any associated endometrial cavity abnormality (as in Case 2). Hysteroscopic metroplasty for a uterine septum or arcuate uterus can be safely performed at the same session as long as submucosal and/or intramural fibroids are not present in the fundal region.

Although transvaginal 2D and 3D US with and without SIH are of great help in determining the treatment plan, the final judgment should be based on the findings on laparoscopy and hysteroscopy [13]. Transvaginal 2D US and 3D US with SIH are the gold standard for determining the type of submucous fibroid according to ESGE [2]. Lasmar et al. introduced a new classification of submucous fibroid in 2005. In this classification, four criteria were considered: (a) the penetration of the nodule into the myometrium, (b) the extension of the base of the nodule with respect to the wall of the uterus, (c) the size of the nodule, and (d) the topography of the nodule [14]. They believe that the new classification provides more clues than the standard ESGE classification about the difficulties of a hysteroscopic myomectomy.

More recently Lasmar et al. renamed the new classification as STEPW [15]. In a multicentric study, they correlated the ESGE and STEPW classifications with complete and incomplete hysteroscopic removal of a submucosal fibroid and concluded that STEPW permits greater correlation [15]. In Case 4, a large type II submucous fibroid (ESGE classification) was found. It was 8 cm in diameter, involving the entire myometrium and reaching and stretching the serosal layer. We believe that the option of hysteroscopic myomectomy is inapplicable to such a case. In fact, in our patient hysteroscopic myomectomy was tried once at another hospital without any significant reduction in the size of the tumor. The fibroid scored an 8 (STEPW classification), and according to this classification, Lasmar et al. recommended an alternative non-hysteroscopic technique [15]. Also in Case 1, the fundal submucous fibroid scored 7 using the STEPW classification, a value at which Lasmar et al. recommended an alternative non-hysteroscopic technique [15]. Traditionally, a large type II submucous fibroid has been dealt with via laparotomy and myomectomy. Robotic assisted laparoscopic myomectomy can now be used successfully to treat such cases [16]. However, the da Vinci robot is not available in many countries and the cost associated with the procedure can be prohibitive. In addition, the introduction of the bidirectional barbed suture may allow experienced endoscopic surgeons to repair the myometrial defect seen in our patient adequately and safely [17].

The technique of minimally invasive surgery for treatment of large type II submucous uterine fibroids described in Case 3 can be performed successfully by a gynecologist with adequate laparoscopic training but limited laparoscopic suturing abilities. It is safe, effective, and avoids the need for traditional laparotomy in most cases of uterine fibroids. This technique was described by our group [18,19] and similar techniques were described by others [20–22].

Transvaginal 2D US is very useful in the diagnosis of pelvic hematoma after any abdominal surgery. It has been shown to be very useful in the diagnosis of hematoma in a myomectomy scar [23]. Its value in the diagnosis of a myometrial abscess, a rare complication after myomectomy, is well illustrated in Case 4. Transvaginal 2D US was also essential during the follow-up on the size of the abscess, ensuring continuous drainage and resolution, which helped successful management of such a rare complication with a minimally invasive technique.

The presence of large broad ligament fibroids usually presents challenges to the gynecologist, even if hysterectomy is the planned surgical procedure. This is as a result of distortion of pelvic anatomy and in turn the possibility of injury to important structures, especially the ureters. During myomectomy, the possibility of injury to the uterine vessels and hemorrhage that can lead to hysterectomy is a major concern in patients who would like to preserve their reproductive potential. The larger the size of the broad ligament fibroid, the greater is the challenge. Therefore, it is very important to choose the correct surgical procedure to perform myomectomy in patients who wish to preserve their reproductive potential. In both Cases 5 and 6, transvaginal 2D US (with and without Doppler flow study) played a major role in the choice of the appropriate surgical procedure. Laparotomy must be performed in the presence of a huge broad ligament fibroid and/or whenever there is increased vascularity in the area where the fibroid is attached to the uterus (as in Case 5). On the other hand, laparoscopic myomectomy [24] or robotic assisted laparoscopic myomectomy can be performed if the broad ligament fibroid is of reasonable size and/or whenever there is minimal vascularity in the area where the fibroid is attached to the uterus (as in Case 6).

References

1. Prayson RA, Hart WR. Pathologic considerations of uterine smooth muscle tumors. *Obstet Gynecol Clin North Am* 1995; **22**: 637–657.

2. Wamsteker K, Emanuel MH, de Kruif JH. Transcervical hysteroscopy resection of submucous fibroids for abnormal uterine bleeding: results regarding the degree of intramural extension. *Obstet Gynecol* 1993; **82**: 736–740.

3. Daly DC, Maier D, Soto-Albers C. Hysteroscopic metroplasty: six years' experience. *Obstet Gynecol* 1989; **73**: 201–205.

4. Eldar-Geva T, Meagher S, Healy DL, et al. Effect of intramural, subserosal, and submucosal uterine fibroids on the outcome of assisted reproductive technology treatment *Fertil Steril* 1998; **70**(4): 687–691.

5. Stovall DW, Parrish SB, Van Voorhis BJ, et al. Uterine leiomyomas reduce the efficacy of assisted reproduction cycles: results of a matched follow-up study. *Hum Reprod* 1998; **13**(1): 192–197.

6. Haney AF. Leiomyomata. In: Gibb RS, et al. *Danforth's Obstetrics and Gynecology*, 10th edn. Philadelphia, PA: Wolters Kluwer Health Lippincott Williams & Wilkins; 2008: 916.

7. Lippman SA, Warner M, Samuels S, et al. Uterine fibroids and gynecologic pain symptoms in a population-based study. *Fertil Steril* 2003; **80**(6): 1488–1494.

8. Sylvestre C, Child TJ, Tulandi T, Tan SL. A prospective study to evaluate the efficacy of two-and three-dimensional sonohysterography in women with intrauterine lesions. *Fertil Steril* 2003; **79**(5): 1222–1225.

9. Fernandez H, Sefrioui O, Virelizier C, et al. Hysteroscopic resection of submucosal myomas in patients with infertility. *Hum Reprod* 2001; **16**(7): 1489–1492.

10. Grimbizis G, Camus M, Clasen K, et al. Hysteroscopic septum resection in patients with recurrent abortions or infertility. *Hum Reprod* 1998; **13**: 1188–1193.

11. Fedele L, Arcaini L, Parazzini F, et al. Reproductive prognosis after hysteroscopic metroplasty in 102 women: lifetable analysis. *Fertil Steril* 1993; **59**: 768–772.

12. Javaid H, Abuzeid M. Surgical dilemma of managing concurrent uterine factors in a patient with recurrent miscarriages. *J Min Invas Gynecol* 2011; **18**(6): Suppl S154.

13. Salim R, Lee C, Davies A, et al. A comparative study of three-dimensional saline infusion sonohysterography and diagnostic hysteroscopy for the classification of submucous fibroids. *Hum Reprod* 2005; **20**(1): 253–257.

14. Lasmar R, Barrozo P, Dias e Marco R, Oliveira A. Submucous fibroids: a new presurgical classification to evaluate the viability of hysteroscopic surgical treatment – preliminary report. *J Min Invas Gynecol* 2005; **12**: 308–311.

15. Lasmar RB, Xinmei Z, Indman PD, et al. Feasibility of a new system of classification of submucous myomas: a multicenter study. *Fertil Steril* 2011; **95**(6): 2073–2077.

16. Bedient CE, Magrina JF, Noble BN, Kho RM. Comparison of robotic and laparoscopic myomectomy. *Am J Obstet Gynecol* 2009; **201**(6): 56.

17. Einarsson JI, Vellinga TT, Twijnstra AR, et al. Bidirectional barbed suture: an evaluation of safety and clinical outcomes *JSLS* 2010; **14**(3): 321–324.

18. Odogwu MH, Agarwal K, Ashraf M, Abuzeid M. A new method of minimally invasive surgery for large uterine fibroids – laparoscopic myomectomy followed by mini-laparotomy for repair of uterine defect. *J Min Invas Gynecol* 2009; **16**(6): Suppl S80.

19. Singh R, Joseph S, Abuzeid M, Ashraf M. Management dilemma of large type II sub mucous fibroid extending up to serosa. *J Min Invas Gynecol* 2010; **17**(6) Suppl: 156–157.

20. Nezhat C, Nezhat F, Bess O, et al. Laparoscopically assisted myomectomy: a report of a new technique in 57 cases. *Int J Fertil Menopausal Stud* 1994; **39**(1): 39.

21. Wood C, Maher P. New strategies for treating myomas. *Diag Ther Endosc* 1996; **2**: 129–134.

22. Catenacci M, Attaran M, Falcone T. Laparoscopic assisted myomectomy. *Fertil Steril* 2011; **96**(3; Suppl V): 11.

23. Sizzi O, Rossetti A, Malzoni M, et al. Italian multicenter study on complications of laparoscopic myomectomy. *J Min Invas Gynecol* 2007; **14**: 453–462.

24. Theodoridis TD, Zepiridis L, Grimbizis G, Bontis J. Laparoscopic management of broad ligament leiomyoma. *J Min Invas Gynecol* 2005; **12**: 4695.

Chapter

10

Pelvic floor ultrasound

Hans Peter Dietz

The assessment of women with symptoms of pelvic floor and lower urinary tract dysfunction has, to date, been limited to the clinical evaluation of surface anatomy. This is clearly insufficient. As a result, imaging of pelvic floor function and anatomy is moving from the fringes to the mainstream of obstetrics and gynecology. This is mainly due to the realization that pelvic floor trauma in labor is common, is generally overlooked, and is a major factor in the causation of pelvic organ prolapse.

Modern imaging methods such as magnetic resonance and three-dimensional (3D) ultrasound have enabled us to diagnose such abnormalities reliably and accurately, most commonly in the form of an avulsion of the puborectalis muscle off its insertion on the os pubis. However, ultrasound has other advantages in the assessment of pelvic organ prolapse, most notably in the differential diagnosis of posterior compartment prolapse, which can be due to at least five different conditions. In addition, ultrasound is the method of choice for imaging mesh and sling implants, since they are not radiopaque and are very difficult to identify on magnetic resonance imaging.

In this chapter I will summarize the methodology of pelvic floor assessment by translabial ultrasound and describe the most common abnormalities and their consequences.

Introduction

To date, the clinical assessment of pelvic organ prolapse has been limited to documenting surface anatomy. While significant progress has been made with the introduction of the Pelvic Organ Prolapse Quantification system (ICS POP-Q), developed by the International Continence Society almost 20 years ago [1], we still describe only the surface. And even that approach is flawed by including essentially normal findings as stage I prolapse of the anterior and posterior compartment [2,3]. It is time for us to look into tissues, rather than just at surface anatomy.

A clinical rectocele may be due to a true rectocele, i.e. a defect of the rectovaginal septum, or due to perineal hypermobility, or an enterocele, or rectal intussusception – or even just a deficient perineum with increased downward displacement of vaginal mucosa. All it requires to make this differential diagnosis is a simple 2D B-mode ultrasound system with a 3–6 MHz

curved array transducer, representing the technology of the mid-1980s. Placement of such a transducer on the perineum will visualize the entire pelvic floor in the midsagittal plane, including the urethra, bladder neck, vagina, cervix, rectal ampulla, and anal canal, as shown in Fig. 10.1. However, many colleagues working in urogynecology still regard ultrasound imaging as investigational, experimental, or optional [4].

Basic methodology

2D imaging

Basic requirements for translabial pelvic floor ultrasound include a B-mode capable 2D ultrasound system with cine loop function, a 3.5–6 MHz curved array transducer, and a video-printer. Such systems have been available since the early 1990s and are cheap and universally available. A midsagittal view is obtained by placing a transducer (usually a curved array with frequencies between 3.5 and 8 MHz) on the perineum (see Fig. 10.1), after covering the transducer with a glove, condom, or thin plastic wrap. Sterilization as for intracavitary transducers is usually considered unnecessary. We use mechanical cleaning and alcoholic wipes.

Powdered gloves can impair imaging quality due to reverberations. It may be necessary to test locally available gloves or probe covers for their effect on image quality. Imaging is usually performed in dorsal lithotomy, with the hips flexed and slightly abducted, or in the standing position. Patient position does not seem to have much effect on maximal organ descent [5], but it sometimes is necessary to scan the patient upright to avoid levator co-activation [6]. The pelvic tilt can be improved by asking the patient to place her heels close to her buttocks and then moving her hips towards her heels. Bladder filling should be specified; usually prior voiding is preferable.

The presence of a full rectum can impair diagnostic accuracy and sometimes necessitates a repeat assessment after bowel emptying. Parting of the labia can improve image quality, which generally is best in pregnancy and poorest in menopausal women with marked atrophy, most likely due to vary-

Ultrasonography in Gynecology, ed. Botros R. M. B. Rizk and Elizabeth E. Puscheck. Published by Cambridge University Press. © Cambridge University Press 2015.

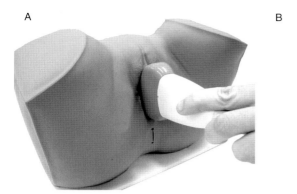

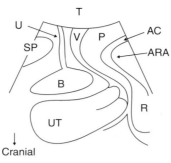

Fig. 10.1 Transducer placement on the perineum (left) with schematic representation of the resulting midsagittal field of vision. T = transducer, SP = symphysis pubis, U = urethra, V = vagina, P = perineal body, R = rectum, B = bladder, UT = uterus, AC = anal canal, ARA = anorectal angle, AC = anal canal. From Dietz HP. Pelvic floor ultrasound: a review. *Am J Obstet Gynecol* 2010; 202: 321–334, with permission.

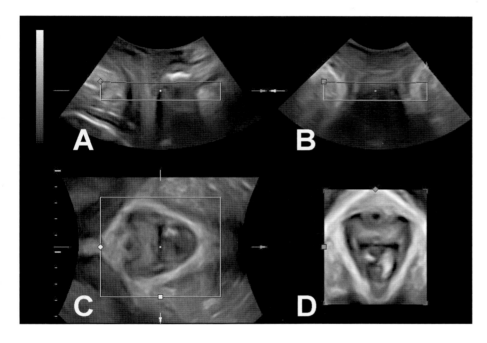

Fig. 10.2 Standard representation of female pelvic floor structures on translabial/perineal ultrasound. The midsagittal plane is shown in (A), the coronal in (B), the axial in (C). A rendered volume (i.e. the semi-transparent representation of all pixels in the "region of interest," the box seen in A–C) in the axial plane is given in (D). Often, A and D are of the most interest and are combined, leaving out B and C. In D the patient's right-hand side is represented on the left, as if the pelvic floor were viewed from below. From Dietz HP. Pelvic floor ultrasound. In: *Sonography in Obstetrics and Gynecology: Principles and Practice.* 7th edn. Fleischer AC et al., McGraw Hill 2010, with permission.

ing hydration of tissues. Vaginal scar tissue can also impair visibility. Obesity is rarely a problem.

The transducer can usually be placed firmly on the perineum and the symphysis pubis without causing discomfort, unless there is marked atrophy. The resulting image includes the symphysis anteriorly, the urethra and bladder neck, the vagina, cervix, rectum, and anal canal (see Fig. 10.1). Posterior to the anorectal junction, a hyperechogenic area indicates the central portion of the levator plate, i.e. the puborectalis muscle. The cul-de-sac may also be seen, filled with a small amount of fluid, echogenic fat, or peristalsing small bowel. Parasagittal or transverse views may yield additional information, e.g. enabling assessment of the pubovisceral muscle and its insertion on the arcus tendineus of the levator ani and for imaging of implants.

While there has been disagreement regarding image orientation in the midsagittal plane, the author prefers an orientation as on conventional transvaginal ultrasound (cranioventral aspects to the left, dorsocaudal to the right). The latter also seems more convenient when using 3D/4D systems.

3D/4D imaging

The introduction of 4D ultrasound has had a major impact on pelvic floor imaging. This is mainly due to the fact that 4D ultrasound gives access to the axial plane to a degree and with an ease that far surpasses what was possible using intracavitary transducers in the past. A single volume obtained at rest with an acquisition angle of 70 degrees or higher will include the entire levator hiatus with symphysis pubis, urethra, paravaginal tissues, the vagina, anorectum, and pubovisceral (puborectalis/pubococcygeus part of the levator ani) muscle from the pelvic sidewall in the area of the arcus tendineus of the levator ani (ATLA) to the posterior aspect of the anorectal junction.

Any system that allows satisfactory 3D/4D imaging using an abdominal obstetric probe will be suitable, provided the acquisition angle is sufficient to include the entire levator hiatus (i.e. between 70 and 85 degrees). Fig. 10.2 demonstrates the two basic display modes currently in use on 3D ultrasound systems. The multiplanar or orthogonal display mode shows

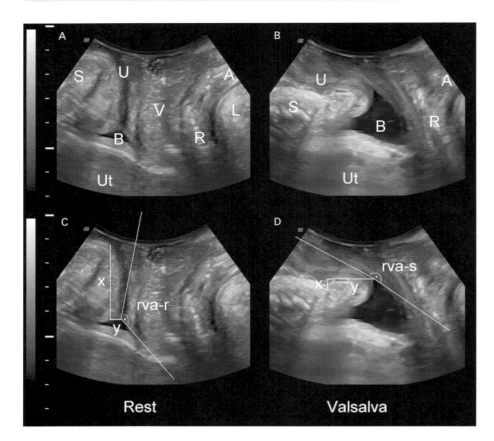

Fig. 10.3 Determination of bladder neck descent and retrovesical angle: Ultrasound images showing the midsagittal plane at rest (A, C) and on Valsalva (B, D). S = symphysis pubis, U = urethra, B = bladder, Ut = uterus, V = vagina, A = anal canal, R = rectal ampulla, L = levator ani. The lower images demonstrate the measurement of distances between inferior symphyseal margin and bladder neck (vertical, x; horizontal, y) and the retrovesical angle at rest (rva-r) and on Valsalva (rva-s). From Dietz HP. Pelvic floor imaging in incontinence: What's in it for the surgeon? *Int Urogynecol J* 2011; 22(9): 1085–1097, with permission.

cross-sectional planes through the volume in question. For pelvic floor imaging, this usually means the midsagittal (A), the coronal (B), and the axial plane (C). The three orthogonal images are complemented by a "rendered image," i.e. a semitransparent representation of all voxels in an arbitrarily definable "box." Fig. 10.2D shows a standard rendered image of the levator hiatus, with the rendering direction set from caudally to cranially.

The ability to perform a real-time 3D (or 4D) assessment of pelvic floor structures makes the technology superior to magnetic resonance imaging. Prolapse assessment by magnetic resonance requires ultra-fast acquisition [7], which is of limited availability and will not allow optimal resolutions. Alternatively, some systems allow imaging of the sitting or erect patient, but again accessibility will be limited for the foreseeable future. The sheer physical characteristics of magnetic resonance imaging systems make it much harder for the operator to ensure efficient maneuvers, as over 50% of all women will not perform a proper pelvic floor contraction when asked [8], and a Valsalva is often confounded by concomitant levator activation [6]. Without real-time imaging, these confounders are impossible to control. Therefore, ultrasound has major potential advantages when it comes to describing prolapse, especially when associated with fascial or muscular defects and in terms of defining functional anatomy. Offline analysis packages allow distance, area, and volume measurements in any user-defined plane (oblique or orthogonal), which is superior

to what is possible with DICOM viewer software on a standard set of single-plane magnetic resonance images.

Functional assessment

Valsalva

The Valsalva maneuver, i.e. a forced expiration against a closed glottis and contracted diaphragm and abdominal wall, is routinely used to document downward displacement of pelvic organs, reveal the symptoms and signs of female pelvic organ prolapse, and demonstrate distensibility of the levator hiatus. The result is a dorsocaudal displacement of urethra and bladder neck that can be quantified using a system of coordinates based on the inferoposterior symphyseal margin (see Fig. 10.3). There also is downward movement of the uterine cervix and the rectal ampulla, and frequently the development of a rectocele, i.e. a sacculation of the anterior wall of the rectal ampulla towards the vaginal introitus or beyond (see below). In the axial plane the hiatus is distended, and the posterior aspect of the levator plate is displaced caudally, resulting in varying degrees of perineal descent. One ought to take care to let the transducer move with the tissues, avoiding undue pressure on the perineum, which would prevent full development of a prolapse.

In young nulliparous women, a Valsalva is frequently confounded by levator activation [6] as any obstetrician is able to observe on a daily basis. Levator co-activation during Valsalva is highly inconvenient – not just in the labor ward during the

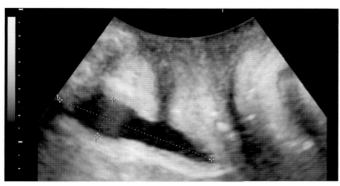

Fig. 10.4 Determination of postvoid residual urine volume by translabial ultrasound. Measurements obtained along the two longest axes placed vertical to each other are 5.99 × 1.47 cm. The volume is calculated as $X \times Y \times 5.6$ = residual urine in mL, which equates to 49.3 mL. From Dietz HP, Velez D, Shek KL, Martin A. Determination of postvoid residual by translabial ultrasound. *Int Urogynecol J* 2012; 23: 1749–52, with permission.

expulsive phase of a woman's first vaginal delivery, but also when we assess women for pelvic floor dysfunction and prolapse. Levator co-activation is visible as a reduction in the anteroposterior diameter of the levator hiatus on Valsalva. It has to be avoided in order to obtain an accurate assessment of pelvic organ descent. Any imaging assessment of organ descent requires real-time observation of the effect of a Valsalva maneuver in order to correct suboptimal efforts, especially if leakage from bladder or bowel is likely.

At times, levator co-activation can prevent adequate assessment in the supine position, in particular in women with a strong, intact levator shelf. Sometimes it is necessary to repeat imaging in the standing position, which seems to increase the likelihood of an adequate bearing-down effort. Other confounders are bladder filling [9], duration of Valsalva maneuver (which should be continued for at least 5 seconds) [10], and abdominal pressure. The latter is the one most commonly mentioned, but it seems that the vast majority of patients are able to generate pressures that are sufficient for a reproducible assessment [48].

Pelvic floor muscle contraction

Ultrasound is a highly useful tool in the assessment of the pelvic floor musculature, both in purely anatomical terms (see below) and for function. A levator contraction will reduce the size of the levator hiatus in the sagittal plane and elevate the anorectum, changing the angle between levator plate and symphysis pubis. As an indirect effect, other pelvic organs such as uterus, bladder, and urethra are displaced cranially, and there is compression of urethra, vagina, and anorectal junction, explaining the importance of the levator ani for urinary and fecal continence as well as for sexual function.

In its most basic form, transabdominal B-mode imaging can demonstrate elevation of the bladder base on pelvic floor muscle contraction (PFMC), but quantification is difficult and repeatability lower than for translabial ultrasound [11]. The latter has been employed for the quantification of pelvic floor

muscle function, both in women with stress incontinence and in continent controls [12] as well as before and after childbirth [13,14]. A cranioventral shift of pelvic organs imaged in a sagittal midline orientation is taken as evidence of a levator contraction. The resulting displacement of the internal urethral meatus is measured relative to the inferoposterior symphyseal margin. Care has to be taken to avoid concomitant activation of the abdominal muscles, especially the rectus abdominis or the diaphragm, as this would tend to cause caudal displacement of the bladder neck.

Another means of quantifying levator activity is to measure reduction of the levator hiatus in the midsagittal plane, or to determine the changing angle of the hiatal plane relative to the symphyseal axis. The method can also be utilized for pelvic floor muscle exercise teaching by providing visual biofeedback [15] and has helped validate the concept of "the knack," i.e. of a reflex levator contraction immediately prior to increases in intra-abdominal pressure, such as those resulting from coughing [16]. Correlations between cranioventral shift of the bladder neck on the one hand and palpation/perineometry on the other hand have been shown to be good [17].

Anatomical assessment

Anterior compartment

As any assessment for female pelvic organ prolapse should be performed after bladder emptying to maximize descent, one can obtain a residual urine measurement at the same time (see Fig. 10.4), using the formula $X \times Y \times 5.6$ = residual urine in mL, where X and Y are the two maximal bladder diameters, vertical to each other, measured in the midsagittal plane [18].

Bladder neck mobility

Bladder neck position and mobility can be assessed with a high degree of reliability [3]. Points of reference are the central axis of the symphysis pubis [19] or its inferoposterior margin [20]; see Fig. 10.3. The full bladder is less mobile [9] and may prevent complete development of pelvic organ prolapse. It is essential not to exert undue pressure on the perineum so as to allow full development of pelvic organ descent. Measurements of bladder neck position are performed at rest and on maximal Valsalva, and the difference yields a numerical value for bladder neck descent.

On Valsalva, the proximal urethra may be seen to rotate in a postero-inferior direction. The extent of rotation can be measured by comparing the angle of inclination between the proximal urethra and any other fixed axis. Some investigators measure the retrovesical angle (RVA or posterior urethrovesical angle, PUV) between proximal urethra and trigone, others determine the angle γ between the central axis of the symphysis pubis and a line from the inferior symphyseal margin to the bladder neck [21]. The reproducibility of bladder neck descent seems good, with intraclass correlations between 0.75 and 0.98, indicating "excellent" agreement [22].

There is no definition of "normal" for bladder neck descent, although cut-offs of 20 and 25 mm have been proposed to define hypermobility. Bladder filling, patient position, and catheterization all have been shown to influence measurements (see Dietz [23] for an overview) and it can occasionally be quite difficult to obtain an effective Valsalva maneuver, especially in nulliparous women who routinely co-activate the levator muscle [6]. Perhaps not surprisingly, publications to date have presented widely differing reference measurements in nulliparous women. The author has obtained measurements of 1.2–40.2 mm (mean 17.3 mm) in a group of 106 stress-continent nulligravid young women of 18–23 years of age [3].

The etiology of increased bladder neck descent is likely to be multifactorial. The wide range of values obtained in young nulliparous women suggests a congenital component. Vaginal childbirth is probably the most significant environmental factor [24,25], with a long second stage of labor and vaginal operative delivery associated with increased postpartum descent. This association between increased bladder descent and vaginal parity is also evident in older women with symptoms of pelvic floor dysfunction [26]. Most recently, it has been shown that it is mid-urethral mobility, not mobility of the bladder neck, which is most important for continence [27].

Funneling and stress incontinence

In patients with stress incontinence, but also in asymptomatic women, funneling of the internal urethral meatus may be observed on Valsalva and sometimes even at rest [28]. Funneling is often (but not necessarily) associated with leakage and an open retrovesical angle. In women with urodynamic stress incontinence, 2.5–4 cm of bladder neck descent and funneling is the most common finding [29] (see Fig. 10.3). Other indirect signs of urine leakage on B-mode real-time imaging are weak grayscale echoes ("streaming") and the appearance of two linear ("specular") echoes defining the lumen of a fluid-filled urethra. However, funneling may also be observed in urge incontinence and cannot be used to prove urodynamic

stress incontinence. Its anatomical basis is unclear. Marked funneling has been shown to be associated with poor urethral closure pressures [30,31] and recurrence after colposuspension [32] and tension-free vaginal tape [33].

Cystocele

Clinical examination is limited to grading anterior compartment prolapse, which we call "cystocele." In fact, imaging can identify a number of entities that are difficult, if not impossible, to tell apart clinically. Pelvic floor ultrasound enables us to distinguish between two types of cystocele with very different functional implications [34]. A cystocele with intact retrovesical angle (first described on X-ray cystourethrography as Green type III in the 1960s [35]) is generally associated with voiding dysfunction, a low likelihood of stress incontinence, and major trauma to the levator ani, while a cystourethrocele (Green type II) is associated with above average flow rates and urodynamic stress incontinence [34] (Fig. 10.5). While it is possible to distinguish the two types clinically [36], on clinical examination these two very different entities are grouped together, which may well be why studies of voiding dysfunction and prolapse have yielded such varying results. In addition, occasionally a cystocele will turn out to be due to a urethral diverticulum (Fig. 10.6), a Gartner duct cyst (Fig. 10.7), or an anterior enterocele, all rather likely to be missed on clinical examination. Exclusion of a urethral diverticulum is a frequently forgotten benefit of pelvic floor ultrasound. It is difficult to understand why magnetic resonance is commonly seen as the diagnostic method of choice [37].

Implants

Another major argument in favor of pelvic floor ultrasound imaging is the popularity and undoubted utility of suburethral slings. These synthetic implants, usually of wide-weave polypropylene mesh, are highly echogenic and easily identified in the anterior vaginal wall. For once, there is absolutely no doubt as to which imaging method is most appropriate, since those implants cannot be seen with plain X-ray, CT, or magnetic

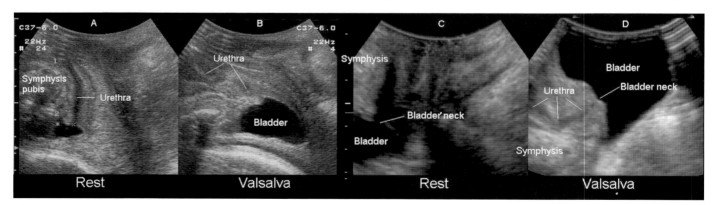

Fig. 10.5 The two most common presentations of cystocele. The left image pair (A and B) shows typical findings in a patient with mild stress urinary incontinence and anterior vaginal wall descent (clinically a cystourethrocele grade II). The right image pair (C and D) demonstrates appearances in a patient with a cystocele with intact retrovesical angle. On the left the bladder neck is part of the leading edge of the cysto(urethro)cele, on the right the leading edge of the cystocele is about 4 cm caudad to the bladder neck. From Dietz HP. Pelvic Floor Imaging in prolapse: What's in it for the surgeon? *Int Urogynecol J* 2011; 22(9): 1085–1097, with permission.

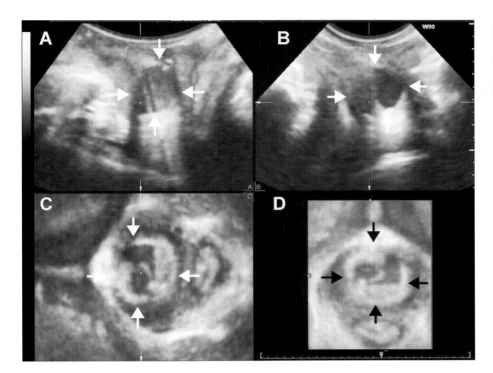

Fig. 10.6 Urethral diverticulum masquerading as a second-degree cystocele. The diverticulum is outlined by arrows and visible in the midsagittal (A), coronal (B), and axial plane, (C), as well as in a rendered volume (D). From Dietz HP The role of 2D and 3D dynamic ultrasound in pelvic organ prolapse. *J Min Inv Gynecol* 2010; 17: 282–294, with permission.

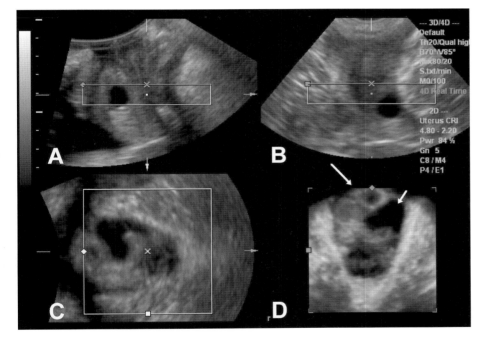

Fig. 10.7 Orthogonal and rendered views of Gartner duct cysts. The pathognomonic feature is the observation of an intact urethral rhabdosphincter (long arrow in D), clearly separate from the cyst (short arrow in D). From Dietz HP The role of 2D and 3D dynamic ultrasound in pelvic organ prolapse. *J Min Inv Gynecol* 2010; 17: 282–294, with permission.

resonance [38–40]. These new procedures, the first of which is the tension-free vaginal tape, are highly successful in most hands. The therapeutic effect, i.e. dynamic compression at times of increased intra-abdominal pressure, is easily observed on real-time ultrasound [41]. However, at times such slings may result in substantial complications, the diagnosis and management of which is greatly helped by imaging. Ultrasound can confirm the presence of such a sling (Fig. 10.8) or detect one in women who are not aware of the type of previous surgery, distinguish between transobturator and retropubic slings [42],

and even allow an educated guess regarding the exact type and material of the sling [43] (Fig. 10.9) in some cases, although different types of wide-weave polypropylene slings are impossible to distinguish if their anatomical course is the same [42,44].

In addition, it is easy to confirm whether the sling is placed at the conventional mid-urethral level, although the importance of this factor is disputed [45–47], and whether it remains outside the urethral rhabdosphincter. Perforation or near-perforation are readily apparent (see Fig. 10.10). Such findings will inform clinical audit and may have substantial consequences

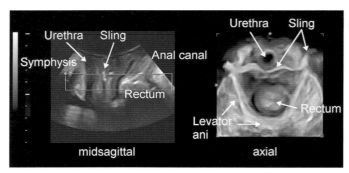

Fig. 10.8 A transobturator sling as imaged in the midsagittal plane (left) and in an axial rendered volume (right). From Dietz HP. Pelvic floor ultrasound. In: *Sonography in Obstetrics and Gynecology: Principles and Practice*. 7th edn. Fleischer AC et al., McGraw Hill 2010, with permission.

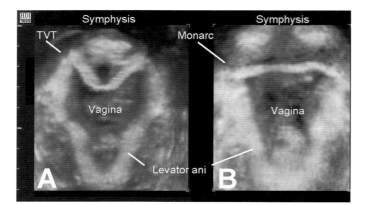

Fig. 10.9 The distinction between retropubic (A) and transobturator tape (B) can often only be made in the axial plane, as here in rendered volumes showing the course of the implant ventrally (A) and laterally (B). From Dietz HP. Pelvic floor ultrasound. *Australasian Society for Ultrasound Medicine Bulletin* 2007; 10: 17–23, with permission.

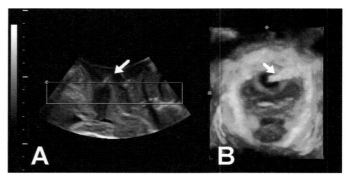

Fig. 10.10 A tension-free vaginal tape that has perforated the urethra as imaged in the midsagittal plane (A) and in an axial rendered volume (B), indicated by arrow. Part of the tape on the patient's right (the left-hand side of the image) has already been removed to alleviate obstruction. From Dietz HP. Pelvic floor imaging in incontinence: What's in it for the surgeon? *Int Urogynecol J* 2011; 22(9): 1085–1097, with permission.

for patient care. In addition, the functional impact of a suburethral sling can be assessed on Valsalva maneuver. The appearance of the sling (straight line, angled line, or c-shape) can be quantified with the "tape angle" [47] and will suggest the degree of tension. The "sling-pubis gap" on Valsalva seems to be a highly reproducible and valid parameter of sling "tightness" [47]; see Fig. 10.11.

A tight c-shaped appearance at rest and a sling-pubis gap of less than 7 mm on Valsalva makes functional obstruction very likely and suggests that tape division would be beneficial in a patient with worsened symptoms of bladder irritability or clinically significant voiding dysfunction. On the other hand, a wide sling-pubis gap and a tape that remains a straight line on Valsalva suggests insufficient tension, or a failure of sling anchoring. Many women would have been spared the suboptimal outcomes of several recently developed mini-slings if manufacturers had used ultrasound outcome measures of sling tension and anchoring in their pre-marketing clinical studies.

Finally, ultrasound is useful for confirming the success of sling division, especially if there are persistent symptoms. It is not always easy to divide a suburethral sling, and some surgeons fail in such an endeavor. Successful sling division results in a clear

separation of the two halves of the implant, and the resulting gap is seen to widen on Valsalva, usually to at least 5–7 mm.

The above remarks regarding the choice of diagnostic method for the evaluation of slings also apply to synthetic mesh implants used in prolapse surgery. These implants are not visible on X-ray, CT, or magnetic resonance, but are easily seen on ultrasound (Fig. 10.12). Cranial aspects of such mesh implants are sometimes difficult to image, especially if they are suspended to the sacrospinous ligaments. However, failure of mesh suspension, or a detachment of organs from a well-suspended mesh, is easily apparent on Valsalva and transvaginal imaging can be added if superior mesh aspects need to be assessed. Biological materials, on the other hand, are usually not that echogenic, and some seem to simply disappear over time.

In clinical audit series on many hundreds of anterior and posterior compartment meshes, we have observed several different forms of prolapse recurrence due to suspension failure [128]. Some authors seem to deny that mesh failure is a significant problem, and in general the focus in women after mesh implantation has been on erosion/mesh exposure and chronic pain syndromes [49]. Others blame supposed mesh contraction [50], a phenomenon that probably does not exist beyond the period of physiological wound healing [51,52]. We have found no evidence of mesh shrinkage or contraction in an observation period of almost 60 woman-years [52] after Perigee implantation.

Either way, there are very few references in the literature to mesh anchoring failure, and no advice on how to deal with such cases. Amazingly, rather than focus on how to deal with complications and failures after procedures that have become widely accepted, everyone seems to chase after the latest innovation in mesh technology. On the incessant prompting of industry, many colleagues start using devices for which there is minimal outcome data, even before we have decent independent medium-term results for the first generation of implants.

The best information we currently have is on success and failure of transobturator meshes, of which the Perigee is the

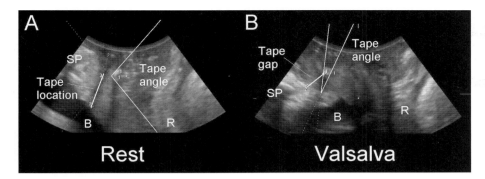

Fig. 10.11 Parameters of tape "tightness." The most useful such parameter seems to be the gap between the posterior symphyseal margin and the sling on Valsalva ("sling pubis gap" or "tape gap"). Tape gaps of less than 7 mm are very likely to be obstructive, and those over 15 mm are much less likely to provide sufficient dynamic compression, leaving the patient stress incontinent. SP = symphysis pubis, B = bladder, R = rectal ampulla. From Dietz HP. Pelvic floor imaging in incontinence: What's in it for the surgeon? *Int Urogynecol J* 2011; 22(9): 1085–1097, with permission.

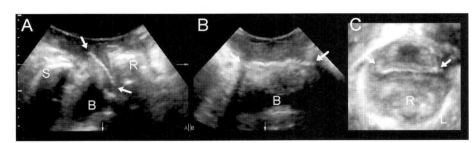

Fig. 10.12 Translabial imaging of a transobturator anterior compartment mesh on Valsalva, seen in the midsagittal plane (A), coronal plane (B), and axial plane (C). The mesh is seen posterior to proximal urethra and bladder neck in the midsagittal plane (arrows). S = symphysis pubis, B = bladder, R = rectocele, L = levator ani. From Dietz HP, Erdmann M, Shek KL. Mesh contraction: myth or reality? *Am J Obstet Gynecol* 2011; 204(2): 173.e1–4, with permission.

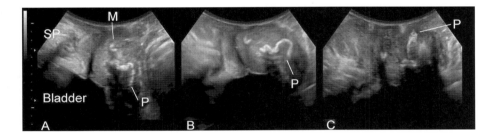

Fig. 10.13 Translabial imaging of a transobturator anterior compartment mesh. A shows the mesh at rest, B halfway through a Valsalva, and C at maximal Valsalva. It is evident that the superior mesh arms have pulled out, resulting in the failure of apical support and a recurrent cystocele, similar in appearances to a high cystocele after Burch colposuspension. SP = symphysis pubis, M = Monarc sling, P = Perigee mesh (cranial aspect).

prototype, invented by Rane and Fraser in 2004, with the Anterior Prolift largely comparable from a functional anatomy point of view [53]. There seem to be three distinct forms of mesh suspension failure, the prevalence of which seems to vary with mesh types and patient factors [128]. Dislodgment of the superior (cranial) anchoring arms is not uncommon and was first described in 2006 [54] (Fig. 10.12). It is not surprising that the superior arms should be more vulnerable, if one considers that the anterior vaginal wall may be seen as a lever arm, anchored to the fulcrum of the symphysis pubis. The further from the fulcrum any support structure is placed, the greater the moment exerted on this structure by forces generated by increases in intra-abdominal pressure. Patients with higher degrees of ballooning [55] or levator avulsion seem to be at an increased risk of support failure, which may be explained by a longer effective lever arm and higher moment.

Dislodgment of the superior arms seems to occur in about 10% of both Anterior Prolift and Perigee, resulting in the appearance of a "high cystocele," similar to what is sometimes observed after an otherwise anatomically successful Burch colposuspension (Fig. 10.13). There currently is no advice on how to deal with such a situation if symptomatic, but apical suspension, by whatever route, may well be necessary. Anterior

compartment meshes that provide apical anchoring to the sacrospinous ligaments may not be subject to this type of suspension failure.

Dislodgment of all arms will require re-suspension of the entire anterior compartment, e.g. by a second mesh placed deep to the first, possibly after removal of some or all of the failed mesh (personal communication, A. Rane). We have begun to suture anchoring arms to the inferior pubic ramus, but in high-risk patients there clearly is some need for more reliable apical suspension, e.g. to the sacrospinous ligaments.

In some instances, meshes are insufficiently secured to the bladder base. This may result in a large sonographic gap between symphysis and mesh, a situation that is associated with postoperative stress urinary incontinence [56]. Occasionally, this gap may become so large that a cystourethrocele develops ventral to a well-supported mesh. This situation, if symptomatic, is easy to correct by mobilizing the posterior bladder base off the mesh and then reconnecting the mesh to the bladder neck [128].

The most recent modifications of mesh systems have abandoned transobturator arms in favor of anchors in the arcus tendineus and the sacrospinous ligaments (e.g. Anterior Elevate or Pinnacle), or in favor of vaginal splinting (Prosima), but such

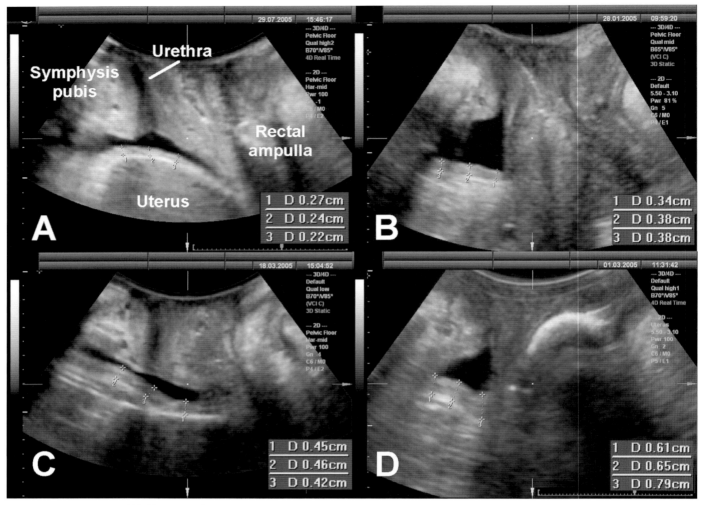

Fig. 10.14 Measurement of bladder wall thickness at the dome in four women with non-neuropathic bladder dysfunction. Images A–C show normal measurements below 5 mm, image D shows abnormal detrusor wall thickness at an average of 6.8 mm. In all cases residual urine is well below 50 mL. From Lekskulchai O, Dietz HP. Detrusor wall thickness as a test for detrusor overactivity in women. *Ultrasound Obstet Gynecol* 2008; 32: 535–539, with permission.

systems may not be suitable for level II support due to inferior sidewall anchoring [58]. Ultrasound will provide information on the relative merit of different anchoring systems and help us deal with the novel forms of iatrogenic pathology that will inevitably result.

Other findings

On a more general note, translabial ultrasound may detect unexpected foreign bodies or bladder tumors [23,57] and can be used to determine residual urine [18]. While detrusor wall thickness (DWT) has probably been overrated as a diagnostic tool in the context of detrusor overactivity [59,60], increased DWT is very likely associated with symptoms of the overactive bladder [60,61] and may be a predictor of postoperative de novo urge incontinence and/or detrusor overactivity after anti-incontinence procedures [62] (Fig. 10.14). Colposuspensions create a typical appearance on translabial ultrasound [32,63,64] and over-elevation is readily apparent [65].

Uterine descent

Generally, uterine prolapse is obvious clinically, as is vault descent. An unusually low cervix is isoechoic, its distal margin evident as a specular line, and it often causes acoustic shadowing. In premenopausal women the cervix often contains nabothian follicles (Fig. 10.15), which are evident as cystic spaces within the cervix and can occasionally measure several centimeters in diameter. A Valsalva maneuver will result in relative movement, distinguishing a nabothian follicle from Gartner duct cysts or urethral diverticula. A low uterus may compress the posterior compartment sufficiently to hide a rectocele or even a recto-enterocele, reducing the diagnostic accuracy of imaging methods.

Translabial ultrasound can graphically show the effect of an anteriorized cervix in women with an enlarged, retroverted uterus, explaining symptoms of voiding dysfunction and supporting surgical intervention in order to improve voiding in a patient with a retroverted fibroid uterus. On the other hand, mild descent of an anteverted uterus may result in compression and inversion of the rectal ampulla, explaining symptoms of obstructed defecation – a situation that is termed a "colpocele" on defecation proctography. The result is a rectal intussusception, with the intussuscipiens propelled not by sigmoid or (as usual) small bowel, but by the cervix.

Vault prolapse

It is frequently possible to image vault descent in women after hysterectomy, but just as often the thin iso- to hypoechoic structure of the vaginal wall is obscured by a descending rectocele or enterocele, which limits the usefulness of assessing the position of the vault.

Posterior compartment

Clinically we diagnose posterior compartment descent as "rectocele," ignoring that at least five different conditions may lead to apparent or actual prolapse of the posterior vaginal wall.

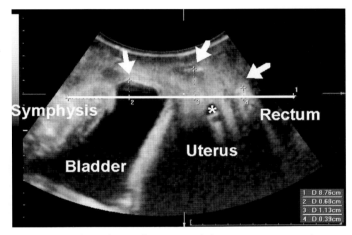

Fig. 10.15 Midsagittal view of a patient with three-compartment prolapse. Arrows indicate the leading edge of the bladder (left), uterus (middle), and rectum (right). In contrast to bladder and rectum the uterus is isoechoic, and frequently a nabothian cyst (*) helps with identifying the cervix. A horizontal line is placed through the inferoposterior margin of the symphysis pubis, providing a line of reference against which pelvic organ descent is measured. From Dietz HP (2010) The role of 2D and 3D dynamic ultrasound in pelvic organ prolapse. *J Min Inv Gynecol* 17: 282–294, with permission.

A second-degree rectocele could be due to a true rectocele, i.e. a defect of the rectovaginal septum (most common, and associated with symptoms of prolapse, incomplete bowel emptying, and straining at stool) [66], due to an abnormally distensible, intact rectovaginal septum (common and associated only with prolapse symptoms), a combined recto-enterocele (less common), an isolated enterocele (uncommon), or just a deficient perineum giving the impression of a "bulge" [67]. Occasionally a "rectocele" turns out to be due to rectal intussusception, a condition that we assume to be an early stage of rectal prolapse, where the wall of the rectum is inverted and enters the anal canal on Valsalva.

Rectocele

An anterior rectocele is evident as a diverticulum of the anterior wall of the rectal ampulla into the vagina, generally much more obvious on Valsalva than at rest. Posterior rectoceles are very uncommon in adult women and may rather be a form of intussusception than an actual rectocele. A rectocele usually contains iso- to hyperechoic feces, and often there is bowel gas as well, resulting in specular echoes and reverberations. Occasionally, there is no stool in the ampulla that could be propelled into the rectocele, and as a result it remains smaller and filled only with rectal mucosa. Since distension of a rectocele will depend on the presence and quality of stool, appearances may vary considerably from one day to the next. Colorectal surgeons and gastroenterologists have used ultrasound gel as contract medium [68,69], sometimes after bowel preparation, which may result in more reproducible findings. However, usually hyperechogenic stool provides for all the contrast required.

The severity of a rectocele can be quantified by measuring maximal descent relative to the inferior symphyseal margin, and by determining the maximal depth of the sacculation as seen in Fig. 10.16, which compares ultrasound and radiological findings in a patient with rectocele.

Enterocele

An enterocele is visualized as downward displacement of abdominal contents into the vagina, ventral to the anal canal. Small bowel may be identifiable due to its peristalsis, and

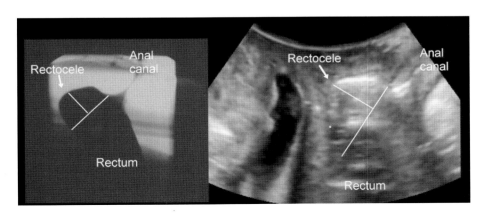

Fig. 10.16 A typical true rectocele as seen on defecation proctogram (left) and translabial ultrasound (right). Whether such a rectocele is symptomatic may depend on stool quality, and other factors, and many such patients are asymptomatic. From Perniola G, Dietz HP, Shek KL, Chew S, Cartmill J, Chong C. Defecation proctography and translabial ultrasound in the investigation of defecatory disorders. *Ultrasound Obstet Gynecol* 2008; 31: 567–571, with permission.

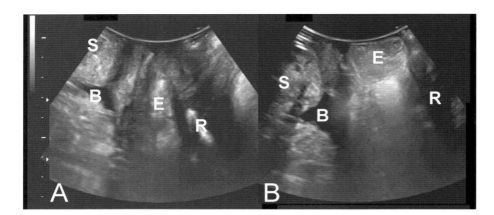

Fig. 10.17 Enterocele filled with small bowel, as seen in the midsagittal plane, at rest (left, A) and during Valsalva (right, B). S = symphysis pubis, B = bladder, R = rectum, E = enterocele. From Dietz HP. Pelvic floor imaging in prolapse: What's in it for the surgeon? *Int Urogynecol J* 2011; 22(9): 1085–1097, with permission.

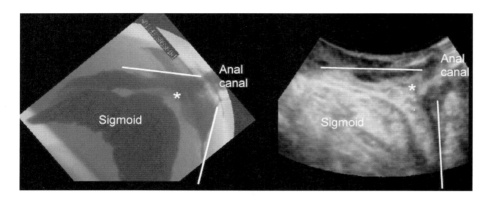

Fig. 10.18 A rectal intussusception (indicated by *) due to a sigmoid enterocele as seen on defecation proctogram (left) and translabial ultrasound (right). It is generally not possible to distinguish which part of the small or large bowel propels the intussuscipiens, although the coarse appearances of the intussuscipiens are suggestive of large rather than small bowel. From Perniola G, Dietz HP, Shek KL, Chew S, Cartmill J, Chong C. Defecation proctography and translabial ultrasound in the investigation of defecatory disorders. *Ultrasound Obstet Gynecol* 2008; 31: 567–571, with permission.

sometimes intraperitoneal fluid outlines the apex of the enterocele. Distal shadowing is much less common than with rectocele, and often contents have an irregular isoechoic or ground-grass-like appearance (Fig. 10.17). A sigmoid enterocele tends to show coarser patterns, as seen in Fig. 10.18.

Rectal intussusception and prolapse

An intussusception is seen as splaying of the normally tubular anal canal, with the anterior wall of the rectal ampulla (and occasionally the posterior wall as well) being inverted and propelled into the opening anal canal. Fig. 10.18 shows a comparison of radiological and ultrasound findings in a patient with rectal intussusception. Usually, a rectal intussusception is due to an enterocele of small bowel that progresses down the anal canal, but other abdominal contents such as sigmoid (as in Fig. 10.18), omentum, and even the uterus can act in a similar way. Ultimately, rectal mucosa and muscularis may protrude from the anus, resulting in rectal prolapse. Intussusception seems associated with avulsion of the puborectalis and with excessive distensibility of the hiatus ("ballooning") [70].

When a rectocele or rectal intussusception is identified on translabial imaging, it makes sense to provide the patient with visual biofeedback. Demonstrating that straining at stool is obviously counterproductive (propelling feces not into the anal canal but into the vagina, or propelling not feces but small bowel) may help in modifying behavior. Ultrasound is much better tolerated than defecation proctography, and of course

it is much cheaper. As a result, it is likely that ultrasound will replace the radiological technique in the initial investigation of women with defecation disorders. If there is a rectocele or a rectal intussusception/prolapse on ultrasound, this condition is very likely to be found on X-ray imaging [71–73]. In addition, anismus may be evident as an inability to relax the levator ani, which can be diagnosed qualitatively or by measuring the anorectal angle [74], although it is often not clear whether observations on diagnostic imaging bear any relation to what happens during defecation.

Clinical consequences of ultrasound diagnosis

It is a useful clinical rule that one should be wary of underestimating prolapse on clinical examination. All too often, findings in theatre show more significant degrees of prolapse than what was observed in the office or outpatient department. To a large degree, this is due to confounding factors that are immediately apparent on translabial ultrasound. A full bladder and/or rectum will tamponade the levator hiatus and prevent downward development of prolapse, especially of the central compartment. In addition, women with an intact pelvic floor often co-activate the levator ani when asked to perform a Valsalva maneuver, reducing the size of the levator hiatus and impeding full development of the prolapse. In nulliparous women, this occurs in almost half and is sometimes difficult to overcome [6], unless one performs the assessment in the standing position. Dynamic real-time imaging demonstrates levator

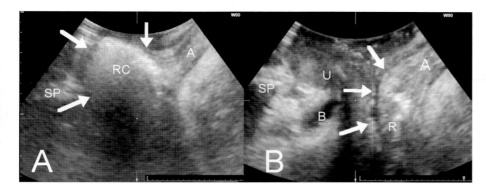

Fig. 10.19 Large rectocele (RC) before (left image, A) and 3 months after defect-specific rectocele repair (right image, B). SP = symphysis pubis, A = anal canal, RC = rectocele, B = bladder, U = urethra, R = rectal ampulla. The defect-specific repair was carried out by closing a transverse defect in the rectovaginal septum, approximating the inferior free margin of the septum to the cervix and the vaginosacral fibers of the uterosacral ligaments, using a row of six single sutures of delayed absorbable material.

co-activation and can help avoid false-negative examination results, reducing the likelihood of unpleasant surprises in theatre. Much less commonly, ultrasound will avoid unnecessary surgery or potential complications, such as the inadvertent opening of a urethral diverticulum or a Gartner cyst that was misdiagnosed as cystocele.

In the posterior compartment, ultrasound will identify defects of the rectovaginal septum and suggest a defect-specific repair as the most appropriate approach. Perineal hypermobility may be reduced by plication of the rectovaginal septum and/or levatorplasty. An enterocele may suggest a different surgical approach and alert to a potential need for apical support, while identification of a rectal intussusception may suggest the need for a colorectal referral.

However, no diagnostic finding is going to help our patients much, unless the surgeon knows what to make of it. This requires a degree of consensus as regards pathophysiology and patho-anatomy. The author feels that defects of the rectovaginal septum can be reliably identified by ultrasound and repaired by a defect-specific approach first popularized by Cullen Richardson [75]. Closure of such a defect is usually very obvious postoperatively (see Fig. 10.19 for an example), and such closure cannot be achieved with colporrhaphy or mesh surgery or stapled trans-anal resection (STARR procedure).

However, at the moment there is no agreement on whether the rectovaginal septum actually exists, let alone how to repair it. Not surprisingly, gynecologists and colorectal surgeons employ a multitude of different techniques to repair posterior compartment prolapse, some of them very unlikely to effect anatomical restitution, and all with very limited outcome data. Ultrasound imaging will in the future allow us to identify the most appropriate intervention in the individual patient, and it is highly likely that some of the techniques used at present will soon become obsolete.

Assessment of the levator muscle and hiatus

One of the most important capabilities of translabial/perineal/introital ultrasound lies in the assessment of the lower aspects of the levator ani muscle. The topic of pelvic floor assessment is increasingly attracting attention from gynecologists, colorectal surgeons, urologists, and physiotherapists. This is largely due to the growing availability of 4D ultrasound, which allows cross-

sectional imaging in the axial plane, facilitating the diagnosis of delivery-related pelvic floor trauma. The integrity of the levator ani, or more specifically the integrity of the puborectalis muscle, which defines the vaginal high pressure zone [76] and the levator hiatus [77], is the best-defined etiological factor in the pathogenesis of female pelvic organ prolapse, especially as regards cystocele and uterine prolapse. As a result, any diagnostic assessment of a patient with prolapse is incomplete without evaluation of the puborectalis muscle.

We now know that "pelvic floor trauma" is much more than what we have been taught to identify and repair in the delivery suite. In 10–30% of all women who have given birth normally, the puborectalis component of the levator ani muscle is disconnected from its insertion, a form of trauma that has been termed "avulsion" [78–81]. Puborectalis avulsion is particularly common in women after forceps delivery [79,82], and it seems that predictors of obstructed labor, such as length of second stage and fetal size, also predict avulsion [83]. This is a recent discovery that has not yet found its way into most textbooks.

The levator ani is a muscular plate surrounding a central V-shaped hiatus, forming the caudal part of the abdominal envelope. As such, it encloses the largest potential hernial portal in the human body, the "levator hiatus," containing the urethra, vagina, and anorectum. Its peculiar shape and function is a compromise between priorities that are difficult to reconcile. On the one hand, abdominal contents have to be secured against gravity, on the other hand, solid and liquid wastes have to be evacuated. In addition, and most importantly, there are the requirements of reproduction: intercourse and childbirth. The latter is the most extreme of tasks required of the pelvic floor, in particular in view of the size of the baby's head. There are other mammalian species for whom giving birth is fraught with danger, but surely *Homo sapiens* ranks near the top of the list when it comes to the hazards of reproduction.

The levator ani is thought to consist of several major subdivisions, and there is considerable confusion in the literature regarding nomenclature and distinctions between pubococcygeus, pubovaginalis, puboperinealis, puborectalis, and iliococcygeus muscles. Since these muscles cannot consistently be distinguished either clinically or on ultrasound or magnetic resonance imaging or even cadaver dissection, the author

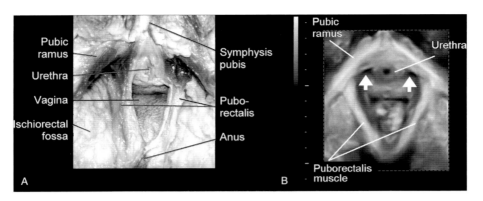

Fig. 10.20 Intact puborectalis muscle in a fresh cadaver, dissected from caudally (A). The vulva, mons pubis, clitoris, perineal muscles, and perineum to the anus, as well as peri- and postanal skin and the fibrofatty tissue of the ischiorectal fossa, have been removed to allow access to the puborectalis muscle. (B) The same representation on axial plane rendered volume in a patient with normal pelvic floor. This quality can be reached with a temporal resolution of 2 Hz or higher.

considers only the puborectalis muscle (as the V-shaped muscle originating on the os pubis/the inferior pubic ramus and surrounding the anorectal angle posteriorly) and the iliococcygeus muscle. The latter is a sheet of muscle that acts as a continuation of the puborectalis cranially and laterally. While the fiber direction is different from the puborectalis, on vaginal palpation the iliococcygeus is palpable as a continuation of the puborectalis above the inferior pubic ramus in the lateral vagina, extending from the pelvic sidewall to the ischial spine and the coccyx. It is possible to distinguish between puborectalis and iliococcygeus on palpation if one considers that the first inserts on the inferior pubic ramus and the second on the arcus tendineus of the levator ani, coursing over the obturator internus muscle.

Fig. 10.20A shows a fresh cadaver dissection of the levator ani muscle, with the puborectalis forming a V-shaped structure about as thick as a fifth finger, anchored to the inferior pubic ramus and the body of the os pubis ventrally. This dissection approach demonstrates the muscle as seen from below or caudally. The left side of the image is the patient's right side, the symphysis pubis is at the top. Fig. 10.20B demonstrates the appearance of the puborectalis muscle on 3D pelvic floor ultrasound, in a "rendered volume," i.e. a semitransparent representation of volume data. The arrows indicate the gap between muscle insertion and urethra, which is important for palpation.

The pelvic floor in childbirth

The levator ani muscle has to distend enormously [84,85] in childbirth. In about half of all women, there is no appreciable change in distensibility or morphological appearance after vaginal delivery [81], but over 40% seem to suffer either frank tears or irreversible overdistension of the hiatus, which has been termed "microtrauma" [86]. 3D/4D pelvic floor ultrasound is a highly useful, repeatable method for assessing the hiatus [77,87–89]. It is not understood how the puborectalis can remain intact after the excessive strain suffered in childbirth, but we assume that it is somehow due to protective hormonal effects of pregnancy and parturition. Childbirth affects the pelvic floor, but the same is likely to be true in the obverse.

The biomechanical properties of this muscle might have some effect on the progress of labor: a more elastic muscle seems to be associated with a shorter second stage of labor and possibly also with delivery mode [90,91].

Trauma to the puborectalis muscle as a consequence of childbirth was first reported in 1943, only to be forgotten for 60 years. It is difficult to believe, but this major form of maternal birth trauma, easily palpable vaginally and occasionally visible in the delivery suite in women with large vaginal tears [92] (Fig. 10.21), is missing from our obstetric and midwifery textbooks, and has only recently been rediscovered by imaging specialists using magnetic resonance and 3D/4D ultrasound. Vaginal operative delivery, length of second stage, and fetal size are likely to be risk factors [78,79,82,86,93,94]. Most commonly, appearances are those of an "avulsion," that is, a traumatic dislodgment of the muscle from its bony insertion. This appearance has also been confirmed in cadavers [95].

There are other forms of localized or generalized morphological abnormalities, but they are much less common and it seems that partial trauma has a much smaller effect on pelvic organ support [96]. Women with a highly dysfunctional pelvic floor often show an avulsion rather than pudendal neuropathy [97], which now appears unlikely to be a major factor in pelvic floor dysfunction [98], but which in the past was considered the main etiological factor in pelvic floor dysfunction [99,100]. "Healing" of muscular trauma seems unlikely, but there have been clearly documented instances of improved imaging appearances after 2–4 years [101].

Diagnosis of avulsion by ultrasound imaging

While palpation can be used to detect levator trauma [102–104], it seems that the diagnosis of levator trauma is more repeatable when undertaken by imaging. Magnetic resonance was the first method used to assess the levator ani [105], but it suffers from a number of obvious shortcomings: cost, accessibility, the inability to use magnetic resonance in women with ferrous implants, issues with claustrophobia in some women, the lack of dynamic imaging, and problems with defining correct planes, since very few currently used systems allow true volume imaging. Most of those

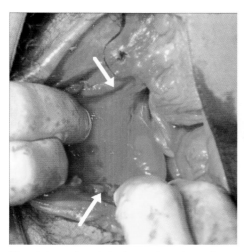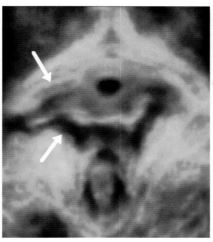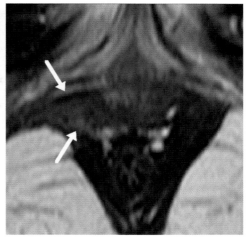

Fig. 10.21 Right-sided puborectalis avulsion after normal vaginal delivery at term. The left-hand image shows appearances immediately postpartum, with the avulsed muscle exposed by a large vaginal tear. The middle image shows a rendered volume (axial plane, translabial 3D ultrasound) 3 months postpartum, and the right-hand image shows magnetic resonance findings (single slice in the axial plane) at 3.5 months postpartum. Top arrows indicate the site of avulsion on the inferior pubic ramus, bottom arrows show the retracted stump of puborectalis. With permission, from Dietz HP, Gillespie A, Phadke P. Avulsion of the pubovisceral muscle associated with large vaginal tear after normal vaginal delivery at term. A case report. *Aust N Z J Obstet Gynaecol* 2007; 47: 341–44.

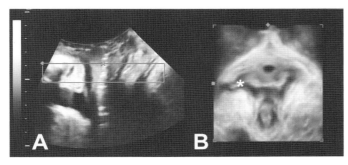

Fig. 10.22 Identification of a typical right-sided avulsion after normal vaginal delivery in a rendered volume, axial plane. The midsagittal plane (A) shows the location of the region of interest (ROI, the "box"), with the ROI of 1.5 cm thickness and placed so as to contain the plane of minimal dimensions. B shows the rendered volume in the axial plane, clearly identifying the avulsion defect (*).

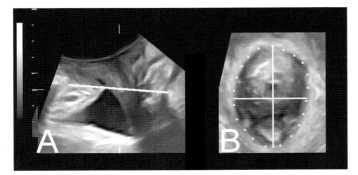

Fig. 10.23 Identification of the plane of minimal hiatal dimensions in an oblique axial plane (B) as identified in the midsagittal plane (A), in a patient with normal levator anatomy and function. This plane, while not always sufficient to diagnose avulsion injury, defines the levator hiatus, is used to determine hiatal dimensions and distensibility, and serves as a convenient reference plane for tomographic ultrasound imaging.

shortcomings do not apply to ultrasound, especially not to translabial 3D/4D ultrasound. This method uses technology that was developed for fetal imaging and that is now almost universally available. While transvaginal ultrasound has been used to image the levator ani [91,106,107], this requires side-firing endoprobes, which are not in general use and rarely found in imaging departments.

The diagnosis of levator trauma by transperineal (or perineal or introital) ultrasound was first described in 2004 [108] on "rendered volumes," that is, semitransparent representations of blocks of volume ultrasound data (Fig. 10.22), using Voluson-type systems and 3D/4D curved array volume transducers that were developed for fetal imaging. Acceptable quality can be obtained with acquisition angles of up to 85 degrees, encompassing the entire levator hiatus even on maximal Valsalva in a patient with severe prolapse, and at a volume frequency of up to 4 Hz. At lower acquisition angles, up to 20 Hz can be reached. This implies that temporal resolution in any plane is superior to magnetic resonance, while spatial resolution of structures within the levator hiatus up to about 4 cm depth is comparable to magnetic resonance, especially considering the better tissue discrimination of ultrasound on distinguishing vaginal muscularis and levator ani.

The diagnosis of avulsion by 3D ultrasound has been shown to be highly reproducible, in particular as compared with palpation [80,82,102]. Modern 3D ultrasound systems commonly allow tomographic imaging, i.e. serial cross-sections at arbitrarily variable inter-slice intervals and angles. Diagnosis by tomographic ultrasound is probably currently the most repeatable technique [109]. Fig. 10.23 shows identification of the plane of minimal dimensions as a reference plane and measurement of hiatal dimensions, while Fig. 10.24 demonstrates a tomographic representation of the entire puborectalis muscle based on this reference plane.

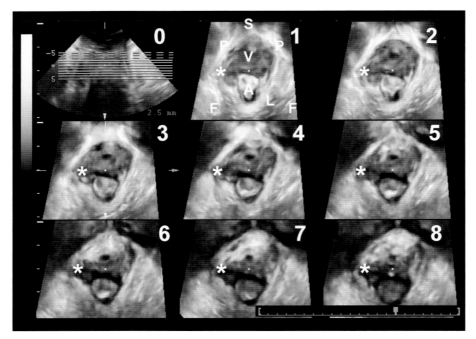

Fig. 10.24 Assessment of the puborectalis muscle by tomographic or multislice ultrasound in a patient with a complete right-sided avulsion. The top left-hand image (0) represents a reference image in the coronal plane. Images 1–8 show slices parallel to the plane of minimal hiatal dimensions. Slices 1 and 2 are 5 and 2.5 mm below this plane, slice 3 represents the plane of minimal dimensions, and slices 4–8 are 2.5–12.5 mm above this plane, likely encompassing the entire puborectalis muscle. The avulsion is identified by (*). S = symphysis pubis, P = inferior pubic ramus, V = vagina, L= levator ani, A = anus, F = ischiorectal fossa. From Dietz H (2007) Quantification of major morphological abnormalities of the levator ani. *Ultrasound Obstet Gynecol* 29:329–334. with permission.

Tomographic ultrasound is probably best performed by bracketing the area of interest, with the lowermost slice just below the insertion of the puborectalis muscle [110]. The three central slices of a tomographic set (i.e. the plane of minimal hiatal dimensions and the two slices 2.5 and 5 mm cranial to that plane) are sufficient to diagnose a full avulsion. Neither caudal nor more cranial slices add to diagnostic accuracy expressed as the odds ratio of symptoms or signs of prolapse [96], and the likelihood of a false-positive diagnosis seems very low [112].

Avulsion can in fact be diagnosed with 2D ultrasound, using the simplest and most commonly available abdominal curved array transducers. However, since there is no clearly identifiable point of reference for parasagittal translabial planes, it is more difficult to be certain of a complete avulsion, and, as a result, repeatability is probably inferior [113].

Regardless of which imaging method is used, clinical examination by palpation and imaging are best seen as complementary, rather than mutually exclusive. Frequently, one method will allow a better appreciation of findings obtained by the other method. The palpating finger provides biomechanical information on tone and contractility that is not currently available on imaging. On the other hand, imaging information is more objective and reproducible, and it provides information on deeper structures that are not accessible on palpation.

Consequences of levator trauma

Levator avulsion is associated with anterior and central compartment prolapse and likely represents the missing link (or a large part of the missing link) between childbirth and prolapse [114]. The larger a defect is, both in width and depth, the more likely are symptoms and/or signs of prolapse [109] are. Levator avulsion seems to at least triple the risk of significant anterior and central compartment prolapse [114], with much less of an effect on posterior compartment descent. This effect seems largely independent of ballooning [115] or abnormal distensibility of the levator hiatus, which also is associated with prolapse [55].

Many laypeople and medical practitioners as well as physiotherapists and continence nurse practitioners assume that urinary incontinence is a sign of a weak pelvic floor. This may not be true. We have recently shown that levator avulsion is *negatively* associated with stress urinary incontinence and urodynamic stress incontinence, and this association remained negative even after controlling for eight potential confounders, including all forms of female pelvic organ prolapse [116]. These findings are counterintuitive, but have been confirmed in a study using magnetic resonance [117].

The second major clinical symptom that has at times been attributed to an abnormal puborectalis muscle (via an opening of the anorectal angle) is fecal incontinence, but we have found no significant association between this symptom and levator trauma [118]. However, in a recent study using magnetic resonance there was a trend towards more fecal incontinence in women after anal sphincter tear who had also suffered levator trauma [119].

Finally, it seems likely that avulsion, especially if bilateral, would have some effect on sexual function. Many women note a reduction in pelvic floor muscle function after vaginal childbirth, and the degree of change is associated with sonographically documented trauma [120]. However, this effect seems to be limited to perceptions of vaginal laxity and reduced muscle strength [111]. Considering the popularity of cosmetic genitoplasty procedures aiming to "tighten" the vagina, this may become an important consideration in the future. In some women the site of the avulsion remains tender, even after decades, and some women and their partners notice a marked difference in sexual relations after the birth of their first child. Other couples, however, do not notice any change. For obvious reasons, this is not an issue that is easy to investigate.

Major morphological abnormalities of the levator ani probably affect surgical outcomes. A study using magnetic resonance imaging demonstrated that recurrence after anterior colporrhaphy was much more likely in women with an abnormal pelvic floor [121]. The author's unit has recently shown that avulsion is associated with prolapse after hysterectomy, anti-incontinence operations, and prolapse operations, especially after anterior repair [122,123]. It seems that, while an anterior colporrhaphy in a patient with intact levator ani results in good anterior compartment support in about 80% at 4 years, this is the case in only 20% of women with levator avulsion [124]. In view of the current, often acrimonious discussion regarding the use of mesh implants in reconstructive surgery, this association may turn out to be of major clinical importance. Anterior compartment mesh seems associated with reduced recurrence rates [125,126], especially in women with avulsion [127].

Is there anything we can do to repair avulsion injury, either immediately after childbirth, or at a later date? From a plastic surgery point of view, surgical failure due to suture dislodgment seems very likely in the postpartum setting, given the quality of the tissues and the fact that there is no opportunity for splinting or immobilization. It is not surprising that intrapartum attempts at avulsion repair have been unsuccessful [92]. Direct repair may have to wait several months and may have to utilize autologous fascia or mesh. The author has developed a direct repair technique through a lateral distal colpotomy, but in a series of 20 avulsion repairs in 17 women (3 bilateral) we have found that the effect on recurrence and hiatal dimensions is disappointing [129]. This is consistent with mathematical modeling [130] and probably due to coexistent microtrauma [86] and/or contralateral trauma.

In a different approach, the author's unit has developed a minimally invasive concept that may partly compensate for avulsion defects and over distension of the levator muscle [131], addressing "ballooning" directly. Unfortunately, avulsion represents only a fraction of the damage sustained by the levator ani in childbirth [86]. Either way, it likely will be many years

before any reconstructive surgical approach can be regarded as proven and ready for general use.

References

1. Bump RC, Mattiasson A, Bo K, et al. The standardization of terminology of female pelvic organ prolapse and pelvic floor dysfunction. *Am J Obstet Gynecol* 1996; **175**: 10–17.
2. O'Boyle AL, Woodman PJ, O'Boyle JD, et al. Pelvic organ support in nulliparous pregnant and nonpregnant women: a case control study. *Am J Obstet Gynecol* 2002; **187**: 99–102.
3. Dietz H, Eldridge A, Grace M, Clarke B. Pelvic organ descent in young nulliparous women. *Am J Obstet Gynecol* 2004; **191**: 95–99.
4. Dalpiaz O, Curti P. Role of perineal ultrasound in the evaluation of urinary stress incontinence and pelvic organ prolapse: a systematic review. *Neurourol Urodyn* 2006; **25**: 301–306.
5. Dietz HP, Clarke B. The influence of posture on perineal ultrasound imaging parameters. *Int Urogynecol J* 2001; **12**: 104–106.
6. Oerno A, Dietz H. Levator co-activation is a significant confounder of pelvic organ descent on Valsalva maneuver. *Ultrasound Obstet Gynecol* 2007; **30**: 346–350.
7. Yang A, Mostwin JL, Rosenshein NB, Zerhouni EA. Pelvic floor descent in women: dynamic evaluation with fast MR imaging and cinematic display. *Radiology* 1991; **179**: 25–33.
8. Bo K, Larson S, Oseid S, et al. Knowledge about and ability to do correct pelvic floor muscle exercises in women with urinary stress incontinence. *Neurourol Urodyn* 1988; **7**: 261–262.
9. Dietz HP, Wilson PD. The influence of bladder volume on the position and mobility of the urethrovesical junction. *Int Urogynecol J* 1999; **10**: 3–6.
10. Orejuela F, Shek K, Dietz H. The time factor in the assessment of prolapse and levator ballooning. *Int Urogynecol J* 2010; **21**: S365–367.
11. Thompson JA, O'Sullivan PB, Briffa K, et al. Assessment of pelvic floor movement using transabdominal and transperineal ultrasound. *Int Urogynecol J* 2005; **16**: 285–292.
12. Wijma J, Tinga DJ, Visser GH. Perineal ultrasonography in women with stress incontinence and controls: the role of the pelvic floor muscles. *Gynecol Obstet Invest* 1991; **32**: 176–179.
13. Peschers UM, Schaer GN, DeLancey JO, Schuessler B. Levator ani function before and after childbirth. *Br J Obstet Gynaecol* 1997; **104**: 1004–1008.
14. Dietz H. Levator function before and after childbirth. *Aust N Z J Obstet Gynaecol* 2004; **44**: 19–23.
15. Dietz HP, Wilson PD, Clarke B. The use of perineal ultrasound to quantify levator activity and teach pelvic floor muscle exercises. *Int Urogynecol J Pelvic Floor Dysfunction* 2001; **12**: 166–168; discussion 168–169.
16. Miller JM, Perucchini D, Carchidi LT, et al. Pelvic floor muscle contraction during a cough and decreased vesical neck mobility. *Obstet Gynecol* 2001; **97**: 255–260.
17. Dietz HP, Jarvis SK, Vancaillie TG. The assessment of levator muscle strength: a validation of three ultrasound techniques. *Int Urogynecol J* 2002; **13**: 156–159.

18. Dietz HP, Velez D, Shek KL, Martin A. Determination of postvoid residual by translabial ultrasound. *Int Urogynecol J* 2012; **23**: 1749–1752.

19. Schaer GN, Koechli OR, Schuessler B, Haller U. Perineal ultrasound for evaluating the bladder neck in urinary stress incontinence. *Obstet Gynecol* 1995; **85**: 220–224.

20. Dietz HP, Wilson PD. Anatomical assessment of the bladder outlet and proximal urethra using ultrasound and videocystourethrography. *Int Urogynecol J* 1998; **9**: 365–369.

21. Martan A, Masata J, Halaska M, Voigt R. Ultrasound imaging of the lower urinary system in women after Burch colposuspension. *Ultrasound Obstet Gynecol* 2001; **17**: 58–64.

22. Dietz HP, Eldridge A, Grace M, Clarke B. Pelvic organ descent in young nulligravid women. *Am J Obstet Gynecol* 2004; **191**: 95–99.

23. Dietz H. Ultrasound Imaging of the pelvic floor. Part 1: 2D aspects. *Ultrasound Obstet Gynecol* 2004; **23**: 80–92.

24. Peschers U, Schaer G, Anthuber C, et al. Changes in vesical neck mobility following vaginal delivery. *Obstet Gynecol* 1996; **88**: 1001–1006.

25. Dietz HP, Bennett MJ. The effect of childbirth on pelvic organ mobility. *Obstet Gynecol* 2003; **102**: 223–228.

26. Dietz HP, Clarke B, Vancaillie TG. Vaginal childbirth and bladder neck mobility. *Aust N Z J Obstet Gynaecol* 2002; **42**: 522–525.

27. Pirpiris A, Shek K, Dietz H. Urethral mobility and urinary incontinence. *Ultrasound Obstet Gynecol* 2010; **36**: 507–511.

28. Huang WC, Yang JM. Bladder neck funneling on ultrasound cystourethrography in primary stress urinary incontinence: a sign associated with urethral hypermobility and intrinsic sphincter deficiency. *Urology* 2003; **61**: 936–941.

29. Nazemian K, Shek K, Martin A, Dietz H. Can urodynamic stress incontinence be diagnosed by ultrasound? *Int Urogynecol J* 2011; **22**: S19–20.

30. Masata J, Martan A, Halaska M, et al. Ultrasound imaging of urethral funneling. *Int Urogynecol J* 1999; **10**:S62.

31. Dietz HP, Clarke B. The urethral pressure profile and ultrasound parameters of bladder neck mobility. *Neurourol Urodynam* 1998; **17**: 374–375.

32. Dietz HP, Wilson PD. Colposuspension success and failure: a long-term objective follow-up study. *Int Urogynecol J* 2000; **11**: 346–351.

33. Harms L, Emons G, Bader W, et al. Funneling before and after anti-incontinence surgery – a prognostic indicator? Part 2: tension-free vaginal tape. *Int Urogynecol J* 2007; **18**: 189–294.

34. Eisenberg V, Chantarasorn V, Shek KL, Dietz HP. Does levator ani injury affect cystocele type? *Ultrasound Obstet Gynecol* 2010; **36**: 618–623.

35. Greenwald SW, Thornbury JR, Dunn LJ. Cystourethrography as a diagnostic aid in stress incontinence. *Obstet Gynecol* 1967; **29**: 324–327.

36. Chantarasorn V, Dietz H. Diagnosis of cystocele type by clinical examination and pelvic floor ultrasound. *Ultrasound Obstet Gynecol* 2012; **39**: 710–714.

37. Giannitsas K, Athanasopoulos A. Female urethral diverticula: from pathogenesis to management. An update. *Exp Rev Obstet Gynecol* 2010; **5**: 57–66.

38. Schuettoff S, Beyersdorff D, Gauruder-Burmester A, Tunn R. Visibility of the polypropylene tape after TVT (tension-free vaginal tape) procedure in women with stress urinary incontinence – a comparison of introital ultrasound and MRI in vitro and in patients. *Ultrasound Obstet Gynecol* 2006; **27**: 687–692.

39. Kaum HJ, Wolff F. TVT: on midurethral tape positioning and its influence on continence. *Int Urogynecol J* 2002; **13**: 110–115.

40. Fischer T, Ladurner R, Gangkofer A, et al. Functional cine MRI of the abdomen for the assessment of implanted synthetic mesh in patients after incisional hernia repair: initial results. *Eur Radiol* 2007; **17**: 3123–3129.

41. Dietz H, Wilson P. The Iris Effect: how 2D and 3D volume ultrasound can help us understand anti-incontinence procedures. *Ultrasound Obstet Gynecol* 2004; **23**: 267–271.

42. Dietz H, Barry C, Lim Y, Rane A. TVT vs Monarc: a comparative study. *Int Urogynecol J* 2006; **17**: 566–569.

43. Dietz HP, Barry C, Lim YN, Rane A. Two-dimensional and three-dimensional ultrasound imaging of suburethral slings. *Ultrasound Obstet Gynecol* 2005; **26**: 175–179.

44. Dietz HP, Foote AJ, Mak HL, Wilson PD. TVT and Sparc suburethral slings: a case-control series. *Int Urogynecol J* 2004; **15**: 129–131.

45. Kociszewski J, Rautenberg O, Kolben S, et al. Tape functionality: position, change in shape, and outcome after TVT procedure – mid-term results. *Int Urogynecol J* 2010; **21**: 795–800.

46. Ng CC, Lee LC, Han WH. Use of three-dimensional ultrasound scan to assess the clinical importance of midurethral placement of the tension-free vaginal tape (TVT) for treatment of incontinence. *Int Urogynecol J* 2005; **16**: 220–225.

47. Chantarasorn V, Shek K, Dietz H. Sonographic appearance of transobturator slings: implications for function and dysfunction. *Int Urogynecol J* 2011; **22**: 493–498.

48. Mulder F, Shek KL, Dietz HP. The pressure factor in the assessment of pelvic organ mobility. *Aust NZ J Obstet Gynaecol* 2012; **52**: 282–285.

49. Feiner B, Jelovsek J, Maher C. Efficacy and safety of transvaginal mesh kits in the treatment of prolapse of the vaginal apex: a systematic review. *Br J Obstet Gynaecol* 2009; **116**: 15–24.

50. Velemir L, Amblard J, Fatton B, et al. Transvaginal mesh repair of anterior and posterior vaginal wall prolapse: a clinical and ultrasonographic study. *Ultrasound Obstet Gynecol* 2010; **35**(4): 474–480.

51. Svabik K, Martan A, Masata J, Elhaddad R, Hubka P. Ultrasound appearances after mesh implantation – evidence of mesh contraction or folding? *Int Urogynecol J* 2011; **22**(5): 529–533.

52. Erdmann M, Shek K, Dietz HP. Mesh contraction: myth or reality? *Am J Obstet Gynecol* 2011; **204**(2): 173.e1–4.

53. Shek K, Rane A, Goh J, Dietz H. Perigee versus Anterior Prolift in the treatment of cystocele. *Int Urogynecol J* 2008; **19**: S88.

54. Shek K, Dietz HP, Rane A, Balakrishan S. Transobturator mesh repair for large and recurrent cystocele. *Ultasound Obstet Gynecol* 2008; **3**: 82–86.

55. Dietz H, De Leon J, Shek K. Ballooning of the levator hiatus. *Ultrasound Obstet Gynecol* 2008; **31**: 676–680.

56. Shek K, Rane A, Goh J, Dietz H. Stress urinary incontinence after transobturator mesh for cystocele repair. *Int Urogynecol J* 2009; **20**: 421–425.

57. Tunn R, Petri E. Introital and transvaginal ultrasound as the main tool in the assessment of urogenital and pelvic floor dysfunction: an imaging panel and practical approach. *Ultrasound Obstet Gynecol* 2003; **22**: 205–213.

58. Wong V, Shek KL, Dietz HP. A comparison of two forms of mesh anchoring. *Aust NZ J Obstet Gynaecol* 2014; in print.

59. Yang JM, Huang WC. Bladder wall thickness on ultrasonographic cystourethrography: affecting factors and their implications. *J Ultrasound Med* 2003; **22**: 777–782.

60. Lekskulchai O, Dietz H. Detrusor wall thickness as a test for detrusor overactivity in women. *Ultrasound Obstet Gynecol* 2008; **32**: 535–539.

61. Robinson D, Anders K, Cardozo L, et al. Can ultrasound replace ambulatory urodynamics when investigating women with irritative urinary symptoms? *Br J Obstet Gynaecol* 2002; **109**: 145–148.

62. Robinson D, Khullar V, Cardozo L. Can bladder wall thickness predict postoperative detrusor overactivity? *Int Urogynecol J* 2005; **16**: S106.

63. Dietz H, Wilson P. Long-term success after open and laparoscopic colposuspension: a case control study. *Gynaecol Endoscopy* 2002; **11**: 81–84.

64. Dietz H, Wilson P. Laparoscopic colposuspension vs. urethropexy: a case control series. *Int Urogynecol J* 2005; **16**: 15–18.

65. Bombieri L, Freeman RM. Do bladder neck position and amount of elevation influence the outcome of colposuspension? *Br J Obstet Gynaecol* 2003; **110**: 197–200.

66. Dietz HP, Korda A. Which bowel symptoms are most strongly associated with a true rectocele? *Aust N Z J Obstet Gynaecol* 2005; **45**: 505–508.

67. Dietz HP, Steensma AB. Posterior compartment prolapse on two-dimensional and three-dimensional pelvic floor ultrasound: the distinction between true rectocele, perineal hypermobility and enterocele. *Ultrasound Obstet Gynecol* 2005; **26**: 73–77.

68. Beer-Gabel M, Teshler M, Schechtman E, Zbar AP. Dynamic transperineal ultrasound vs. defecography in patients with evacuatory difficulty: a pilot study. *Int J Colorect Dis* 2004; **19**: 60–67.

69. Zbar A, Beer-Gabel M. Dynamic transperineal ultrasonography. In: Pescatori M, Regadas F, Murad Regadas S, Zbar A, eds. *Imaging Atlas of the Pelvic Floor and Anorectal Diseases*. Milan: Springer Italia; 2008.

70. Rodrigo N, Shek K, Dietz H. Rectal intussusception is associated with abnormal levator structure and morphometry. *Tech Coloproctol* 2011; **15**(1): 39–43.

71. Perniola G, Shek K, Dietz H, et al. Can ultrasound replace xray proctography in women with obstructed defecation? *Ultrasound Obstet Gynecol* 2007; **30**(4): 446.

72. Steensma AB, Oom DMJ, Burger CW, Schouten WR. Comparison of defecography and 3D/4D translabial ultrasound in patients with pelvic organ prolapse and/or evacuation disorders. *Ultrasound Obstet Gynecol* 2007; **30**: 447.

73. Konstantinovic ML, Steensma AB, Domali E, et al. Correlation between 3D/4D translabial ultrasound and colpocystodefecography in diagnosis of posterior compartment prolapse. *Ultrasound Obstet Gynecol* 2007; **30**: 448.

74. Grasso R, Piciucchi S, Quattrocchi C, et al. Posterior pelvic floor disorders: a prospective comparison using introital ultrasound and colpocystodefecography. *Ultrasound Obstet Gynecol* 2007; **30**: 86–94.

75. Richardson AC. The rectovaginal septum revisited: its relationship to rectocele and its importance in rectocele repair. *Clin Obstet Gynecol* 1993; **36**: 976–983.

76. Jung S, Pretorius D, Padda B, et al. Vaginal high-pressure zone assessed by dynamic 3-dimensional ultrasound images of the pelvic floor. *Am J Obstet Gynecol* 2007; **197**: 52.e1–7.

77. Dietz H, Shek K, Clarke B. Biometry of the pubovisceral muscle and levator hiatus by three-dimensional pelvic floor ultrasound. *Ultrasound Obstet Gynecol* 2005; **25**: 580–585.

78. Dietz H, Lanzarone V. Levator trauma after vaginal delivery. *Obstet Gynecol* 2005; **106**: 707–712.

79. Kearney R, Miller J, Ashton-Miller J, Delancey J. Obstetric factors associated with levator ani muscle injury after vaginal birth. *Obstet Gynecol* 2006; **107**: 144–149.

80. Dietz HP, Steensma AB. The prevalence of major abnormalities of the levator ani in urogynaecological patients. *Br J Obstet Gynaecol* 2006; **113**: 225–230.

81. Shek K, Dietz H. The effect of childbirth on hiatal dimensions: a prospective observational study. *Obstet Gynecol* 2009; **113**: 1272–1278.

82. Krofta L, Otcenasek M, Kasikova E, Feyereisl J. Pubococcygeus-puborectalis trauma after forceps delivery: evaluation of the levator ani muscle with 3D/4D ultrasound. *Int Urogynecol J* 2009; **20**: 1175–1181.

83. Valsky DV, Lipschuetz M, Bord A, et al. Fetal head circumference and length of second stage of labor are risk factors for levator ani muscle injury, diagnosed by 3-dimensional transperineal ultrasound in primiparous women. *Am J Obstet Gynecol* 2009; **201**: 91.e1–91.e7.

84. Lien KC, Mooney B, DeLancey JO, Ashton-Miller JA. Levator ani muscle stretch induced by simulated vaginal birth. *Obstet Gynecol* 2004; **103**: 31–40.

85. Svabik K, Shek K, Dietz H. How much does the levator hiatus have to stretch during childbirth? *Br J Obstet Gynaecol* 2009; **116**: 1657–1662.

86. Shek K, Dietz H. Intrapartum risk factors of levator trauma. *Br J Obstet Gynaecol* 2010; **117**: 1485–1492.

87. Yang J, Yang S, Huang W. Biometry of the pubovisceral muscle and levator hiatus in nulliparous Chinese women. *Ultrasound Obstet Gynecol* 2006; **26**: 710–716.

88. Kruger J, Dietz H, Murphy B. Pelvic floor function in elite nulliparous athletes and controls. *Ultrasound Obstet Gynecol* 2007; **30**: 81–85.

89. Hoff Braekken I, Majida M, Ellstrom Engh M, et al. Test-retest and intra-observer repeatability of two-, three- and four-dimensional perineal ultrasound of pelvic floor muscle anatomy and function. *Int Urogynecol J* 2008; **19**: 227–235.

90. Lanzarone V, Dietz H. 3Dimensional ultrasound imaging of the levator hiatus in late pregnancy and associations with delivery outcomes. *Aust N Z J Obstet Gynaecol* 2007; **47**: 176–180.

91. Balmforth J, Toosz-Hobson P, Cardozo L. Ask not what childbirth can do to your pelvic floor but what your pelvic floor can do in childbirth. *Neurourol Urodyn* 2003; **22**: 540–542.

92. Dietz H, Gillespie A, Phadke P. Avulsion of the pubovisceral muscle associated with large vaginal tear after normal vaginal delivery at term. *Aust N Z J Obstet Gynaecol* 2007; **47**: 341–344.

93. Cassado Garriga J, Pessarodona Isern A, Espuna Pons M, et al. Tridimensional sonographic anatomical changes on pelvic floor muscle according to the type of delivery. *Int Urogynecol J* 2011;**22**(8): 1011–1018.

94. Falkert A, Endress E, Weigl M, Seelbach-Göbel B. Three-dimensional ultrasound of the pelvic floor 2 days after first delivery: influence of constitutional and obstetric factors. *Ultrasound Obstet Gynecol* 2010; **35**: 583–588.

95. Wallner C, Wallace C, Maas C, et al. A high resolution 3D study of the female pelvis reveals important anatomical and pathological details of the pelvic floor. *Neurourol Urodyn* 2009; **28**: 668–670.

96. Dietz H, Bernardo M, Kirby A, Shek K. Minimal criteria for the diagnosis of avulsion of the puborectalis muscle by tomographic ultrasound. *Int Urogynecol J* 2011; **22**(6): 699–704.

97. Sarma S, Hersch M, Siva S, et al. Women who cannot contract their pelvic floor muscles: avulsion or denervation? *Neurourol Urodyn* 2009; **28**: 680–681.

98. Dietz H, Habtemariam T, Williams G. Pelvic floor structure in women with vesicovaginal fistula. *J Urol* 2012; **188**(5): 1772–1777.

99. Swash M, Snooks SJ, Henry MM. Unifying concept of pelvic floor disorders and incontinence. *J R Soc Med* 1985; **78**: 906–911.

100. Allen RE, Hosker GL, Smith AR, Warrell DW. Pelvic floor damage and childbirth: a neurophysiological study. *Br J Obstet Gynaecol* 1990; **97**: 770–779.

101. Shek K, Chantarsorn V, Langer S, Dietz HP. Does levator trauma heal? *Ultrasound Obstet Gynecol* 2012; **40**(5) 570–575.

102. Dietz HP, Shek KL. Validity and reproducibility of the digital detection of levator trauma. *Int Urogynecol J* 2008; **19**: 1097–1101.

103. Dietz HP, Shek C. Levator avulsion and grading of pelvic floor muscle strength. *Int Urogynecol J* 2008; **19**: 633–636.

104. Kearney R, Miller JM, Delancey JO. Interrater reliability and physical examination of the pubovisceral portion of the levator ani muscle, validity comparisons using MR imaging. *Neurourol Urodyn* 2006; **25**: 50–54.

105. Debus-Thiede G. Magnetic resonance imaging (MRI) of the pelvic floor. In: Schuessler B, Laycock J, Norton P, Stanton SL, eds. *Pelvic Floor Reeducation – Principles and Practice*. London: Springer; 1994.

106. Toosz- Hobson P, Athanasiou S, Khullar V, et al. Does vaginal delivery damage the pelvic floor? *Neurourol Urodyn* 1997; **16**: 385–386.

107. Athanasiou S, Chaliha C, Toozs-Hobson P, et al. Direct imaging of the pelvic floor muscles using two-dimensional ultrasound: a comparison of women with urogenital prolapse versus controls. *Br J Obstet Gynaecol* 2007; **114**: 882–888.

108. Dietz H. Ultrasound imaging of the pelvic floor: 3D aspects. *Ultrasound Obstet Gynecol* 2004; **23**: 615–625.

109. Dietz H. Quantification of major morphological abnormalities of the levator ani. *Ultrasound Obstet Gynecol* 2007; **29**: 329–334.

110. Dietz H. Tomographic ultrasound of the pelvic floor: which levels matter most? *Ultrasound Obstet Gynecol* 2009; **33**: 698–703.

111. Thibault-Gagnon S, Yusuf S, Langer S, Wong V, Shek KL, Dietz HP. Do women notice the impact of childbirth-related levator trauma on pelvic floor and sexual function? Results of an observational ultrasound study. *Int Urogynecol J* 2014; in print.

112. Adi Suroso T, Shek KL, Dietz HP. Tomographic imaging of the pelvic floor in nulliparous women: limits of normality. *Ultrasound Obstet Gynecol* 2012; **39**: 698–703.

113. Dietz HP, Shek KL. Levator defects can be diagnosed by 2D translabial ultrasound. *Int Urogynecol J* 2009; **20**: 807–811.

114. Dietz H, Simpson J. Levator trauma is associated with pelvic organ prolapse. *Br J Obstet Gynaecol* 2008; **115**: 979–984.

115. Abdool Z, Shek K, Dietz H. The effect of levator avulsion on hiatal dimensions and function. *Am J Obstet Gynecol* 2009; **201**: 89.e1–89.e5.

116. Dietz H, Kirby A, Shek K, Bedwell P. Does avulsion of the puborectalis muscle affect bladder function? *Int Urogynecol J* 2009; **20**: 967–972.

117. Morgan D, Cardoza P, Guire K, et al. Levator ani defect status and lower urinary tract symptoms in women with pelvic organ prolapse. *Int Urogynecol J* 2010; **21**: 47–52.

118. Chantarasorn V, Shek KL, Dietz HP. Sonographic detection of puborectalis muscle avulsion is not associated with fecal incontinence. *Aust NZ J Obstet Gynaecol* 2011; **51**: 130–135.

119. Heilbrun M, Nygaard I, Lockhart ME, et al. Correlation between levator ani muscle injuries on magnetic resonance imaging and fecal incontinence, pelvic organ prolapse, and urinary incontinence in primiparous women. *Am J Obstet Gynecol* 2010; **202**: 488.e1–6.

120. Dietz H, Shek K, Chantarasorn V, Langer S. Do women notice the effect of levator trauma? *Aust NZ J Obstet Gynecol* 2012; **52**: 277–281.

121. Adekanmi OA, Freeman R, Puckett M, Jackson S. Cystocele: does anterior repair fail because we fail to correct the fascial defects? A clinical and radiological study. *Int Urogynecol J* 2005; **16**: S73.

122. Dietz HP, Chantarasorn V, Shek KL. Levator avulsion is a risk factor for cystocele recurrence. *Ultrasound Obstet Gynecol* 2010; **36**: 76–80.

123. Model A, Shek KL, Dietz HP. Levator defects are associated with risk of prolapse after pelvic floor surgery. *Eur J Obstet Gynecol Reprod Biol* 2010; **153**: 220–223.

124. Dietz HP, Chantarasorn V, Shek KL. Levator avulsion is a risk factor for cystocele recurrence. *Ultrasound Obstet Gynecol* 2010; **36**: 76–80.

125. Wong V, Shek K, Goh J,Rane A,Dietz HP. Cystocele recurrence after anterior colporrhaphy with and without mesh use. *EJOGRB* 2014; **172**: 131–5.

126. Altman D, Väyrynen T, Ellström Engh M, et al. Anterior colporrhaphy versus transvaginal mesh for pelvic-organ prolapse. *N Engl J Med* 2011; **364**: 1826–1836.

127. Wong V, Shek K, Rane A, Goh J, Krause H, Dietz HP. Is levator avulsion a predictor of recurrence after anterior compartment mesh? *UOG* 2013; **42**(2): 230–234.

128. Shek KL, Wong V, Lee J, Rosamilia A, Rane AJ, Krause H, Goh H, Dietz HP. Anterior compartment mesh: a descriptive study of mesh anchoring failure. *Ultrasound Obstet Gynecol* 2013; **42**(6): 699–704.

129. Dietz H, Shek K, Daly O, Korda A. Can levator avulsion be repaired surgically? *Int Urogynecol J* 2013; **24**: 1011–1015.

130. Dietz HP, Bhalla R, Chantarasorn V, Shek KL. Avulsion of the puborectalis muscle causes asymmetry of the levator hiatus. *Ultrasound Obstet Gynecol* 2011; **37**: 723–726.

131. Dietz H, Korda A, Benness C, Wong V, Shek KL, Daly O. Surgical reduction of levator hiatus. *Neurourol Urodyn* 2012; **31**(6): 872–873.

Ultrasound imaging in endometriosis

Luciano G. Nardo, Sree Durga Patchava and Spyridon Chouliaras

Introduction

Endometriosis remains an enigmatic disease, which causes significant morbidity in reproductive-age women with a detrimental impact on their quality of life. Endometriosis is characterized by the presence of functional endometrial glands and stroma in extrauterine sites [1,2]. It remains a challenging condition for clinicians and patients alike owing to its etiology, pathophysiology, and progression. Several factors seem to favor development of the disease, such as early menarche, nulliparity, Asian or European ethnic origin, and a family history of endometriosis [3]. Various estimates suggest that between 6–44% of women of reproductive age have endometriosis [4]. This wide variation in the reported prevalence of endometriosis often reflects investigators' biases at the time of studies [5].

Clinical characteristics

Endometriosis is essentially a disease of symptoms and clinical signs are difficult to elicit. Surprisingly, it may be asymptomatic as noted in one-fifth of women in the Brisbane series [6], in whom the disease was coincidentally diagnosed during other surgical procedures. Considerable diagnostic delay of up to 8 years from presenting symptoms has been reported, which often confers a heavy economic and social burden [7].

Dysmenorrhea is the cardinal symptom of endometriosis and occurs in 85% of women with this condition. There is a congestive phase of pelvic discomfort often felt for several days, gradually increasing during the second half of the menstrual cycle from the time of ovulation. The actual incidence of dysmenorrhea is difficult to assess and depends on many complex and variable factors, including prevailing social and sexual attitudes in different societies.

The pain during intercourse is felt in any coital position that facilitates deep penetration in 25–40% of women. The pain is fairly localized and can be quite severe, especially in women with deposits in the rectovaginal space and uterosacral ligaments, causing significant disruption to sex life.

The existence of pain on defecation (also known as dyschezia) at the time of menstruation should always be investigated in women who experience deep dyspareunia. Nonspecific pelvic pain unrelated to the menstrual cycle occurred in 16% of women with endometriosis. It is important to realize that the severity of the pain is not related to the score on the revised scale of the AFS (American Fertility Society) scale [8].

Some authors have suggested that the relationship of mild endometriosis with infertility is casual rather than causal [9]. There is little doubt that severe endometriosis with large endometriomas of the ovary and gross distortion of the fallopian tube that is invariably patent, but unable to function effectively because of swelling and stretching over the ovary, is causally linked to infertility.

Classification

Laparoscopy is the gold standard for the diagnosis and classification of pelvic endometriosis. During laparoscopy, endometriosis is classified according to the revised American Fertility Society classification r-AFS [8]. The r-AFS classification is based on a number of points given for the presence of ovarian or peritoneal endometriosis (subdivided into superficial and deep), the presence of adhesions, and posterior cul-de-sac obliteration. On the basis of the overall score women are categorized as having minimal, mild, moderate, or severe disease. Due to fair reproducibility [10] and absent correlation between stage of disease, various pain symptoms [11], and the severity of disease [12], the clinical value of the actual classification remains a matter of debate [12,13].

Types

Endometriosis [14] involves many peritoneal and extraperitoneal sites [15]. The most frequent locations are in the pelvic area, with other sites having a lesser frequency [14,15].

- Pelvic endometriosis: this refers to lesions located in the ovaries, the rectovaginal space, or the pelvic peritoneum [3,5]. Pelvic endometriosis presents as superficial, ovarian, and deep-infiltrating [2].
- Superficial endometriosis: endometriotic foci in the peritoneal serosa may present according to their

Ultrasonography in Gynecology, ed. Botros R. M. B. Rizk and Elizabeth E. Puscheck. Published by Cambridge University Press. © Cambridge University Press 2015.

activity as purple/black spots, red lesions, adhesions, or yellowish dots.

- Endometrioma or cystic endometriosis: hemorrhagic ovarian cysts with an inner wall of endothelial mucosa.
- Deep infiltrating endometriosis: endometriotic lesions that penetrate at least 5 mm into the retroperitoneal space.
- Extrapelvic endometriosis: this refers to all the other implants, including the gastrointestinal and urinary systems, the liver, pancreas, spleen, lungs, the extremities, the skin, and the nervous system [14].

Diagnosis

The diagnosis of endometriosis still presents several problems, resulting from similarities in clinical symptoms to other benign or malignant gynecological diseases. These gynecological symptoms may, however, be of diagnostic help in the suspicion of endometriosis, which should be included in the differential diagnosis in any patient presenting with worsening dysmenorrhea, pelvic pain, dyspareunia, or other cycle-associated symptoms related particularly to the bowel or bladder, with or without infertility.

Physical findings of endometriosis are nonspecific. Localized tenderness along the uterosacral ligaments and the cul-de-sac is often present. Thickened or nodular ligamental or rectovaginal masses may be palpated. Adnexal tenderness or masses may be found and felt if there is ovarian involvement. Pelvic organs may be fixed from adhesions, with the uterus often fixed in a retroverted position [1]. The physical examination should be performed during early menses because implants are more likely to be large and tender at this time in the cycle. However, most women with endometriosis have normal or nonspecific results from physical examinations.

With the current practice of combining diagnostic and operative procedures in laparoscopy, the risk exists that unexpected operative findings may lead to under-treatment or unnecessary surgery. Unfortunately, laparoscopy is a costly, invasive procedure, requiring general anesthesia, and it is inevitably associated with rare, but potentially severe complications [16]. Noninvasive imaging techniques are therefore becoming increasingly important to preoperatively determine the presence and extent of the surgical pathology. Whenever possible, with the use of noninvasive techniques, the decision to operate or not should be based on accurate preoperative diagnosis and proper assessment of the extent of the disease. Imaging techniques currently and commonly used to diagnose endometriosis are ultrasound scan (USS) and magnetic resonance imaging (MRI).

USS for diagnosis of superficial endometriosis

Pelvic endometriotic peritoneal implants are difficult to detect by conventional ultrasonography. They are usually very small in size and their identification in the serosa or uterosacral

ligaments is limited. However, recent experimental work in animals with high-resolution ultrasound imaging using a frequency of 40 MHz and a focal depth of 6 mm enabled the in vivo analysis of intraperitoneal endometriotic lesions [17]. Development of this technique may provide a new dimension in the noninvasive diagnosis of peritoneal endometriosis.

USS for diagnosis of endometriomas

The ultrasonographic findings most commonly associated with endometriosis are endometriotic cysts of the ovary. Historically, these have been described as early as in 1921 by Sampson who introduced the term "chocolate cysts," due to the cyst's content usually being old clotted blood [18]. The endometrioma can be unilateral or bilateral in up to half of the cases. Unilateral endometriomas occur more frequently in the left ovary [19]. They rarely exceed 15 cm in diameter and can be unilocular or multilocular. The cyst wall is usually smoothed, thick, and fibrotic.

Transabdominal (TA) and even more so transvaginal (TV) USS performs well in detecting endometriomas. In a systematic review of six studies using grayscale TV ultrasound imaging, the positive (7.6–29.8) and negative (0.1–0.4) likelihood ratios suggested that ultrasound can accurately confirm and exclude the diagnosis. In these studies the diameter of the endometriomas, when reported, was greater than 18 mm. Therefore, the diagnosis of smaller endometriomas with conventional grayscale imaging has not been validated [20].

The use of high-frequency transducers in TV sonography and the continuous advancement in the technology of ultrasonographic equipment results in improved delineation of pelvic structures and anatomy. There are always pitfalls and diagnostic challenges, as endometriomas can mimic sonographically different structures (Table 11.1). Multilocular endometriomas can manifest a variety of characteristics as a result of the continuous process of resolution of the cyst's content.

The typical image of an endometrioma has been described as demonstrating diffuse low-level homogeneous internal echoes with a "ground-glass" texture (Fig. 11.1A). In one study, 95% of the endometriomas had this appearance [21]; however, in other studies, slightly different definitions for the "classic" appearance of an endometrioma have been used [22,23].

Patel et al. [21] in an original paper analyzed the sonographic features associated with endometriomas, giving specific consideration to the examination of the endometriotic cyst wall:

(a) *Hyperechoic wall foci* within the cyst wall were observed in approximately one-third of the cases, being the highest single predictor for the presence of an endometrioma. These should be discriminated from true wall nodularity as they are more echogenic and smaller. Although the pathologic basis of these echogenic foci has not been well described, it is speculated that they arise from the accumulation of cholesterol deposits in the endometriotic cyst wall over time. For that reason, it has been suggested that they can help in estimating the age of the cyst as they are very rarely seen in newly formed endometriomas [24].

(b) *Wall nodularity* is characterized as solid masses protruding from the endometrioma wall into the cyst lumen. Morphologically, these appeared as papillary projections; therefore, neoplasia should be excluded.

(c) *Wall thickness* has not been shown to be helpful in distinguishing between endometriomas and other ovarian masses.

Multilocularity with the presence of internal septations as a feature, in addition to low-level echoes, and in the absence of neoplastic characteristics strongly suggests the diagnosis of an endometrioma. The internal septa within a multilocular endometrioma may be thin or thick [25].

Hemorrhagic cysts can demonstrate diffuse low-level internal echoes and need to be differentiated from endometriomas. They will usually appear more heterogeneous with fibrinous strands and retracting clots, suggesting recent hemorrhage, a feature not common in endometriomas. The hemorrhagic area will tend to be more central in location [21].

Fibrin strands, when compared with septations, are thinner and weaker reflectors, giving a fishnet appearance and do not traverse the entire cyst [26].

However, still the strongest feature to enable the differentiation of a hemorrhagic cyst from an endometrioma is the evolution over time of its internal structure, thus necessitating a follow-up examination [27].

Due to the fact that in the process of the disease adhesions are usually formed, endometriomas can be atypically located in the pelvis. Adhesions may be revealed by the "sliding organ signs" when there is absence of free movement of the pelvic organs following gentle pressure with the vaginal probe. This may also reproduce symptoms of deep dyspareunia. Bilateral endometriomas can be found adherent to each other in the pouch of Douglas or even above the uterus (known as kissing ovaries; see Fig. 11.1B) [24].

The value of Doppler ultrasound in the diagnosis of endometriomas is still not well established. Guerriero et al. [23] suggested that color Doppler energy (CDE) imaging or power Doppler imaging could be a useful "secondary test" for the characterization of endometriomas in premenopausal women.

Endometriomas are considered relatively avascular, whereas other adnexal masses, and particularly malignant tumors, are characterized by abundant vascularization or the presence of color flow in the internal septations or the papillary projections of the cyst wall. Typically, a pattern of vascular distributions in the endometrioma showed vessels at the level of the ovarian hilus [28].

USS for the diagnosis of deep infiltrating endometriosis (DIE)

Endometriosis is considered to be infiltrative when lesions reach a depth of >5 mm into the peritoneum, and may be situated in the pouch of Douglas, in the vesico-uterine pouch and in other

Table 11.1 Differential ultrasound scan diagnosis of endometrioma

Dermoid or teratomas
Fibroid
Ovarian abscess
Hemorrhagic corpora lutea
Pyosalpinx
Torsion of adnexal mass
Ovarian adenofibroma
Unspecified benign ovarian cyst
Mucinous and serous cystadenoma

A
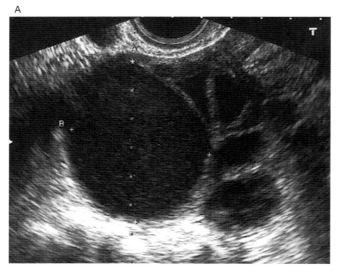

B
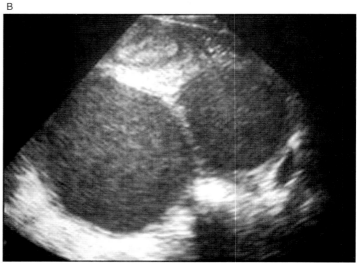

Fig. 11.1 (A) Endometrioma. Presence of a regular cyst with diffuse low-level homogeneous internal echoes with a ground-glass texture. (B) Kissing endometriomas. Bilateral endometriomas adherent to each other.

areas of the pelvis [29]. DIE presents dominantly as a nodular, myoproliferative lesion interspersed with a sparse amount of glandular and stromal tissue and micro-endometriomas. Similar to uterine adenomyosis, these lesions have no capsule and are in continuity with the surrounding fibromuscular and/or muscular structures as well as vessels.

One of the most frequent locations of DIE is the uterosacral ligaments (USL) [30] and the torus uterinus, defined anatomically as a small transverse thickening joining the insertion of the USLs to the posterior wall of the uterus. Involvement of these structures by endometriotic implants produces a discrete sheet-like or stellate hypoechoic nodule with irregular outer margins, usually located in close proximity to the uterine cervix.

A normal USL is barely detectable on TVS, but when harboring DIE, it thickens and becomes visible [31]. Simultaneous comparison of the left and right USLs will easily depict a nodule if it is unilateral; asymmetry between the two ligaments and irregularity of their profiles are more specific for the presence of endometriosis than is a simple thickness measurement [31]. Deep endometriotic implants are fixed and painful under pressure from the transvaginal probe.

The other common location of DIE is the lower gastrointestinal tract. Endometriotic implants of the gastrointestinal tract are estimated to occur in 12–37% of patients with severe pelvic endometriosis [25]. It most commonly affects those segments of bowel in the dependent portion of the pelvis and is rarely found proximal to the terminal ileum [32]. The most commonly affected areas in decreasing order of frequency are the rectosigmoid colon, appendix, cecum, and distal ileum [32,33].

Rectovaginal septum endometriosis is a misnomer as involvement of this structure rarely occurs. The nodule can eventually reach the upper extremity of the rectovaginal septum. The lesion frequently extends laterally into the parametrium and, if larger than 3 cm, may involve the ureters [26]. A number of studies strongly suggest that excisional radical surgery is highly effective in treating DIE and leads to long-term curative effects regarding associated symptoms and subfertility [34,35]. Adequate assessment of patients with symptoms suggestive of endometriosis is of major importance. It not only reduces diagnostic delay, but also enables the clinician to discuss and plan appropriate surgical treatment options, especially in cases of advanced disease, and to counsel the patient regarding the complication potential.

Clinical examination is of limited use in establishing both the presence and the extent of DIE lesions [36], so preoperative imaging modalities are often required when DIE is suspected. Although advanced imaging techniques such as MRI or computed tomography (CT) have been shown to be valuable tools for noninvasive diagnosis of DIE [37,38], these modalities are equally time-consuming and expensive, hence of limited use as easy-at-hand primary assessment tools in the outpatient clinical setting.

These issues are partly overcome by the use of TV sonography. The use of TV ultrasound for diagnosing rectal infiltration in women with rectovaginal endometriosis was originally proposed by Gorell and colleagues [39]. More recently, in a series of six women with rectovaginal endometriosis, Koga et al. [40] demonstrated that both TV and transrectal (TR) ultrasonography provide characteristic ultrasonographic images of rectosigmoid nodules; however, the authors did not determine the sensitivity and specificity of these techniques in estimating bowel infiltration.

By using TV sonography, Bazot et al. [41] diagnosed endometriotic infiltration of the rectal muscularis propria in 21 out of 22 cases. The exam had a sensitivity of 95.5%, a specificity of 100%, a PPV (positive predictive value) of 100%, and an NPV (negative predictive value) of 88.9%. By combining TV USS with a retrograde bowel preparation performed one hour before the examination, Abrao et al. [42] obtained a sensitivity of 95.4%, a specificity of 96.4%, a PPV of 95.4%, and an NPV of 96.5% in diagnosing rectal infiltration in 110 women with DIE. In a series of 46 patients, "sonovaginography," a technique combining TV USS with the introduction of a saline solution in the vagina, was demonstrated to diagnose rectovaginal endometriosis more accurately than TV USS alone. It is noteworthy that only three patients included in the study had infiltration of the rectal wall, which means that the value of this technique in the diagnosis of rectal infiltration remains unclear [43].

More recently, "tenderness-guided" TV sonography has been proposed for the detection of deep endometriosis. This technique, which consists of the introduction of 12 mL of ultrasound transmission gel in the probe cover, was proved to be accurate in the diagnosis of deep endometriosis [44]. Unfortunately, only four patients with infiltration of the rectal wall were included in the study; therefore, the value of the tenderness-guided TV approach in determining bowel involvement remains to be determined. Abrao et al. [36] compared the use of bimanual examination, TV USS, and MRI for detection of DIE of the rectosigmoid and/or "retrocervical sites" as defined by the authors, demonstrating higher sensitivity, specificity, NPV, and PPV for TV sonography in cases of rectal DIE when compared with MRI and clinical examination. Although the presence of gas and stool can potentially raise difficulties in viewing images of rectal DIE, the sensitivities, specificities, PPVs, and NPVs of TV sonography with respect to diagnosis of rectal endometriosis do not differ from the results of recent studies using bowel preparation previous to USS [36].

Histologically, the endometriotic nodule progressively infiltrates the serosal surface of the bowel and then reaches the muscularis propria, forming a bulky nodule composed of smooth muscle cells, collagen, fibroblasts, and islands of scattered endometrial stroma and glands [40]. The submucosal and mucosal layers are rarely affected, which explains the high proportion of false negatives on colonoscopy [38]. Inflammatory response to cyclic hemorrhage can lead to adhesions, bowel stricture, and obstruction.

On TV USS, a normal rectal wall exhibits a thin (<3 mm) hypoechoic smooth muscle layer and a hyperechoic internal

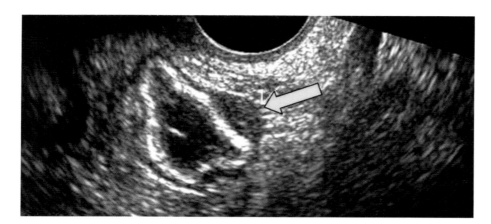

Fig. 11.2 Bowel endometriosis. Presence of a hypoechoic fixed endometriotic nodule (arrow) in direct contact with the hyperechoic submucosa and mucosa layers (courtesy of Dr. L. Pardini Chamie, Brazil).

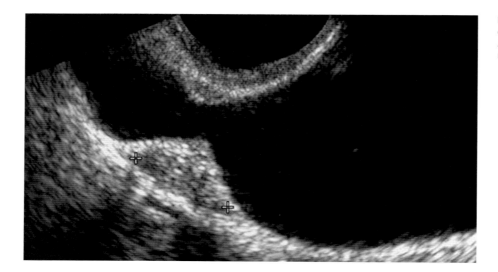

Fig. 11.3 Bladder endometriosis. Presence of an endometriotic nodule projecting into the bladder. Anechoic "bubble-like" areas are seen within the nodule (courtesy of Dr. L. Pardini Chamie, Brazil).

layer corresponding to the rectal submucosa, and mucosa. Diagnosis of bowel endometriosis on TVS is straightforward when a hypoechoic fixed nodule is seen (Fig. 11.2). The external margins of the nodule are hyperechoic due to the presence of congested adipose tissue, submucosa, and mucosa. Some nodules manifest internal hyperechoic spots, probably due to calcified portions; power Doppler invariably shows few blood vessels within and around the nodule. Moreover, as most of the nodules obliterate the pouch of Douglas, TV sonography is recommended as a dynamic examination by evaluating the sliding of the cervix along the rectum by gently pushing the vaginal probe while looking for the presence of DIE.

When intestinal DIE is found, the examiner should be aware that, in up to 93% of cases, there is a second DIE location (USL, vagina, bladder and/or ureter) [45,46]. TVS is of limited value in locating DIE in the sigmoid colon, above the level of the uterine fundus far from the tip of the probe. These lesions are difficult to visualize, especially if air and stool are interposed. Moreover, on TVS it is very difficult to accurately measure the distance between the lower limit of the lesion and the anal canal.

USS for the diagnosis of endometriosis of the genitourinary tract

Involvement of the urinary tract occurs in approximately 1–2% of patients with endometriosis and in 90% of these cases, the bladder is involved followed by the ureters [47]. Once considered a rare pathological condition, bladder endometriosis is probably underdiagnosed because of its nonspecific symptoms. Only scattered cases of renal or urethral involvement have been reported [48]. When the bladder is involved, endometriotic implants are often confined to the serosal surface, but can infiltrate the muscle and appear as mural masses projecting into the bladder lumen (Fig. 11.3).

Typically, it is found in patients with dysmenorrhea associated with urinary symptoms such as micturition frequency. In order to identify the presence of bladder endometriosis, the transducer should be positioned in the anterior vaginal fornix and tilted upward to visualize the vesico-uterine space and the bladder, using both longitudinal and transverse sections. In these planes, the bladder wall is visualized easily if a moderate amount of urine is present.

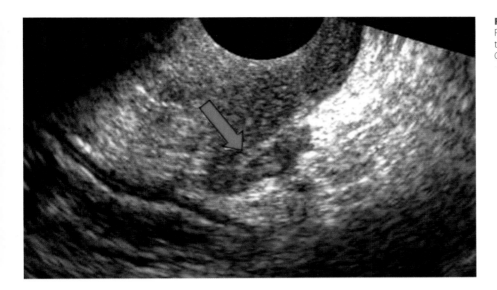

Fig. 11.4 Rectovaginal space endometriosis. Presence of an irregular fixed nodule (arrow) in the posterior cul-de-sac (courtesy of Dr. L. Pardini Chamie, Brazil).

Diagnostic criteria suggestive of a bladder endometriotic nodule include the presence of a hypo- or isoechogenic nodule within the bladder wall and the presence of a nodule with heterogeneous echo-structure containing numerous anechoic ("bubble-like") areas [49]. As with other locations, patients with bladder endometriosis report pain under pressure from the TV probe. Color Doppler studies may detect low to moderate vascularity, and mild pressure with the vaginal probe often elicits focal pain [50]. These masses are typically near the dome of the bladder and can be seen during excretory urography or with USS, CT, and MR imaging.

USS for the diagnosis of endometriosis of the vagina and rectovaginal space

The vagina is considered to be involved when its wall is thickened or when a nodule with an irregular outer contour and spiculations are seen attached to it. The most frequently affected portion of the vaginal canal is the posterior fornix (Fig. 11.4). Typical symptoms correspond to dyschezia during menstruation and dyspareunia. Diagnosis is usually clinical and identified at physical examination in 80% of cases [16]. The sensitivity of ultrasound is reported to be as low as 29% [31]. This difficulty is due to the configuration of TV ultrasound probes with the receiver oriented toward the vaginal fornix. Orientation of the probe toward the posterior vaginal wall can be limited by the symphysis pubis and associated pelvic pain.

Dessole et al. [43] have described an increase in the sensitivity of TV ultrasound when a saline solution is instilled in the vagina. In this series sonovaginography identified 91% of the pathologically confirmed lesions compared with 44% with conventional TV sonography alone, with a specificity of 86% and 50%, respectively.

The problem with vaginal lesions is not the diagnosis, but the choice of the appropriate surgical option. For this purpose,

other questions such as location, extension, and infiltration of the vaginal lesion are more important than the identification of the lesion. Results of MRI have been described by Bazot et al. [51] in 15 patients, with a sensitivity of 80% and a specificity of 93%. Therefore, MRI represents the ideal complement to ultrasound and physical examination to predict lesion extension higher upward and posteriorly when planning surgery.

USS for the diagnosis of rare locations of endometriosis

Ectopic endometrial glands and stroma can develop at the site of prior gynecological surgery, such as scars from a prior cesarean section or laparoscopy or spontaneously within the abdominal wall at the recti abdomini [52]. Clinical symptoms include cyclic pain and swelling of a subcutaneous nodule or permanent lower abdominal pain. On ultrasound scan a subcutaneous nodule demonstrates irregular borders and a heterogeneous texture with internal scattered hyperechoic echoes surrounded by a hyperechoic ring of variable width and vascularity on color Doppler imaging.

Conclusions

Endometriosis of the pelvis demonstrates a large distribution of lesion locations and imaging features. The goal of surgical treatment of deep endometriotic lesions is to achieve complete resection of all symptomatic deep lesions during a one-step multidisciplinary surgical procedure. The efficiency of surgical management depends on how radical the exeresis is [53]. Although MRI is able to diagnose all sites of endometriosis [51], TV USS should be the initial imaging modality due to immediate availability, costs, and easy access. The accuracy of TV sonography has greatly improved over recent years as knowledge has increased regarding the various sonographic aspects of endometriosis. The performance of ultrasound is heavily operator dependent, which is both a limitation and a strength of this diagnostic approach.

The diagnoses of endometriomas and bladder endometriosis by TV ultrasound are reliable. In women with chronic dysmenorrhea, dyspareunia, clinical suspicion of deep endometriosis, or inconclusive sonographic findings, MRI will identify endometriosis with a high degree of accuracy, particularly at the torus uterinus, uterosacral ligaments, upper vagina, and lower gastrointestinal tract.

References

1. Olive DL, Schwartz LB. Endometriosis. *N Engl J Med* 1993; **328**: 1759–1769.

2. Brosens IA. Endometriosis. Current issues in diagnosis and medical management. *J Reprod Med* 1998; **43**: 281–286.

3. Nargund G. Ovarian pathology. In: Nargund G, ed. *Advanced Ultrasound in Reproductive Medicine: A Theoretical and Practical Workshop*. London: HER Trust; 2006: 10–14.

4. Vercellini P, Crosignani PG. Epidemiology of endometriosis. In: Brosens IA, Donnez J, eds. *The Current Status of Endometriosis: Research and Management. Proceedings of the 3rd World Congress on Endometriosis*; June 1–31992. Brussels, Belgium. Carnforth: CRC Press-Parthenon Publishing Group;1993.

5. Haney AF. The pathogenesis and etiology of endometriosis. In: Thomas EJ, Rock J, eds. *Modern Approaches to Endometriosis*. Lancaster: Kluwer Academic Publishers; 1991: 113–128.

6. O'Connor DT. Clinical features and diagnosis of endometriosis. In: O'Connor DT, ed. *Endometriosis*. London: Churchill Livingstone; 1987: 68–84.

7. Ballard K, Lowton K, Wright J. What's the delay? A qualitative study of women's experiences of reaching a diagnosis of endometriosis. *Fertil Steril* 2006; **86**: 1296–1301.

8. Revised American Society For Reproductive Medicine classification of endometriosis: 1996. *Fertil Steril* 1997; **67**: 817–821.

9. Lilford RJ, Dalton ME. Effectiveness of treatment for infertility. *Br Med J (Clin Res Ed)* 1987; **295**: 6591–6592.

10. Rock JA. The revised American Fertility Society classification of endometriosis: reproducibility of scoring. ZOLADEX Endometriosis Study Group. *Fertil Steril* 1995; **63**: 1108–1110.

11. Vercellini P, Trespidi L, De Giorgi O, et al. Endometriosis and pelvic pain: relation to disease stage and localization. *Fertil Steril* 1996; **65**: 299–304.

12. Chapron C, Fauconnier A, Dubuisson JB, et al. Deep infiltrating endometriosis: relation between severity of dysmenorrhoea and extent of disease. *Hum Reprod* 2003; **18**: 760–766.

13. Damario MA, Rock JA. Classification of endometriosis. *Semin Reprod Endocrinol* 1997; **15**: 235–244.

14. Woodward PJ, Sohaey R, Mezzetti TP Jr. Endometriosis: radiologic–pathologic correlation. *Radiographics* 2001; **21**: 193–216.

15. Candiani GB. *La clinica ostetrica e ginecologica*. Milan: Masson Ed; 1996.

16. Chapron C, Dubuisson JB, Pansini V, et al. Routine clinical examination is not sufficient for diagnosing and locating deeply infiltrating endometriosis. *J Am Assoc Gynecol Laparosc* 2002; **9**: 115–119.

17. Laschke MW, Korbel C, Rudzitis-Auth J, et al. High-resolution ultrasound imaging: a novel technique for the noninvasive in vivo analysis of endometriotic lesion and cyst formation in small animal models. *Am J Pathol* 2010; **176**: 585–593.

18. Sampson JA. Perforating hemorrhagic [chocolate] cysts of the ovary. *Arch Surg* 1921; **2**: 245–323.

19. Vercellini P, Aimi G, De Giorgi O, et al. Is cystic ovarian endometriosis an asymmetric disease? *Br J Obstet Gynaecol* 1998; **105**: 1018–1021.

20. Moore J, Copley S, Morris J, et al. A systematic review of the accuracy of ultrasound in the diagnosis of endometriosis. *Ultrasound Obstet Gynecol* 2002; **20**: 630–634.

21. Patel MD, Feldstein VA, Chen DC, et al. Endometriomas: diagnostic performance of US. *Radiology* 1999; **210**: 739–745.

22. Alcazar JL, Laparte C, Jurado M, Lopez-Garcia G. The role of transvaginal ultrasonography combined with color velocity imaging and pulsed Doppler in the diagnosis of endometrioma. *Fertil Steril* 1997; **67**: 487–491.

23. Guerriero S, Ajossa S, Mais V, et al. The diagnosis of endometriomata using colour Doppler energy imaging. *Hum Reprod* 1998; **13**: 1691–1695.

24. Savelli L. Transvaginal sonography for the assessment of ovarian and pelvic endometriosis: how deep is our understanding? *Ultrasound Obstet Gynecol* 2009; **33**: 497–501.

25. Clement PB. Diseases of the peritoneum. In: Kurman RJ, ed. *Blaustein's Pathology of the Female Genital Tract*, 4th edn. New York, NY: Springer-Verlag; 1994: 660–680.

26. Brown DL, Dudiak KM, Laing FC. Adnexal masses: US characterization and reporting. *Radiology* 2010; **254**: 342–354.

27. Derchi LE, Serafini G, Gandolfo N, et al. Ultrasound in gynecology. *Eur Radiol* 2001; **11**: 2137–2155.

28. Kupesic S, Kurjak A. Normal and abnormal ovarian circulation. In Kurjak A, ed. *Ultrasound and the Ovary*. Carnforth: Parthenon Publishing; 1994: 189–210.

29. Cornillie FJ, Oosterlynck D, Lauweryns JM, Koninckx PR. Deeply infiltrating pelvic endometriosis: histology and clinical significance. *Fertil Steril* 1990; **53**: 978–983.

30. Bazot M, Malzy P, Cortez A, et al. Accuracy of transvaginal sonography and rectal endoscopic sonography in the diagnosis of deep infiltrating endometriosis. *Ultrasound Obstet Gynecol* 2007; **30**: 994–1001.

31. Bazot M, Thomassin I, Hourani R, et al. Diagnostic accuracy of transvaginal sonography for deep pelvic endometriosis. *Ultrasound Obstet Gynecol* 2004; **24**: 180–185.

32. Gedgaudas-McClees RK. Gastrointestinal complications of gynecologic diseases. In: *Textbook of Gastrointestinal Radiology*. Philadelphia, PA: Saunders; 1994: 2559–2567.

33. Zwas FR, Lyon DT. Endometriosis: an important condition in clinical gastroenterology. *Dig Dis Sci* 1991; **36**: 353–364.

34. Sutton CJ, Pooley AS, Ewen SP, Haines P. Follow-up report on a randomized controlled trial of laser laparoscopy in the treatment of pelvic pain associated with minimal to moderate endometriosis. *Fertil Steril* 1997; **68**: 1070–1074.

35. Ferrero S, Abbamonte LH, Giordano M, et al. Deep dyspareunia and sex life after laparoscopic excision of endometriosis. *Hum Reprod* 2007; **22**: 1142–1148.

36. Abrao MS, Goncalves MO, Dias JA Jr, et al. Comparison between clinical examination, transvaginal sonography and magnetic resonance imaging for the diagnosis of deep endometriosis. *Hum Reprod* 2007; **22**: 3092–3097.

37. Kinkel K, Chapron C, Balleyguier C, et al. Magnetic resonance imaging characteristics of deep endometriosis. *Hum Reprod* 1999; **14**: 1080–1086.

38. Kinkel K, Frei KA, Balleyguier C, Chapron C. Diagnosis of endometriosis with imaging: a review. *Eur Radiol* 2006; **16**: 285–298.

39. Gorell HA, Cyr DR, Wang KY, Greer BE. Rectosigmoid endometriosis. Diagnosis using endovaginal sonography. *J. Ultrasound Med* 1989; **8**: 459–461.

40. Koga K, Osuga Y, Yano T, et al. Characteristic images of deeply infiltrating endometriosis on transvaginal and transrectal ultrasonography. *Hum Reprod* 2003; **18**: 1328–1333.

41. Bazot M, Detchev R, Cortez A, Amouyal P, Uzan S, Darai E. Transvaginal sonography and rectal endoscopic sonography for the assessment of pelvic endometriosis: a preliminary comparison. *Hum Reprod.* 2003; **18**: 1686–1692.

42. Abrao MS, Goncalves MO, Gonzales M, Dias JA Jr. Is it possible to evaluate deeply infiltrating endometriosis with transvaginal ultrasound. *Eur J Obstet Gynecol Reprod Biol* 2005; **123**(Suppl 1): S14.

43. Dessole S, Farina M, Rubattu G, et al. Sonovaginography is a new technique for assessing rectovaginal endometriosis. *Fertil Steril* 2003; **79**: 1023–1027.

44. Guerriero S, Ajossa S, Gerada M, et al. "Tenderness-guided" transvaginal ultrasonography: a new method for the detection of deep endometriosis in patients with chronic pelvic pain. *Fertil Steril* 2007; **88**: 1293–1297.

45. Chapron C, Fauconnier A, Goffinet F, et al. Laparoscopic surgery is not inherently dangerous for patients presenting with benign gynaecologic pathology. Results of a meta-analysis. *Hum Reprod* 2002; **17**: 115–119.

46. Piketty M, Chopin N, Dousset B, et al. Preoperative work-up for patients with deeply infiltrating endometriosis: transvaginal ultrasonography must definitely be the first-line imaging examination. *Hum Reprod* 2009; **24**: 602–607.

47. Nezhat CH, Malik S, Osias J, et al. Laparoscopic management of 15 patients with infiltrating endometriosis of the bladder and a case of primary intravesical endometrioid adenosarcoma. *Fertil Steril* 2002; **78**: 872–875.

48. Savelli L, Manuzzi L, Pollastri P, et al. Diagnostic accuracy and potential limitations of transvaginal sonography for bladder endometriosis. *Ultrasound Obstet Gynecol* 2009; **34**: 595–600.

49. Fedele L, Bianchi S, Raffaelli R, Portuese A. Pre-operative assessment of bladder endometriosis. *Hum Reprod* 1997; **12**: 2519–2522.

50. Brosens J, Timmerman D, Starzinski-Powitz A, Brosens I. Noninvasive diagnosis of endometriosis: the role of imaging and markers. *Obstet Gynecol Clin North Am* 2003; **30**: 96–114.

51. Bazot M, Darai E, Hourani R, et al. Deep pelvic endometriosis: MR imaging for diagnosis and prediction of extension of disease. *Radiology* 2004; **232**: 379–389.

52. Balleyguier C, Chapron C, Chopin N, et al. Abdominal wall and surgical scar endometriosis: results of magnetic resonance imaging. *Gynecol Obstet Invest* 2003; **55**: 220–224.

53. Garry R. Laparoscopic excision of endometriosis: the treatment of choice? *Br J Obstet Gynaecol* 1997; **104**: 513–551.

Chapter

12

Ultrasound imaging of uterine fibroids: evaluation and management

Gautam N. Allahbadia and Rubina Merchant

Uterine fibroids are benign, estrogen-dependent smooth muscle tumors; they are most common among women of reproductive age and can even occur in pregnancy (Fig. 12.1). Though the pathophysiology and epidemiology of fibroids is not well understood, recent evidence suggests that genetic predisposition, mutations, steroid hormones, and growth factors may play an important role in the fibrotic processes and angiogenesis observed during the formation and growth of these tumors. High-resolution ultrasound and magnetic resonance imaging (MRI) are noninvasive, high-quality diagnostic procedures that may be used to accurately evaluate the histology, position, and size of fibroids to direct management options and evaluate treatment outcomes. Advanced, sophisticated treatment options, such as laparoscopic and vaginal myomectomy, uterine artery embolization (UAE), magnetic-resonance-guided focused ultrasound surgery (MRgFUS), hysteroscopic resection, myolysis by heat, cold coagulation and laser, laparoscopic uterine artery occlusion, and temporary transvaginal uterine artery occlusion are newer, minimally invasive, and effective alternatives to conventional surgery. However, the pros, cons,

cost–benefit ratio, and long-term efficacy of these techniques, based on a thorough knowledge of the nature, number, and location of fibroids, their impact on fertility, and the possible treatment outcome, is essential prior to deciding the appropriate mode of management.

Introduction

Uterine fibroids are the most common benign tumors of the uterus in women of reproductive age and affect 20–30% of women older than 35 years [1,2]. At least 1 in 4 women will develop one or more fibroids during their lifetime, the incidence of uterine fibroid tumors increases as women grow older, and they may occur in more than 30% of women between the ages of 40 and 60 [3]. Approximately 50% of women of reproductive age have fibroids, and at least 50% of these women have significant symptoms [4]. Fibroids are also a common occurrence in pregnancy; however, the true incidence of fibroids during pregnancy is unknown and reported rates vary from as low as 0.1% of all pregnancies to as high as 12.5% [5]. The prevalence rates vary with race, being three times more common in women of Afro-Caribbean descent than in Caucasian women. Risk factors for the development of fibroids include age, nulliparity, race, family history, obesity [5], and prolonged (>5 years) estrogen and progestogen therapy (EPT), which is associated with a 1.7-fold increased risk of subsequent leiomyomas (95% CI 0.9–3.3), particularly limited to the subset of women with low body mass index [6].

Though fibroids may be asymptomatic in two-thirds of cases, especially if they are small and may not require treatment, they often present with abnormal uterine bleeding and menorrhagia, acute pelvic pain due to torsion of a pedunculated fibroid, pelvic mass, increasing girth, pressure symptoms (urinary frequency and/or constipation), pelvic or urinary obstructive symptoms, infertility, and pregnancy loss when enlarged [3,7]. Uterine fibroids, specifically submucosal and intramural myomas, negatively impact fertility and are associated with adverse obstetric outcomes such as abdominal pain, miscarriage, preterm labor, placental abruption, malpresentation, postpartum

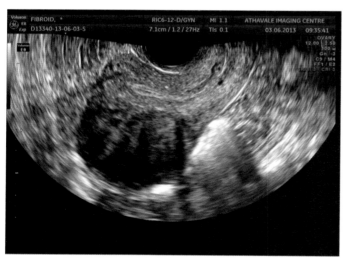

Fig. 12.1 Ultrasound image of a fibroid (courtesy of Dr. Umesh Athavale, Athavale Imaging Centre, Mumbai, India).

Ultrasonography in Gynecology, ed. Botros R. M. B. Rizk and Elizabeth E. Puscheck. Published by Cambridge University Press. © Cambridge University Press 2015.

hemorrhage, and cesarean section [8]. The size, location, and number of fibroids and their relation to the placenta are critical factors [5]. Transvaginal ultrasonography, MRI, sonohysterography, and hysteroscopy are available to evaluate the size and position of tumors. Ultrasonography should be used initially because it is the least invasive and most cost-effective investigation [3]. Saline infusion sonohysterography (SIS) is most valuable in the detection of focal intracavitary lesions [9].

Many advances have been made in the management of uterine myomas. Watchful waiting, medical therapy, hysteroscopic myomectomy, endometrial ablation, laparoscopic myomectomy, abdominal myomectomy, abdominal, vaginal, and laparoscopic hysterectomy, UAE, uterine artery occlusion, and focused ultrasound are now available [10]. Treatment must be individualized based on such considerations as the presence and severity of symptoms, the patient's desire for definitive treatment, the desire to preserve childbearing capacity, the importance of uterine preservation, infertility related to uterine cavity distortions, and previous pregnancy complications related to fibroid tumors [3].

Clinical discussion

Evaluation of fibroids

A thorough history and gynecologic examination is a mandatory step in the initial evaluation of uterine fibroids and this may be followed by imaging techniques to confirm the diagnosis and plan further management.

Transvaginal sonography (TVS)

Transvaginal sonography is a safe, noninvasive method for the detection of abnormal endometrial pathology in perimenopausal women with abnormal uterine bleeding, with a high incidence of detection for focal lesions as fibroids [11], after excluding other causes of abnormal vaginal bleeding including endometrial cancer [1]. When combined with color Doppler, TVS is the cornerstone of initial management of abnormal uterine bleeding in both pre- and postmenopausal women and, in experienced hands, can reliably exclude the most common intracavitary pathologies, including endometrial polyps and submucosal fibroids. To allow for reliable evaluation of the endometrium, TVS must be performed before endometrial sampling. TVS with or without SIS can provide enough information to avoid an unnecessary hysteroscopy. In postmenopausal women, the endometrial thickness reliably selects those who need further testing. If a thin and regular endometrium is visualized, malignancy is most unlikely [9].

Ultrasound scanning plays a key role in diagnosing and monitoring fibroids during pregnancy and in determining the position of the fibroids relative to the placenta. It is equally useful for detecting heterogeneous echo patterns associated with the appearance of pain in pregnancy. Color flow Doppler scanning differentiates fibroids from myometrial thickening, which may be mistaken for fibroids [5]. Pregnancies with myomas are known to have an increased risk for complications, such as placental abruption, dysfunctional labor, growth of the tumor, necrosis, and delivery problems, but prediction is still difficult based on clinical and real-time ultrasound evaluations alone. Doppler results may give insights into the typical pathophysiologic sequences and help with the management; however, the clinical role of Doppler flow analysis in pregnancies with myomas needs to be further evaluated [12].

Hysteroscopy and hysterosonography may be recommended if ultrasonography is not sufficiently informative or if medical treatment fails. MRI is recommended as a second-line investigation (in cases of multiple uterine fibroids, or suspected adenomyosis, and if an arterial embolization is required) [13].

Magnetic resonance imaging

The Australasian CREI Consensus Expert Panel on Trial evidence (ACCEPT) recommends that fibroids with suspected cavity involvement be defined by MRI, sonohysterography, or hysteroscopy because modalities such as TVS and hysterosalpingography lack appropriate sensitivity and specificity [14]. Although laparoscopy, hysteroscopy, hysterosalpingography, and TVS are the most effective techniques for evaluation of pelvic disorders related to female infertility, MRI offers an accurate, noninvasive diagnosis of leiomyoma and helps to predict the outcome of conservative treatment for leiomyomas, leading to the selection of better treatment plans and management [15].

Though in-office TVS reinforces the clinical diagnosis of uterine myomas, it often fails in the detection of their number, resulting in a poor preoperative characterization of patients. Fambrini et al. [16] reported a 59.4% sensitivity of TVS in revealing the exact number of myomas, with at least one myoma missed at TVS in 35.2% cases with a preoperative diagnosis of ≤3 myomas, while 26.4% patients diagnosed with one myoma at preoperative TVS had two or more myomas at the end of surgery. They suggested that the fact that one myoma may be overlooked in one-third of patients theoretically eligible for laparoscopic conservative surgery may motivate the implementation of ultrasound diagnosis when laparoscopic myomectomy is considered [16].

The superb contrast resolution and multiplanar capabilities of MRI make it particularly valuable for characterizing these tumors, which usually show low signal intensity similar to that of smooth muscle on T2-weighted images. The radiologist's recognition of this and other characteristic features may help steer the clinician towards timely, appropriate management and away from unnecessary, potentially harmful treatment [2]. Moreover, MRI analysis for leiomyoma quantity, size and location, uterine volume, and the presence of potential contraindications to UAE has been cited as more accurate than pelvic ultrasound for characterizing uterine leiomyomas and is capable of identifying findings missed by ultrasound (such as adenomyosis and a pedunculated subserosal leiomyoma) which, in a small but statistically insignificant number of cases, changed management [17].

In a comparative evaluation of MRI and sonography for uterine size, fibroid size and location (categorized as para-endometrial, intramural, subserosal, or pedunculated) of the four largest fibroids in each patient, and the total number of fibroids present in the preliminary evaluation for fibroid embolization, MRI and sonography were well correlated for the volume of the single largest fibroid in each patient ($R = 0.87$), but poorly correlated for fibroid location ($R = 0.17$) [18]. Discrepancy in the total number of fibroids was noted, with additional fibroids found on MRI in 31 of 49 patients and erroneously suspected on sonography in 5 of 49 patients. Pelvic MRI affected management in 11 of 49 patients, leading to cancellation of UAE in 4 patients. Spielmann et al. [18] concluded that MRI provides considerable additional information compared with sonography and affects clinical decision making in a substantial number of patients. Hence, MRI should be considered in all patients being evaluated for UAE [18].

Preoperative pelvic MRI is reported to have a high sensitivity (94%) and a low specificity (33%) for diagnosing leiomyomas and a high specificity (91%) and a low sensitivity (38%) for diagnosing adenomyosis. Positive and negative predictive values of MRI for leiomyoma were 95% and 27%, respectively, with 90% accuracy. Positive and negative predictive values of MRI for adenomyosis were 52% and 85%, respectively, with 80% accuracy. However, due to the high cost and technical variations, Moghadam et al. [19] suggested that MRI be used only as an adjunctive diagnostic tool when ultrasound is not conclusive and differentiation between the two pathologies ultimately affects patient management [19].

Endometrial biopsy

Some authors [20] consider histological diagnosis as the gold standard, particularly important to exclude adenomyosis or malignancies and for an accurate preoperative diagnosis in the management of fibroids when procedures such as UAE are planned. TVS-guided gun biopsy of the uterus or ovaries has been considered a safe, simple office-based effective technique to obtain a tissue sample for histological confirmation of the preliminary ultrasound findings [20].

Complications

Uterine leiomyomas are common tumors in women, and most of their complications are well known. Rupture of a uterine leiomyoma due to spontaneous rupture of a leiomyoma vessel or secondary to abdominal trauma is an unusual source of severe hemoperitoneum, warranting a subtotal laparotomic hysterectomy [21].

Management of fibroids

Fibroid management is surrounded by considerable controversy and uncertainty. Consensus on the evidence concerning the impact and management of fibroids in infertility, developed by a group of Australasian subspecialists in reproductive endocrinology and infertility (the ACCEPT group), suggests

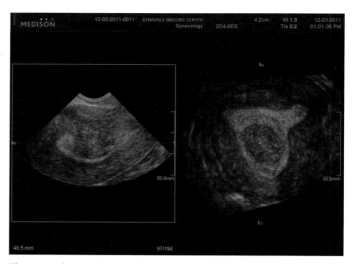

Fig. 12.2 Ultrasound image of a submucosal fibroid (courtesy of Dr. Umesh Athavale, Athavale Imaging Centre, Mumbai, India).

that: (i) the location of a fibroid within the uterus influences its effect on fertility; (ii) subserosal fibroids do not appear to impact fertility outcomes; (iii) intramural (IM) fibroids may be associated with reduced fertility and an increased miscarriage rate; however, there is insufficient evidence to inform whether myomectomy for IM fibroids improves fertility outcomes; (iv) submucosal fibroids are associated with reduced fertility and an increased miscarriage rate, and myomectomy for submucosal fibroids appears likely to improve fertility outcomes; and (v) the relative effect of multiple or different-sized fibroids on fertility outcomes is uncertain, as is the relative usefulness of myomectomy in these situations [14].

Several approaches are available for the treatment of uterine fibroids. These include pharmacologic options, such as hormonal therapies and gonadotropin-releasing hormone (GnRH) agonists, surgical approaches, such as hysterectomy, myomectomy, myolysis by heat, cold coagulation and laser, laparoscopic uterine artery occlusion, MRI-guided focused ultrasound surgery (MRgFUS), and UAE. However, the choice of approach may be dictated by factors such as the patient's desire for future conception, the importance of uterine preservation, symptom severity, and tumor characteristics [22] such as the number, size, and location of fibroids and may accordingly influence the pregnancy outcome. Subserosal myomas (up to 5–7 cm in diameter) seem to have little, if any, effect on reproductive outcome. Intramural myomas (<4–5 cm in diameter) that do not encroach upon the endometrium also can be considered to be relatively harmless to reproduction. Myomas that compress the uterine cavity with an intramural portion (submucous myoma type II) and submucous myomas, which significantly reduce pregnancy rates, should be removed before assisted reproductive techniques are used [23].

While the management of submucous myomas (Fig. 12.2) requires a hysteroscopic approach, intramural (Fig. 12.3) and subserous myomas in women who opt for nonsurgical treatment could be treated with UAE, high-intensity focused ultrasound

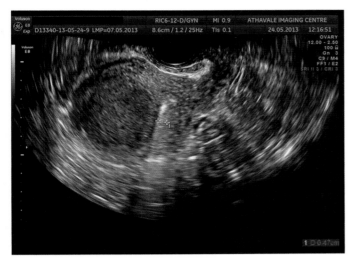

Fig. 12.3 Ultrasound image of an intramural fibroid (courtesy of Dr. Umesh Athavale, Athavale Imaging Centre, Mumbai, India).

(HIFU), or medical treatment such as selective GnRH agonists, progesterone receptor modulators, or aromatase inhibitors [1]. Asymptomatic myomas may be managed by reassurance and careful follow-up. Medical therapy may be tried as first-line treatment for symptomatic myomas, with surgical treatment reserved only for appropriate indications [24]. However, with such a wide range of new and emerging treatment options, it is important for providers to understand which fibroids are likely to respond optimally to a specific treatment in order to individualize appropriate and effective management for patients [8].

Medical management

For women who do not desire surgery, medical management of myomas with GnRH agonists may be considered; however, newer medications such as progesterone antagonists, selective progesterone receptor modulators, and aromatase inhibitors with fewer side effects have all shown promise as effective therapies [8]. Conservative treatment with GnRH analogues (GnRHa; leuprolide acetate), 3.75 mg per month for 6 months, may help to achieve successful pregnancy in cases of diffuse uterine leiomyomatosis with innumerable small fibroids (4–42 mm in size) and a symmetrically enlarged uterus (131 × 80 × 60 mm), clinically corresponding to that of 12 weeks of gestation and presenting with menorrhagia and infertility [25]. Cabergoline (0.5 mg, once a week for 6 weeks) has been shown to be as effective as triptorelin (Diphereline; 3.75 mg, four times every 28 days) in the shrinkage of myomas, accompanied by improvement in the sonographic, clinical, and intraoperative outcomes without any adverse pathological changes, and could be a good medical regimen as an adjunct to surgical management [26]. Asoprisnil (25 mg), a novel, orally active, selective progesterone receptor modulator for the management of symptomatic uterine leiomyomas, when administered daily for a 12-week period, moderately reduces uterine artery blood flow, which may contribute, in part, to the clinical effects of asoprisnil. The treatment is

well tolerated without serious adverse events [27]. Tropeano et al. [28] have also shown promising results following the use of mifepristone and asoprisnil in randomized controlled trials [28]. Medical therapy with medroxyprogesterone acetate (Depo Provera;150 mg/month) for 6 months in premenopausal women with symptomatic fibroids causes significant improvement in bleeding pattern as well as a reduction in the fibroid volume measured sonographically [29].

Surgical management

Myomectomy

Medication can only be used to improve symptoms and/or shrink the fibroids prior to surgery. Women with fibroids >3 cm in diameter causing significant symptoms, pain, or pressure and wishing to retain their uterus may consider myomectomy [7]. Current evidence suggests that myomectomy, which may be performed successfully in carefully selected patients without jeopardizing the pregnancy outcome, with appropriate surveillance and supportive management for a successful pregnancy and delivery, is the treatment of choice in women desiring to conceive [8] and among the few treatment options available for fibroids in pregnancy [5]. Though the treatment for fibroids in pregnant women is primarily conservative, in cases of failure, a myomectomy cannot be avoided [30]. Hysteroscopic myomectomy has been considered the gold standard for the treatment of submucous myomas, while abdominal myomectomy or laparoscopic myomectomy – when the experience of the surgeon and the facilities are sufficient – are the best alternatives for other myomas with increased pregnancy rates and decreased miscarriage rates [23]. Myomectomy, performed for submucosal and intramural fibroids, significantly improves fertility outcome [8]. Preoperative GnRH analog treatment before myomectomy decreases the size and vascularity of the myoma, but may render the capsule more fibrous and difficult to resect [24].

Laparoscopic myomectomy may be used for the excision of myoma(s), myometrium repair, and removal of the myoma from the abdomen, with ultrasound imaging and Doppler velocimetry to assess uterine scars after myomectomy [31]. Laparoscopic myomectomy has provided a minimally invasive alternative to laparotomy for intramural and subserous myomas, associated with faster postoperative recovery and potentially reduced risk of postoperative adhesions as compared with laparotomy with good surgical experience, and a comparable risk of perioperative complications with conventional surgery. According to Altgassen et al. [32], laparoscopic myomectomy for the treatment of fibroids >5.3 cm among women who wish to retain their uterus without improving fertility is an effective technique that can be offered to all women, with a low morbidity rate (intraoperative complication rate: 2.6% and postoperative complication rate: 5.7%) and an encouraging ongoing pregnancy rate of 57.1% [32].

However, though laparoscopic myomectomy offers several benefits to patients compared with laparotomic myomectomy, it remains a challenging technical procedure with demanding laparoscopic suturing [1,4] and is associated with high surgical morbidity, such as spontaneous uterine rupture, which although uncommon, is still a concern, a higher risk of recurrence compared with laparotomic myomectomy, and a high incidence of blood transfusion [31,33]. Though robotic-assisted laparoscopic myomectomy can help to overcome the technical demands of the conventional laparoscopic approach [1], the cost–benefit ratio of the former must be worked out prior to using it as a treatment option. As in vaginal myomectomy, there are limitations on the size and number of fibroids that can be treated by this modality [4]. The laparoscopic approach may not be justified for very large myomas, that may necessitate a uterine-conserving procedure via laparotomy, facilitated by preoperative and intraoperative measures that aim to minimize or replace operative blood loss and morbidity [34], especially in the case of large intramural fibroids [31]. Although laparoscopic myomectomy is minimally invasive in terms of the wound, it remains an advanced and invasive procedure that requires an appropriate management strategy for each patient, and careful discussion and counseling regarding all the issues are necessary [31].

Solitary myomectomy has been associated with lower rates of leiomyoma recurrence compared with patients with multiple leiomyomas (11% vs. 74%; $P = 0.011$). Smaller (≤ 10 menstrual weeks) intraoperative uterine size has been associated with lower rates of leiomyoma recurrence after myomectomy compared with >10 menstrual weeks (46% vs. 82%; $P = 0.032$) at 5 years cumulative probability of recurrence. Subsequent parity is associated with a lower probability of recurrence (26% vs. 76.0%; $P = 0.010$), but the cause and effect relationship between these two variables is unclear [35].

Hysterectomy

Hysterectomy provides a permanent cure for uterine fibroids but may be a treatment option only in case of multiple fibroids, in women with symptomatic fibroids who have not improved with medical treatment, and when the woman's family is complete [7]. UAE is only recommended if surgery was planned for symptomatic fibroids and if the fibroids are <20 weeks in size. Referral is recommended in the following cases: (i) submucous fibroid and abnormal bleeding; (ii) fibroids >3 cm in diameter, uterus palpable abdominally or >12 cm in size on scan; (iii) persistent intermenstrual bleeding; and (iv) age >45 where treatment has failed or been ineffective. Sarcomatous change within fibroids is rare and is normally associated with rapid growth. Such cases should be referred urgently [7].

Laparoscopic uterine artery coagulation (LUC)

Laparoscopic uterine artery coagulation is a cost-effective and low-morbidity option in the management of symptomatic myomas with low complication rates (fever, infection), no requirement for hysterectomy due to complications, and 90% patient satisfaction with the procedure compared with conventional approaches, such as myomectomy or hysterectomy [36]. Simsek et al. [36] reported a 57% reduction in bleeding at 12 months (303 ± 30.4 mL [95% CI 284–328] baseline vs. 173.5 ± 17.8 mL

[95% CI 164–184] after treatment; $P < 0.05$), mean reduction in uterine volume (pre- to post-LUC) of 195 ± 24.3 cm³, as documented by ultrasonography and MRI, mean operating time of 52.1 ± 7.2 minutes (95% CI 49.8–55.4), and a mean hospitalization time of 32.3 ± 6.6 hours (95% CI 29.2–35.4) following LUC. However, though these results are encouraging, more research is needed to validate the cost-effectiveness and long-term results [36].

Preliminary data following laparoscopic uterine artery occlusion suggest that outcomes are similar to those with UAE, but these data are derived from studies involving relatively small numbers. Temporary uterine artery occlusion is also promising, but has yet to be evaluated robustly [4]. If the patient's predominant complaint is the feeling of a mass and/or bleeding, alternative treatment options should be explored [36]. Other treatment modalities, such as laparoscopic myolysis or MRgFUS, should be monitored and evaluated thoroughly before they are applied as routine procedures [23].

Transvaginal temporary uterine artery occlusion

A 40–50% reduction in fibroid volume has been demonstrated following transvaginal temporary uterine artery occlusion in 75 women in five feasibility studies [28].

Bilateral uterine artery ligation

Bilateral uterine artery ligation by the vaginal route for the management of myomas is a safe, inexpensive, and effective therapeutic option for the treatment of symptomatic uterine fibroids with significantly reduced mean uterine and fibroid volumes at 6 and 12 months, a consistent pattern of decreased duration of menstrual blood flow, and high patient satisfaction with treatment outcome at completion of follow-up. However, these results need to be buttressed in a larger study [37]. Uterine depletion by ligation of the uterine arteries, performed by either an abdominal or a laparoscopic approach before myomectomy, for the management of patients with symptomatic fibroids who wished to retain their uteri, has been reported to result in a complete resolution of fibroid-related menorrhagia with reduced blood loss during the operation, the potential to prevent fibroid recurrence, and without compromising fertility capacity [38].

Laparoscopic cryomyolysis

In an open, one-arm pilot study in 20 patients, Zupi et al. [39] reported directed laparoscopic cryomyolysis to be a minimally invasive, effective, and safe technique for the treatment of symptomatic uterine myomas (4–10 cm) in menstruating women, providing rapid symptom relief with a steady mean shrinkage volume of approximately 60% (61.9% ± 11.9%) 12 months after surgery and at least 12 months' effectiveness in the treatment of symptomatic uterine leiomyomas. Power color Doppler ultrasound was performed preoperatively and postoperatively to demonstrate the effectiveness of the technique in reducing or eliminating the primary blood supply to the myomas, as well as documenting regression of the myomas [39].

Alternative management

Efforts to develop alternatives to surgery for management of symptomatic uterine fibroids have provided new techniques and new medications [28]. Non-pharmacologic treatments such as UAE and MRI-guided ultrasound have emerged as effective treatments for uterine fibroids [8].

Uterine artery embolization

UAE, which involves the complete occlusion of both the uterine arteries with particulate emboli, has, on the basis of case controlled studies and case reports, been reported to be an effective and safe alternative in the treatment of menorrhagia and other fibroid-related symptoms in women not desiring future fertility [40]. It is a new and attractive treatment for patients with symptomatic fibroids that provides excellent relief for abnormal bleeding, pelvic pain, and bulk-related symptoms [33], particularly in women with large symptomatic myomas who are poor surgical risks or wish to avoid major surgery [24]. Case studies report 50–60% reduction in fibroid size and 85–95% relief of symptoms following UAE. The largest of these studies reported an in-hospital complication rate of 2.7% (90 of 3041 patients) and a post-discharge complication rate of 26% (710 of 2729 patients) [28].

UAE versus surgery

Several randomized controlled trials comparing UAE with conventional surgery (hysterectomy/myomectomy) have demonstrated that UAE is associated with a shorter hospital stay, a rapid recovery time, and quicker resumption of activities compared with hysterectomy/myomectomy [28,40,41], laparoscopic myomectomy [33], and abdominal hysterectomy [42] for symptomatic uterine fibroids. Tropeano et al. [28] reported a hospital stay of 1–2 days vs. 5–5.8 days, recovery time of 9.5–28 days vs. 36.2–63 days, and similar major complication rates (2–15% vs. 2.7–20%) following UAE and surgery, respectively [28]. A recent study comparing UAE and myomectomy and their impact on quality of life suggests that both the procedures result in significant and equal improvements in quality of life by 1 year, though UAE allows a shorter hospital stay (2 vs. 6 days, $P <0.001$) [43] and fewer major complications (2.9% vs. 8%), but with a higher rate of reintervention (14.0% vs. 2.7%) by 2 years [43]. These views also have been confirmed in a recent contemporary study by van der Kooij et al. [41], who reported similar mid- and long-term benefits with regard to health-related quality of life and patient satisfaction, but a higher reintervention rate after UAE [41]. Stovall [42] reported that after uterine fibroid embolization, up to 20% of women need a second procedure. Randomized controlled trials, analyzing the cost-effectiveness of UAE with conventional surgery, found UAE more cost-effective than surgery [28].

Two randomized controlled trials comparing UAE with abdominal hysterectomy in 234 women with a minimum follow-up of 6 months (mean: 17 ± 9.3 months) reported an 85% decrease in menstrual loss in the UAE group with a decrease in the mean dominant fibroid volume by 30–46%, and no differences in major complication between the two groups [40]. A systematic review and meta-analysis of four randomized clinical trials, including 515 patients, comparing UAE with hysterectomy/myomectomy in premenopausal women with heavy menstrual bleeding caused by symptomatic uterine fibroids, also reported lower blood loss [41]. However, UAE was associated with a higher rate of minor post-procedural complications, such as vaginal discharge, post-puncture hematoma, and post-embolization syndrome (pain, fever, nausea, vomiting), as well as higher unscheduled visits and readmission rates after discharge, as compared with hysterectomy. Three women in the myomectomy trial had elevated follicle-stimulating hormone (FSH) levels post UAE, indicating possible ovarian dysfunction. The authors concluded that, though UAE offers an advantage over hysterectomy with regard to a shorter hospital stay and a quicker return to routine activities, there is no evidence of a benefit of UAE compared with surgery (hysterectomy/myomectomy) for satisfaction. The higher minor complications rate after discharge in the UAE group as well as the unscheduled visits and readmission rates require more longer-term follow-up trials to comment on its effectiveness and safety profile [40].

Follow-up studies on the efficacy of UAE have demonstrated that it is an efficient therapy in the management of symptomatic myomas and a valid alternative to surgery with an average reduction of 55% in dominant myoma volume at 6 months and 70% at 1-year follow-up at ultrasonic examination, with amenorrhea and fibroid sloughs being the only principal complications [44]. A recent long-term follow-up after UAE for symptomatic uterine leiomyomas on 96 patients treated at a median age of 43 years (range 23–59 years), with the median size of the largest myoma being 69 mm (range 20–170 mm), reported full recovery from symptoms in 53% patients and some effect on symptoms in 36% patients after a median of 8.9 years (range 8–9.4 years). Overall, 25% of the women reported a need for further treatment. The rate of eventual hysterectomy was 22%. The authors confirmed that UAE is among the established treatment options for symptomatic uterine leiomyoma that is safe and well tolerated, with a proven effect on the size of leiomyomas and high long-term satisfaction rate [45].

UAE prior to myomectomy has been shown to be more effective than myomectomy alone, with a lower mean operating time (138 min vs. 240 min; $P < 0.01$), lower mean estimated blood loss (250 mL vs. 690 mL; $P < 0.01$), absence of transfusion requirement (0% vs.13%), lower mean hospital stay (5 days vs. 8 days), and no complications (0% vs. 20% subsequent hysterectomy and bowel/bladder injuries) and a positive pregnancy outcome [46].

Though UAE has been widely used in the United States and Western Europe, and has been recommended by the National Institute for Health and Care Excellence (NICE) in the United Kingdom as an alternative therapy to hysterectomy, it is associated with a range of complications, including premature ovarian failure, chronic vaginal discharge, and pelvic sepsis, and may have limited efficacy when the fibroids are large [4]. Although there are a number of reports of successful pregnancy following UAE, there is insufficient evidence regarding fertility and pregnancy outcome after UAE, the experience is limited, and research is required in this area [4,24,28]. Serial follow-up without surgery for growth and/or development of symptoms is advisable for asymptomatic women, particularly those approaching menopause [24]. Good quality evidence supports the safety and effectiveness of UAE for women with symptomatic fibroids; however, the available data are insufficient to routinely offer UAE to women who wish to preserve or enhance their fertility [28].

USG-guided ablation of fibroids

Real-time USG-guided ablation of fibroids under conscious sedation has been reported to result in a significant reduction in fibroid volume ($76 \pm 24\%$ to $45 \pm 21\%$ at 3 months and $59 \pm 26\%$ at 6 months; $P < 0.05$) and a 92% improved symptom score, with 84.6% patients showing more than 50% volume reduction at 6 months. The ratio of ablated area and volume reduction of fibroids were periodically assessed by MRI, symptom improvements were evaluated by uterine fibroid symptom (UFS), and complications were analyzed by guidelines of the Society of International Radiation (SIR) [47]. Medical management of fibroids delays efforts to conceive and is not recommended for the management of infertility associated with fibroids. Newer treatments such as UAE, radiofrequency ablation, bilateral uterine artery ligation, MRgFUS surgery, and fibroid myolysis require further investigation prior to their establishment in the routine management of fibroid-associated infertility [14]. No increased incidence of complications in women with large-diameter fibroids (≥ 10 cm) or uterine volumes (≥ 750 cm³) has been observed, suggesting that UAE should be offered to women with large fibroids and uterine volumes [48].

Percutaneous sonographically guided radiofrequency ablation

Percutaneous sonographically guided radiofrequency ablation alone in premenopausal women with symptomatic submucosal or intramural uterine myomas is a feasible and efficient procedure in the management of medium-sized uterine myomas [49].

Hydrothermablation

The hydrothermablator is a simple and efficient endometrial ablation technique for patients suffering from menometrorrhagias that can be used in those with uterine myomas and irregular uterine cavity, with good patient satisfaction and results, with pelvic pain as the most common postoperative complication. Hydrothermablation, following a histological evaluation, must be carried out under hysteroscopic control to enable the assessment of treatment success at the end of the intervention [50]. Stovall [42] has reported high (90–95%) patient satisfaction scores after endometrial ablation, but lower amenorrhea rates (15–60%) [42].

Magnetic resonance-guided focused ultrasound surgery (MRgFUS)

MRgFUS is a novel, noninvasive technique of thermoablation for the treatment of symptomatic uterine leiomyomas [51]. It uses MRI for target definition, treatment planning, and closed-loop control of energy deposition. Integrating focused ultrasound surgery and MRI as a therapy delivery system enables the clinician to localize, target, and monitor in real time, and thus, to ablate targeted tissue without damaging normal structures. This precision makes MRgFUS an attractive alternative to surgical resection or radiation therapy of benign and malignant tumors. A disruptive technology, MRgFUS provides new therapeutic approaches and may cause major changes in patient management [52].

A multicenter study, evaluating the pregnancies to date after MRgFUS for the conservative treatment of clinically significant uterine fibroids in reproductive-age women, reported 54 pregnancies in 51 women, following a mean time to conception of 8 months after treatment, 20% ongoing pregnancies beyond 20 gestational weeks, a 41% live birth rate, 28% spontaneous abortion rate, and 64% vaginal delivery rate [53]. Leiomyoma symptom relief after focused ultrasound therapy at 1 year postprocedure is high (85–95%) [42].

Clinical advantages of MRgFUS for symptomatic uterine leiomyomas include sustained symptomatic relief, as measured by the symptom severity score at 24 months, with significantly greater improvement with more complete ablation ($P < 0.001$), a significant reduction in the percentage of women undergoing additional leiomyoma treatment ($P = 0.001$) in the high nonperfused volume group, and a low incidence of adverse events. The nonperfused volume ratio after treatment, calculated from gadolinium-enhanced MRI and the best measure of tissue necrosis after treatment to assess outcome based on completeness of leiomyoma ablation, demonstrated a mean shrinkage and residual nonperfused volume ratio significantly above zero at 6 months in the high nonperfused volume group ($P < 0.001$). For women with minimal treatment, the risk of additional procedures was high [54].

An evaluation of the learning curve effect of MRgFUS on the outcomes of patients treated for uterine fibroids showed that the learning process and accumulation of data on MRgFUS enable the optimization of treatments in order to safely achieve large nonperfused volume ratios, an evaluation of the extent of fibroid ablation and, hence, treatment success and sustained clinical benefit [55].

The use of a 3-month course of GnRH agonist therapy prior to MRgFUS has been shown to improve the thermoablative treatment effect of leiomyomas (>10 cm in diameter) with a reported 45% reduction in median symptom severity score at 6 months and 48% at 12 months post-treatment, with 83% of women achieving at least a 10-point reduction in symptom scoring at 6 months and 89% at 12 months ($P < 0.001$). There was an average reduction in target leiomyoma volume of 21% overall at 6 months ($P < 0.001$) and 37% at 12 months ($P < 0.001$). No serious infective complications or emergency operative interventions were recorded [51].

Magnetic resonance-guided focused ultrasound versus total abdominal hysterectomy

A multicenter contemporaneous and comparative assessment of the safety of MRgFUS (109 women) versus total abdominal hysterectomy (83 women) showed that MRgFUS treatment of uterine leiomyomas leads to clinical improvement with fewer significant clinical complications and adverse events compared with hysterectomy at 6 months' follow-up [56].

According to an estimated economic model of the management of uterine fibroids among premenopausal women receiving treatment with MRgFUS, UAE, abdominal myomectomy, hysterectomy, or pharmacotherapy, MRgFUS was in the range of currently accepted criteria for cost-effectiveness, along with hysterectomy and UAE. Myomectomy was more costly and less effective than both MRgFUS and UAE [57]. However, despite the numerous advantages of MRgFUS, the treatment may not be available to some women for multiple reasons, including leiomyoma size, desire for fertility, and, most commonly, financial limitations. With increasing clinical experience, further research, and broadened insurance coverage, it may be possible to increase accessibility and expand eligibility criteria for this minimally invasive therapy [58].

Electroacupuncture

Electroacupuncture has been reported as a useful, alternative, and relatively noninvasive tool for the management of submucous fibroids with menorrhagia as a severe complaint and decreased blood flow of the uterine artery on Doppler ultrasonographic assessment [59].

Assisted reproduction

Any distortion of the endometrial cavity seriously affects in vitro fertilization (IVF) outcomes. Fibroid location, followed by size, is the most important factor determining the impact of fibroids on IVF outcomes. Although several medical therapies may reduce fibroid volume or decrease menorrhagia, myomectomy remains the standard of care for future fertility and should also be considered for patients with large fibroids, and for patients with unexplained unsuccessful IVF cycles [60]. Myomas that compress the uterine cavity with an intramural portion (submucous myoma type II) and submucous myomas significantly reduce pregnancy rates and should be removed before assisted reproductive technology (ART) is used [61]. Submucosal fibroids have the strongest association with lower ongoing pregnancy rates primarily through decreased implantation [62], while significantly higher pregnancy rates have been reported among patients with submucosal (43.3% vs. 27.2%) and submucosal-intramural (40.0% vs. 15.0%) fibroids who underwent myomectomy as compared with those patients who did not undergo surgical treatment [63]. No statistically significant differences in ART outcomes have been reported in patients with subserosal or intramural leiomyomas, particularly those <4 cm, not encroaching on the uterine cavity [61,63,64]. While some authors report an increase in miscarriage rates in patients with intramural fibroids (20.4%

vs. 12.9%) [62], it is suggested that endometrial receptivity and implantation are not affected by the presence of uterine intramural leiomyomas [61] and they might not require myomectomy prior to ART [64]. However, according to others, the position of the uterine fibroids for infertility may be significant and patients benefit from their removal before attempting conception [63].

Conclusion

In light of several advanced techniques for the evaluation and management of symptomatic uterine fibroids that may serve as effective alternatives to the conventional surgical management, it is absolutely mandatory to adopt an individualized patient-tailored strategy with accurate diagnostic and therapeutic power to maximize the benefits of these techniques. A thorough diagnostic evaluation of the histology, size, and position of the fibroids, symptom severity, the impact on future fertility, and patient preferences with regard to future fertility must be conducted to enable a directed treatment approach that will ensure the achievement of treatment goals and patient satisfaction and minimize reintervention. While TVS, laparoscopy, HSG, hysteroscopy, and hysterosonography are effective first-line diagnostic options, MRI offers an accurate assessment of the number and type of fibroid, occasionally missed by some of these procedures with the potential to direct the management option and outcome.

Medical management may be used as a first-line therapeutic option, but only to improve symptoms and/or shrink the fibroids prior to surgery. Surgical myomectomy for myoma excision is an effective management option for preserving fertility that may be adopted even in the pregnant uterus; however, disadvantages include invasiveness, operative complications, and high technical skills, especially with laparoscopic myomectomy. Hysteroscopic resection, UAE, HIFU, myolysis by heat, cold coagulation and laser, laparoscopic uterine artery occlusion, and temporary transvaginal uterine artery occlusion are minimally invasive procedures for women who opt for nonsurgical treatment. However, they are technically demanding and limited in application by the nature and size of fibroid. The use of hysteroscopic resection is restricted to submucous fibroids, while UAE and HIFU may be more effective for intramural and subserous myomas. UAE and MRgFUS are attractive, minimally invasive, and effective treatment alternatives to surgical resection or radiation therapy with diagnostic and therapeutic potential. However, the incidence of reintervention and complications of UAE and the technical and financial demands of MRgFUS limit their use. Assisted reproduction may be an option following myomectomy for large fibroids with cavity involvement and for intramural and submucosal fibroids that are associated with reduced fertility and increased miscarriage rates. Hysterectomy may be adopted as a last resort in the event of failure of medical and/or surgical options and when there is no desire for future fertility. Larger, comparative, prospective randomized controlled trials, evaluating the long-term efficacy with regard to the nature of fibroids, symptom severity and quality of life, the cost–benefit ratio, and the learning curve of the newer methods of intervention compared to surgery are warranted.

References

1. Agdi M, Tulandi T. Minimally invasive approach for myomectomy. *Semin Reprod Med* 2010; **28**(3):228–234.

2. Fasih N, Prasad Shanbhogue AK, Macdonald DB, et al. Leiomyomas beyond the uterus: unusual locations, rare manifestations. *Radiographics* 2008; **28**(7): 1931–1948.

3. Evans P, Brunsell S. Uterine fibroid tumors: diagnosis and treatment. *Am Fam Physician* 2007; **75**(10): 1503–1508.

4. Istre O. Management of symptomatic fibroids: conservative surgical treatment modalities other than abdominal or laparoscopic myomectomy. *Best Pract Res Clin Obstet Gynaecol* 2008; **22**(4): 735–747.

5. Cooper NP, Okolo S. Fibroids in pregnancy – common but poorly understood. *Obstet Gynecol Surv* 2005; **60**(2): 132–138.

6. Reed SD, Cushing-Haugen KL, Daling JR, et al. Postmenopausal estrogen and progestogen therapy and the risk of uterine leiomyomas. *Menopause* 2004; **11**(2): 214–222.

7. King R, Overton C. Management of fibroids should be tailored to the patient. *Practitioner* 2011; **255**(1738): 19–23, 2–3.

8. Cook H, Ezzati M, Segars JH, McCarthy K. The impact of uterine leiomyomas on reproductive outcomes. *Minerva Ginecol* 2010; **62**(3): 225–236.

9. Bignardi T, Van den Bosch T, Condous G. Abnormal uterine and post-menopausal bleeding in the acute gynaecology unit. *Best Pract Res Clin Obstet Gynaecol* 2009; **23**(5): 595–607.

10. Parker WH. Uterine myomas: management. *Fertil Steril* 2007; **88**(2): 255–271.

11. Najeeb R, Awan AS, Bakhtiar U, Akhter S. Role of transvaginal sonography in assessment of abnormal uterine bleeding in perimenopausal age group. *J Ayub Med Coll Abbottabad* 2010; **22**(1): 87–90.

12. Gojnic M, Pervulov M, Mostic T, Petkovic S. Doppler ultrasound as an additional parameter for the evaluation of myomas and the indication of myomectomy during pregnancy. *Fetal Diagn Ther* 2004; **19**(5): 462–464.

13. Gervaise A. [Hierarchy for diagnostic and etiological management in menometrorrhagia].[Article in French]. *J Gynecol Obstet Biol Reprod (Paris)* 2008; **37**(Suppl 8): S349–355.

14. Kroon B, Johnson N, Chapman M, et al; on behalf of the Australasian CREI Consensus Expert Panel on Trial evidence (ACCEPT) group. Fibroids in infertility – consensus statement from ACCEPT (Australasian CREI Consensus Expert Panel on Trial evidence). *Aust N Z J Obstet Gynaecol* 2011; **51**(4): 289–295.

15. Imaoka I, Wada A, Matsuo M, et al. MR imaging of disorders associated with female infertility: use in diagnosis, treatment, and management. *Radiographics* 2003; **23**(6): 1401–1421.

16. Fambrini M, Tondi F, Scarselli G, et al. Comparison of the number of uterine myomas detected by in-office transvaginal ultrasonography removed by laparotomic myomectomy: preoperative work-up concerns. *Clin Exp Obstet Gynecol* 2009; **36**: 97–101.

17. Rajan DK, Margau R, Kroll RR, et al. Clinical utility of ultrasound versus magnetic resonance imaging for deciding to proceed with uterine artery embolization for presumed symptomatic fibroids. *Clin Radiol* 2011; **66**(1): 57–62.

18. Spielmann AL, Keogh C, Forster BB, et al. Comparison of MRI and sonography in the preliminary evaluation for fibroid embolization. *Am J Roentgenol* 2006; **187**(6): 1499–1504.

19. Moghadam R, Lathi RB, Shahmohamady B, et al. Predictive value of magnetic resonance imaging in differentiating between leiomyoma and adenomyosis. *JSLS* 2006; **10**(2): 216–219.

20. Walker J. Transvaginal ultrasound guided biopsies in the diagnosis of pelvic lesions. *Minim Invasive Ther Allied Technol* 2003; **12**(5): 241–244.

21. Estrade-Huchon S, Bouhanna P, Limot O, et al. Severe life-threatening hemoperitoneum from posttraumatic avulsion of a pedunculated uterine leiomyoma. *J Minim Invasive Gynecol* 2010; **17**(5): 651–652.

22. Levy BS. Modern management of uterine fibroids. *Acta Obstet Gynecol Scand* 2008; **87**(8): 812–823.

23. Kolankaya A, Arici A. Myomas and assisted reproductive technologies: when and how to act? *Obstet Gynecol Clin North Am* 2006; **33**(1): 145–152.

24. Duhan N. Current and emerging treatments for uterine myoma – an update. *Int J Womens Health* 2011; **3**: 231–241.

25. Purohit R, Sharma JG, Singh S. A case of diffuse uterine leiomyomatosis who had two successful pregnancies after medical management. *Fertil Steril* 2011; **95**(7): 2434.e5–6.

26. Sayyah-Melli M, Tehrani-Gadim S, Dastranj-Tabrizi A, et al. Comparison of the effect of gonadotropin-releasing hormone agonist and dopamine receptor agonist on uterine myoma growth. Histologic, sonographic, and intra-operative changes. *Saudi Med J* 2009; **30**(8): 1024–1033.

27. Wilkens J, Chwalisz K, Han C, et al. Effects of the selective progesterone receptor modulator asoprisnil on uterine artery blood flow, ovarian activity, and clinical symptoms in patients with uterine leiomyomata scheduled for hysterectomy. *J Clin Endocrinol Metab* 2008; **93**(12): 4664–4671.

28. Tropeano G, Amoroso S, Scambia G. Non-surgical management of uterine fibroids. *Hum Reprod Update* 2008; **14**(3): 259–274.

29. Venkatachalam S, Bagratee JS, Moodley J. Medical management of uterine fibroids with medroxyprogesterone acetate (Depo Provera): a pilot study. *J Obstet Gynaecol* 2004; **24**(7): 798–800.

30. Suwandinata FS, Gruessner SE, Omwandho CO, Tinneberg HR. Pregnancy-preserving myomectomy: preliminary report on a new surgical technique. *Eur J Contracept Reprod Health Care* 2008; **13**(3): 323–326.

31. Lee CL, Wang CJ. Laparoscopic myomectomy. *Taiwan J Obstet Gynecol* 2009; **48**(4): 335–341.

32. Altgassen C, Kuss S, Berger U, et al. Complications in laparoscopic myomectomy. *Surg Endosc* 2006; **20**(4): 614–618.

33. Falcone T, Bedaiwy MA. Minimally invasive management of uterine fibroids. *Curr Opin Obstet Gynecol* 2002; **14**(4): 401–407.

34. Parker WH. Laparoscopic myomectomy and abdominal myomectomy. *Clin Obstet Gynecol* 2006; **49**(4): 789–797.

35. Hanafi M. Predictors of leiomyoma recurrence after myomectomy. *Obstet Gynecol* 2005; **105**(4): 877–881.

36. Simsek M, Sadik S, Taskin O, et al. Role of laparoscopic uterine artery coagulation in management of symptomatic myomas: a prospective study using ultrasound and magnetic resonance imaging. *J Minim Invasive Gynecol* 2006; **13**(4): 315–319.

37. Akinola OI, Fabamwo AO, Ottun AT, Akinniyi OA. Uterine artery ligation for management of uterine fibroids. *Int J Gynaecol Obstet* 2005; **91**(2): 137–140.

38. Liu WM, Tzeng CR, Yi-Jen C, Wang PH. Combining the uterine depletion procedure and myomectomy may be useful for treating symptomatic fibroids. *Fertil Steril* 2004; **82**(1): 205–210.

39. Zupi E, Marconi D, Sbracia M, et al. Directed laparoscopic cryomyolysis for symptomatic leiomyomata: one-year follow up. *J Minim Invasive Gynecol* 2005; **12**(4): 343–346.

40. Gupta JK, Sinha AS, Lumsden MA, Hickey M. Uterine artery embolization for symptomatic uterine fibroids. *Cochrane Database Syst Rev* 2006; **25**(1): CD005073.

41. van der Kooij SM, Bipat S, Hehenkamp WJ, et al. Uterine artery embolization versus surgery in the treatment of symptomatic fibroids: a systematic review and meta-analysis. *Am J Obstet Gynecol* 2011; **205**(4): 317.e1–18.

42. Stovall DW. Alternatives to hysterectomy: focus on global endometrial ablation, uterine fibroid embolization, and magnetic resonance-guided focused ultrasound. *Menopause* 2011; **18**(4): 437–444.

43. Manyonda IT, Bratby M, Horst JS, et al. Uterine artery embolization versus myomectomy: impact on quality of life-results of the FUME (Fibroids of the Uterus: Myomectomy versus Embolization) trial. *Cardiovasc Intervent Radiol* 2012; **35**(3): 530–536.

44. Ravina JH, Aymard A, Ciraru-Vigneron N, et al. [Uterine fibroids embolization: results about 454 cases].[Article in French] *Gynecol Obstet Fertil* 2003; **31**(7–8): 597–605.

45. Poulsen B, Munk T, Ravn P. Long-term follow up after uterine artery embolization for symptomatic uterine leiomyomas. *Acta Obstet Gynecol Scand* 2011; **90**(11): 1281–1283.

46. Üstünsöz B, Uğurel MS, Bozlar U, et al. Is uterine artery embolization prior to myomectomy for giant fibroids helpful? *Diagn Interv Radiol* 2007; **13**(4): 210–212.

47. Chen WZ, Tang LD, Yang WW, et al. [Study on the efficacy and safety of ultrasound ablation in treatment of uterine fibroids.] [Article in Chinese] *Zhonghua Fu Chan Ke Za Zhi* 2010; **45**(12): 909–912.

48. Parthipun AA, Taylor J, Manyonda I, Belli AM. Does size really matter? Analysis of the effect of large fibroids and uterine volumes on complication rates of uterine artery embolisation. *Cardiovasc Intervent Radiol* 2010; **33**(5): 955–959.

49. Recaldini C, Carrafiello G, Laganà D, et al. Percutaneous sonographically guided radiofrequency ablation of medium-sized fibroids: feasibility study. *Am J Roentgenol* 2007; **189**(6): 1303–1306.

50. Guillot E, Omnes S, Yazbeck C, et al. [Endometrial ablation using hydrothermablator: results of a French multicenter study]. [Article in French] *Gynecol Obstet Fertil* 2008; **36**(1): 45–50.

51. Smart OC, Hindley JT, Regan L, Gedroyc WG. Gonadotrophin-releasing hormone and magnetic-resonance-guided ultrasound surgery for uterine leiomyomata. *Obstet Gynecol* 2006; **108**(1): 49–54.

52. Jolesz FA. MRI-guided focused ultrasound surgery. *Annu Rev Med* 2009; **60**: 417–430.

53. Rabinovici J, David M, Fukunishi H, et al; MRgFUS Study Group. Pregnancy outcome after magnetic resonance-guided focused ultrasound surgery (MRgFUS) for conservative treatment of uterine fibroids. *Fertil Steril* 2010; **93**(1): 199–209.

54. Stewart EA, Gostout B, Rabinovici J, et al. Sustained relief of leiomyoma symptoms by using focused ultrasound surgery. *Obstet Gynecol* 2007; **110**(2 Pt 1): 279–287.

55. Okada A, Morita Y, Fukunishi H, et al T. Non-invasive magnetic resonance-guided focused ultrasound treatment of uterine fibroids in a large Japanese population: impact of the learning curve on patient outcome. *Ultrasound Obstet Gynecol* 2009; **34**(5): 579–583.

56. Taran FA, Tempany CM, Regan L, et al; MRgFUS Group. Magnetic resonance-guided focused ultrasound (MRgFUS) compared with abdominal hysterectomy for treatment of uterine leiomyomas. *Ultrasound Obstet Gynecol* 2009; **34**(5): 572–578.

57. O'Sullivan AK, Thompson D, Chu P, et al. Cost-effectiveness of magnetic resonance guided focused ultrasound for the treatment of uterine fibroids. *Int J Technol Assess Health Care* 2009; **25**(1): 14–25.

58. Behera MA, Leong M, Johnson L, Brown H. Eligibility and accessibility of magnetic resonance-guided focused ultrasound (MRgFUS) for the treatment of uterine leiomyomas. *Fertil Steril* 2010; **94**(5): 1864–1868.

59. Cakmak YÖ, Akpınar IN, Yoldemir T, Cavdar S. Decreasing bleeding due to uterine fibroid with electroacupuncture. *Fertil Steril* 2011; **96**(1): e13–15.

60. Rackow BW, Arici A. Fibroids and in-vitro fertilization: which comes first? *Curr Opin Obstet Gynecol* 2005; **17**(3): 225–231.

61. Kolankaya A, Arici A. Myomas and assisted reproductive technologies: when and how to act? *Obstet Gynecol Clin North Am* 2006; **33**(1): 145–152.

62. Klatsky PC, Tran ND, Caughey AB, Fujimoto VY. Fibroids and reproductive outcomes: a systematic literature review from conception to delivery. *Am J Obstet Gynecol* 2008; **198**(4): 357–366.

63. Casini ML, Rossi F, Agostini R, Unfer V. Effects of the position of fibroids on fertility. *Gynecol Endocrinol* 2006; **22**(2): 106–109.

64. Oliveira FG, Abdelmassih VG, Diamond MP, et al. Impact of subserosal and intramural uterine fibroids that do not distort the endometrial cavity on the outcome of in vitro fertilization-intracytoplasmic sperm injection. *Fertil Steril* 2004; **81**(3): 582–587.

Chapter

13

Uterine artery embolization for the treatment of uterine fibroids

Shawky Z. A. Badawy, Harold Henning and Bruce Singer

Introduction

Leiomyomas or fibroids of the uterus are the most common benign uterine tumors in women. They affect about 20–50% of women during their reproductive years [1]. The etiology of these benign tumors is not known. However, genetic predisposition has been suggested since members of families have been reported to be affected with these tumors [2]. A high incidence has been found in African American women, nulliparous women, and obese women [3].

Leiomyomas are mostly present in the corpus uteri and less than 0.4% are present in the cervix of the uterus. These tumors can be subserosal, intramural, or submucous in their location.

A cut section in these myomas shows that they are firm in consistency and represent a whorled appearance because of the presence of muscle fibers as well as connective tissue fibers. Subserous myomas sometimes enlarge and develop a pedicle, and are then known as pedunculated tumors [4].

Leiomyomas are subject to develop various kinds of degeneration, including hyaline degeneration, cystic degeneration, and vascular necrosis. Rarely, fibroids or leiomyomas have been found in the ovary, fallopian tube, round ligament, and broad ligament.

Pathogenesis

Leiomyomas have been found to have receptors for estrogens and progesterone, and they have also been found to be rich in growth factors, including transforming growth factor beta 3, fibroblast growth factor, epidermal growth factor, and insulin-like growth factor 1 [5–8].

Steroidal oral contraceptives may affect leiomyomas by stimulating their growth or they may have no effect [9]. However, during pregnancy with high levels of estrogens and progesterone, these tumors grow to a large size and may undergo degeneration. They also affect the pregnancy in the form of miscarriages, premature labor, and malpresentations. The incidence of cesarean section might be higher, especially if these tumors are located in the lower segment where they may interfere with vaginal delivery [10]. These tumors also regress with onset of menopause due to loss of the ovarian function and very low levels of estrogens and progesterone.

Clinical picture

Many of these fibroid tumors are asymptomatic and they are discovered during routine clinical evaluation. In other groups of women, the fibroids lead to symptoms that may affect the quality of life. These symptoms include menorrhagia, which is heavy and/or prolonged bleeding during menses. In severe longstanding cases, it may lead to anemia and may require blood transfusion. Many of these patients present to the Emergency Room or offices of their physicians because of this heavy bleeding. The heavy bleeding is due to an increase in blood supply to these fibroids and an increase in the surface area of the endometrial cavity; and therefore bleeding will be heavier during the menstrual cycle. Some of these patients present with pelvic pain which is related to the tumor degeneration that may occur or due to association with endometriosis in the same patient. In cases of fibroids that are occupying the lower part of the uterus or the cervix, pressure on the bladder will occur leading to increased frequency of urination or difficulty in urination. Large pelvic fibroids may put pressure on the pelvic colon and cause constipation [11].

Diagnosis

The clinical picture and the pelvic examination usually lead to the diagnosis of pelvic masses that are firm in consistency, attached to the uterus. However, in order to differentiate these fibroids from ovarian neoplasms, the use of ultrasound studies and various radiologic techniques, including CT scan and MRI, will help in confirming the diagnosis.

Ultrasound by the use of abdominal or endovaginal probe usually helps in making the proper diagnosis. It shows the uterus and the fibroids with their locations, whether subserous, intramural, or submucous. The ovaries are usually detected very easily. We believe that ultrasound methodology is much more informative than CT scans and MRI for the diagnosis of pelvic conditions.

Ultrasonography in Gynecology, ed. Botros R. M. B. Rizk and Elizabeth E. Puscheck. Published by Cambridge University Press. © Cambridge University Press 2015.

Management

Expectant management

Small fibroids, less than 4 cm in diameter, and at the same time asymptomatic by the fact that they were discovered during routine pelvic examination, could be followed up expectantly with pelvic examination every 6 months to one year. This might be supplemented with an ultrasound evaluation. This usually has no deleterious effect on the health of the patient or her wellbeing.

Symptomatic fibroids causing menorrhagia, pelvic pain, and/or discomfort should be actively treated, according to the following modalities.

1. Medical treatment

Various medications have been used in either prospective or controlled studies and have been shown to be effective in reducing the size of the fibroid. Aromatase inhibitors act on aromatase present locally in the fibroids. The use of aromatase inhibitors has been shown to reduce the size of the fibroid without reduction in the level of estradiol or changes in follicle-stimulating hormone (FSH) level. This is because aromatase inhibitors act on aromatase enzymes within the myoma itself [12,13].

In a placebo-controlled study, the antiprogesterone mifepristone has been used to treat fibroids. Mifepristone use resulted in a decrease in menstrual blood loss and an increase in hemoglobin level, and 84.2% of patients became amenorrheic. The myoma size was reduced by 26.6% as compared with the placebo-treated group. Mifepristone acts by decreasing the progesterone receptors in the fibroids directly. One of the side effects of the use of mifepristone is the development of endometrial hyperplasia without atypia in some patients [14,15]

GnRH agonists have been used to reduce the size of the myomas and also to reduce uterine bleeding and correct anemia in some patients who suffer from heavy uterine bleeding. It has been the custom with many gynecologists to use GnRH agonists for 3 months prior to surgery, thus dealing with smaller myomas and reducing blood flow, which makes the operation easier and also improves the recovery rate. One side effect of the use of GnRH agonists may be vasomotor symptoms as a result of hypoestrogenism. If that is the case, then an add-back therapy using a progestin or even estrogen and progestin will alleviate all these problems. Use of GnRH agonists in medical treatment of fibroids for 3–6 months will not be very effective in the long term. This is due to the fact that, once the medication is discontinued, the fibroids will start growing back again and the various symptoms will return. Therefore, GnRH agonists are not suitable for long-term therapy of myomas, except for cases that are eventually going to surgery [16].

2. Surgical treatment

Surgical treatment depends on the needs of the patient as relates to fertility potential. For young patients who would like to have pregnancies in the future and their fibroids are symptomatic, myomectomy will be an appropriate surgical treatment. Myomectomy can be done by laparotomy, laparoscopy, or robotic surgery. Each one of these technologies will need good experience. The amount of blood loss during myomectomy can be high, and therefore the experience of the surgeon is very important. The use of agents to control bleeding during surgery is advisable. One method is the use of diluted vasopressin solution, which is injected intramurally into the myoma and around the myoma to constrict blood supply. Surgery will be done by incising the capsule and extracting the myoma, then reconstructing the uterine wall with several sutures. In order to prevent postoperative adhesions, usually a barrier method is used, specifically, Interceed or Seprafilm, to cover the surgical incision in the uterus. The recurrence rate after myomectomy varies with the number of myomas removed and also the length of time since myomectomy. It also varies with the technique used, whether abdominal myomectomy or laparoscopic surgery.

Abdominal myomectomy is used for large uterine myomas that are symptomatic and which may be intramural or subserous. The surgery traditionally can be done through laparotomy and evaluation of the myoma. To control the bleeding during myomectomy, usually the capsule of the myoma is injected with diluted Pitressin solution. Following myomectomy, the uterine wall is constructed.

Recently, myomectomy has also been performed through laparoscopic surgery and also robotic surgery. These technological advances need proper training for the removal of the myoma and reconstruction of the uterine wall.

Following myomectomy, the pregnancy rate is usually in the range of 50–60%[17]. However, the recurrence rate is estimated to be about 60% [17]. Patients who do not desire pregnancy and are symptomatic may require hysterectomy. However, in order to avoid major surgery, an alternative would be uterine artery embolization (UAE) [17–20].

Hysteroscopic myomectomy is reserved for cases of submucous myomas. In these cases, a resectoscope is used with a distension medium using glycine and the myoma is resected piecemeal until the capsule is reached. The success rate depends on the circumference of the myoma in the uterine cavity and the wall of the uterus. Larger myomas that project into the uterine cavity have a better success rate than when the myoma is mostly intramural and only a small portion is in the uterine cavity. Therefore, preoperative assessment with ultrasound evaluation is essential [21].

Uterine artery embolization

UAE for the management of uterine leiomyomas was first reported by Ravina et al. in 1995 [22]. The procedure was done first in France and then it was introduced in the United States by Goodwin and Walker in 1998 [23]. Since that time, many cases have been treated with this methodology.

UAE has become a widely accepted alternative to hysterectomy and myomectomy, with approximately 25 000 UAE procedures performed annually worldwide. Since 1999, the Fibroid Registry for Outcomes Data has enrolled 2000 patients. The clinical response rate was 86%. There was a 14.4% recurrence rate after 3 years [24].

Inclusion criteria for UAE are similar for patients that would have had surgical treatment. However, UAE is limited to patients who have up to a 20-week-sized uterus or a dominant fibroid less than 12 cm. Patients with pedunculated leiomyomas have been successfully treated with UAE [25]. However, pedunculated leiomyomas with a narrow stalk may best be treated with myomectomy. Often, UAE is performed 3 weeks prior to myomectomy to facilitate leiomyoma bulk reduction and to reduce bleeding complications. Patients have an endometrial biopsy to exclude neoplasm if there is a history of menstruation lasting longer than 10 days or there is postmenopausal bleeding.

The technique of UAE requires selective catheterization of each uterine artery using contralateral and/or ipsilateral femoral artery approaches. Often a flush pelvic arteriogram is obtained to provide a roadmap to the uterine arteries. This step is not needed if pelvic magnetic resonance angiogram (MRA) has been obtained. Routine use of MRI with MRA prior to UAE is essential to map the leiomyoma burden and characterize the types of fibroids that will be embolized.

Transvaginal and transabdominal ultrasound underrepresents the leiomyoma burden and does not allow accurate localization of leiomyomas, especially when they are subserosal. MRI displays degenerated leiomyomas that will not respond well to UAE. MRI also reveals occult internal iliac vein thrombus, which has been reported to cause subacute pulmonary emboli after UAE. Uterine volume reduction decompressed the internal iliac vein and allowed the thrombus to embolize [26]. MRI also convincingly identifies coexisting adenomyosis, which has a symptom complex that overlaps leiomyomas. UAE has been shown to be effective for adenomyosis, but the duration of response is approximately 50% after 3 years [27].

MRI is essential to define the size and number of submucosal and cervical leiomyomas. Most interventional radiologists will refer patients for endometrial myomectomy if the leiomyoma is smaller than 3–4 cm. UAE is not effective for cervical leiomyomas because of the collateral blood supply from the cervicovaginal arteries.

Four- or 5-French catheters are used to select the internal uterine arteries. Most interventional radiologists employ coaxial 3-French microcatheters to select the uterine arteries (Fig. 13.1). Coaxial microcatheters are much less likely to induce spasm of the uterine arteries. Initially, UAE was performed with gelfoam and polyvinyl alcohol particles. Now, precisely sized gelatin microspheres, typically 500–700 μm, are slowly injected with contrast to occlude the arterioles that feed the leiomyomas. Angiographers desire a "pruned tree" endpoint to UAE to preserve patency of the main uterine artery branches while occluding the larger leiomyoma arterioles (Fig. 13.2). Overembolization of the uterine arteries causes uterine infarction and increased pain for the patient. Uterine

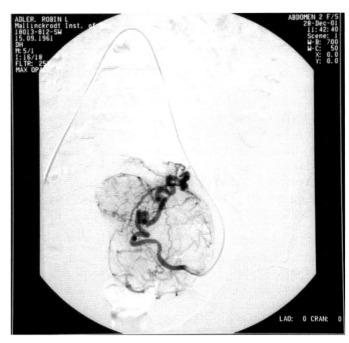

Fig. 13.1 Selective arteriogram of the left uterine artery showing hypervascular leiomyomas.

infarction is associated with a higher risk of endometritis that may require hysterectomy.

Evaluation of the ovarian arteries is important in revealing collateral arterial supply to the leiomyomas. Failure to look for ovarian artery collaterals is a main reason for UAE failure. Ovarian artery embolization is usually performed with gelfoam pledgets that temporarily occlude the proximal uterine arteries. UAE can induce menopause in a selected number of patients. For this reason, FSH levels are obtained routinely in UAE patients to identify the perimenopausal patient.

Patients typically have post-embolization pain and a low-grade fever following UAE. A common sequela of UAE is prolonged watery vaginal discharge. Rarer complications include prolonged pain, pyometria, endometritis, urinary tract infection, and urinary retention. There have been reports of death from sepsis, pulmonary embolism, uterine necrosis, and non-target embolization [24]. Patients with submucosal leiomyomas are at increased risk for transcervical expulsion of the fibroid. Patients are counseled that leiomyoma expulsion can occur up to 2 years after UAE. Patients are typically treated in a 23-hour outpatient scenario. Some interventional radiologists discharge patients the same day. Patients are given prescriptions for narcotics and NSAIDs for the next 7–10 days. Post-embolization follow-up consists of a pelvic MRI in 3–6 months to evaluate response to therapy (Fig. 13.3). Most patients are able to resume normal activity within one week.

Pathologic effects on the leiomyomas after UAE include hyaline degeneration and necrosis. The leiomyoma involutes and improved bulk and bleeding symptoms are noticed within 2 weeks. The pathologic impact on leiomyomas from UAE mimics menopause. At 3 months after UAE, MRI imaging showed

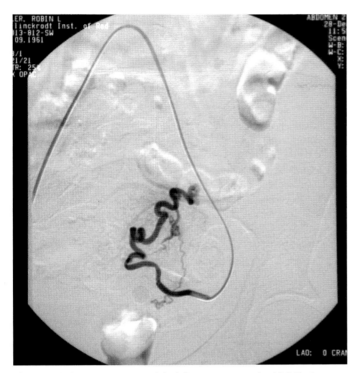

Fig. 13.2 Selective angiogram of the left uterine artery after UAE. Notice devascularized leiomyomas with preserved uterine perfusion.

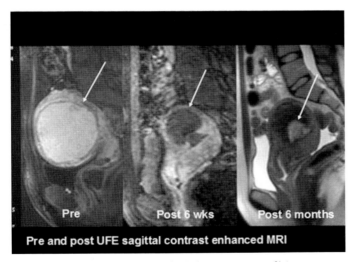

Pre and post UFE sagittal contrast enhanced MRI

Fig. 13.3 Sagittal contrast-enhanced MRI depicts response of leiomyoma (arrows) to UAE.

that 98.8% of patients had decreased leiomyoma volume [28]. There was a mean of 52.6% leiomyoma volume reduction. After one year, there was a 73.3% reduction in leiomyoma volume. Submucosal leiomyomas showed the greatest volume reduction while subserosal leiomyomas showed the least volume reduction [28]. Many patients have transient amenorrhea. Three percent of patients less than 45 years old and 20–40% of patients over 45 years old become menopausal [24].

Myomectomy has been the standard therapy in patients desiring pregnancy. However, the operative morbidity and increased incidence of abnormal placental implantation make UAE an attractive alternative. UAE has been prospectively studied in patients desiring pregnancy with 2-year pregnancy rates of 50%, abortion rate of 64%, and delivery rate of 19% [29]. The myomectomy cohort had a pregnancy rate of 78%, abortion rate of 23%, and delivery rate of 48%. Therefore, myomectomy remains the standard of care because of the increased rate of spontaneous abortion, preterm delivery, and abnormal placental implantation after UAE compared with myomectomy [29].

UAE of symptomatic leiomyomas has come of age since 1995, with durable success rates and worldwide clinical acceptance.

Long-term effect of uterine artery embolization

UAE has been reported since 1995 for treatment of symptomatic leiomyomas and clinical studies related to pregnancy after UAE were subsequently reported in 2008 [30]. Initially, UAE was not used in women who desired future childbearing because of the potential and unknown risks associated with changing the blood flow to the uterus. Additional concerns included potential effects on the circulation to the ovaries, which theoretically could lead to devastating effects on the germ cells, causing premature menopause, decreasing ovulation rates, or increased miscarriage rates.

More data are available about the long-term effects of UAE on fibroids (excluding pregnancy issues); therefore, this subject will be addressed first, followed by the effects of UAE on fertility and pregnancy.

Long-term outcomes for the treatment of leiomyomas via UAE are available from the FIBROID Registry reported in 2008, which was a 3-year study [31]. Short-term outcomes, including baseline comparisons as well as complications of UAE, were reported in 2005 from the same study [32– 34]. The long-term 3-year study resulted in a significant improvement in quality of life in the majority of women. This represented a diverse set of practices across the country at 27 sites and included 2112 symptomatic women; 1916 women remained in the study, but only 1278 completed the study survey, thought to be due to consent issues and extending the end point a number of years [31].

A 2005 study by Spies et al. addressed long-term outcome over a 5-year period [35,36]. Of the 200 women initially treated with UAE, 182 completed the study and of those women, 73% had successful control of their symptoms. Twenty percent of women studied had symptom control failure or their symptoms recurred, of which 13.7% had a hysterectomy performed. These results support using UAE in symptomatic women with leiomyomas because the majority (73–85%) had successful outcomes.

The largest study addressing pregnancy after UAE, complications of pregnancy, and pregnancy outcomes was recorded with analyses and pregnancy outcomes from the FIBROID Registry [31]. Two studies published in 2008 were designed to evaluate pregnancies in women who had previously undergone UAE using tris-acryl gelatin microspheres [30,37]. The first study included 100 women who had symptomatic fibroids and a desire to preserve their fertility. They were advised to wait 6 months after UAE before attempting pregnancy. Five patients were lost to follow-up and one patient became pregnant twice. None of the women who were older than age 40 conceived after UAE. Eleven pregnancies were documented in 10 patients with eight live births and three miscarriages in two patients, giving a pregnancy rate of 12% and a live birth rate of 8.4%. However, only 39 of 95 patients were less than 40 years of age and some of them did not want to conceive after their UAE procedure, explaining the overall low rate of pregnancy and live births.

The second study was actually a prospective, cohort-controlled comparative study of the reproductive outcomes after laparoscopic uterine artery occlusion (LUAO) and UAE. Thirty-nine patients were treated with UAE and 20 conceived with a 51.2% pregnancy rate, but a 56% miscarriage rate, as compared with an 11.1% miscarriage rate for those patients treated with LUAO [37].

A potential reason for the higher miscarriage rate could be an abnormal endometrial cavity, as demonstrated via hysteroscopic evaluation after UAE as compared with LUAO [38]. There was also a higher incidence of necrosis in the uterine cavity of patients having UAE performed (43.2%) compared with patients after LUAO (2.7%) [38]. Another study compared patients treated with UAE versus patients having fibroid-containing pregnancies, matched for age and fibroid location, with a miscarriage rate of 35.2% in the UAE pregnancies as compared with 16.5% in the matched fibroid containing controls [39]. Also in that study the UAE patients were more likely to be delivered by cesarean section and to experience postpartum hemorrhage (PPH).

A 2005 study by Greene, Schnatz, and Hallisey stated that the American College of Obstetricians and Gynecologists Committee on Gynecologic Practice considered UAE investigational in women wishing to retain their fertility [40]. They selected 60 women for UAE who had symptomatic fibroids and wanted to retain their potential for future fertility. Of those patients, 22 were reachable by telephone and only 3 had conceived. Two had delivered singleton gestations and one was again pregnant with twins. One patient was yet undelivered at the time of publication and one of the pregnant patients presented with placenta previa. They stated that many studies at that time showed little to no effect of UAE on future fertility, but that more data were needed to support this conclusion [40].

Tulandi and Salamah in a 2010 study stated that women who wish to conceive should not be treated with UAE due to the possibility of decreased ovarian function as well as increased pregnancy complications [41]. Another prospective cohort 5-year study published in the same year suggested, however, that UAE does not lead to an accelerated decline in ovarian reserve in younger patients (26–39 years of age) [42]. Tulandi and Salamah went on to state that myomectomy is preferred over UAE because it preserves ovarian function, making it the preferable intervention in reproductive-age women [41].

References

1. Buttram Jr VC, Reiter RC. Leiomyomata: etiology, symptomatology and management. *Fertil Steril* 1981; **36**: 433–445.

2. Vikhlyaeva EM, Khogehaeva ZS, Fantszhenko ND. Familial predisposition to uterine leiomyomas. *Int J Gynecol Obstet* 1995; **51**(2): 127–131.

3. Flake GP, Andersen J, Dixon D. Etiology and pathogenesis of uterine leiomyomas: a review. *Environ Health Perspect* 2003; **111**(8): 1037–1054.

4. Robboy SJ, Bentley RC, Butnor K, Anderson MC. Pathology and pathophysiology of uterine smooth muscle tumors. *Environ Health Perspect* 2000; **108**(S5): 779–784.

5. Vrandon DD, Erickson TE, Keenan EG, et al. Estrogen receptor gene expression in human uterine leiomyomata. *J Clin Endocrinol Metab* 1985; **80**: 1876–1881.

6. Vrandon DD, Bethea CL, Stawn EY, et al. Progesterone receptor messenger ribonucleic assay and protein are over expressed in human uterine leiomyomas. *Am J Obstet Gynecol* 1993; **169**: 78–85.

7. Boehn KD, Daimon M, Gorodeski IG, et al. Expression of insulin-like and platelet derived growth factor genes in human uterine tissues. *Mol Reprod Def* 1990; **27**: 93–101.

8. Asahara T, Bauters T, Zheng LP, et al. Synergistic effect of vascular endothelial growth factor and basic fibroblast growth factor on angiogenesis in vivo. *Circulation* 1995; **92**(2): 365–371.

9. Parazzini F, Netri T, Lavecchia C, et al. Oral contraceptive use and risk of uterine fibroids. *Obstet Gynecol* 1992; **79**: 430–433.

10. Bromberg JV, Goltberg J, Rychlak K, et al. The effect of uterine fibroids on pregnancy outcome. *Am J Obstet Gynecol* 2004; **191**: 18–21.

11. Evans P, Brunsell S. Uterine fibroid tumors: diagnosis and patency. *J Am Acad Family Phys* 2007; **75**(10): 1503–1508.

12. Kaunitz AM. Aromatase inhibitor therapy for uterine bleeding in a postmenopausal woman with leiomyomata. *Menopause* 2007; **14**(5): 941–943.

13. Hilario SG, Bozzini N, Borsari R, Baracat EC. Action of aromatase inhibitor for treatment of uterine leiomyoma in perimenopausal patients. *Fertil Steril* 2009; **91**(1): 240–243.

14. Engman M, Grandberg S, Williams ARW, et al. Misepristone for treatment of uterine leiomyoma – a perspective randomized placebo-controlled trial. *Hum Reprod* 2009; **24**(8): 1870–1879.

15. Vagaria M, Suneja A, Vaid ND, et al. Low dose misepristone in treatment of uterine leiomyoma – a randomized double-blind placebo controlled clinical trial. *Aust N Z J Obstet Gynecol* 2009; **49**: 77–83.

16. Defalco M, Tollio F, Pontillo M, et al. GNRH agonists and antagonists in the preoperative therapy of uterine fibroids – literature review. *Minerva Gynecol* 2006; **58**(6): 553–560.

17. Goldberg J, Pereira L. Pregnancy outcomes following treatment for fibroids: uterine fibroid embolization vs. laparoscopic myomectomy. *Curr Opin Obstet Gynecol* 2006; **18**(4): 402–406.

18. Dillon T. Control of blood loss during gynecologic surgery. *Obstet Gynecol* 1962; **19**: 428.

19. Iverson R, Chelmow D. Relative morbidity of abdominal hysterectomy and myomectomy for management of uterine leiomyomas. *Obstet Gynecol* 1996; **88**: 415.

20. Dubuisson JB, Lecuru F, Foulo CH, et al. Myomectomy by laparoscopy, preliminary report of forty three cases. *Fertil Steril* 1991; **56**: 828.

21. Neuwrth RS. Hysteroscopic management of symptomatic submucous fibroids. *Obstet Gynecol* 1993; **62**: 509.

22. Ravina JH, Bouret JM, Fried D, et al. Value of preoperative embolization of uterine fibroma; report of a multicenter series of 31 cases. *Contracept Fertil Sex* 1995; **23**: 45–49.

23. Goodwin SC, Walker WJ. Uterine artery embolization for the treatment of uterine fibroids. *Curr Opin Obstet Gynecol* 1998; **10**: 315–320.

24. Stokes LS, Wallace MJ, Godwin RB, et al. Quality improvement guidelines for uterine artery embolization for symptomatic leiomyomas. *J Vasc Inter Radiol* 2010; **21**: 1153–1161.

25. Smeets AJ, Nijenhuis RJ, Beikkooi PF, et al. Safety and effectiveness of UAE in patients with pedunculated fibroids. *J Vasc Interv Radiol* 2009; **20**: 1172–1175.

26. Lanocita R, Frigerio LF, Patelli G, et al. A fatal complication of percutaneous transcatheter embolization for treatment of uterine fibroids [abstract]. Presented at: 11th Annual Meeting of the Society for Minimally Invasive Therapy. 1999; Boston, MA; Abstract UAE-04.

27. Kim MD, Kim S, Kim NK, et al. Long-term results of UAE for symptomatic adenomyosis. *Am J Roentgenol* 2007; **188**: 176–181.

28. Naguib NN, Mbalisike E, Nour-Eldin NA, et al. Leiomyoma volume changes at follow-up after UAE: correlation with the initial leiomyoma volume and location. *J Vasc Interv Radiol* 2010; **21**: 490–495.

29. Verma SK, Bergin D, Gonsalves CF, et al. Midterm clinical and first reproductive results of a randomized controlled trial comparing uterine artery embolization and myomectomy. *Cardiovasc Intervent Radiol* 2008; **31**: 73–85.

30. Pabon IP, Magret JP, Unzurrunzaga EA, et al. Pregnancy after uterine fibroid embolization: follow-up of 100 patients embolized using tris-acryl gelatin microspheres. *Fertil Steril* 2008; **90**: 2356–2359.

31. Goodwin S, Spies J, Worthington-Kirsch R, et al. Uterine artery embolization for treatment of leiomyomata: the FIBROID Registry. *Obstet Gynecol* 2008; **111**: 22–33.

32. Myers E, Goodwin S, Landow W, et al. Prospective data collection of a new procedure by a specialty society: the FIBROID Registry. *Obstet Gynecol* 2005; **106**: 44–51.

33. Spies J, Myers ER, Worthington-Kirsch Mulgund J, et al. The FIBROID Registry: symptom and quality-of-life status 1 year after therapy. *Obstet Gynecol* 2005; **106**: 1309–1318.

34. Worthington-Kirsch R, Spies J, Myers E, et al. The Fibroid Registry for Outcomes Data (FIBROID) for Uterine Artery Embolization: short term outcomes [published erratum appears in Obstet Gynecol 2005; 106: 869]. *Obstet Gynecol* 2005; **106**: 52–59.

35. Spies J, Bruno J, Czeyda-Peommersheim F, et al. Long-term outcome of uterine artery embolization of leiomyomata. *Obstet Gynecol* 2005; **106**: 933–939.

36. Hoeldtke N. Letters to the Editor and In Reply: *Obstet Gynecol* 2006; **107**: 741–742.

37. Holub Z, Mara M, Kuzel D, et al. Pregnancy outcomes after uterine artery occlusion: prospective multicentric study. *Fertil Steril* 2008; **90**: 1886–1891.

38. Kuzel D, Mara M, Horak P, et al. Comparative outcomes of hysteroscopic examinations performed after uterine artery embolization or laparoscopic uterine artery occlusion to treat leiomyomas. *Fertil Steril* 2011; **95**(6): 2143–2145.

39. Homer H, Saridogan E. Uterine artery embolization for fibroids is associated with an increased risk of miscarriage. *Fertil Steril* 2011; **95**: 872–876.

40. Greene J, Schnatz P, Hallisey M. Fertility outcomes after uterine artery embolization. *Obstet Gynecol* 2005; **105**(4): 67S–68S.

41. Tulandi T, Salamah K. Fertility and uterine artery embolization. *Obstet Gynecol* 2010; **115**: 857–860.

42. Tropeoano G, Stasi C, Amoroso S, et al. Long-term effects of uterine fibroid embolization on ovarian reserve: a prospective cohort study. *Fertil Steril* 2010; **94**: 2296–2300.

Ectopic pregnancy: ultrasound diagnosis and management

Botros R. M. B. Rizk, Sheri A. Owens, John LaFleur and Mostafa I. Abuzeid

Introduction

Ultrasonography is the cornerstone of the diagnosis and management of ectopic pregnancy [1–3]. Ectopic pregnancies account for 1–2% of all reported pregnancies and result in 10–18% of all maternal deaths annually. In the United States, more than 125 000 ectopic pregnancies occur every year [4]. The death rate from ectopic pregnancy is less than 1 per 1000; ectopic pregnancy has a risk of death 10 times greater than that of childbirth and 50 times greater than legally induced abortion. The death rate from ectopic pregnancy has declined by more than tenfold as a result of early diagnosis by ultrasonography. However, it is still a leading cause of mortality in the first trimester of pregnancy [5–9].

The majority of ectopic pregnancies, 90–95%, are located in the fallopian tubes named after Gabriel Fallopio (Latin name Falloppius; Figs 14.1 and 14.2). The majority of these tubal pregnancies are located in the ampullary region of the fallopian tube and less commonly in the isthmical region. In 2–4%, the pregnancy implants in the intramural portion of the fallopian tube, termed interstitial. Cervical pregnancy is rare; the gestational sac implants in the cervix. Abdominal ectopic pregnancy is a very rare form of ectopic pregnancy in which the gestational sac implants in the peritoneal cavity. Heterotopic pregnancy refers to the coexistence of intrauterine and extrauterine pregnancies at the same time [10–19].

Tubal ectopic pregnancy

The increased prevalence of pelvic inflammatory disease and the use of assisted reproductive technology (ART) have increased the incidence of ectopic pregnancy over the past three decades [10–12] (Figs 14.3–14.20). Rare forms of ectopic pregnancy have been reported following the widespread use of ART. Rizk et al. in 1990 reported four bilateral tubal pregnancies and one unilateral tubal twin pregnancy [11].

Clinical presentation of ectopic tubal pregnancy

The classic presentation of ectopic pregnancy includes the triad of pelvic pain, abnormal vaginal bleeding, and an adnexal mass.

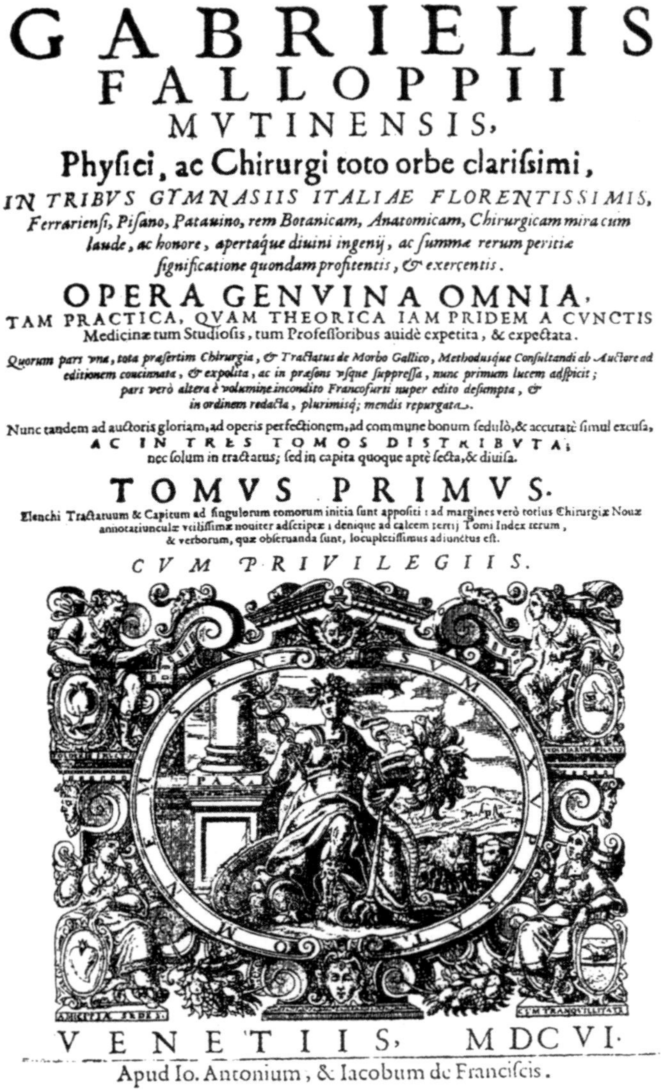

Fig. 14.1 The frontispiece of the Falloppius book.

This classic triad is less commonly seen today. More commonly, abnormal vaginal bleeding or pelvic tenderness is encountered

Ultrasonography in Gynecology, ed. Botros R. M. B. Rizk and Elizabeth E. Puscheck. Published by Cambridge University Press. © Cambridge University Press 2015.

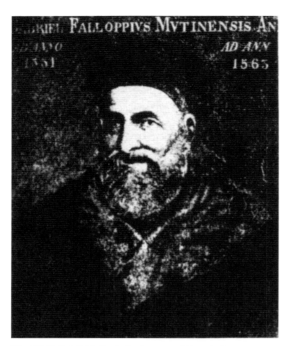

Fig. 14.2 Gabriel Fallopio (Latin name Falloppius).

as the leading presenting symptom. Abdominal pain has been reported in 90–100% of ectopic pregnancies, and frequently begins far in advance of tubal rupture. Abnormal vaginal bleeding or amenorrhea is associated with 75% of cases. The possibility of ectopic pregnancy should be considered in all women with lower abdominal pain and a positive pregnancy test.

The most common clinical finding on physical examination is adnexal tenderness, which has been reported to occur in 75–90% of ectopic pregnancies. Internal hemorrhage may be severe enough to cause hypovolemic shock, particularly if there has been a delay in diagnosis.

The differential diagnosis includes threatened or incomplete abortion, pelvic inflammatory disease, adnexal torsion, degeneration of a uterine leiomyoma, endometriosis, or appendicitis.

Ultrasonographic appearance of tubal ectopic pregnancy

Ultrasonography is the primary modality for the diagnosis of ectopic pregnancy (Figs 14.21–14.41). Transvaginal ultrasonography has revolutionized female pelvic imaging [20–26]. If a woman of reproductive age presents with pelvic pain, vaginal bleeding, and a positive pregnancy test, ultrasonography should be performed immediately to determine if the pregnancy is inside or outside the uterus. The optimal approach for the evaluation of suspected ectopic pregnancy is to focus on the uterus in an effort to detect an intrauterine pregnancy [8]. Approximately 90% of women with a positive pregnancy test referred to rule out an ectopic pregnancy are ultimately shown to have an intrauterine pregnancy. This frequency combined

with the knowledge that coexistent intrauterine and extrauterine pregnancies are rare makes it initially logical to search for an intrauterine pregnancy [7–9].

The visualization of a fluid-filled sac outside the uterine cavity that contains an embryo with or without cardiac activity or a yolk sac is definitive for ectopic pregnancy (Figs 14.21–14.38). Stiller et al. [20] and Fleischer et al. [21] observed that approximately one-sixth to one-third of ectopic pregnancies develop to yolk sac formation or cardiac activity. These strict criteria have the highest specificity (100%), but the lowest sensitivity (20%) in identifying an ectopic pregnancy. A more common ultrasonographic finding in a woman with ectopic pregnancy is a complex adnexal mass [7–9]. The presence of this finding has a sensitivity of 20–80% and a specificity of 93–99%.

Brown and Doubilet [25] concluded that, based on the results of 10 studies, the most useful criterion was the presence of any noncystic adnexal ovarian mass. This criterion, which includes living ectopics, tubal rings, and common solid or cystic masses, had a high specificity (99%), positive predictive value (96%), sensitivity (84%), and negative predictive value (95%). Therefore, in the absence of an intrauterine pregnancy, the ultrasonographic visualization of a complex adnexal mass that is separate from the ovary can be used to diagnose an ectopic pregnancy (Figs 14.26–14.31). However, in 15–35% of patients with ectopic pregnancies, no adnexal masses will be identified despite meticulous ultrasonographic technique [25].

Ultrasonography of the uterus in ectopic pregnancy

The endometrium varies in appearance and thickness in tubal pregnancy (Figs 14.25, 14.31, 14.38). There is no specific endometrial pattern or thickness that can be used to suggest an ectopic pregnancy, or to differentiate the endometrial appearance in women subsequently shown to have an ectopic pregnancy versus a normal or abnormal intrauterine pregnancy. However, in patients presenting with a positive pregnancy test and an ultrasound scan showing an empty endometrial cavity, especially in the absence of a period or significant vaginal bleeding, the diagnosis should be ectopic pregnancy until proven otherwise.

Pseudogestational sac

The uterine cavity may contain secretions or blood and what is often termed a pseudogestational sac because it can be mistaken for a true gestational sac. However, a pseudogestational sac does not have the actual characteristics of a true gestational sac. It lacks the double echogenic ring around it and has no embryo or yolk sac within it [7–9]. The double decidual sac sign has been suggested as a finding that characterizes an early intrauterine pregnancy and reliably discriminates an intrauterine gestational sac from the pseudogestational sac of an ectopic pregnancy before being able to visualize either the yolk sac or the embryo [7]. The double sac, which consists of two concentric rings surrounding a portion of the gestational sac, was thought to represent the decidua parietalis (vera) adjacent to the decidua capsularis. Filly [7] observed by endovaginal

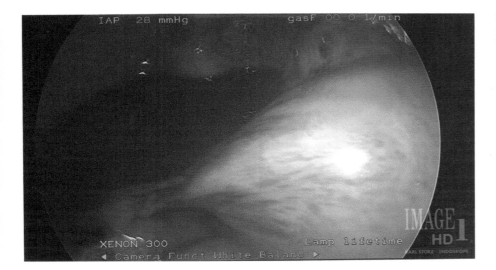

Fig. 14.3 Hemoperitoneum in the anterior and posterior cul-de-sac as well as pelvic sidewall prior to salpingectomy for left ectopic pregnancy.

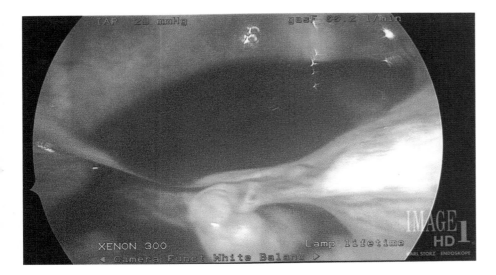

Fig. 14.4 Hemoperitoneum in the anterior and posterior cul-de-sac as well as pelvic sidewall prior to salpingectomy for left ectopic pregnancy.

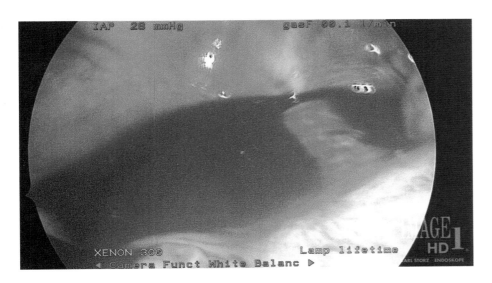

Fig. 14.5 Hemoperitoneum in the anterior and posterior cul-de-sac as well as pelvic sidewall prior to salpingectomy for left ectopic pregnancy.

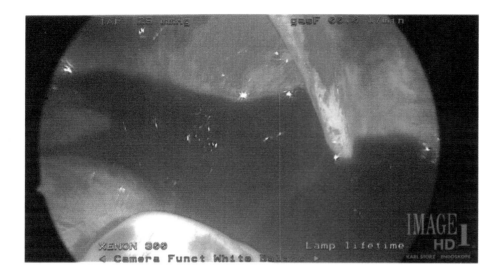

Fig. 14.6 Hemoperitoneum in the anterior and posterior cul-de-sac as well as pelvic sidewall prior to salpingectomy for left ectopic pregnancy.

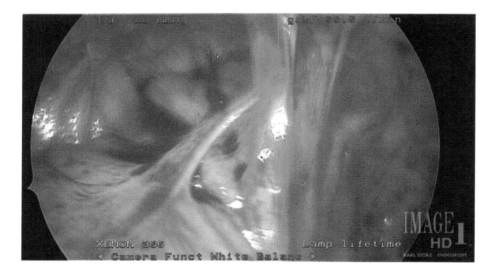

Fig. 14.7 Adhesions between ascending colon and abdominal wall.

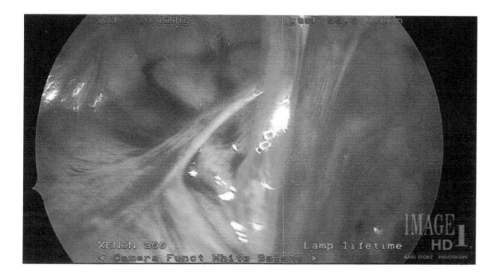

Fig. 14.8 Adhesions between ascending colon and abdominal wall.

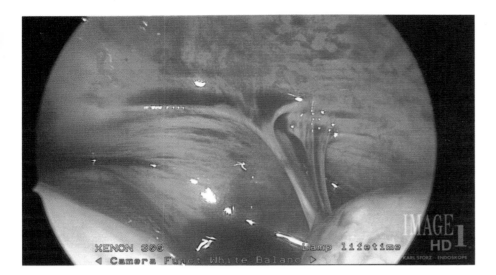

Fig. 14.9 Adhesions.

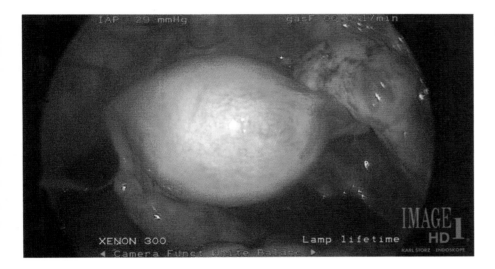

Fig. 14.10 Adhesion of right ovary and pelvic sidewall.

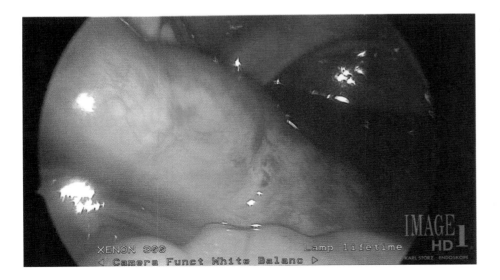

Fig. 14.11 Fallopian tube and blood in the cul-de-sac.

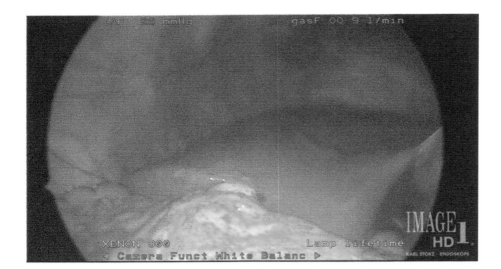

Fig. 14.12 Liver.

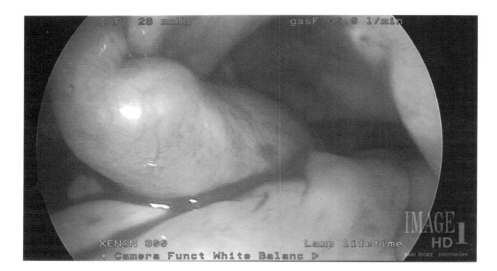

Fig. 14.13 Left ampullary ectopic pregnancy.

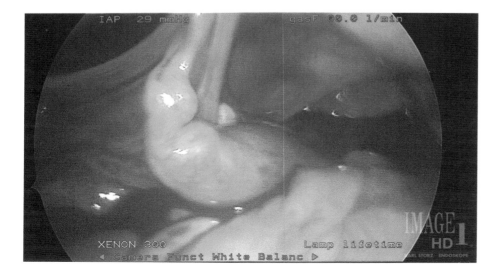

Fig. 14.14 Left ampullary ectopic pregnancy.

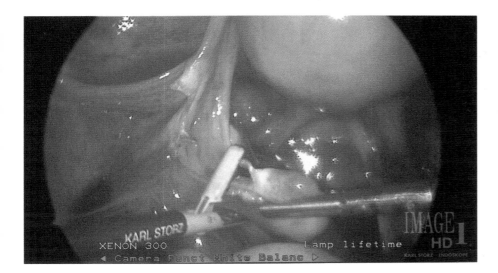

Fig. 14.15 Left salpingectomy for ectopic pregnancy.

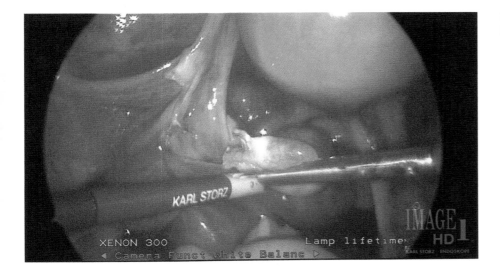

Fig. 14.16 Left salpingectomy for ectopic pregnancy.

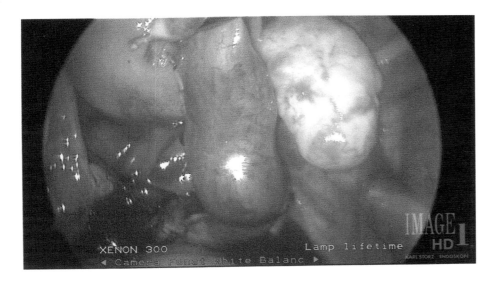

Fig. 14.17 Laparoscopic salpingectomy for left ectopic pregnancy.

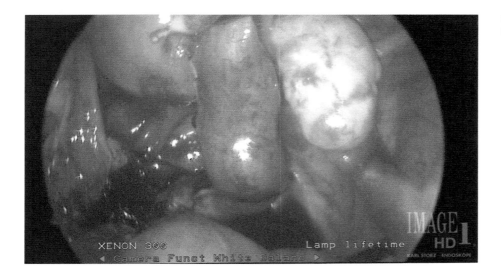

Fig. 14.18 Laparoscopic salpingectomy for left ectopic pregnancy.

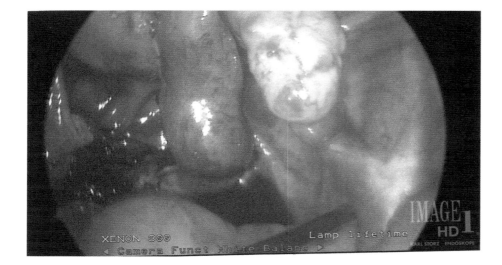

Fig. 14.19 Left ectopic pregnancy.

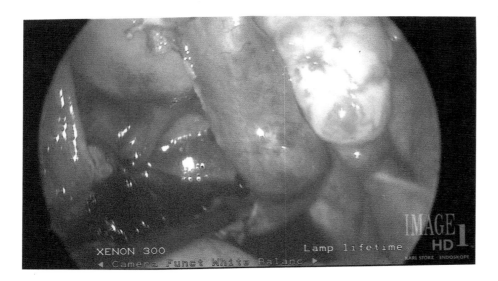

Fig. 14.20 Left ectopic pregnancy.

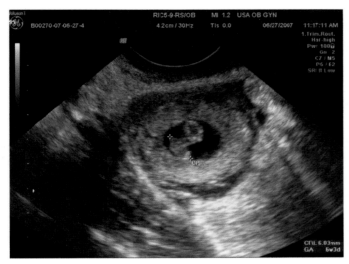

Fig. 14.21 Ectopic pregnancy with an extrauterine gestational sac containing a live embryo. The figure shows the measurement of the crown–rump length (calipers) and the echogenic ring of the ectopic pregnancy. Reproduced with permission from Rizk B, Abuzeid M, et al. Ectopic pregnancy. In: Rizk B (Ed.) *Ultrasonography in Reproductive Medicine and Infertility*. Cambridge University Press, 2010. Chapter 31, 260.

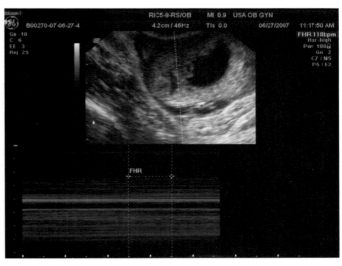

Fig. 14.23 Ectopic pregnancy with an extrauterine gestational sac; the embryo has cardiac activity documented by M-mode (dotted line on image). Calipers measure a single heartbeat. Reproduced with permission from Rizk B, Abuzeid M, et al. Ectopic pregnancy. In: Rizk B (Ed.) *Ultrasonography in Reproductive Medicine and Infertility*. Cambridge University Press, 2010. Chapter 31, 260.

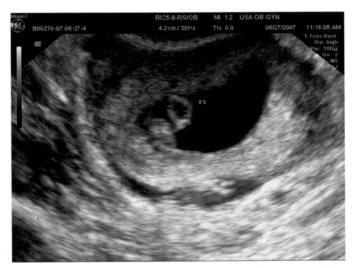

Fig. 14.22 Ectopic pregnancy with an extrauterine gestational sac containing a yolk sac and fetal pole. Reproduced with permission from Rizk B, Abuzeid M, et al. Ectopic pregnancy. In: Rizk B (Ed.) *Ultrasonography in Reproductive Medicine and Infertility*. Cambridge University Press, 2010. Chapter 31, 260.

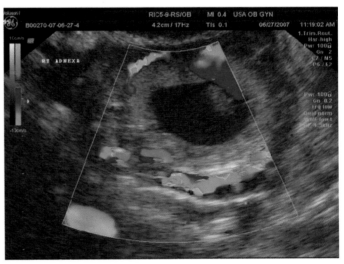

Fig. 14.24 Ectopic pregnancy with an extrauterine gestational sac with color Doppler demonstrating considerable blood flow. Reproduced with permission from Rizk B, Abuzeid M, et al. Ectopic pregnancy. In: Rizk B (Ed.) *Ultrasonography in Reproductive Medicine and Infertility*. Cambridge University Press, 2010. Chapter 31, 260.

sonography that the inner ring is composed of the chorionic villi proliferating around the developing gestation, while the outer ring is the deeper and more echogenic layer of the decidua vera. When the decidua vera is uniformly echogenic throughout its entire thickness, a true double decidual sac sign cannot be demonstrated [6]. In contrast, the pseudoges-tational sac is composed of an echogenic ring surrounding an intraendometrial fluid collection. However, Filly cautioned that the double decidual sac sign does not absolutely exclude a pseudogestational sac, nor does its presence confirm that an intrauterine pregnancy is normal [7].

Evaluation of intrauterine contents beyond exclusion of an intrauterine pregnancy does not improve diagnostic accuracy. A pseudogestational sac may be present in 5–35% of ectopic pregnancies.

Doppler ultrasonography in the diagnosis of adnexal masses and ectopic pregnancy

The use of color and pulsed Doppler could improve the sensitivity of making the diagnosis of ectopic pregnancy. The rationale for using Doppler is to detect high-velocity,

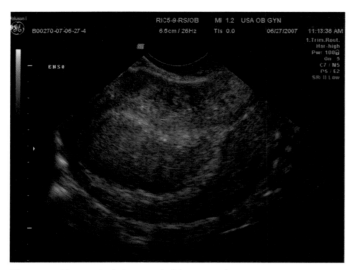

Fig. 14.25 Transvaginal ultrasound of the uterus showing no intrauterine gestational sac. Reproduced with permission from Rizk B, Abuzeid M, et al. Ectopic pregnancy. In: Rizk B (Ed.) *Ultrasonography in Reproductive Medicine and Infertility.* Cambridge University Press, 2010. Chapter 31, 260.

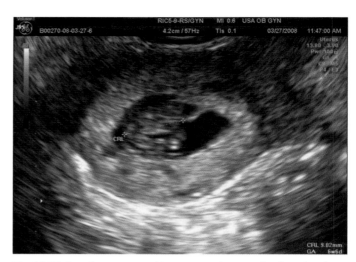

Fig. 14.27 Ectopic pregnancy with an extrauterine gestational sac showing the crown–rump length (CRL) of the embryo (calipers). Reproduced with permission from Rizk B, Abuzeid M, et al. Ectopic pregnancy. In: Rizk B (Ed.) *Ultrasonography in Reproductive Medicine and Infertility.* Cambridge University Press, 2010. Chapter 31, 261.

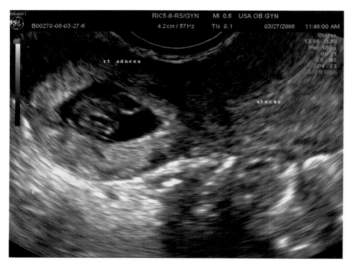

Fig. 14.26 Ectopic pregnancy with an extrauterine gestational sac containing a live embryo and the uterus. Reproduced with permission from Rizk B, Abuzeid M, et al. Ectopic pregnancy. In: Rizk B (Ed.) *Ultrasonography in Reproductive Medicine and Infertility.* Cambridge University Press, 2010. Chapter 31, 261.

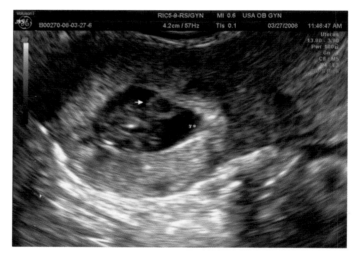

Fig. 14.28 Ectopic pregnancy with an extrauterine gestational sac showing the embryo and yolk sac (arrow). Reproduced with permission from Rizk B, Abuzeid M, et al. Ectopic pregnancy. In: Rizk B (Ed.) *Ultrasonography in Reproductive Medicine and Infertility.* Cambridge University Press, 2010. Chapter 31, 261.

low-resistance arterial flow pattern within the trophoblastic tissue in the ectopic pregnancy (Figs 14.23, 14.24, 14.29, 14.30, 14.35, 14.36). Once color flow identifies a possible ectopic pregnancy, the use of pulsed Doppler and determining the resistance index could differentiate an ectopic pregnancy from a corpus luteum [26]. There is an overlap in the resistance index of the ectopic pregnancy and corpus luteum. The blood flow around the ectopic pregnancy is sometimes referred to as the "ring of fire." In contrast, the lack of flow cannot be used to exclude an ectopic pregnancy.

Pellerito et al. [27] performed endovaginal sonography and endovaginal imaging in 155 patients with clinical suspicion of ectopic pregnancy. Sixty-five patients, 42%, had surgically confirmed ectopic pregnancies. They diagnosed 36 of the ectopic pregnancies with endovaginal sonography alone, the criteria being an extrauterine gestational sac or an ectopic fetus (sensitivity, 54%). Endovaginal color flow imaging diagnosed 62 ectopic pregnancies when an ectopic fetus or sac was visualized or placental flow was identified in an adnexal mass separate from the uterus, with a sensitivity of 95%. The authors concluded that the use of color Doppler flow imaging in addition to vaginal sonography increased the sensitivity in the detection of ectopic pregnancy. They utilized a low-impedance pattern separate from the ovary to suggest or diagnose placental flow. Several of the early or dead ectopic pregnancies demonstrated no evidence of placental flow. All of the avascular ectopic pregnancies demonstrated serum human chorionic gonadotropin

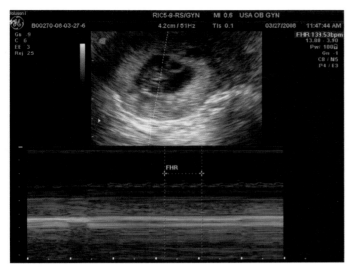

Fig. 14.29 Ectopic pregnancy with an extrauterine gestational sac; the embryo has cardiac activity documented by M-mode (dotted line). Calipers measure a single heartbeat. Reproduced with permission from Rizk B, Abuzeid M, et al. Ectopic pregnancy. In: Rizk B (Ed.) *Ultrasonography in Reproductive Medicine and Infertility*. Cambridge University Press, 2010. Chapter 31, 261.

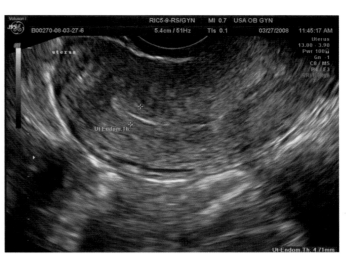

Fig. 14.31 Transvaginal ultrasonography of the uterus; sagittal view of uterus reveals no evidence of an intrauterine gestational sac. Reproduced with permission from Rizk B, Abuzeid M, et al. Ectopic pregnancy. In: Rizk B (Ed.) *Ultrasonography in Reproductive Medicine and Infertility*. Cambridge University Press, 2010. Chapter 31, 261.

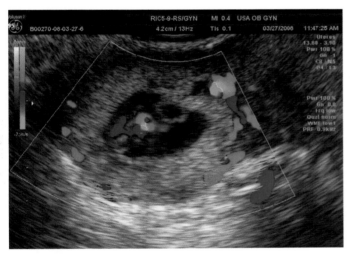

Fig. 14.30 Color Doppler imaging demonstrating blood flow in the embryo and surrounding gestational sac. Reproduced with permission from Rizk B, Abuzeid M, et al. Ectopic pregnancy. In: Rizk B (Ed.) *Ultrasonography in Reproductive Medicine and Infertility*. Cambridge University Press, 2010. Chapter 31, 261.

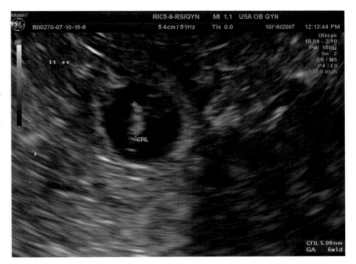

Fig. 14.32 Ectopic pregnancy with an extrauterine gestational sac demonstrating crown–rump length (CRL) and coronal view of the left ovary. Reproduced with permission from Rizk B, Abuzeid M, et al. Ectopic pregnancy. In: Rizk B (Ed.) *Ultrasonography in Reproductive Medicine and Infertility*. Cambridge University Press, 2010. Chapter 31, 262.

(hCG) levels of less than 6000 mIU/mL. Only 1 of the 65 ectopic pregnancies, 1.5%, was a solid avascular mass. Doppler may provide additional information about some adnexal masses [3]. However, the actual diagnosis depends on the grayscale features and Doppler should not be considered mandatory during the evaluation of an ectopic pregnancy [7–9].

Endometrial Doppler in the diagnosis of ectopic pregnancy

The application of color and duplex Doppler to the endometrium has been used to differentiate a true gestational sac from a pseudogestational sac. The rationale for using Doppler with an early intrauterine pregnancy is to identify a high-velocity, low-resistant arterial flow associated with developing chorionic villi [7–9]. The resistance index should be <0.6. The specificity of this application remains to be determined because a failed intrauterine pregnancy may or may not demonstrate blood flow in the developing trophoblast.

Free fluid in ectopic pregnancy

Free intraperitoneal fluid is not diagnostic for ectopic pregnancy. Isolated free fluid has been observed in 15% of patients with ectopic pregnancy. The fluid may result from active bleeding from the fimbriated end of the fallopian tube or rupture of the fallopian tube. A ruptured corpus luteum or hemorrhagic

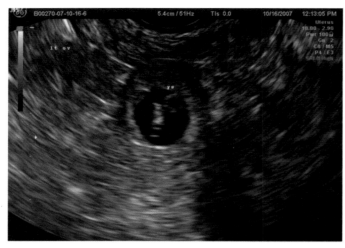

Fig. 14.33 Ectopic pregnancy with an extrauterine gestational sac revealing yolk sac and a coronal view of the left ovary. Reproduced with permission from Rizk B, Abuzeid M, et al. Ectopic pregnancy. In: Rizk B (Ed.) *Ultrasonography in Reproductive Medicine and Infertility*. Cambridge University Press, 2010. Chapter 31, 262.

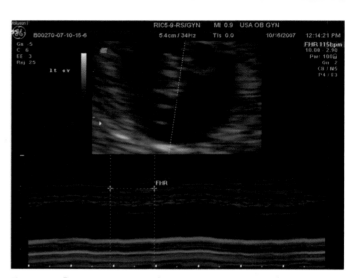

Fig. 14.35 Ectopic pregnancy with an extrauterine gestational sac; the embryo has cardiac activity documented by M-mode (dotted line). Caliper reveals single heartbeat. Reproduced with permission from Rizk B, Abuzeid M, et al. Ectopic pregnancy. In: Rizk B (Ed.) *Ultrasonography in Reproductive Medicine and Infertility*. Cambridge University Press, 2010. Chapter 31, 262.

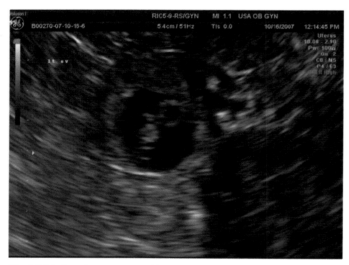

Fig. 14.34 Ectopic pregnancy with an extrauterine gestational sac revealing the embryo and the yolk sac and a coronal section of the left ovary. Reproduced with permission from Rizk B, Abuzeid M, et al. Ectopic pregnancy. In: Rizk B (Ed.) *Ultrasonography in Reproductive Medicine and Infertility*. Cambridge University Press, 2010. Chapter 31, 262.

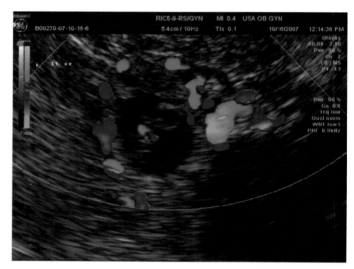

Fig. 14.36 Transvaginal color Doppler of an ectopic pregnancy demonstrating blood flow within the embryo and considerable blood flow surrounding the gestational sac. Reproduced with permission from Rizk B, Abuzeid M, et al. Ectopic pregnancy. In: Rizk B (Ed.) *Ultrasonography in Reproductive Medicine and Infertility*. Cambridge University Press, 2010. Chapter 31, 262.

ovarian cyst could also be the source of the intraperitoneal fluid. The echogenicity of the intraperitoneal fluid may also help to suggest the absence or presence of hemoperitoneum (Figs 14.3–14.6).

Ultrasonography and human chorionic gonadotropin (hCG) levels in the diagnosis and management of ectopic pregnancy

If an ectopic pregnancy cannot be clearly visualized by transvaginal sonography, and in the absence of an intrauterine gestational sac, it is imperative to determine the quantitative serum level of β-hCG. In normal pregnancy, hCG levels double every 48 hours during the first 6 weeks and using sensitive radioimmunoassay, the serum level can be determined 23 days after the last normal menstrual period, which is approximately 8 days after ovulation. If the result of the hCG test is negative, a developing pregnancy is excluded. A chronic, nonliving ectopic pregnancy is a rare exception to this rule. If the pregnancy test is positive, the serum β-hCG level should be determined and correlated with the findings of transvaginal ultrasonography.

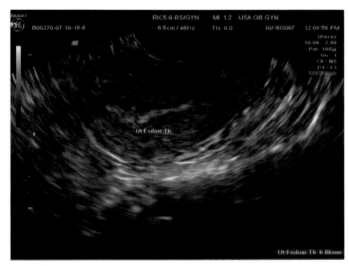

Fig. 14.37 Transvaginal sagittal view of the uterus revealing a thin endometrium (6 mm) and no gestational sac. Reproduced with permission from Rizk B, Abuzeid M, et al. Ectopic pregnancy. In: Rizk B (Ed.) *Ultrasonography in Reproductive Medicine and Infertility*. Cambridge University Press, 2010. Chapter 31, 262.

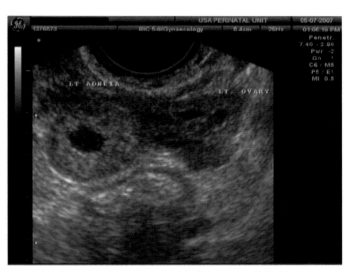

Fig. 14.39 Transvaginal coronal view of the left ovary and left adnexa demonstrating an extrauterine gestational sac with an echogenic ring but no fetal pole or fetal heart. Reproduced with permission from Rizk B, Abuzeid M, et al. Ectopic pregnancy. In: Rizk B (Ed.) *Ultrasonography in Reproductive Medicine and Infertility*. Cambridge University Press, 2010. Chapter 31, 263.

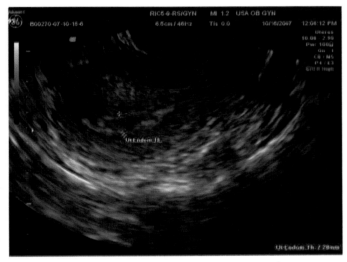

Fig. 14.38 Transvaginal view of uterus revealing no gestational sac. Reproduced with permission from Rizk B, Abuzeid M, et al. Ectopic pregnancy. In: Rizk B (Ed.) *Ultrasonography in Reproductive Medicine and Infertility*. Cambridge University Press, 2010. Chapter 31, 263.

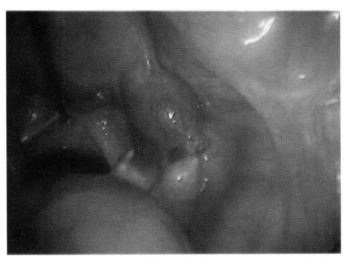

Fig. 14.40 Laparoscopic view of isthmical ectopic pregnancy. Reproduced with permission from Rizk B, Abuzeid M, et al. Ectopic pregnancy. In: Rizk B (Ed.) *Ultrasonography in Reproductive Medicine and Infertility*. Cambridge University Press, 2010. Chapter 31, 263.

Human chorionic gonadotropin discriminatory zone

A normal intrauterine gestational sac should be visualized by ultrasonography when the level is 1000 mIU/mL or greater [28]. Failure to identify a normal intrauterine gestational sac when this discriminatory zone is reached suggests either an abnormal intrauterine pregnancy with a spontaneous abortion or an ectopic pregnancy [28]. If the β-hCG level is increasing on further evaluation and still no intrauterine gestational sac is identified, an ectopic pregnancy is suggested, except if the patient has experienced a spontaneous abortion. The history is often crucial for suggesting the correct diagnosis. The process may be distressing and about half of the suspected cases require four or more visits to confirm or exclude the diagnosis of an ectopic pregnancy. In about 40% of cases, the initial diagnosis of ectopic pregnancy is erroneous and a nonviable intrauterine pregnancy is found [29,30]. Rizk et al. [15] cautioned that in multiple pregnancy, where the β-hCG level would be greater than for the expected gestational age, hCG levels should be interpreted, taking into consideration the multiplicity as determined by the ultrasonographic appearance.

Management of ectopic pregnancy

Ultrasonography has revolutionized the management of tubal ectopic pregnancy [21–26]. Early diagnosis allows medical

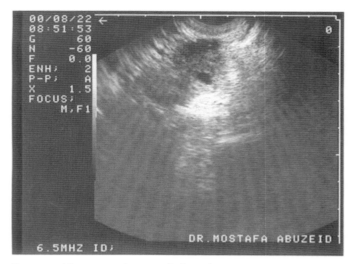

Fig. 14.41 Ultrasonographic view of isthmical ectopic pregnancy. Reproduced with permission from Rizk B, Abuzeid M, et al. Ectopic pregnancy. In: Rizk B (Ed.) *Ultrasonography in Reproductive Medicine and Infertility* Cambridge University Press, 2010. Chapter 31, 263.

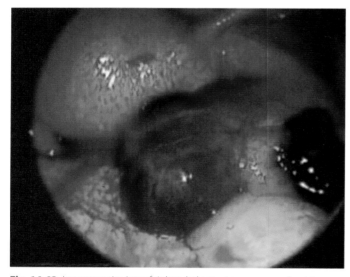

Fig. 14.42 Laparoscopic view of right tubal ectopic pregnancy about to rupture and hemoperitoneum. Courtesy of John LaFleur.

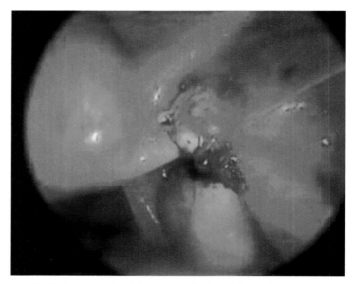

Fig. 14.43 Laparoscopic salpingectomy of right tubal ectopic pregnancy. Courtesy of John LaFleur.

treatment to be the first-line choice in appropriately selected cases [31]. Medical management of ectopic pregnancy with methotrexate has more than tripled in the United States in the last decade, from 11% in 2002 to 35% in 2007 [32].

The Practice Committee of the American Society for Reproductive Medicine considers the following conditions to be relative contraindications for medical therapy in ectopic pregnancy: a high initial hCG concentration (>5000 mIU/mL), ectopic pregnancy >4 cm in size as imaged on transvaginal ultrasound scan, and the presence of embryonic cardiac activity on transvaginal ultrasound scan. Cepni et al. [33] challenged that concept and suggested that transvaginal ultrasound-guided aspiration of the fetus followed by local and systemic methotrexate administration can be used successfully to treat 92% of patients. However, this was a small study (13 cases of unruptured ectopic pregnancy). Therefore, more studies are required to confirm this finding.

Ectopic pregnancies are surgically managed by laparoscopy (Figs 14.40–14.43), laparotomy, and ultrasound-guided aspiration. Surgical management of ectopic pregnancies has declined in the United States from 74% in 2002 to 65% in 2007, with 21.5% laparotomies and 43.5% laparoscopies. More than a century ago, Lawson-Tate reported the successful surgical management of ectopic pregnancy by salpingectomy in four women in Great Britain. Conservative management has been considered for more than a century. One of the earliest reports of conservative treatment, vaginal puncture to treat ectopic pregnancy instead of laparotomy, was reported by Kelly in 1896 in the Johns Hopkins Hospital bulletin [34]. Once encouraged by his success, he treated 10 other cases using vaginal puncture. Mahfouz in 1938 presented a comprehensive and elegant management of a series of ectopic pregnancies in Cairo, Egypt, where he debated the role of salpingostomy versus salpingectomy [35]. O'Dowd and Philipp reviewed the milestones of laparoscopic tubal surgery in the management of ectopic pregnancy in their fascinating book on the history of obstetrics and gynecology [36]. In the United States, Hope (1937) described the use of the laparoscope in the diagnosis of extrauterine pregnancy. Shapiro and Adler (1973) reported laparoscopic salpingectomy using electrocoagulation followed by excision for ectopic pregnancy. Gomel (1977) pioneered the laparoscopic treatment of hydrosalpinges. Soderstrom (1981) used the snare technique for salpingectomy. DeCherney (1981) proposed linear salpingostomy using a cutting current for the removal of the ectopic pregnancy and conservation of the fallopian tube [36]. Minimally invasive surgery is widely used for the management of ectopic pregnancy as it has the advantages of quicker recovery, less postoperative pain, shorter hospital stay, and reduced costs. There is no significant difference in future reproductive outcome when laparoscopy is compared to laparotomy. Salpingostomy could be followed by residual trophoblastic tissue and also recurrence of ectopic pregnancy. On the other hand, a better fertility outcome has been reported with salpingostomy in women with contralateral tubal pathology. In patients with the diagnosis of heterotopic tubal pregnancy, laparoscopic salpingectomy is the treatment of choice.

Many modalities of ultrasonographic guided treatment have been reported including injection of potassium chloride in the fetal heart of the ectopic gestation or methotrexate in the ectopic gestational sac. Feichtinger and Kemeter [37] treated unruptured ectopic pregnancies by needling and injection of methotrexate or prostaglandin (PGE2) under transvaginal sonography control. Timor-Tritsch et al. [38] used transvaginal salpingocentesis for treatment of ectopic pregnancy. Rizk et al. [11] utilized potassium chloride for the treatment of the extrauterine pregnancy for selected cases of heterotopic pregnancies after in vitro fertilization at Bourn Hall Clinic.

Conclusion

Ectopic pregnancy represents 2% of pregnancies, but contributes to 11.6% of maternal mortality. Tubal pregnancy represents 90–95% of all ectopic pregnancies. The majority of tubal pregnancies are located in the ampullary region of the fallopian tube. Transvaginal ultrasonography revolutionized the diagnosis and management of ectopic pregnancy. A combination of transvaginal sonography and hCG determination is the best approach for the early diagnosis of ectopic pregnancy. The visualization of a fluid-filled sac outside the uterine cavity that contains an embryo with or without cardiac activity or a yolk sac is definitive for ectopic pregnancy. This strict criterion has the highest specificity (100%), but the lowest sensitivity (20%) in identifying an ectopic pregnancy. A more common ultrasonographic finding in a woman with an ectopic pregnancy is an adnexal mass. Despite meticulous ultrasonography, no adnexal mass will be identified in 15–35% of patients with ectopic pregnancies. A pseudogestational sac may be present in 5–35% of ectopic pregnancies, and if mistaken for a true uterine gestation, the diagnosis could be delayed. Doppler ultrasound may provide useful information about adnexal masses; however, the final diagnosis depends on the grayscale features. If an ectopic pregnancy is diagnosed by transvaginal sonography, systemic methotrexate is the first line of treatment. Laparoscopic management by salpingostomy or salpingectomy remains a very effective modality of treatment in patients not suitable for medical management or who have failed medical management [39–41]. Conservative management of ectopic pregnancy could also be achieved by transvaginal salpingocentesis, injection of methotrexate into the sac, or injection of potassium chloride into the fetal heart [42].

References

1. Rizk B, Abuzeid M, Rizk C. Ectopic pregnancy. In: Rizk B (Ed.) *Ultrasonography in Reproductive Medicine and Infertility*. Cambridge University Press: 2010: 259–270.

2. Marcus SF, Dimitry ES, Dimitry M, et al. Heterotopic pregnancy and assisted reproduction. In: Rizk B (Ed.) *Ultrasonography in Reproductive Medicine and Infertility*. Cambridge University Press; 2010: 271–275.

3. Moustafa HF, Rizk B, Brooks N, et al. Cervical pregnancy. In: Rizk B (Ed.) *Ultrasonography in Reproductive Medicine and Infertility*. Cambridge University Press; 2010: 276–282.

4. Seror V, Gelfucci F, Garbaud L, et al. Care pathways for ectopic pregnancy: a population-based cost-effectiveness analysis. *Fertil Steril* 2007; **87**: 737–748.

5. Centers for Disease Control and Prevention. Ectopic pregnancy: United States 1990–92 Morbidity and Mortality Weekly Report MMWR. *Obstet Gynecol* 1995; **44**: 46.

6. Dorfman SF, Grimes DA, Cates W Jr, et al. Ectopic pregnancy, United States clinical aspects: 1979–1980. *Obstet Gynecol* 1984; **64**: 386.

7. Filly RA. Ectopic pregnancy. In: Callen P (Ed.) *Ultrasonography in Obstetrics and Gynecology*, 3rd edn. London, Philadelphia: WB Saunders Company; 1994: 641–659.

8. Laing FC. Ectopic pregnancy. In: Timor-Tritsch IE, Goldstein SR (Eds.) *Ultrasound in Gynecology*, 2nd edn. Philadelphia: Churchill, Livingstone, Elsevier; 2007: 161–175.

9. Doubilet PM, Benson CB. Ectopic pregnancy. In: Doubilet PM, Benson CB (Eds.). *Atlas of Ultrasound in Obstetrics and Gynecology: A Multimedia Reference*. Philadelphia: Lippincott Williams and Wilkins; 2003: 318–330.

10. Dimitry ES, Subak-Sharpe R, Mills M, et al. Nine cases of heterotopic pregnancies in 4 years of in-vitro fertilization. *Fertil Steril* 1990; **53**: 107–110.

11. Rizk B, Morcos S, Avery S, Elder K, et al. Rare ectopic pregnancies after *in-vitro* fertilization: One unilateral twin and four bilateral tubal pregnancies. *Hum Reprod* 1990; **5**(8): 1025–1028.

12. Rizk B, Tan SL, Morcos S, et al. Heterotopic pregnancies following in-vitro fertilization and embryo transfer. *Am J Obstet Gynecol* 1991; **164**(1): 161–164.

13. Dimitry ES, Rizk B. Ectopic pregnancy: epidemiology, advances in diagnosis and management. *Br J Clin Pract* 1992; **46**(1): 52–54.

14. Rizk B, Brinsden PR. Total abdominal and pelvic ultrasound: incidental findings and the comparison between out-patient and general practice referrals in 1000 cases. *Br J Radiol* 1990; **63**: 501–502.

15. Rizk B, Dimitry ES, Morcos S, et al. A multicentre study on combined intrauterine and extrauterine pregnancy after IVF. *European Society for Human Reproduction and Embryology meeting*, 1990; Milan, Italy. *Hum Reprod* 1990; abstract.

16. Marcus SF, Macnamee M, Brinsden P. Heterotopic pregnancies after in vitro fertilization and embryo transfer. *Hum Reprod* 1995; **10**(5): 1232–1236.

17. Marcus SF, Brinsden PR. Analysis of the incidence and risk factors associated with ectopic pregnancy following in-vitro fertilization and embryo transfer. *Hum Reprod* 1995; (1): 199–120.

18. Rizk B. The impact of pelvic inflammatory disease and tubal damage on heterotopic pregnancy following in vitro fertilization and embryo transfer. *J Clin Pract Sexuality* 1996; **11**(3/4): 46–51.

19. Marcus S, Rizk B, Fountain S, Brinsden PR. Tuberculous infertility and in vitro fertilization. *Am J Obstet Gynecol* 1994; **171**(6): 1593–1596.

20. Stiller RJ, de Regt RH, Blair E. Transvaginal ultrasonography in patients at risk for ectopic pregnancy. *Am J Obstet Gynecol* 1989; **161**: 930–933.

21. Fleischer AC, Pennell RG, McKee MS, et al. Ectopic pregnancy: features at transvaginal sonography. *Radiology* 1990; **174**: 375–378.

22. Rizk B, Steer C, Tan SL, et al. Vaginal versus abdominal ultrasound guided oocyte retrieval in IVF. *Br J Radiology* 1990; **63**: 638.

23. Steer C, Rizk B, Tan SL, et al. Vaginal versus abdominal ultrasound for obtaining uterine artery Doppler flow velocity waveforms. *Br J Radiol* 1990; **63**: 398–399.

24. Steer C, Rizk B, Tan SL, et al. Vaginal color Doppler assessment of uterine artery impedance in a subfertile population. *Br J Radiol* 1990; **63**: 638.

25. Brown DL, Doubilet PM. Transvaginal sonography for diagnosing ectopic pregnancy: positivity criteria and performance characteristics. *J Ultrasound Med* 1994; **13**: 259–266.

26. Kurjak A, Zalud I, Schulman H. Ectopic pregnancy: transvaginal color Doppler of trophoblastic flow in questionable adnexa. *J Ultrasound Med* 1991; **10**: 685–689.

27. Pellerito JS, Taylor KJW, Quedens-Case C, et al. Ectopic pregnancy: evaluation with endovaginal color flow imaging. *Radiology* 1992; **183**: 407–411.

28. Cacciatore B. Can the status of tubal pregnancy be predicted with transvaginal sonography? A prospective comparison of sonographic, surgical, and serum hCG findings. *Radiology* 1990; **177**: 481–484.

29. Wedderburn CJ, Warner P, Graham B, et al. Economic evaluation of diagnosing and excluding ectopic pregnancy. *Hum Reprod* 2010; **25**: 328–333.

30. Barnhart KT, Katz I, Hummel A, et al. Presumed diagnosis of ectopic pregnancy. *Obstet Gynecol* 2002; **100**: 505–510.

31. Verma U, Jacques E. Conservative management of live tubal pregnancies by ultrasound guided potassium chloride injection and systemic methotrexate treatment. *J Clin Ultrasound* 2005; **33**: 460–463.

32. Hoover KW, Tao G, Kent CK. Trends in the diagnosis and treatment of ectopic pregnancy in the United States. *Obstet Gynecol* 2010; **115**: 495–502.

33. Cepni I, Gurapl O, Ocal P, et al. An alternative treatment option in tubal ectopic pregnancies with fetal heartbeat: aspiration of the embryo followed by single-dose methotrexate administration. *Fertil Steril* 2011; **96**(1): 79–83.

34. Kelly H. Treatment of ectopic pregnancy by vaginal puncture. *Johns Hopkins Medical Bulletin, Proceedings of Societies, The Johns Hopkins Medical Society Meeting*, 1896; **68–69**(Nov–Dec): 209–210.

35. Mahfouz N. Ectopic pregnancy. *J Obstet Gynaecol Br Empire* 1938; **45**(2): 201–230.

36. O'Dowd M, Philipp E. *The History of Obstetrics and Gynecology*. London: The Parthenon Publishing Group; 1994.

37. Feichtinger W, Kemeter P. Treatment of unruptured ectopic pregnancy by needling of sac and injection of methotrexate or PG E2 under transvaginal sonography control. *Arch Gynecol Obstet* 1989; **246**: 85–89.

38. Timor-Tritsch IE, Baxi L, Peisner DB. Transvaginal salpingocentesis: a new technique for treating ectopic pregnancy. *Am J Obstet Gynecol* 1989; **160**: 459–461.

39. Eyvazzadeh A, Levine D. Ultrasonographic evaluation of acute pelvic pain. In: Rizk B (Ed.) *Ultrasonography in Reproductive Medicine and Infertility*. Cambridge University Press; 2010: 176–186.

40. Rizk B, Holliday CP, Abuzeid M. Challenges in the diagnosis and management of interstitial and cornual ectopic pregnancies. *Middle East Fertil Society J* 2013; **18**: 235–240.

41. Rizk B, Holliday CP, Owens S, Abuzeid M. Cervical and cesarean scar ectopic pregnancies: diagnosis and management. *Middle East Fertil Society J* 2013;**18**: 67–73.

42. Rizk B, Holliday CP, Abuzeid M. Interstitial ectopic pregnancies: laparoscopy vs. laparotomy. *Egyptian Fertil Society J* 2013; **17**(1).

Chapter

15

Ultrasound diagnosis of interstitial, cornual and angular pregnancy

Botros R. M. B. Rizk, John LaFleur, Nicolette Holliday and Mostafa I. Abuzeid

Introduction

Interstitial pregnancy

Interstitial ectopic pregnancy is a pregnancy that implants in the interstitial or intramural portion of the fallopian tube (Figs 15.1–15.24). The interstitial portion of the fallopian tube is tortuous, 0.7 mm in diameter, and 1–2 cm in length [1]. Implantation within the interstitial segment of the fallopian tube is associated with the same risk factors as tubal ectopic pregnancies. Interstitial pregnancies account for 2–4% of ectopic pregnancies [2–15].

The interstitial segment of the tube is a relatively thick segment with a greater capacity to expand than the distal segment of the fallopian tube [15]. It is commonly stated that, in contrast to a tubal ectopic pregnancy which may rupture at 6 to 8 weeks of gestation, an interstitial ectopic pregnancy may progress without symptoms until a rupture occurs at 12–16 weeks. A study by the Society for Reproductive Surgeons (SRS) has questioned this statement [1]. The SRS study analyzed 32 cases of interstitial pregnancy reported to the Registry between 1999 and 2002. Fourteen of 32 patients experienced rupture at less than 12 weeks of gestation. Thus, the authors concluded that interstitial pregnancies could rupture earlier than assumed [1].

Cornual pregnancy

Cornual pregnancy is a term that is frequently used interchangeably with interstitial pregnancy (Figs 15.25–15.27). However, the term should be strictly reserved for pregnancies that develop in a rudimentary uterine horn, a unicornuate uterus (Fig. 15.25), the cornual region of septate uterus (Fig. 15.26), a uterus didelphys (Fig. 15.27) or bicornuate uterus. The interchangeable use of these terms in clinical practice can create problems for clinicians interpreting ultrasound reports, as the clinical course and management differ markedly between intrauterine cornual gestations and ectopic interstitial gestations [2].

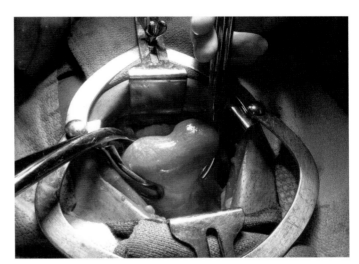

Fig. 15.1 Left interstitial ectopic pregnancy.

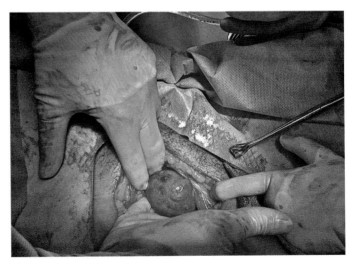

Fig. 15.2 Interstitial ectopic pregnancy.

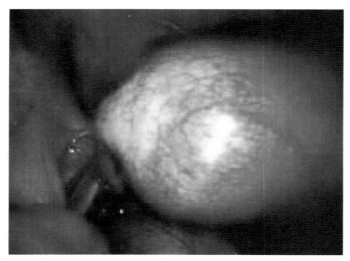

Fig. 15.3 Laparoscopic view of interstitial ectopic pregnancy. Reproduced with permission from Rizk B, Abuzeid M, et al. Ectopic pregnancy. In: Rizk B (Ed.) *Ultrasonography in Reproductive Medicine and Infertility*. Cambridge University Press, 2010; Chapter 31, 264.

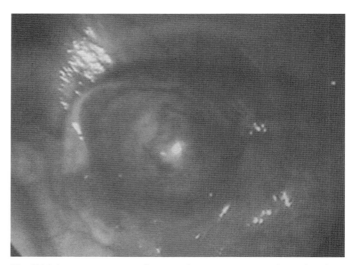

Fig. 15.6 Laparoscopic view of interstitial ectopic pregnancy. Reproduced with permission from Abuzeid M, et al. Ectopic pregnancy. In: Rizk B (Ed.) *Ultrasonography in Reproductive Medicine and Infertility*. Cambridge University Press 2010; Chapter 31, 264.

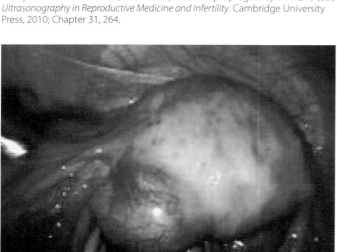

Fig. 15.4 Laparoscopic view of interstitial ectopic pregnancy after Pitressin injection. Reproduced with permission from Rizk B, Abuzeid M, et al. Ectopic pregnancy. In: Rizk B (Ed.) *Ultrasonography in Reproductive Medicine and Infertility*. Cambridge University Press, 2010; Chapter 31, 264.

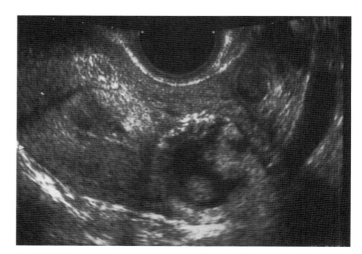

Fig. 15.7 Ultrasonographic view of interstitial ectopic pregnancy. Reproduced with permission from Abuzeid M, et al. Ectopic pregnancy. In: Rizk B (Ed.) *Ultrasonography in Reproductive Medicine and Infertility*. Cambridge University Press, 2010; Chapter 31, 264.

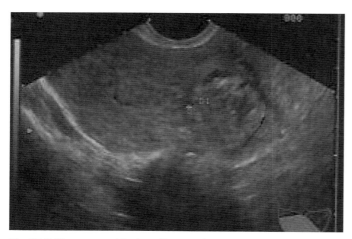

Fig. 15.5 Ultrasonographic view of interstitial ectopic pregnancy. Reproduced with permission from Rizk B, Abuzeid M, et al. Ectopic pregnancy. In: Rizk B (Ed.) *Ultrasonography in Reproductive Medicine and Infertility*. Cambridge University Press 2010; Chapter 31, 264.

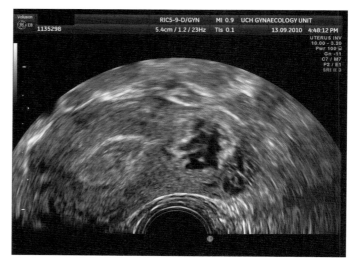

Fig. 15.8 Interstitial ectopic pregnancy. Reproduced with permission from Day A, Jurkovic D, The role of ultrasound in early pregnancy after assisted conception. In: Jauniaux ERM, Rizk B (Eds.) *Pregnancy after Assisted Reproductive Technology*. Cambridge University Press, 2012; Chapter 3, 24.

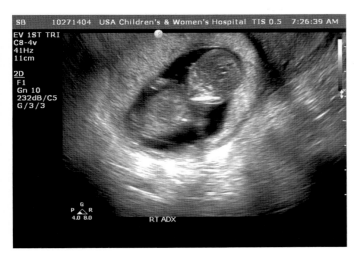

Fig. 15.9 Interstitial ectopic pregnancy.

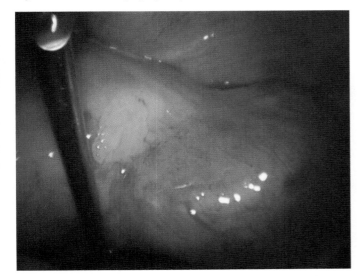

Fig. 15.10 Laparoscopic view of right interstitial ectopic pregnancy after Pitressin injection. Courtesy of Mostafa Abuzeid.

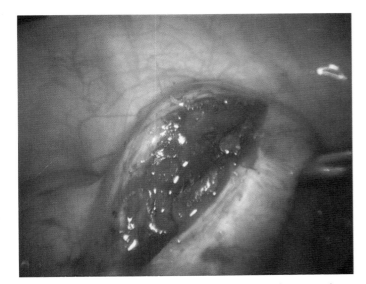

Fig. 15.11 Laparoscopic view of cornuostomy incision in right interstitial ectopic pregnancy. Courtesy of Mostafa Abuzeid.

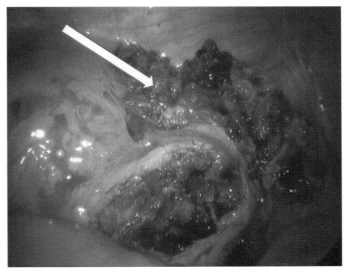

Fig. 15.12 Laparoscopic view of cornuostomy in right interstitial ectopic pregnancy after trimming the edges of the incision. Products of conception seen on anterior surface of the right broad ligament (arrow). Courtesy of Mostafa Abuzeid.

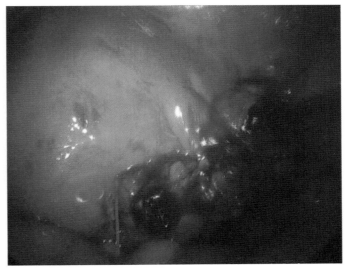

Fig. 15.13 Laparoscopic view of cornuostomy in right interstitial ectopic pregnancy after repair with a few interrupted figure-of-8 sutures with 0-Vicryl sutures. Courtesy of Mostafa Abuzeid.

Angular pregnancy

Angular pregnancies are implanted in one of the lateral angles of the uterine cavity, medial to the uterine junction. Asymmetric enlargement of the uterus is noted. The distinction between an interstitial ectopic pregnancy and an angular pregnancy can be made at the time of laparoscopy. The laparoscopic appearance of the bulge of an interstitial pregnancy is lateral to the round ligament, whereas the bulge of an angular pregnancy is medial to the round ligament and displaces the round ligament laterally [14]. Early miscarriage is common in angular pregnancies. When pregnancy continues, vaginal

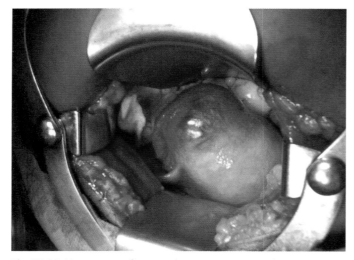

Fig. 15.14 Management of interstitial ectopic pregnancy at laparotomy.

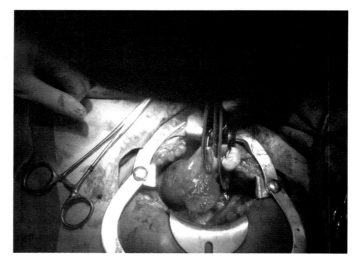

Fig. 15.15 Management of interstitial ectopic pregnancy at laparotomy.

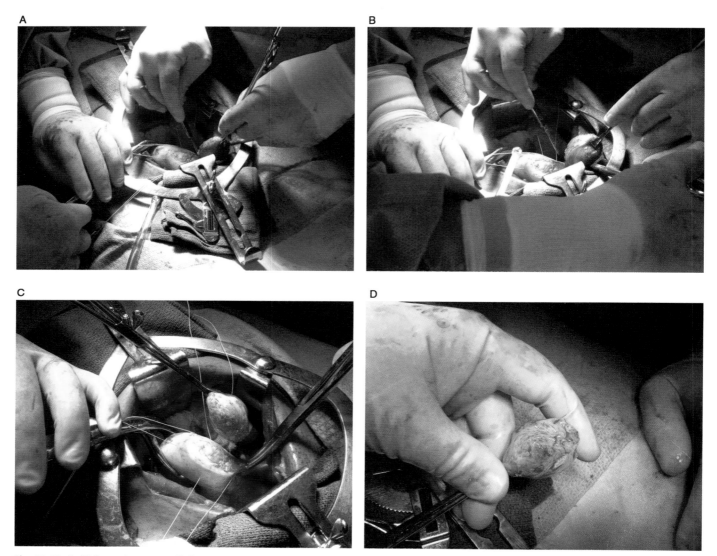

Fig. 15.16 (A–D) Cornual resection of left interstitial pregnancy and stay sutures in place. Courtesy of John LaFleur.

A

B

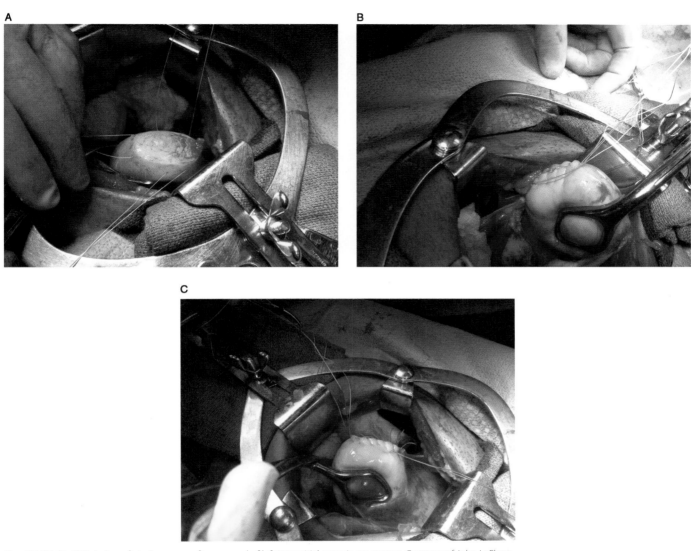

C

Fig. 15.17 (A–C) Suturing of uterine cornu after removal of left interstitial ectopic pregnancy. Courtesy of John LaFleur.

A

B

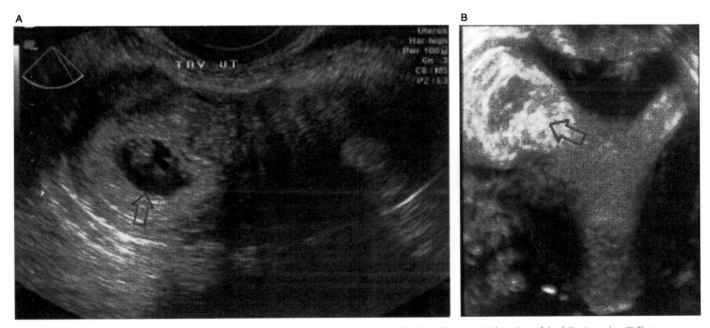

Fig. 15.18 (A) Transverse transvaginal ultrasound appearance of an ectopic pregnancy within the right interstitial portion of the fallopian tube. (B) Three-dimensional transvaginal ultrasound rendered coronal appearance of a right interstitial ectopic pregnancy. Arrows show interstitial line sign. Parts A and B reproduced with permission from Flystra DL. *Am J Obstet Gynecol* 2012; **206(4)**: 294.

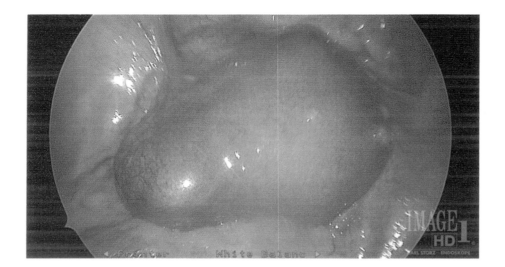

Fig. 15.19 Interstitial ectopic pregnancy.

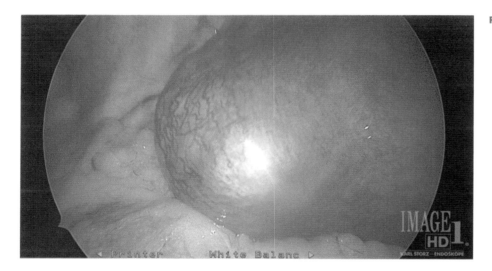

Fig. 15.20 Interstitial ectopic pregnancy.

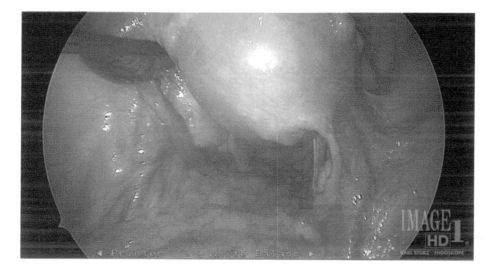

Fig. 15.21 Interstitial ectopic pregnancy.

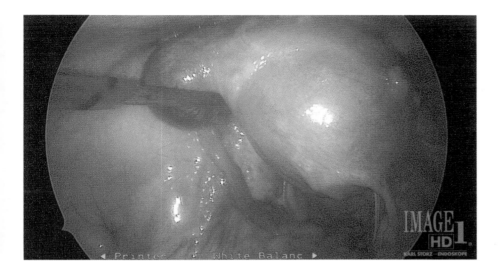

Fig. 15.22 Interstitial ectopic pregnancy.

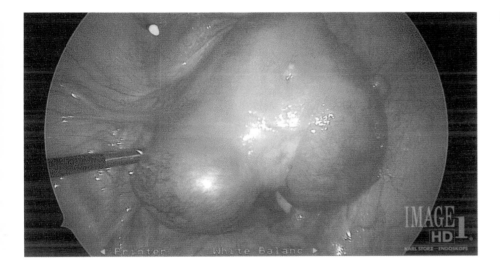

Fig. 15.23 Interstitial ectopic pregnancy.

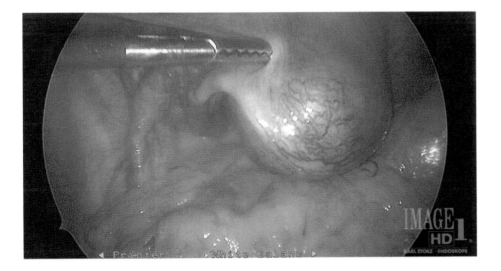

Fig. 15.24 Interstitial ectopic pregnancy.

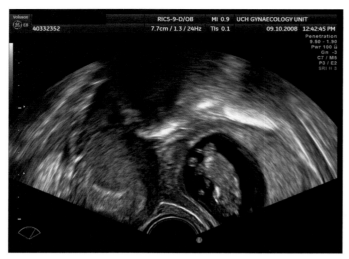

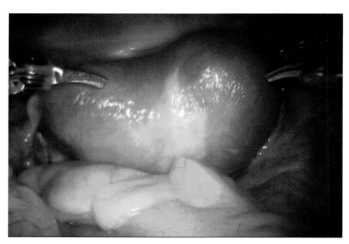

Fig. 15.26 Cornual pregnancy in a septate uterus.

Fig. 15.25 Cornual ectopic pregnancy. Reproduced with permission from Day A, Jurkovic D, The role of ultrasound in early pregnancy after assisted conception. In: Jauniaux ERM, Rizk B (Eds.) *Pregnancy after Assisted Reproductive Technology*. Cambridge, University Press, 2012; Chapter 3, 24.

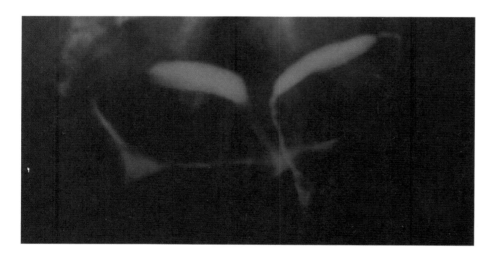

Fig. 15.27 Hysterosalpingogram of uterus didelphys. Reproduced with permission from Badaway S, Singer S, et al. Hysterosalpingography. In: Rizk B (Ed.) *Ultrasonography in Reproductive Medicine and Infertility*. Cambridge University Press, 2010; Chapter 3, 25.

pelvic pain and vaginal bleeding may occur. After delivery, placental retention may occur and uterine rupture may be rarely encountered [14].

Ultrasonography of interstitial pregnancy

The diagnosis of interstitial pregnancy should be suspected when ultrasonography demonstrates eccentric implantation of the gestational sac at the superior fundal level of the uterus (Figs 15.6–15.9). Ultrasonographic diagnosis of interstitial pregnancy is possible at an early stage before rupture (Figs 15.5, 15.7–15.8). Timor-Tritsch et al. [3] used three sonographic criteria for diagnosis of interstitial pregnancy: (1) an empty uterine cavity; (2) a chorionic sac seen separately 1 cm from the most lateral edge of the uterine cavity; and (3) a thin myometrial layer surrounding the chorionic sac.

The interstitial line sign is another useful ultrasound diagnostic criterion [3]. It is an echogenic line that extends into the upper regions of the uterine horn and borders the margins of the intrauterine gestational sac. Ackerman et al. [4] suggested that the thin echogenic line likely represents the interstitial portion of the fallopian tube. This sign had 80% sensitivity and 98% specificity for the ultrasonographic diagnosis of interstitial pregnancy [4]. Coronal images generated by 3D ultrasonography are very helpful in identifying these features (Fig. 15.18).

Distinguishing between interstitial ectopic pregnancy and an eccentrically located intrauterine pregnancy can present a diagnostic dilemma [4]. The appearance of myometrium around the sac appears to be the most useful ultrasonographic feature in making the distinction. Three-dimensional ultrasonography could also be very useful in differentiating a questionable ectopic from an eccentrically located intrauterine pregnancy [5]. In a subseptate uterus, the eccentric location of the pregnancy might make it difficult to distinguish it from a cornual pregnancy [5].

Magnetic resonance imaging

Magnetic resonance imaging (MRI) could be helpful if ultrasound imaging is inconclusive. MRI criteria for the diagnosis of interstitial ectopic pregnancy are identical to those of ultrasonography. These criteria can be clearly visualized: the gestational sac is eccentric, myometrial tissue surrounds the entire gestational sac with a thickness of 5 mm, and an interstitial line connects the gestational sac to the endometrial cavity.

Management of interstitial pregnancy

The management of interstitial pregnancy depends on whether the ectopic pregnancy has ruptured and whether the patient is stable or not. Diagnosis after rupture most commonly requires laparotomy, and frequently, hysterectomy [14]. Ultrasonography and a high index of suspicion have made it possible for early diagnosis of interstitial pregnancy and have increased the success of conservative management.

Conservative management has been used with laparoscopy (Figs 15.3–15.5, 15.10–15.13), laparotomy (Figs 15.2, 15.14, 15.15), hysteroscopy, or medical treatment. Tanaka et al. introduced medical treatment with methotrexate in 1982 [6]. However, medical treatment with methotrexate has been associated with a failure rate ranging from 9% to 65% [1, 14, 16–18]. Conservative surgical management via laparotomy with cornual resection (Fig. 15.16) or cornuostomy [9] has been advocated over the past two decades. Reich et al. reported the first case of laparoscopic management in 1988 [7]. Since then many cases of laparoscopic cornuostomy have been described in the literature [19–25]. Various hemostatic techniques have been used laparoscopically, including intramyometrial injection of diluted Pitressin (Figs 15.4, 15.10), purse-string suture or endoloop [25] or stay sutures (Figs 15.3, 15.4, 15.10–15.13) [9], electrocauterization, ultrasonic cutting and coagulating surgical device (Harmonic scalpel), and fibrin glue. Warda et al. described a simplified technique of laparoscopic cornuostomy for interstitial ectopic using intramyometrial injection of diluted Pitressin (20 units in 100 mL of normal saline) and adequate laparoscopic suturing [26,27]. Timor-Tritsch et al. [3] treated cornual pregnancy using local injection of methotrexate and, in a case of heterotopic pregnancy, local injection of potassium chloride.

In addition, Katz et al. (two patients) [28] and Meyer and Mitchell (1989) (one patient) [8] reported successful hysteroscopically guided evacuation of interstitial pregnancies under laparoscopic visualization and ultrasound guidance, respectively. Zhang et al. [29] have also reported three cases of large interstitial pregnancies that were successfully treated with transcervical curettage under laparoscopic guidance. Diagnostic hysteroscopy was performed in all three patients before proceeding with transcervical curettage under laparoscopic guidance. These authors stressed that such procedures can only be performed when the interstitial ectopic pregnancy is situated in the proximal portion of the interstitium, preferably with dilated proximal tubal ostium, by a very experienced endoscopic surgeon, in a patient who is hemodynamically stable.

Management of subsequent pregnancy after interstitial pregnancy

Most authorities advocate cesarean section (CS) delivery when pregnancy occurs after conservative surgery. Su et al. [24] reported a case of uterine rupture at the scar of prior laparoscopic cornuostomy after vaginal delivery of a full-term healthy infant. In the two patients reported by Kulkarni et al. [9] a favorable reproductive outcome was achieved after CS without rupture of uterine scar.

Conclusion

Interstitial pregnancy represents 2–4% of ectopic pregnancies. However, interstitial pregnancies may be catastrophic because of rupture. Rupture of interstitial pregnancy has been thought to occur between 12 and 16 weeks. Having said that, at least one-third could rupture between 8 and 12 weeks. Three-dimensional ultrasonography is very helpful in distinguishing interstitial pregnancy and eccentrically located intrauterine pregnancy. Conservative management of interstitial pregnancy was achieved successfully by laparoscopic cornuostomy, hysteroscopy, or methotrexate injection [30]. Laparoscopic management of interstitial pregnancy requires careful hemostatic measures such as electrocoagulation, diluted Pitressin injection, and laparoscopic suturing [31]. The latter also ensures an adequate uterine scar, thus reducing the risk of rupture during subsequent pregnancy.

References

1. Tulandi T, Al-Jaroudi D. Interstitial pregnancy: results generated from the Society of Reproductive Surgeons Registry. *Obstet Gynecol* 2004; **103**: 47–50.

2. Milanowski A, Bates SK. Semantics and pitfalls in the diagnosis of cornual/interstitial pregnancy *Fertil Steril* 2006; **86**(8): 1764. e11–1764.e14.

3. Timor-Tritsch IE, Monteagudo A, Matera C, et al. Sonographic evolution of cornual pregnancies treated without surgery. *Obstet Gynecol* 1992; **79**: 1044–1049.

4. Ackerman TE, Levi CS, Dashefky SC, et al. Interstitial line: sonographic finding in interstitial (cornual) ectopic pregnancy. *Radiology* 1993; **189**: 83–87.

5. Lawrence A, Jurkovic D. Three-dimensional ultrasound diagnosis of interstitial pregnancy. *Ultrasound Obstet Gynecol* 1999; **14**: 292–293.

6. Tanaka T, Hayashi H, Kutsuzawa T, et al. Treatment of interstitial ectopic pregnancy with methotrexate: report of a successful case. *Fertil Steril* 1982; **37**: 851–852.

7. Reich H, Johns DA, DeCaprio J, et al. Laparoscopic management of 109 ectopic pregnancies. *J Reprod Med* 1988; **33**: 885–890.

8. Meyer W, Mitchell DE. Hysteroscopic removal of an interstitial ectopic gestation; a case report. *J Reprod Med* 1989; **34**: 928–929.

9. Kulkarni K, Ashraf M, Abuzeid M. Interstitial ectopic pregnancy: management and subsequent reproductive outcome. American Association of Gynecologic Laparoscopists (AAGL) 37th Global Congress Of Minimally Invasive Gynecology, Las Vegas, NV, October 30–November 1, 2008.

10. Morito Y, Tsutsumi O, Momoeda M. Cornual pregnancy successfully treated laparoscopically with fibrin glue. *Obstet Gynecol* 1997; **90**: 685–690.

11. Choi YS, Eun DS, Cho J, et al. Laparoscopic cornuotomy using a temporary tourniquet suture and a diluted vasopressin injection in interstitial pregnancy. *Fertil Steril* 2009; **91**(5): 1933–1937.

12. Marcus SF, Dimitry ES, Dimitry M, et al. Heterotopic pregnancy. In: Rizk B (Ed.) *Ultrasound in Reproductive Medicine and Infertility*. Cambridge University Press; 2010: 271–275.

13. Rizk B, Abuzeid M, Rizk CB, et al. Ectopic pregnancy. In: Rizk B (Ed.) *Ultrasound in Reproductive Medicine and Infertility*. Cambridge University Press; 2010: 259–270.

14. Fylstra DL. Ectopic pregnancy not within the (distal) fallopian tube: etiology, diagnosis, and treatment. *Am J Obstet Gynecol* 2012; **206**(4): 289–299.

15. Lau S, Tulandi T. Conservative medical and surgical management of interstitial ectopic pregnancy. *Fertil Steril* 1999; **72**: 207–215.

16. Tang A, Baartz D, Khoo SK. A medical management of interstitial ectopic pregnancy: a 5-year clinical study. *Aust N Z J Obstet Gynaecol* 2006; **46**(2): 107–111.

17. Tawfiq A, Agameya AF, Claman P. Predictors of treatment failure for ectopic pregnancy treated with single dose methotrexate. *Fertil Steril* 2000; **74**: 877–880.

18. Potter MB, Lepine LA, Jamieson DJ. Predictors of success with methotrexate treatment of tubal ectopic pregnancy at Grady Memorial Hospital. *Am J Obstet Gynecol* 2003; **188**: 1192–1194.

19. Katz Z, Lurie S. Laparoscopic cornuostomy in the treatment of interstitial pregnancy with subsequent hysterosalpingography. *Br J Obstet Gynecol* 1997; **104**: 955–956.

20. Matsuzaki S, Fukaya T, Murakami T, Yajima A. Laparoscopic cornuostomy for interstitial pregnancy. A case report. *J Reprod Med* 1999; **44**(11): 981–982.

21. Sagiv R, Golan A, Arbel-Alon S, Glezerman M. Three conservative approaches to treatment of interstitial pregnancy. *J Am Assoc Gynecol Laparosc* 2001; **8**(1): 154–158.

22. Pasic RP, Hammons G, Gardner JS, Hainer M. Laparoscopic treatment of cornual heterotopic pregnancy. *J Am Assoc Gynecol Laparosc* 2002: **9**(3): 372–375.

23. Chan LY, Yuen PM. Successful treatment of ruptured interstitial pregnancy with laparoscopic surgery. A report of 2 cases. *J Reprod Med* 2003: **48**(7): 569–571.

24. Su CF, Tsai HJ, Chen GD, Shih YT, Lee MS. Uterine rupture at scar of prior laparoscopic cornuostomy after vaginal delivery of a full-term healthy infant. *J Obstet Gynaecol Res* 2008; **34**(4 Pt 2): 688–691.

25. Moon HS, Choi YJ, Park YH, Kim SG. New simple endoscopic operations for interstitial pregnancies. *Am J Obstet Gynecol* 2000; **182**(1 Pt 1): 114–121.

26. Warda H, Salem H, Abuzeid M. A simplified technique of laparoscopy cornuostomy for interstitial ectopic pregnancy. *J Min Invasiv Gynecol* 2011; **18**(6;Suppl): S114.

27. Warda H, Abuzeid M. Laparoscopic cornuostomy for a large interstitial ectopic pregnancy. The 41st AAGL Global Congress on MIGS, November 5–9, 2012 Las Vegas, Nevada, USA. Video presentation, November 9, 2012.

28. Katz DL, Barrett JP, Sanfilippo JS, Badway DM. Combined hysteroscopy and laparoscopy in the treatment of interstitial pregnancy. *Am J Obstet Gynecol* 2003; **188**: 1113–1114.

29. Zhang X, Xinchang L, Fan H. Interstitial pregnancy and transcervical curettage. *Obstet Gynecol* 2004; **104**(5): 1193–1195.

30. Rizk B, Holliday CP, Abuzeid M. Challenges in the diagnosis and management of interstitial and cornual ectopic pregnancies. *Middle East Fertil Society J* 2013; **18**: 235–240.

31. Rizk B, Holliday CP, Abuzeid M. Interstitial ectopic pregnancies: laparoscopy vs. laparotomy. *Egyptian Fertil Society J* 2013; **17**(1).

Ultrasound diagnosis of cervical pregnancy

Botros R. M. B. Rizk, Kathryn H. Clarke, Candice P. Holliday and Donna C. Bennett

Introduction

Cervical ectopic pregnancy is very rare in naturally conceived pregnancies [1–7]. Its incidence represents 0.15–0.2% of all ectopic pregnancies. Its actual incidence has been estimated to vary from 1 per 1000 to 1 per 20 000 pregnancies. Rizk and Brinsden [8] observed that cervical pregnancy is still very rare following assisted reproduction. In a cervical pregnancy, the pregnancy implants most often in the endocervical canal, although implantation in the fibromuscular layer of the cervix or the ectocervix is possible [9]. Although the causes of cervical pregnancies are unknown, risk factors can include previous manipulation or instrumentation of the endocervical canal, intrauterine devices, endometriosis in the area of the cervix where nidation occurs, anatomic or structural anomalies, endometrial inflammation, in vitro fertilization, and diethylstilbestrol exposure [9].

Clinical presentation of cervical pregnancy

Painless first trimester bleeding is the first presenting symptom in women with a cervical pregnancy. Patients also report abdominal cramping, pelvic discomfort, and back pain. The patient can also present with soft enlargement of her cervix caused by an intracervical mass, a closed internal os, and an open external os [9]. Urinary difficulties have also been reported in patients with more advanced cervical pregnancy. Thus, cervical pregnancies can present as a hemorrhagic mass, a gestational sac, or with the presence of a fetus [9].

Mechanism of cervical pregnancy

Cervical pregnancies can occur in a number of ways. The gestational sac can grow up to the external os, reaching the uterine cavity [9]. In this manner, a normal evolution of pregnancy can occur, even though the placenta implants on the internal uterine os [9]. The gestational sac can also totally develop in the cervical channel, which can be associated with major complications [9]. Transport of the embryo can also be too quick for the potentially immature endometrium to accept [9]. Additionally,

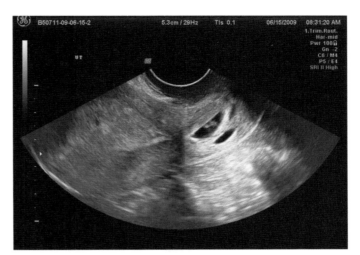

Fig. 16.1 Ultrasonography of a cervical twin pregnancy; sagittal view of the uterus showing thick endometrium and two gestational sacs in the cervix below the internal os. Reproduced with permission from Rizk B (Ed.) *Ultrasonography in Reproductive Medicine and Infertility.* Cambridge University Press, 2010; Chapter 33, 276–282.

fertilization in the cervix can result in implantation in the cervical canal [9].

Ultrasonography

Transvaginal ultrasonography has revolutionized the diagnosis of cervical pregnancy, because it allows for the utilization of conservative options (Figs 16.1–16.7). With the use of ultrasound, the proportion of cases diagnosed preoperatively rose from 35% between 1978 and 1982 to 87% between 1991 and 1994 [1–8].

The exact location of the gestational sac in the cervix and the assessment of the uterine corpus and endometrium are crucial to the diagnosis of cervical pregnancy (Figs 16.1–16.7) [1]. The location of the placenta, the extent of trophoblastic invasion, and blood flow using color Doppler are documented. Typically, the gestational sac is located entirely in the cervix below the level of the internal os [1]. Trophoblastic invasion of the cervix is an important component for the diagnosis of cervical pregnancy.

Ultrasonography in Gynecology, ed. Botros R. M. B. Rizk and Elizabeth E. Puscheck. Published by Cambridge University Press. © Cambridge University Press 2015.

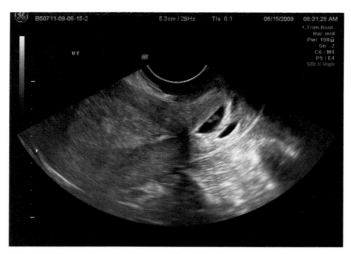

Fig. 16.2 Ultrasonography of a cervical twin pregnancy. Reproduced with permission from Rizk B (Ed.) *Ultrasonography in Reproductive Medicine and Infertility*. Cambridge University Press, 2010; Chapter 33, 276–282.

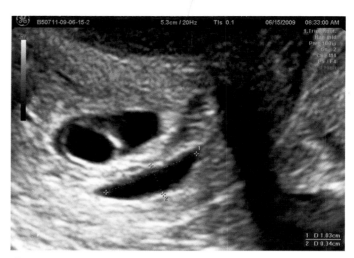

Fig. 16.4 Ultrasonographic diagnosis of cervical twin pregnancy with the second sac a blighted ovum. Reproduced with permission from Rizk B (Ed.) *Ultrasonography in Reproductive Medicine and Infertility*. Cambridge University Press, 2010; Chapter 33, 276–282.

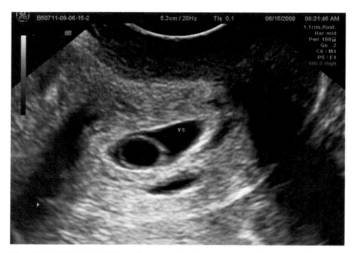

Fig. 16.3 Ultrasonography of a cervical twin pregnancy, demonstrating a yolk sac (YS) in the larger gestational sac. Reproduced with permission from Rizk B (Ed.) *Ultrasonography in Reproductive Medicine and Infertility*. Cambridge, University Press, 2010; Chapter 33, 276–282.

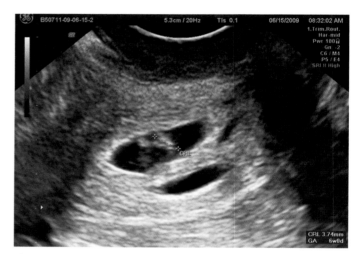

Fig. 16.5 Cervical twin pregnancy showing the crown–rump length (CRL) of the fetus of the first gestational sac. Reproduced with permission from Rizk B (Ed.) *Ultrasonography in Reproductive Medicine and Infertility*. Cambridge University Press, 2010; Chapter 33, 276–282.

A hyperechogenic trophoblastic ring around the implantation site is the classic feature seen on ultrasound (Fig. 16.6). In the absence of signs of trophoblastic invasion, the mere presence of a gestational sac in the cervix may represent only a cervical abortion, where the gestational sac is retained in the cervix before the dilatation of the cervical os [1].

Management of cervical pregnancy

Uncontrollable hemorrhage remains the most serious aspect of medical care and its management has included a variety of innovative options, including angiographic uterine artery embolization, curettage and local prostaglandin injection, hysteroscopic resection, uterine artery ligation and cervicotomy, intracervical injections of vasoconstrictive agents, and Shirodkar-type cervical cerclage [10–25]. For cervical

pregnancy, the success of conservative treatment often depends on the diagnostic accuracy of the initial ultrasound [9].

Systemic chemotherapy

Systemic chemotherapy in the form of methotrexate alone is the first line of treatment in patients with cervical pregnancy whose gestational age is less than 9 weeks and without fetal cardiac activity. Side effects of methotrexate include bone marrow suppression, stomatitis, anorexia, nausea, vomiting, and diarrhea. Systemic methotrexate can be used in a single-dose regimen, 50 mg/m^2, or a multiple dose regimen, 1 mg/kg on days 1, 3, 5, and 7. When multiple doses are used, folinic acid rescue (leucovorin 0.1 mg/kg) should be used on days 2, 4, 6, and 8 to decrease the side effects of the methotrexate.

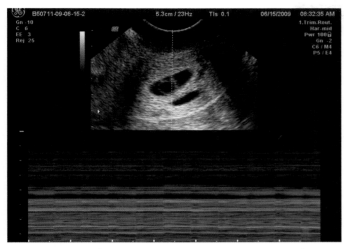

Fig. 16.6 Doppler ultrasound confirming cardiac activity in a cervical pregnancy. Reproduced with permission from Rizk B (Ed.) *Ultrasonography in Reproductive Medicine and Infertility*. Cambridge University Press, 2010; Chapter 33, 276–282.

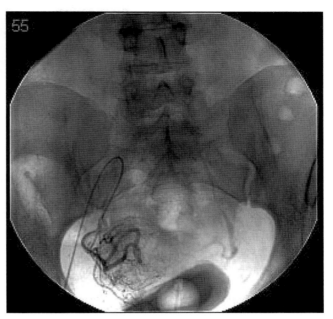

Fig. 16.8 Right uterine artery embolization in a cervical twin pregnancy. Reproduced with permission from Rizk B (Ed.) *Ultrasonography in Reproductive Medicine and Infertility*. Cambridge University Press, 2010; Chapter 33, 276–282.

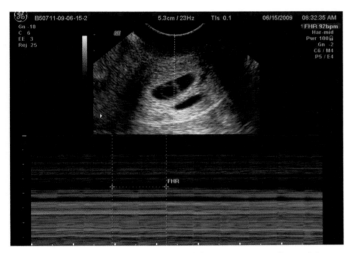

Fig. 16.7 Transvaginal Doppler ultrasound demonstrating cardiac activity in the fetal pole. FHR = fetal heart rate. Reproduced with permission from Rizk B (Ed.) *Ultrasonography in Reproductive Medicine and Infertility*. Cambridge University Press, 2010; Chapter 33, 276–282.

Unlike tubal ectopic pregnancy, there is no contraindication for the use of systemic methotrexate if fetal cardiac activity was seen on ultrasound, even if β-hCG levels are 100 000 mIU/mL or more. However, the success rate tends to decrease and multiple courses may be needed. Multiple-dose regimens are more effective than single-dose regimens at the expense of side effects. Serial hCG measurements are performed on days 4 and 7. The hCG levels may rise or plateau on day 4, especially if cardiac activity was present. This rise is not a sign of treatment failure, but if it persists on or after day 7, methotrexate should be given again or another treatment option considered. On average, it takes about 2 to 4 weeks for a nonviable cervical

pregnancy, and 6 to 8 weeks for a viable cervical pregnancy, to show undetectable levels of hCG. Spontaneous expulsion usually takes place during that time if a dilatation and curettage is not performed.

Uterine artery embolization

Uterine artery embolization (UAE) is currently one of the important interventions in the management of cervical pregnancy (Figs 16.8–16.15). The literature is full of cases proving the efficacy of UAE for the reduction of uterine bleeding and hysterectomy risk [1]. It can be performed in patients who are acutely bleeding or in stable patients who are managed conservatively using methotrexate [21–22]. UAE is usually performed by interventional radiologists using digital subtraction and angiography with low-frequency pulsed fluoroscopy to reduce radiation exposure (Figs 16.8–16.11). After percutaneous catheterization of the femoral artery, a 4-French catheter is used to embolize both uterine arteries using gelatin sponge particles that are injected under fluoroscopy until the descending portion of the uterine artery becomes completely blocked (Figs 16.8–16.11). Upon follow-up, UAE patients typically resume menstruation within 2 months.

UAE is also performed after systemic methotrexate treatment in order to diminish blood loss after the gestational sac is expelled [1]. Moreover, UAE is often used before dilatation and curettage to reduce the excessive bleeding risks from the procedure (Figs 16.12–16.14). Lastly, UAE is also undertaken in patients presenting with acute hemorrhage in an effort to avoid hysterectomy [1].

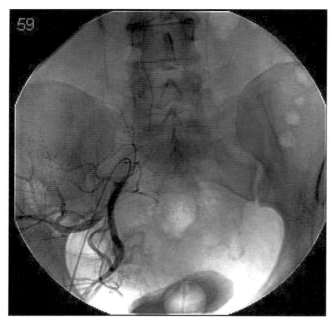

Fig. 16.9 Right uterine artery embolization in a cervical twin pregnancy. Reproduced with permission from Rizk B (Ed.) *Ultrasonography in Reproductive Medicine and Infertility*. Cambridge University Press, 2010; Chapter 33, 276–282.

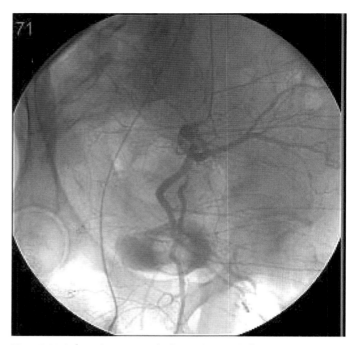

Fig. 16.11 Left uterine artery embolization in a cervical twin pregnancy. Reproduced with permission from Rizk B (Ed.) *Ultrasonography in Reproductive Medicine and Infertility*. Cambridge University Press, 2010; Chapter 33, 276–282.

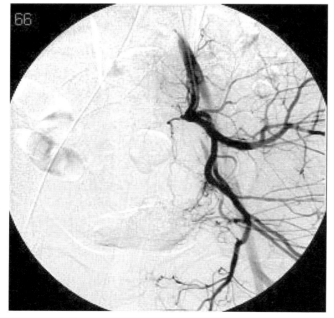

Fig. 16.10 Left uterine artery embolization in a cervical twin pregnancy. Reproduced with permission from Rizk B (Ed.) *Ultrasonography in Reproductive Medicine and Infertility*. Cambridge University Press, 2010; Chapter 33, 276–282.

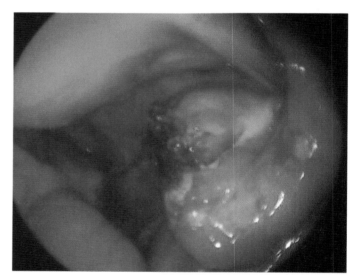

Fig. 16.12 Cervical pregnancy after methotrexate treatment and uterine artery embolization at the time of dilatation and curettage. Reproduced with permission from Rizk B (Ed.) *Ultrasonography in Reproductive Medicine and Infertility*. Cambridge University Press, 2010; Chapter 33, 276–282.

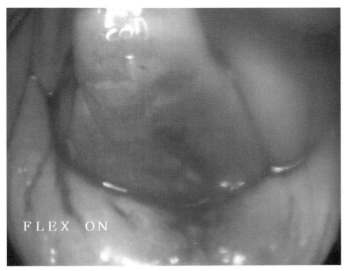

Fig. 16.13 Cervical pregnancy at the time of dilatation and curettage. Reproduced with permission from Rizk B (Ed.) *Ultrasonography in Reproductive Medicine and Infertility*. Cambridge University Press, 2010; Chapter 33, 276–282.

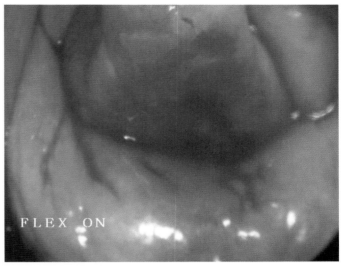

Fig. 16.14 Cervical pregnancy after methotrexate treatment, uterine artery embolization, and dilatation and curettage. Reproduced with permission from Rizk B (Ed.) *Ultrasonography in Reproductive Medicine and Infertility*. Cambridge University Press, 2010; Chapter 33, 276–282.

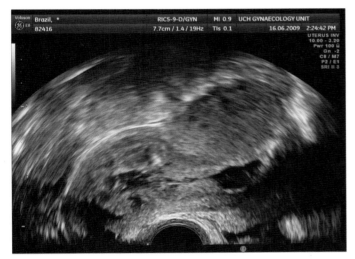

Fig. 16.15 Cervical ectopic pregnancy. Reproduced with permission from Day A, Jurkovic D, The role of ultrasound in early pregnancy after assisted conception. In: Jauniaux ERM, Rizk B, (Eds.) *Pregnancy after Assisted Reproductive Technology*. Cambridge University Press, 2012; Chapter 3, 24.

Foley catheter tamponade

There are other techniques to reduce blood loss from a cervical pregnancy. In many cases, the Foley catheter can be used successfully to manage bleeding. The catheter's bulb is inserted in the cervix and inflated up to 90 mL to manage hemorrhage [1]. The catheter's central lumen can be joined with a suction unit in order to drain the uterus, while the balloon remains inflated for 1–2 days [1]. Particularly in patients with advanced cervical pregnancy (where the patients have significant thinning of the

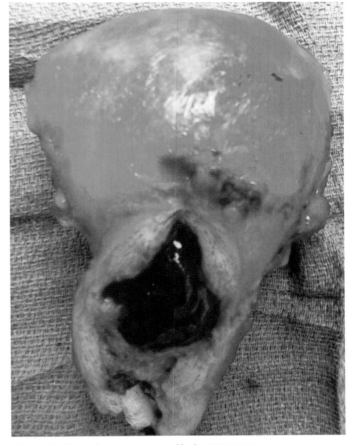

Fig. 16.16 Cervical pregnancy treated by hysterectomy.

cervix), the bulb should be inflated under ultrasound guidance in order to avoid the risk of cervical rupture [26,27]. Although this practice has not been used by the authors, other physicians consider this an attractive option to reduce blood loss [1].

Hysterectomy

Hysterectomy is performed in patients who have completed their families, and are diagnosed with a cervical pregnancy that is actively bleeding (Fig. 16.16). Hysterectomy is becoming less and less popular since many patients wish to maintain their fertility potential.

Conclusion

Cervical pregnancy is rare in naturally conceived pregnancies, and even after IVF it remains a rare occurrence. Painless first trimester bleeding is typically the first presenting symptom; however, abdominal cramping, pelvic discomfort, and back pain can occur. In more advanced cases, urinary difficulties may be encountered.

Transvaginal ultrasonography has revolutionized the diagnosis of cervical pregnancy and has therefore allowed the utilization of conservative treatment options. The proportion of cases diagnosed preoperatively increased from 35% between 1978 and 1982 to 87% between 1991 and 1994. The exact location of the gestational sac in the cervix below the level of the internal os and the absence of a gestational sac in the uterine cavity are essential for the diagnosis. The presence of hyperechogenic trophoblastic tissue around the implantation site is also essential for the diagnosis, and differentiates cervical pregnancy from the cervical stage of abortion, where the gestational sac is retained in the cervix before expulsion.

Uncontrollable hemorrhage remains the most serious concern for medical care and the management of cervical pregnancy. Systemic methotrexate is typically the first line of treatment in patients with cervical pregnancy and less than 9 weeks gestation. UAE is currently widely used to avoid the risk of bleeding, which may be catastrophic. Hysterectomy is offered to patients who have completed their families and who do not wish to keep open the option for future conception.

References

1. Moustafa HF, Rizk B, Brooks N, et al. Cervical pregnancy. In: Rizk B (Ed.) *Ultrasonography in Reproductive Medicine and Infertility*. Cambridge University Press; 2010: 276–282.

2. Dimitry ES, Rizk B. Ectopic pregnancy: epidemiology, advances in diagnosis and management. *Br J Clin Pract* 1992; **46**(1): 52–54.

3. Rizk B, Dimitry ES, Morcos S, et al. A multicentre study on combined intrauterine and extrauterine pregnancy after IVF. European Society for Human Reproduction and Embryology meeting, 1990; Milan, Italy. *Hum Reprod* 1990; abstract.

4. Parente JT, Chau-su O, Levy J, Legatt E. Cervical pregnancy analysis. *Obstet Gynecol* 1983; **62**: 79–82.

5. Ushakov FB, Elchalal U, Aceman PJ, Schenker JG. Cervical pregnancy: past and future. *Obstet Gynecol Surv* 1997; **52**(1): 45–59.

6. Sherer DM, Abramowicz JS, Thompson HO, et al. Comparison of transabdominal and endovaginal sonographic approaches in the diagnosis of a case of cervical pregnancy successfully treated with methotrexate. *J Ultrasound Med* 1991; **10**(7): 409–411.

7. Rizk B, Tan SL, Morcos S, et al. Heterotopic pregnancies following in-vitro fertilization and embryo transfer. *Am J Obstet Gynecol* 1991; **164**(1): 161–164.

8. Rizk B, Brinsden PR. Embryo migration responsible for ectopic pregnancies. *Am J Obstet Gynecol* 1990; **164**(4): 1639.

9. Kraemer B, Abele H, Hahn M, et al. Cervical ectopic pregnancy on the portio: conservative case management and clinical review. *Fertil Steril* 2008; **90**: 2011.e1–4.

10. Shinagawa S, Nagayama M. Cervical pregnancy as a possible sequela of induced abortion. Report of 19 cases. *Am J Obstet Gynecol* 1969; **105**(2): 282–284.

11. Copas P, Semmer J. Cervical ectopic pregnancy: sonographic demonstration at 28 weeks' gestation. *J Clin Ultrasound* 1983; **11**: 328–330.

12. Lin EP, Bhatt S, Dogra VS. Diagnostic clues to ectopic pregnancy. *Radiographics* 2008; **28**(6): 1661–1671.

13. Timor-Tritsch IE, Monteagurdo A, Mandeville EO, et al. Successful management of viable cervical pregnancy by local injection of methotrexate guided by transvaginal ultrasonography. *Am J Obstet Gynecol* 1994; **17**: 737–739.

14. Bennett S, Waterstone J, Parsons J, et al. Two cases of cervical pregnancy following in vitro fertilization and embryo transfer to the lower uterine cavity. *J Assist Reprod Genet* 1993; **10**(1): 100–103.

15. Vas W, Suresh PL, Tang-Barton P, et al. Ultrasonographic differentiation of cervical abortion from cervical pregnancy. *J Clin Ultrasound* 1984; **12**: 553–557.

16. Jurkovic D, Hacket E, Campbell S. Diagnosis and treatment of early cervical pregnancy. *Ultrasound Obstet Gynecol* 1996; **8**: 373–380.

17. Pellerito JS, Taylor KJW, Quedens-Case C, et al. Ectopic pregnancy: evaluation with endovaginal color flow imaging. *Radiology* 1992; **183**: 407–411.

18. Dillon EH, Feyock AL, Taylor KJW. Pseudogestational sacs: Doppler US differentiation from normal or abnormal intrauterine pregnancies. *Radiology* 1990; **176**: 359–364.

19. Mitra AG, Harris-Owens M. Conservative medical management of advanced cervical ectopic pregnancies. *Obstet Gynecol Surv* 2000; **55**(6): 385–389.

20. Aboulghar M, Rizk B. Ultrasonography of the cervix. In: Rizk B, Garcia-Velasco JA, Sallam H, Makrigiannakis A. (Eds.) *Infertility and Assisted Reproduction*. New York, NY: Cambridge University Press;. 2008: 143–151.

21. Honey L, Leader A, Claman P. Uterine artery embolization – a successful treatment to control bleeding cervical pregnancy with a simultaneous intrauterine gestation. *Hum Reprod* 1999; **14**(2): 553–555.

22. Nappi C, D'Elia A, Di Carlo C, et al. Conservative treatment by angiographic uterine artery embolization of a 12 week cervical ectopic pregnancy. *Hum Reprod* 1999; **14**(4): 1118–21.

23. Mashiach S, Admon D, Oelsner G, et al. Cervical Shirodkar cerclage may be the treatment modality of choice for cervical pregnancy. *Hum Reprod* 2002; **17**(2): 493–496.

24. Fylstra DL. Ectopic pregnancy not within the (distal) fallopian tube: etiology, diagnosis, and treatment. *Am J Obstet Gynecol* 2012; **206**(4): 289–299.

25. Rizk B, Holliday CP, Owens S, Abuzeid M. Cervical and cesarean scar ectopic pregnancies: diagnosis and management. *Middle East Fertil Society J* 2013; **18**: 67–73.

26. Kuppuswami N, Vindekilde J, Sethi CM, et al. Diagnosis and treatment of cervical pregnancy. *Obstet Gynecol* 1983; **61**(5): 651–653.

27. Hurley VA, Beischer NA. Cervical pregnancy: hysterectomy avoided with the use of a large Foley catheter balloon. *Aust N Z J Obstet Gynaecol* 1988; **28**: 230–232.

Chapter

17

Ultrasound diagnosis of cesarean scar ectopic pregnancy

Botros R. M. B. Rizk, Rizwan Malik, Kathryn H. Clarke and Mostafa I. Abuzeid

Incidence of cesarean scar pregnancy

The incidence of pregnancy within the scar of a previous cesarean section (CS) is increasing worldwide, as seen in both Western and Chinese literature [1–24]. This increase might have resulted from the higher number of CS deliveries and the increase in diagnosed cases. The incidence of cesarean scar pregnancy (CSP) has been estimated to range from 1 per 1800 to 1 per 2500 of all CSs performed, and constitutes 6.1% of all ectopic pregnancies in patients with a history of at least one CS delivery. The early diagnosis of CSP is possible by ultrasonography (Figs 17.1–17.7).

Pathogenesis of cesarean scar pregnancy

The mechanism of development of CSP is interesting. Fylstra [1] suggested that the disruption of the endometrium and myometrium during a CS and subsequent scarring can predispose a patient to abnormal pregnancy implantation (Fig. 17.2). Trophoblastic invasion is enhanced because of the scant decidualization of the lower uterine segment. A distinction is made between CSP and intrauterine pregnancy with placenta accreta. A CSP is completely surrounded by myometrium and scar tissue and separated from the endometrial cavity or fallopian tube. The time interval between the CS and subsequent pregnancy varies and some of the cases occurred within a few months of the prior CS delivery, with the implication that incomplete healing of the CS is a contributing factor to the occurrence of this type of pregnancy.

Ultrasonographic diagnosis

Early diagnosis is very helpful in CSPs, as it is in all types of ectopic pregnancy [1–4]. It offers different treatment options and avoids hemorrhage and uterine rupture [2–4]. It is sometimes difficult to distinguish between CSP or cervical-isthmic pregnancy and a spontaneous abortion that is still in progress. Fylstra emphasized the necessity for strict criteria for diagnosis of CSP [1]. Ultrasonography should be obtained in a sagittal position and plainly demonstrate a clear uterine cavity and an

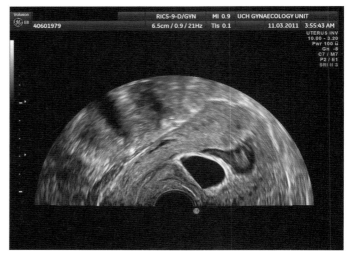

Fig. 17.1 Cesarean scar pregnancy. Reproduced with permission from Day A, Jurkovic D, The role of ultrasound in early pregnancy after assisted conception. In: Jauniaux ERM, Rizk B (Eds.) *Pregnancy after Assisted Reproductive Technology*. Cambridge University Press, 2012; Chapter 3: 51–68.

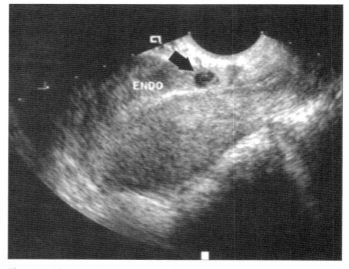

Fig. 17.2 Ultrasound appearance of early cesarean scar pregnancy. Reproduced with permission from Fylstra DL. *Am J Obstet Gynecol*, 2012; 206(4): 293.

Ultrasonography in Gynecology, ed. Botros R. M. B. Rizk and Elizabeth E. Puscheck. Published by Cambridge University Press. © Cambridge University Press 2015.

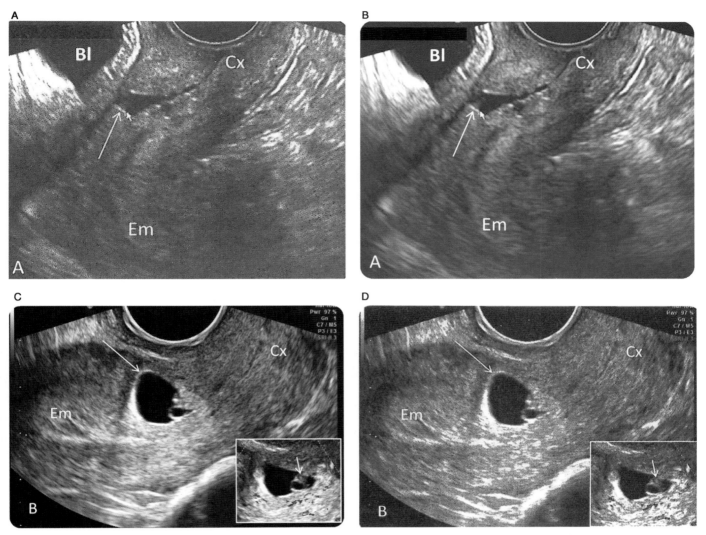

Fig. 17.3 (A) Sonographic image of a niche at the site of the hysterotomy performed at cesarean delivery. (B) Sonographic image of a cesarean section scar pregnancy (arrow) at 6 postmenstrual weeks and 3 days showing the yolk sac and above it the embryonic pole. Parts A and B reproduced with permission from Timor-Tritsch IE, Monteagudo A. Unforeseen consequences of the increasing rate of cesarean deliveries: early placenta accreta and cesarean scar pregnancy. *Am J Obstet Gynecol* 2012; 207: 14–29.

empty cervical canal. The gestational sac typically develops in the anterior part of the uterine isthmus and there should be no myometrium between the gestational sac and the bladder, so as to differentiate it from a cervical pregnancy.

Timor-Tritsch et al. highlighted the difficulty in the diagnoses of CSP [3]. Many of those cases presented with shock, hemoperitoneum, and heavy bleeding for termination of an early pregnancy, or D&C for missed abortion. In some cases, arteriovenous malformations are detected in the placenta within the cesarean scar.

Management of cesarean scar pregnancy

A wide variety of options exist for the management of CSP, highlighting the lack of standard protocol [2–18] (Table 17.1). Treatment should be performed as soon as the diagnosis is confirmed (Table 17.2). In hemodynamically stable patients, two options should be considered: (a) medical, the most

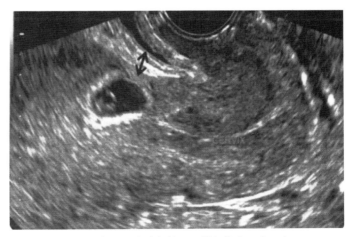

Fig. 17.4 Gestational sac embedded in scar. Thin (1–3 mm) or absent myometrium (arrow) between sac and bladder. Reproduced with permission from Timor-Tritsch IE, et al. The diagnosis, treatment and follow-up of cesarean scar pregnancy. *Am J Obstet Gynecol* 2012: 207: 45.

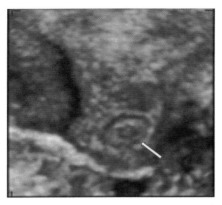

Fig. 17.5 Transvaginal 3D ultrasound picture of cesarean scar pregnancy (arrow).

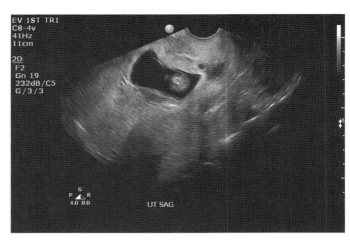

Fig. 17.7 Cesarean scar pregnancy.

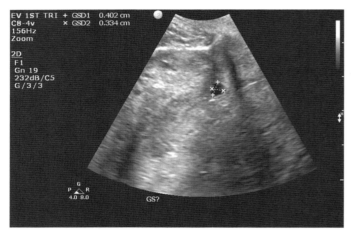

Fig. 17.6 Cesarean scar pregnancy.

successful being local injection of methotrexate, and (b) surgical treatment utilizing laparoscopic aspiration of the gestational sac and repair of the uterus. Both medical and surgical options aim to eliminate the gestational sac and retain the patient's fertility. In the past, laparotomy and hysterectomy were performed, particularly for patients presenting with hemorrhage. With the advancement of laparoscopic surgery, repair of the uterus and resection of the ectopic pregnancy can be accomplished.

Methotrexate treatment

Methotrexate injections have been used both systemically and locally. UAE alone or combined with local methotrexate has also been reported. As the CSP is surrounded by scar tissue, this scar tissue may impede the absorption of methotrexate. Direct injection into the gestational sac may be more useful if this is the chosen method of treatment.

Timor-Tritsch et al. [3] reported a retrospective case series of 26 patients between 6 and 14 menstrual weeks. The diagnosis was confirmed with transvaginal ultrasound. In 19 of the 26 patients, the gestational sac was injected with 50 mg of

methotrexate: 25 mg into the area of the embryo or fetus and 25 mg into the placental area. An additional 25 mg of methotrexate was administered intramuscularly. Serial hCG determinations were performed and then gestational sac volumes and vascularization were assessed by 3D ultrasound. The pregnancies that were treated were followed for 24–177 days without complications.

Seow et al. [24] reviewed 12 cases of CSP, which were diagnosed using transvaginal color sonography, during a 6-year period in Taiwan. The rate of CSP was 6.1% in women with an ectopic pregnancy and at least one previous CS. The time interval from the first CS to diagnosis of CSP ranged from 6 months to 12 years. The 12 patients were treated using a variety of options aiming to preserve fertility. Transvaginal ultrasound-guided methotrexate injection into the gestational sac was performed in three cases and transabdominal ultrasound-guided injection in two cases. Transabdominal ultrasound-guided methotrexate injection into the gestational sac followed by systemic methotrexate was performed in two cases. Systemic methotrexate alone was performed in two patients. Dilatation and curettage (D&C) was performed in two patients and local resection of the gestational sac in one patient. Eleven of the 12 patients preserved their reproductive capacity, while in one patient a hysterectomy was necessary because of profuse bleeding. The authors suggest ultrasound-guided methotrexate injection as the treatment of choice for CSP [24]. Surgical techniques, including D&C, are not recommended due to high morbidity and poor prognosis.

Surgical treatment

Surgical treatment includes laparoscopy and robotic surgery with assisted vaginal repair [6–8]. Donnez et al. [6] performed laparoscopic repair in three patients, one of whom had a successful pregnancy. Yalcinkaya et al. [8] performed a robotic assisted cesarean scar repair. Klemm et al. [7] performed laparoscopic assisted vaginal repair of the scar in five patients.

Table 17.1 First-line treatment choices for cesarean scar pregnancy, with the highest and the lowest complication rates

	Methotrexate alone	Dilation and curettage	Uterine artery embolization	Hysteroscopy	Local injection of methotrexate/KCl (transabdominal or transvaginal ultrasound guidance)
Cases	87	305	64	119	81
Complications	54	189	30	22	8
%	62.1	61.9	46.9	18.4	9.6

Modified with permission from Timor-Tritsch IE, Monteagudo A. *Am J Obstet Gynecol* 2012; 207: 14–29.

Table 17.2 Clinical outcome of patients with cesarean section scar pregnancy as a function of gestational age at first treatment

Gestational age (weeks)	No complications	Complications
5–6	51	12
7	35	16
8	14	26
9	4	6
10–15	4	16

Modified with permission from Timor-Tritsch IE, Monteagudo A. *Am J Obstet Gynecol* 2012; 207: 14–29.

Expectant management

Expectant management has been newly reported in the literature. In one case it resulted in hemorrhage, and hysterectomy was necessary after the delivery of a healthy infant.

Heterotopic cesarean scar and ectopic twin pregnancy after in vitro fertilization (IVF)

Heterotopic CSP is very rare after IVF [19–23]. Wang et al. [22] reported successful management of heterotopic CSP of 7 weeks gestation by transvaginal intracardiac injection of potassium chloride. The pregnancy continued successfully and a healthy infant was delivered 6 months later. Chueh et al. [21] reported two ectopic twin pregnancies in CS scars after IVF. Focused application of high-resolution ultrasound and diagnostic hysteroscopy were used for the prompt management of these rare ectopic twin pregnancies [21,22]. Mitwally et al. [23] reported a case of heterotopic pregnancy that included a normal twin intrauterine pregnancy (IUP) and one ectopic pregnancy in a CS scar, which was diagnosed at 6 weeks gestation. Ultrasound-guided aspiration of the ectopic gestational sac was performed and the concurrent twin IUP was preserved successfully.

Management of cesarean scar molar pregnancy

There is very scant literature on the management of molar CSP. In a recently reported case of molar pregnancy from Hong Kong, a 34-year-old woman presented with persistent symptoms of pregnancy after surgical termination of pregnancy [25]. During ultrasonography, molar CSP pregnancy was suspected. Under ultrasound guidance, suction evacuation was performed. This was followed by oxytocin and manual compression. UAE was necessary to reduce uterine bleeding. The authors emphasized that a high index of suspicion is required to diagnose a molar CSP.

The relation between early intervention and the outcome of cesarean scar pregnancies

It appears that early diagnosis and treatment results in an improved outcome of CSP (Table 17.2). Timor-Tritsch et al. identified the exact diagnoses in only 184 of 751 cases [3,4]. They divided these cases into either a good outcome group (if the patients did not have complications after the initial treatment) and an emergency group (if the patients required emergency surgery or embolization). If elective hysterectomy, UAE, or laparotomy was the primary treatment of choice and there were no complications, then these patients were included in the good outcome group. In the analyses of these groups of patients at 5–15 weeks gestation, there was a trend of improvement in outcome if the diagnosis was made early.

Future obstetric performance after cesarean scar pregnancy

In the review of the literature, Timor-Tritsch and Monteagudo identified and reported on 64 intrauterine pregnancies after treatment of CSP [4]. They speculated that there is significant underreporting, as many authors would not consider a successful pregnancy after CS delivery as worthy of publication.

Conclusion

The incidence of CSP has increased worldwide as a result of increasing incidence of CS deliveries and increased general recognition. Ultrasonography should be performed as early as possible when this type of pregnancy is suspected [14–23]. Ultrasonography should confirm an empty uterine cavity and cervical canal as well as the absence of myometrium between the gestational sac and the bladder. The diagnosis is difficult, and in many patients CSP was often misdiagnosed as cervical pregnancy or miscarriage in process. A correct diagnosis that is made early is associated with a better outcome, even when treatments with slightly higher complication rates were used.

Although there is no consensus regarding treatment of CSP, certain conclusions could be made from the review of the reported cases. D&C should be avoided because it may lead to excessive bleeding, making blood transfusion and, in certain circumstances, laparotomy and hysterectomy necessary. Systemic methotrexate as a single treatment of choice should also be avoided [3]. The time required for methotrexate to work could result in an increase in the size of the fetus and vascularization and thus, more complications from the treatment. Local injection of methotrexate under transvaginal or transabdominal ultrasound guidance, with or without intramuscular methotrexate, as well as hysteroscopic resection carried the lowest complication rate. UAE should be used in cases of significant bleeding or arteriovenous malformations.

References

1. Fylstra DL. Ectopic pregnancy not within the (distal) fallopian tube: etiology, diagnosis, and treatment. *Am J Obstet Gynecol* 2012; **206**(4): 289–299.

2. Jurkovic D, Hillaby K, Woelfer B, et al. First trimester diagnosis and management of pregnancies implanted into the lower uterine segment Cesarean section scar. *Ultrasound Obstet Gynecol* 2003; **21**: 220.

3. Timor-Tritsch IE, Monteagudo A, Santos R, et al. The diagnosis, treatment and follow-up of cesarean scar pregnancy. *Am J Obstet Gynecol* 2012; **207**: 44–46.

4. Timor-Tritsch IE and Monteagudo A. Unforeseen consequences of the increasing rate of cesarean deliveries: early placenta accreta and cesarean scar pregnancy. *Am J Obstet Gynecol* 2012; **207**: 14–29.

5. Holland MG, Bienstock JL. Recurrent ectopic pregnancy in a cesarean scar. *Obstet Gynecol* 2008; **111**: 541–545.

6. Donnez O, Jadoul P, Squiffet J. Laparoscopic repair of wide and deep uterine scar dehiscence after cesarean section. *Fertil Steril* 2008; **89**: 974–980.

7. Klemm P, Koehler C, Mangler M. Laparoscopic and vaginal repair of uterine scar dehiscence following cesarean section as detected by ultrasound. *J Perinat Med* 2005; **33**: 324–331.

8. Yalcinkaya TM, Akar ME, Kammire LD. Robotic assisted laparoscopic repair of symptomatic cesarean scar defect: a report of two cases. *J Reprod Med* 2011; **56**: 265–270.

9. Godin PA, Bassil S, Donnez J. An ectopic pregnancy developing in a previous cesarean section scar. *Fertil Steril* 1997; **67**: 398–400.

10. Herman A, Weinraub Z, Avrech O, et al. Follow up and outcome of isthmic pregnancy located in a previous cesarean section scar. *Br J Obstet Gynaecol* 1995; **102**: 839–841.

11. Fylstra DL. Ectopic pregnancy within a cesarean scar: a review. *Obstet Gynecol Surv* 2002; **57**: 537–543.

12. Fylstra DL, Pound-Chang T, Miller MG, et al. Ectopic pregnancy within a cesarean delivery scar: a case report. *Am J Obstet Gynecol* 2002; **187**: 302–304.

13. Chen CH, Wang PH, Liu WM. Successful treatment of cesarean scar pregnancy using laparoscopically assisted local injection of etoposide with transvaginal ultrasound guidance. *Fertil Steril* 2009; **92**: 1747.e9–e11.

14. Dandawate B, Carpenter T. Caesarean scar pregnancy presenting as anaemia. *Am J Obstet Gynecol* 2009; **29**: 772–773.

15. Ficicioglu C, Attar R, Tildirim G, et al. Fertility preserving surgical management of methotrexate-resistant cesarean scar pregnancy. *Taiwan J Obstet Gynecol* 2010; **49**: 211–213.

16. Rygh AB, Greve OJ, Fjetland L, et al. Arteriovenous malformation as a consequence of a scar pregnancy. *Acta Obstet Gynecol Scand* 2009; **88**: 853–855.

17. Bignardi T, Condous G. Transrectal ultrasound-guided surgical evacuation of cesarean scar ectopic pregnancy. *Ultrasound Obstet Gynecol* 2010; **35**: 481–485.

18. Deviate AJM, Brolmann HA, van der Slikke JW, et al. Therapeutic options of caesarean scar pregnancy: case series and literature review. *J Clin Ultrasound* 2010; **38**: 75–84.

19. Eininkel J, Stumpp O, Kosling S, et al. A misdiagnosed case of cesarean scar pregnancy. *Arch Gynecol Obstet* 2005; **271**: 178–181.

20. Fabunmi L, Perks N. Caesarean section scar ectopic pregnancy following postcoital contraception. *J Fam Plann Reprod Health Care* 2002; **28**: 155–156.

21. Cheuh HY, Cheng PJ, Wang CW, et al. Ectopic twin pregnancy in cesarean scar after IVF/embryo transfer. *Fertil Steril* 2008; **90**(5): 2009.e19–21.

22. Wang CN, Chen CK, Wang HS, et al. Successful management of heterotopic cesarean scar pregnancy combined with intrauterine pregnancy after in vitro fertilization/embryo transfer. *Fertil Steril* 2007; **88**(3): 706,e13–16.

23. Mitwally MF, Hafsa A, Diamond MP, et al. Gestational sac aspiration of heterotopic pregnancy in a cesarean section scar. *J Gynecol Surg* 29(6): 317–320.

24. Seow KM, Huang LW, Lin YH, et al. Cesarean scar pregnancy: issues in management. *Ultrasound Obstet Gynecol* 2004; **23**(3): 247–253.

25. Ko JK, Wan HL, Ngu SF, et al. Cesarean scar molar pregnancy. *Obstet Gynecol* 2012; **119**(2 Pt 2): 449–451.

Ultrasound diagnosis of ovarian and abdominal ectopic pregnancies

Botros R. M. B. Rizk, Candice P. Holliday, Kathryn H. Clarke and John LaFleur

Ovarian pregnancy

Primary ovarian pregnancy is a rare form of ectopic pregnancy [1–6]. Secondary ovarian pregnancy begins as an endometrial or tubal implantation and then reimplants in the ovary [7]. In 1614, Mercier was the first to suggest that pregnancy might occur within the ovary [8,9]. The classic anatomical and histological criteria for the diagnosis of an authentic case of ovarian pregnancy were suggested by Spiegelberg in 1878 [3]. The criteria are: (a) the fallopian tubes, including the fimbria, must be intact and separate from the ovary; (b) the pregnancy must occupy the normal position of the ovary; (c) the ovary must be attached to the uterus through the utero-ovarian ligament; and (d) ovarian tissue must be attached to the pregnancy [7].

Incidence of ovarian pregnancy

The incidence of ovarian pregnancy has been reported to range from as low as 1 in 60 000 to as high as 1 in 2000 [7]. Its occurrence remains rare, despite the different forms of ectopic pregnancy occurring after assisted conception [8]. Even more rarely, ovarian pregnancies can be of a twin ovarian pregnancy or part of a heterotopic pregnancy [10].

Mechanism of ovarian pregnancy

The etiology of ovarian pregnancy is unknown [7]. The likely mechanism causing the occurrence of an ovarian pregnancy is the reverse migration of one of the embryos through the fallopian tube with subsequent implantation in the ovary, although other possibilities cannot be excluded [8]. Such possibilities include an interference with the release of the ovum from the ruptured follicle, malfunction of the fallopian tubes, or inflammatory thickening of the tunica albuginea [7]. Although an ovarian pregnancy can occur in women without any risk factors, there are some associations [10]. Several possible risk factors for ovarian pregnancy include the use of intrauterine devices or assisted reproductive technology, previous abdominal or laparoscopic surgery, endometriosis, pelvic inflammatory disease, and uterine anomalies [7,10].

Clinical picture of ovarian pregnancy

The clinical picture of ovarian pregnancy is indistinguishable from that of tubal pregnancy during early gestation. Most women present with abdominal pain, with or without vaginal bleeding [10]. Most ovarian pregnancies (75–90%) rupture in the first trimester, with two-thirds occurring during the first 8 weeks. Indeed, among the sites in which pregnancy may develop ectopically, the ovary may have the greatest ability to accommodate a pregnancy. Thus, the ovary may offer the highest chance of development to term and survival of the infant. Between 4% and 12% of ovarian pregnancies have been reported to be maintained into the third trimester [9].

Ultrasonography of ovarian pregnancy

The essential ultrasonographic features of an ovarian pregnancy are a more echogenic wide ring on the ovary, as compared with the ovarian tissue, and a yolk sac or fetal parts [7]. When these features are not clearly visualized on ultrasound, however, it is almost impossible to accurately diagnose an ovarian pregnancy [7].

The challenge on ultrasound is to distinguish an ovarian pregnancy from a corpus luteum (Fig. 18.1) or hemorrhagic cyst, because a positive pregnancy test with a cystic adnexal mass and no obvious intrauterine gestation also indicates a corpus luteum in an early or failing intrauterine or tubal pregnancy [10]. Corpus luteum is suggested when ultrasonography notes decreased wall echogenicity compared with the endometrium and an anechoic texture [10].

Management of ovarian pregnancy

Early diagnosis by ultrasonography (Fig. 18.2) allows for the conservation of the ovary [7]. However, ovarian pregnancy may be difficult to manage because preoperative diagnosis is so challenging [10]. Traditionally, oophorectomy or salpingo-oophorectomy was used to treat ovarian pregnancy by laparotomy [7]. However, with the advances in laparoscopy, conservative laparoscopy is now preferred [7] (Figs 18.3, 18.4).

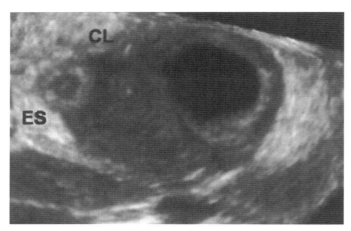

Fig. 18.1 Three-dimensional volume ultrasound of the left ovary: a small mass compatible with "bagel" appearance bulging from the cortex and coexisting with two additional masses is noted. CL, corpus luteum, ES, ectopic sac. Reproduced with permission from Ghi T, Banfi A, Marconi R, et al. Three-dimensional sonographic diagnosis of ovarian pregnancy. *Ultrasound Obstet Gynecol* 2005; 26: 103.

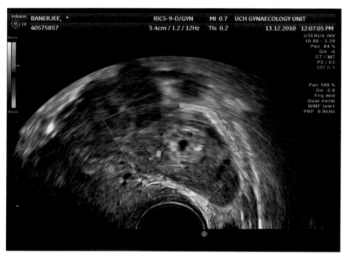

Fig. 18.2 Ovarian ectopic pregnancy. Reproduced with permission from Day A, Jurkovic D, The role of ultrasound in early pregnancy after assisted conception. In: Jauniaux ERM and Rizk B (Eds.) *Pregnancy after Assisted Reproductive Technology*. Cambridge University Press, 2012; Chapter 3.

Thus, surgical excision of trophoblastic tissue and ovarian conservation should be the aim (Fig. 18.5). However, if the excision is accompanied by severe bleeding, ovarian wedge resection or oophorectomy may be necessary [7]. Rizk et al. [11] reported successful surgical removal of an ovarian ectopic pregnancy with ovarian preservation followed by a successful in vitro fertilization (IVF) attempt with a subsequent intrauterine pregnancy.

Kraemer et al. [10] also reported successful laparoscopic wedge resection, where the intact ovarian pregnancy was completely removed (Fig. 18.6). The authors surgically treated the ovarian pregnancy so that a wedge-shaped section of healthy ovarian tissue was removed without initial electrocauterization. On direct examination, the section of ovarian tissue removed

resembled a hemorrhagic cyst. However, the authors were aware of the positive heart rate detected preoperatively and were able to dissect the ectopic pregnancy inside the yolk sac from the ovarian tissue. Although the literature usually states that the ectopic pregnancy's appearance lags in comparison with actual gestational age, that is not always the case [10].

Medical treatment with methotrexate and etoposide has also been reported, but it is not a first-line treatment [7,10,12]. That said, use of medical treatment is less common and failure of methotrexate treatment has been reported [7,10]. This lower rate of medical treatment could also be a result of the American Society for Reproductive Medicine's recommendation that ovarian pregnancy should be definitively diagnosed by surgical exploration [13].

Abdominal pregnancy

Abdominal pregnancy is a rare form of ectopic pregnancy in which the gestational sac implants in the peritoneal cavity of the abdomen or pelvis (Fig. 18.7). The incidence rate ranges from 1 in 3000 to 1 in 10 000 pregnancies [14]. Although most abdominal pregnancies currently are reported in underdeveloped countries, Louisiana and Mississippi have similar rates of incidence [14]. Similar to other ectopic pregnancies, abdominal pregnancies can result from diseased fallopian tubes, congenital anomalies, endometriosis, previous ectopic pregnancies, surgery, and assisted reproductive techniques [14,15].

Abdominal pregnancy may be primary or secondary. In primary abdominal pregnancies, which are rarer than secondary abdominal pregnancies, the pregnancy implants directly in the peritoneal cavity of the abdomen or the pelvis [14]. In secondary abdominal pregnancy, the pregnancy begins as a tubal pregnancy and then reimplants in the peritoneal cavity after the expulsion of the gestational sac from the end of the fallopian tube or after the rupture of the fallopian tube [14].

Maternal mortality in abdominal pregnancy

Maternal mortality is significantly increased in abdominal pregnancy due to the high incidence of internal hemorrhage, sepsis, and renal failure [14,15]. Primary abdominal pregnancies frequently result in spontaneous abortions in the first trimester, which result in hemoperitoneum that often precipitates diagnosis [16]. In many abdominal pregnancies, the fetus dies early in pregnancy. However, the fetus can remain alive to the second or even third trimester. That said, the outcomes for both mother and fetus have improved as a result of imaging techniques that allow for earlier diagnosis and advances in laparoscopy [14].

Ultrasonography of abdominal pregnancy

In the early part of the first trimester, abdominal pregnancy is very difficult to distinguish from tubal pregnancy by ultrasonography [15]. In fact, even with the most expert of ultrasonographers, ultrasonography's sensitivity for abdominal

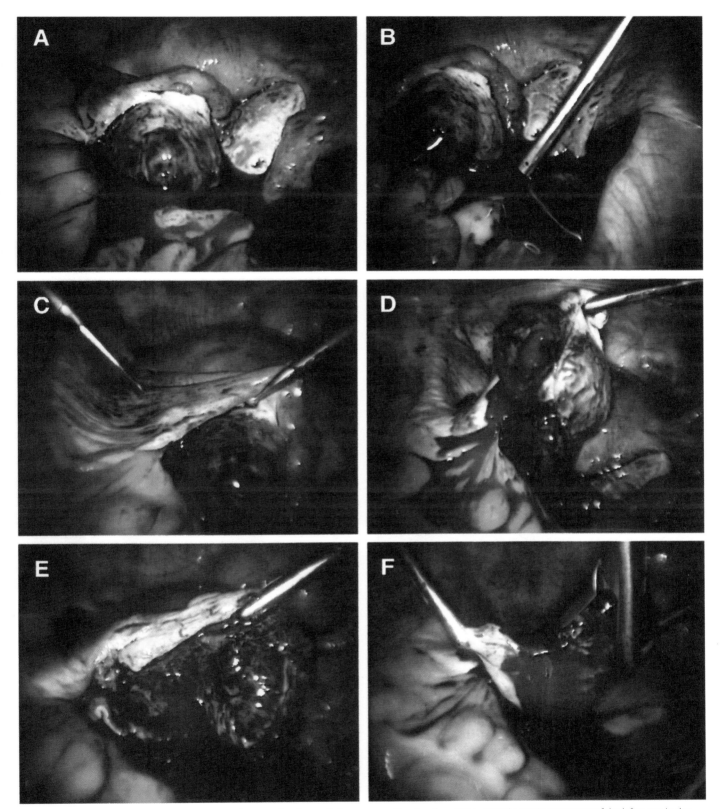

Fig. 18.3 (A) Overview after creating a pneumoperitoneum for diagnostic laparoscopy. Bleeding from the ruptured ectopic pregnancy of the left ovary. In the background, the slightly enlarged uterus and the right ovary with the corpus luteum cyst. (B) Suction of the blood out of the cul-de-sac. (C) Preparation of the left ovary and injection of ornipressin into the infundibulo-pelvic ligament. (D) Blunt preparation and enucleation of the gestational sac from the orthotopic ovarian tissue. Removal of the product of conception by (E) enucleation. Healthy ovarian tissue can be seen on the left. (F) Removal after complete separation of the trophoblast from the ovary. Reproduced with permission from Alkatout I, Stuhlmann-Laeisz C, Mettler L, et al. Organ-preserving management of ovarian pregnancies by laparoscopic approach. *Fertil Steril* 2011; 95(8): 2470.e2.

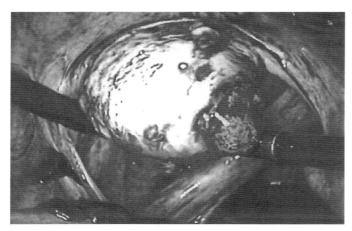

Fig. 18.4 Appearance of left ovary at laparoscopy; a small bleeding bulge on the ovarian surface compatible with a gestational sac is noted. Reproduced with permission from Ghi T, Banfi A, Marconi R, et al. Three-dimensional sonographic diagnosis of ovarian pregnancy. *Ultrasound Obstet Gynecol* 2005; 26: 103.

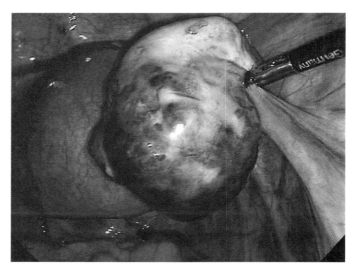

Fig. 18.6 Appearance of right ovarian ectopic pregnancy at laparoscopy. Reproduced with permission from Kraemer B, Kraemer E, Guengoer E, et al. Ovarian ectopic pregnancy: diagnosis, treatment, correlation to Carnegie stage 16 and review based on a clinical case. *Fertil Steril* 2009; 92(1): 392.e14.

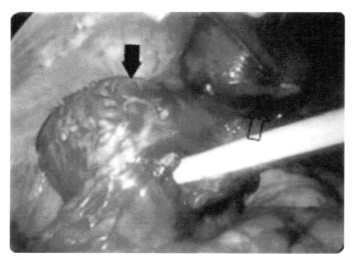

Fig. 18.5 Laparoscopic appearance of an ovarian pregnancy (arrow) after prior subtotal cesarean hysterectomy. Post-hysterectomy vaginal cuff. Reproduced with permission from Fylstra DL. Ectopics not within the (distal) fallopian tube: etiology, diagnosis, and treatment. *Am J Obstet Gynecol* 2012; 206: 296.

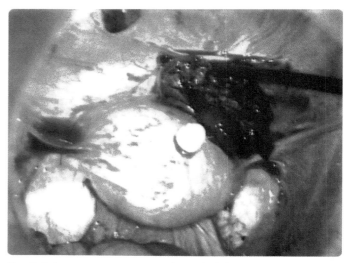

Fig. 18.7 Laparoscopic appearance of an early abdominal pregnancy implanted in the anterior cul-de-sac. Reproduced with permission from Fylstra DL. Ectopics not within the (distal) fallopian tube: etiology, diagnosis, and treatment. *Am J Obstet Gynecol* 2012; 206: 292.

pregnancy ranges from 50% to 90% [17]. In the late part of the first trimester, demonstration of a live fetus outside the uterus is highly suggestive of abdominal pregnancy, because the fallopian tube cannot contain a pregnancy as large as 12 weeks [18,19]. It is important to delineate the margin of the uterus carefully in order to demonstrate that the gestational sac lies outside the uterus [20] (Figs 18.8–18.10). Other important ultrasonographic features of abdominal pregnancy include: (a) oligohydramnios; (b) abnormal fetal lie, usually above the maternal pelvis; (c) extrauterine placental tissue; (d) close approximation of fetal parts to maternal abdominal wall; (e) lack of uterine wall between products of conception and maternal bladder; (f) maternal peritoneal fluid; and (g) fetal death [17].

Management of abdominal pregnancy

For abdominal pregnancies with concurrent intra-abdominal hemorrhage, laparotomy is often the preferred treatment because of delayed diagnosis and the risks of hemorrhage [15,21]. The recent advances in laparoscopic surgery have allowed for successful management of abdominal pregnancies by laparoscopy as well, but laparoscopic management is less successful when extensive intra-abdominal bleeding exists [15,21]. In fact, the rate of laparoscopic treatment for abdominal pregnancy has been reported to be as low as 55% [22]. If the patient is hemodynamically stable and the abdominal pregnancy is situated in an unusual site, such as a cesarean section

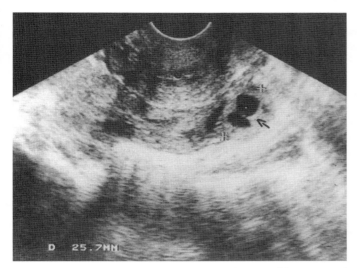

Fig. 18.8 Ultrasonogram showing the extrauterine location of the gestational sac (arrow); U, uterus. Reproduced with permission from Ginath S, Malinger G, Golan A, et al. Successful laparoscopic treatment of a ruptured primary abdominal pregnancy. *Fertil Steril* 2000; 74(3): 602.

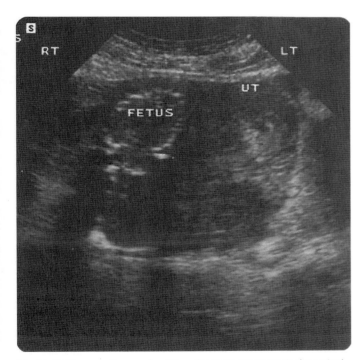

Fig. 18.9 Ultrasound image of an 18-week ectopic pregnancy in the sagittal view. The fetus is noted to be outside an empty uterus (UT). Reproduced with permission from Worley KC, Hnat MD, Cunningham FG. Advanced extrauterine pregnancy: diagnostic and therapeutic challenges. *Am J Obstet Gynecol* 2008; 198(3): 297.e5.

scar or uterovesical fold, laparoscopic management can offer faster recovery, less blood loss, and decreased chance of surgical morbidity [21].

A live fetus is born in 10–20% of advanced abdominal pregnancies. That said, neonatal mortality is very high because of pulmonary hypoplasia and oligohydramnios. Advanced

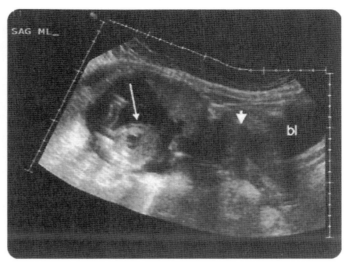

Fig. 18.10 Extended field-of-view ultrasound image of a 20-week rudimentary horn pregnancy. The live fetus (thin arrow) is outside the uterine cavity (thick arrow). The bladder (bl) is noted anterior to the uterus. Reproduced with permission from Worley KC, Hnat MD, Cunningham FG. Advanced extrauterine pregnancy: diagnostic and therapeutic challenges. *Am J Obstet Gynecol* 2008; 198(3): 297.e5.

abdominal pregnancy should be managed by prompt delivery of the fetus and removal of the placenta if it appears that the blood supply can be effectively controlled [16,21]. If the placenta cannot be removed, and there are large vessels involved, the cord should be ligated and the placenta left in situ [16,21]. Methotrexate treatment has been associated with several deaths and should not be considered for abdominal pregnancies [16,23].

Lithopedion

A lithopedion is a rare form of calcified and mummified abdominal pregnancy [24]. The term "lithopedion" is derived from the Greek *lithos*, meaning "stone," and *paedion*, meaning "child." Lithopedions can also result from a tubal pregnancy, an ovarian pregnancy, or a ruptured intrauterine pregnancy [24]. In the event an intra-abdominal fetus dies, four subsequent mechanisms are possible: skeletalization, adipocere formation, suppuration with abscess formation, or lithopedion formation by dehydration and calcification [24]. In order for lithopedion formation to occur, the following factors must be present: (a) the fetus survives at least 3 months to prevent absorption; (b) sterile membranes, fetus, and peritoneum are present; (c) an environment conducive for calcification exists; and (d) failure to detect, diagnose, or otherwise interfere with the pregnancy [24]. Estimating the gestational age of a lithopedion is difficult due to dehydration and shrinkage [24]. In some instances, individual bones can be used to estimate age along with a detailed history.

There are three types of lithopedion: (a) lithokelyphos; (b) lithokelyphopedion; and (c) lithotecnon [24]. A lithokelyphos has calcified membranes alone, forming a calcified shell around the fetus (which may be skeletonized), such that fetal soft parts

A B C

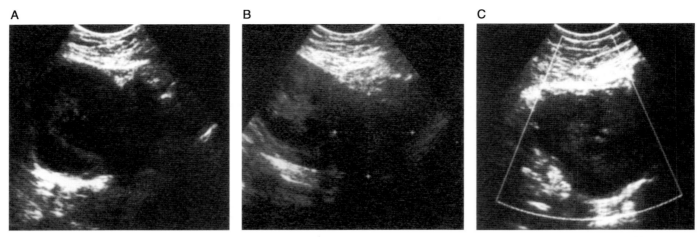

Fig. 18.11 (A–C) Ultrasound of a lithopedion. Reproduced with permission from Rizk B, Gorgy BA, West JD, et al. Calcified pelvic mass in a 75-year-old woman. *Acad Radiol* 1996; 1(1): 3–16.

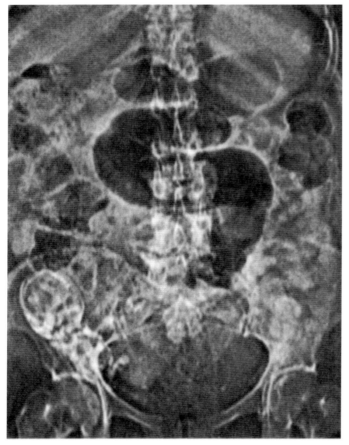

Fig. 18.12 X-ray of pelvis containing lithopedion. Reproduced with permission from Rizk B, Gorgy BA, West JD, et al. Calcified pelvic mass in a 75-year-old woman. *Acad Radiol* 1996; 1(1): 3–16.

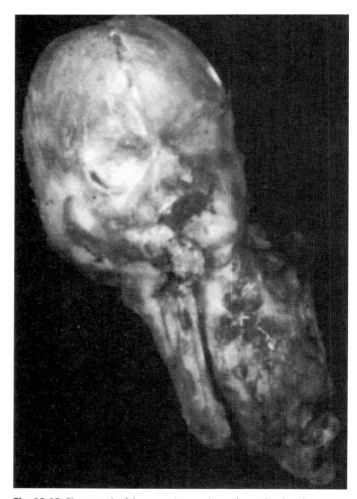

Fig. 18.13 Photograph of the operative specimen shows the shrunken, dehydrated fetus partially covered with fetal membrane, which can be compared easily to the radiographs. (Parts of the lower extremities were lost in the dissection). Reproduced with permission from Rizk B, Gorgy BA, West JD, et al. Calcified pelvic mass in a 75-year-old woman. *Acad Radiol* 1996; 1(1): 3–16.

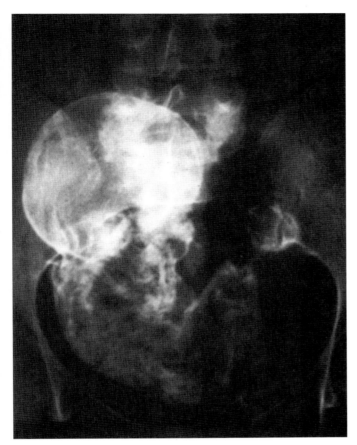

Fig. 18.14 X-ray of lithopedion's head. Reproduced with permission from Rizk B, Gorgy BA, West JD, et al., Calcified pelvic mass in a 75-year-old woman. *Acad Radiol* 1996; 1(1): 3–16.

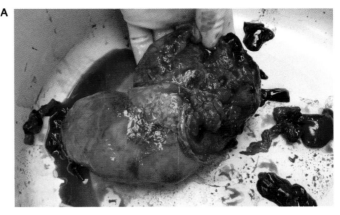

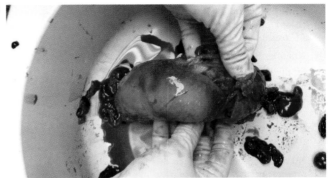

Fig. 18.15 (A and B) Abdominal pregnancy.

are not involved in the process of calcification. A lithokelyphopedion has calcification of both fetus and membranes. In a lithotecnon, only the fetus is calcified. Rizk et al. [24] reported a lithokelyphos type of lithopedion that had been present for almost 50 years after its occurrence in the patient (Figs 18.11–18.14). In that situation, the patient presented with signs of colon cancer and during X-ray and CT scan, a lithopedion was diagnosed, which was 6 months in size [24].

Diagnosing a lithopedion is difficult because of the unusual signs and symptoms. While ultrasonography can demonstrate an echogenic mass, it cannot differentiate such a formation from other calcified masses like ovarian tumors, myomas, or epiploic calcifications [25]. CT scans, however, can identify the position, content, and integration of a calcified mass [25].

Because of increased prenatal care and surveillance, lithopedions have become so rare that they are not commonly included in differential diagnosis considerations [24,26]. That said, it should be considered, particularly in patients from exotic locations [26,27]. Minor nonspecific complaints such as pain with change in position, defecation, or urination or other gastrointestinal or genitourinary disturbances have been cited [24]. Major complaints, while rare, include tissue necrosis,

organ perforation, primary infection, and peritonitis [24,27]. Some women have reported extrusion of fetal parts through every body orifice, as well as the abdominal wall [24].

Conclusion

Both ovarian and abdominal pregnancies are rare forms of ectopic pregnancies (Fig. 18.15A and B). Although ultrasonography can assist in the diagnosis of these pregnancies, it is challenging to diagnose these conditions preoperatively. These types of pregnancy are associated with high morbidity and adverse consequences. For ovarian pregnancies, usually oophorectomy or ovarian wedge resection is the preferred management treatment. For abdominal pregnancies, laparoscopy or laparotomy is the preferred management treatment (Fig. 18.15A and B). In neither ovarian nor abdominal pregnancies is medical treatment a first-line option. Lithopedions are an extremely rare form of abdominal pregnancy where the fetus dies and is calcified within the mother's body.

References

1. Ismail M. Ovarian pregnancy. *J Obstet Gynaecol Br Emp* 1950; **57**: 49–51.
2. Van Tussenbroek C. Un case de grossesse ovarienne. *Ann Gynecol* 1899; **52**: 537.
3. Spiegelberg O. Zur casuistic der ovaialschwangershaft. *Arch Gynaekol* 1878; **13**: 73.

4. Boronow R, McElin TW, West RH, et al. Ovarian pregnancy: report of four cases and a thirteen-year survey of the English literature. *Obstet Gynecol* 1965; **143**: 55–60.

5. Grimes HG, Nosal RA, Gallagher JC. Ovarian pregnancy: a series of 24 cases. *Obstet Gynecol* 1983; **61**: 174–180.

6. Carter JE, Jacobsen A. Reimplantation of a human embryo with subsequent ovarian pregnancy. *Am J Obstet Gynecol* 1986; **155**: 282–283.

7. Koo Y, Choi H, Im K, et al. Pregnancy outcomes after surgical treatment of ovarian pregnancy. *Int'l J Gynecol Obstet* 2011; **114**(2): 97–100.

8. Brown DL, Doubilet PM. Transvaginal sonography for diagnosing ectopic pregnancy: positivity criteria and performance characteristics. *J Ultrasound Med* 1994; **13**: 259–266.

9. Kurjak A, Zalud I, Schulman H. Ectopic pregnancy: transvaginal color Doppler of trophoblastic flow in questionable adnexa. *J Ultrasound Med* 1991; **10**: 685–689.

10. Kraemer B, Kraemer E, Guengoer E, et al. Ovarian ectopic pregnancy: diagnosis, treatment, correlation to Carnegie stage 16 and review based on a clinical case. *Fertil Steril* 2009; **92**(1): 392. e13–392.e15.

11. Rizk B, Lachelin CL, Davies MC, et al. Ovarian pregnancy following in-vitro fertilization and embryo transfer. *Hum Reprod* 1990; **5**: 763–764.

12. Alkatout I, Stuhlmann-Laeisz C, Mettler L, et al. Organ-preserving management of ovarian pregnancies by laparoscopic approach. *Fertil Steril* 2011; **95**(8): 2467–2470.e2.

13. Practice Committee of the American Society for Reproductive Medicine. Medical treatment of ectopic pregnancy. *Fertil Steril* 2006; **86**(5 Suppl 1): S96–S102.

14. Cotler AM. Extrauterine pregnancy: a historical review. *Current Surg* 2000; **57**(5): 484–492.

15. Ginath S, Malinger G, Golan A, et al. Successful laparoscopic treatment of a ruptured primary abdominal pregnancy. *Fertil Steril* 2000; **74**(3): 601–602.

16. Ory SJ. Surgery for ectopic pregnancy. In: Gershenson DM, DeCherney AH, Curry SL, and Brubaker L (Eds.) *Operative Gynecology*. Philadelphia: W. B. Saunders Company; 2001: 655–666.

17. Brandt AL, Tolson D. Missed abdominal ectopic pregnancy. *J Emerg Med* 2006; **30**(2): 171–174.

18. Little KJ, Green MM. Abdominal gestation. *J Emerg Med* 1995; **13**(2): 195–198.

19. Zaki ZMS. An unusual presentation of ectopic pregnancy. *Ultrasound Obstet Gynecol* 1998; **11**: 456–458.

20. Dover RW, Powell MC. Management of a primary abdominal pregnancy. *Am J Obstet Gynecol* 1995; **172**(5): 1603–1604.

21. Young RS, Huang M, Chen C. Successful laparoscopic management of primary abdominal pregnancy in the cul-de-sac. *Taiwanese J Obstet Gynecol* 2005; **44**(2): 172–174.

22. Gorry A, Morelli M, Olowu O, et al. Laparoscopic management of abdominal ectopic pregnancy using FLOSEAL Hemostatic Matrix. *Int J Gynecol Obstet* 2012; **117**(1): 83–84.

23. Worley KC, Hnat MD, Cunningham FG. Advanced extrauterine pregnancy: diagnostic and therapeutic challenges. *Am J Obstet Gynecol* 2008; **198**(3): 297.e1–297.e7.

24. Rizk B, Gorgy BA, West JD, et al. Calcified pelvic mass in a 75-year-old woman. *Acad Radiol* 1996; **1**(1): 3–16.

25. Sun J, Pan Z, Xie X, Li B. Intrauterine and extrauterine lithopedion following cesarean scar rupture. *Int J Gynecol Obstet* 2010; **109**(3): 249–250.

26. Burger NZ, Hung YE, Kalof AN, Casson PR. Lithopedion: laparoscopic diagnosis and removal. *Fertil Steril* 2007; **87**(5): 1208–1209.

27. Acharya S, Barnick C. Retained pregnancy for five years in a rudimentary uterine horn. *Acta Obstet Gynecol Scand* 2003; **82**: 387–388.

Chapter

19

Ultrasound diagnosis of heterotopic ectopic pregnancies

Botros R. M. B. Rizk, Rizwan Malik, Candice P. Holliday and Mostafa I. Abuzeid

Introduction

A heterotopic pregnancy occurs when an intrauterine and ectopic pregnancy simultaneously exist. Although more than 90% of ectopic pregnancies occur in the fallopian tubes, implantation also occurs in the abdomen, cervix, ovary, or previous cesarean scar [1]. Dimitry, Rizk, Marcus, and colleagues were at the forefront of alerting other clinicians to the increased danger of heterotopic pregnancies with the increased use of in vitro fertilization (IVF) [1]. The incidence of heterotopic pregnancy in spontaneously conceived pregnancies is rare and ranges from 1 in 2600 to 1 in 30 000 [1–7]. The risks of a heterotopic pregnancy have significantly increased with the advent of assisted reproductive technology (ART), including IVF, gamete intrafallopian transfer (GIFT), and ovulation induction [1,8–10]. In fact, heterotopic pregnancies happen in 0.75–2.9% of ART pregnancies [8–10]. For IVF specifically, heterotopic pregnancies constitute 15–16% of all ectopic pregnancies resulting from the procedure [10]. Thus, patients receiving two or more embryos in an ART cycle should have a heterotopic pregnancy specifically ruled out [4]. Because the diagnosis of a heterotopic pregnancy is difficult, the rise in the incidence of heterotopic pregnancies is very concerning.

Etiology

Although damage to the fallopian tubes is the main factor in the etiology of heterotopic pregnancy after IVF, other factors exist [1]. One clinician reported that 60% of his patients with heterotopic pregnancy had tubal damage, while another reported 100% [1]. Chronic pelvic infection, appendectomy, tubal surgery, previous ectopic pregnancy, sterilization, and reversal of sterilization are among the causes of tubal damage that lead to ectopic pregnancies (Figs 19.1–19.10). It is ironic given that IVF is used to assist patients with tubal disease to conceive, yet also increases the risk of ectopic pregnancies. In fact, the very first reported IVF and embryo transfer (IVF-ET) resulted in an ectopic pregnancy [1]. Other possible risk factors for heterotopic pregnancy are ovarian stimulation, the dorsal position of the patient with head tilted downward at the time

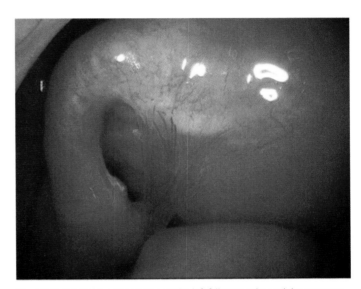

Fig. 19.1 Pelvic adhesions between the left fallopian tube and the uterus at laparoscopy.

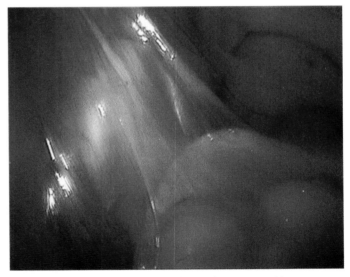

Fig. 19.2 Pelvic adhesions as a result of appendicitis managed by appendectomy.

Ultrasonography in Gynecology, ed. Botros R. M. B. Rizk and Elizabeth E. Puscheck. Published by Cambridge University Press. © Cambridge University Press 2015.

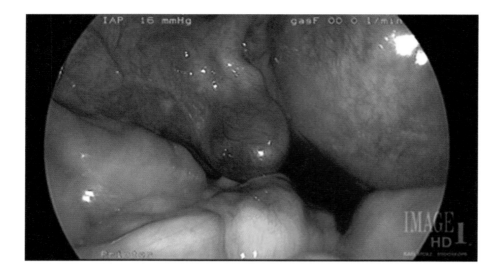

Fig. 19.3 Left ectopic pregnancy and hemoperitoneum. Courtesy of John LaFleur.

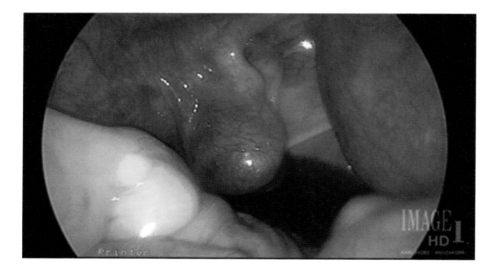

Fig. 19.4 Left ectopic pregnancy and hemoperitoneum. Courtesy of John LaFleur.

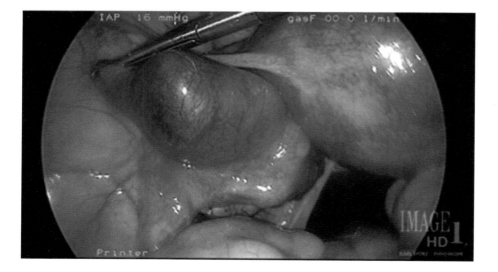

Fig. 19.5 Left ectopic pregnancy and hemoperitoneum. Courtesy of John LaFleur.

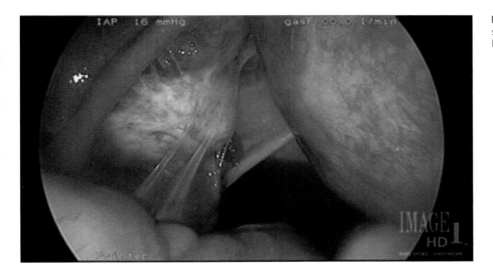

Fig. 19.6 Adhesions between left ovary and pelvic sidewall and hemoperitoneum. Courtesy of John LaFleur.

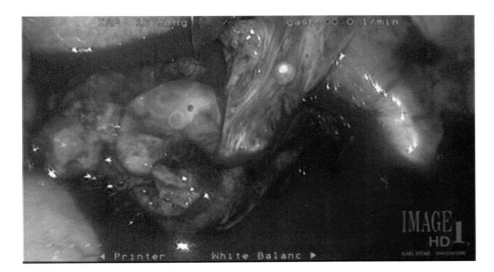

Fig. 19.7 Ruptured ectopic pregnancy with placental tissue and fetus in the cul-de-sac, soaked in hemoperitoneum. Courtesy of John LaFleur.

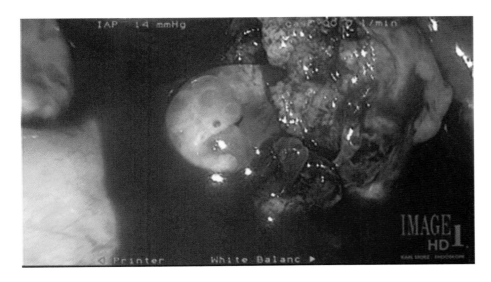

Fig. 19.8 Ruptured ectopic pregnancy with placental tissue and fetus in the cul-de-sac, soaked in hemoperitoneum. Courtesy of John LaFleur.

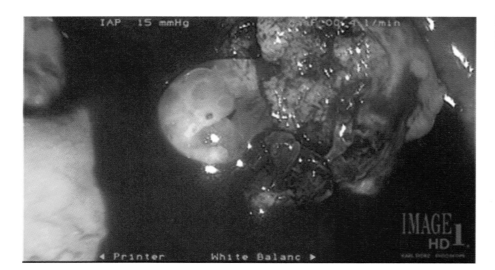

Fig. 19.9 Ruptured ectopic pregnancy with placental tissue and fetus in the cul-de-sac, soaked in hemoperitoneum. Courtesy of John LaFleur.

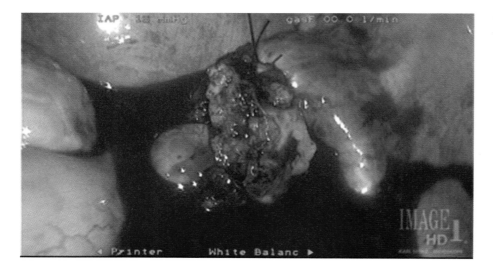

Fig. 19.10 Partial salpingectomy. Courtesy of John LaFleur.

of ET, and high numbers of transferred embryos (although heterotopic pregnancies have resulted from the transfer of two embryos) [1]. Moreover, the actual ET technique itself possibly may result in heterotopic pregnancy [1].

Diagnosis

Patients with a heterotopic pregnancy have varied clinical presentations [1]. Thirty percent of patients are asymptomatic, while 25% have abdominal pain and 30% have both abdominal pain and vaginal bleeding [1] (Table 19.1). In one case where clomiphene citrate (Clomid) was given to a patient, a heterotopic right ectopic pregnancy with in utero dizygotic twins resulted [11]. The patient presented at 19 weeks with right pelvic pain that was severe enough that it was evaluated extensively. However, the pain subsided before she could undergo surgery and she remained clinically stable. At 36 weeks, she elected to have a cesarean section and a right adnexal process was found to be a chronic ectopic pregnancy. On ultrasound,

the sonograms demonstrated two right adnexal fluid locules with complex fluid. In another case, the patient presented at 7.5 weeks with dizziness, abdominal and shoulder pain, but no vaginal bleeding after undergoing ART [11]. Upon ultrasound of the right upper quadrant, a very large amount of free fluid (later found to be hemoperitoneum) was observed. Upon transverse transabdominal ultrasound of the pelvis, a live intrauterine pregnancy was observed along with a second smaller ectopic pregnancy in the right juxtacorneal area. Following surgery, the ectopic pregnancy was found to be ruptured and actively bleeding, and was successfully resected with conservation of the intrauterine pregnancy.

The diagnosis of a heterotopic pregnancy is usually delayed because of the presence of an intrauterine pregnancy, which could be hazardous. For patients with an intrauterine pregnancy who are otherwise asymptomatic, a heterotopic pregnancy should be suspected if their hCG levels are higher than singleton levels [8,12]. At that point, a patient with higher than

Table 19.1. Clinical presentation and ultrasonographic diagnosis of 17 heterotopic pregnancies after IVF

Patient no.	Clinical presentation	Examination type	Ultrasonographic findings			Duration of pregnancy at diagnosis (weeks)	
			Gestational sac in utero	Fetal heart in utero	Ectopic pregnancy	IUP	Ectopic
1	Abdominal pain	Abdominal	1	1	1	6	8
2	Abdominal pain	Abdominal	3	2	0	6	No
3	Abdominal pain	Abdominal	1	0	0	5	No
4	Abdominal pain	Abdominal	1	0	1	6	6
5	Abdominal pain	Abdominal	1	0	0	5	No
6	Abdominal pain	Abdominal	1	0	1	7	7
7	Abdominal pain and bleeding	Abdominal	2	1	1	7	7
8	Abdominal pain and bleeding	Abdominal	1	0	0	7	No
9	Abdominal pain and bleeding	Abdominal	1	0	1	8	8
10	Acute abdominal pain	Abdominal	1	0	0	5	No
11	Acute abdominal pain	Abdominal	2	2	0	8	No
12	Acute abdominal pain	Abdominal	1	1	0	6	No
13	Asymptomatic	Abdominal + vaginal	1	1	1	7	7
14	Asymptomatic	Abdominal + vaginal	2	2	1	7	7
15	Asymptomatic	Abdominal + vaginal	1	1	1	7	7
16	Asymptomatic	Abdominal + vaginal	1	1	1		7
17	Asymptomatic	Abdominal + vaginal	1	1	1	7	7

Reproduced with permission from Marcus SF, Dimitry ES, et al. In: Rizk B (Ed.) *Ultrasonography in Reproductive Medicine and Infertility*. Cambridge University Press; 2010: Chapter 32, 272.

usual levels of hCG should have repeat ultrasounds to rule out a heterotopic pregnancy [3]. Moreover, even if ectopic pregnancy symptoms exist, these symptoms may be initially misattributed to intrauterine pregnancy complications, such as miscarriage [1]. For women who are symptomatic, the differential diagnosis includes acute appendicitis, ruptured corpus luteum cyst or ovarian follicle, spontaneous abortion, threatened miscarriage, ovarian torsion, urinary tract disease, and degenerating fibroids [1].

Because the diagnosis of a heterotopic pregnancy is often delayed, whether due to misdiagnosis or patients otherwise without symptoms, there is an elevated rate of rupture at presentation [13]. Thus, a high index of suspicion is essential for diagnosing heterotopic pregnancies [9,14]. Unfortunately, for patients with delayed diagnosis and treatment, their heterotopic pregnancy can be life-threatening.

Ultrasonography

High-resolution ultrasonography has increased the rate of early diagnosis. Transvaginal ultrasonography has greater resolution and thus is better than transabdominal ultrasonography in early

pregnancies (Figs 19.11 and 19.12). Ultrasonographic findings for heterotopic pregnancies are presented in Table 19.1. The findings include live extrauterine pregnancy, complex adnexal mass, free fluid in the pelvis, and extrauterine gestational sac with or without a fetal pole [1]. It is imperative that careful examination of adnexa occurs on ultrasound [3,15]. When free fluid in the abdomen and the pouch of Douglas is present, it may be incorrectly identified as ascites related to ovarian hyperstimulation syndrome. Transvaginal ultrasound's diagnostic sensitivity and specificity may be improved with color Doppler ultrasonography, particularly when the presence of a gestational sac is uncertain or the gestational sac is absent [1].

Management

Heterotopic pregnancies are difficult to manage. Treatment of heterotopic pregnancies must be individualized because it depends on several factors: location of the ectopic pregnancy, a previous ectopic pregnancy in the same tube, the condition of the contralateral tube, the general condition of the patient, and the status of the pelvis [1]. Methotrexate is contraindicated for managing heterotopic pregnancies because of the simultaneous

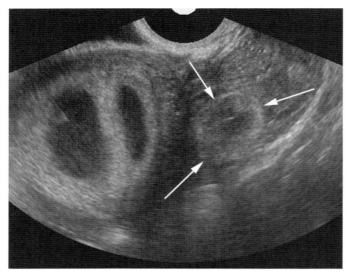

Fig. 19.11 Heterotopic pregnancy with twin intrauterine pregnancy and a concomitant ectopic pregnancy as demonstrated by arrows. Reproduced with permission from Eyvazzadeh A and Levine D. In: Rizk B (Ed.) *Ultrasonography in Reproductive Medicine and Infertility*. Cambridge University Press, 2010; Chapter 32, 273.

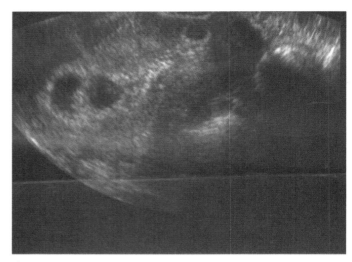

Fig. 19.12 Heterotopic twin pregnancy. Transvaginal ultrasonography showing twin intrauterine pregnancy and ectopic pregnancy (courtesy M. I. Abuzeid). Reproduced with permission from Marcus SF, Dimitry ES, et al. In: Rizk B (Ed.) *Ultrasonography in Reproductive Medicine and Infertility*. Cambridge University Press, 2010; Chapter 32, 273.

viable intrauterine pregnancy [3]. The goal of all treatments is to protect the simultaneous intrauterine pregnancy so conservative management is needed if possible.

Ultrasound-guided management

Ultrasound-guided management is more popular these days because it can be undertaken safely on an outpatient basis. This removes the morbidity related to surgical risks. Patients who are hemodynamically stable with unruptured heterotopic pregnancies are most suitable for ultrasound-guided management. Heterotopic pregnancies are treated by ultrasound-guided aspiration of the gestational sac and potassium chloride injection into the fetal heart with transvaginal ultrasonography [10,16]. Instead of potassium chloride, hyperosmolar glucose or a hypertonic sodium chloride solution can be used [1]. In one study, 55% patients with a heterotopic pregnancy undergoing potassium chloride injection needed a salpingectomy [17]. In the case of a heterotopic cervical pregnancy, suction curettage of the cervical pregnancy was undertaken under abdominal ultrasound guidance [18]. Physicians placed and tightly tied a high cervical cerclage in order to avoid potentially significant cervical bleeding from the cervical pregnancy site [18].

Expectant management

There are some reports of expectant management of patients with a heterotopic pregnancy who were hemodynamically stable [10]. Physicians should be careful in not only selecting patients to be managed expectantly, but also in follow-up and patient education. These patients must be conscious of the risks (tubal rupture, hemorrhage, and subsequent loss of the intrauterine pregnancy) inherent in expectant management.

Selection criteria for expectant management have not been reported. Specifically, β-hCG levels are inapplicable criteria for heterotopic pregnancies [1].

Surgical management

For most patients with a heterotopic pregnancy, laparoscopy is the treatment of choice, specifically laparoscopic salpingectomy [1,3]. Salpingectomy circumvents any issues with subsequent serum hCG levels, which can be affected by persistent trophoblastic tissue after salpingostomy [3]. Physicians should be careful using electrocoagulation during salpingectomy because of the risk of compromising the blood supply to the concomitant intrauterine pregnancy [3]. Laparoscopy allows the physician not only to diagnose the heterotopic pregnancy, but also to assess the pelvis, the presence of hemoperitoneum, and the presence of other conditions, such as ovarian cysts and ovarian torsion [1]. Moreover, the use of laparoscopy is associated with notably decreased blood loss, need for analgesia, economic cost, hospital time, and recovery time.

For the most part, laparotomy during the first trimester is not used because it risks the intrauterine pregnancy. However, for patients with cornual ectopic pregnancies or patients who are not hemodynamically stable, laparotomy may be used [1]. Laparotomy is also used when the physician is more comfortable with laparotomy than laparoscopy or when the patient is not a good candidate for laparoscopy [1].

Salpingostomy in patients with heterotopic tubal pregnancy is not recommended because it involves the risk of a persistent active trophoblast, which serial serum hCG measurements cannot be used to detect. Surgery when the ectopic pregnancy is situated on the cervix, ovary, or interstitial or cornual segment of the fallopian tube has an increased risk of hemorrhage [1]. For patients with a heterotopic pregnancy located on a cesarean scar, surgical management is by wedge resection via laparotomy, laparoscopy, or hysterectomy [1].

Conclusion

Heterotopic ectopic pregnancies are a major health issue. Around 50–66% of patients with a heterotopic pregnancy miscarry the simultaneous intrauterine pregnancy [10,13,19]. Interestingly, when comparing patients with a spontaneously conceived heterotopic pregnancy to those with an ART-conceived heterotopic pregnancy, Han et al. reported that the spontaneous patients had a lower live birth rate than the ART group (20% vs. 47.8%) [20]. Regardless, the incidence of heterotopic pregnancies is markedly higher in ART patients than in patients who spontaneously conceive. Heterotopic pregnancies are not easy to diagnose before clinical symptoms occur. Clinical suspicion and ultrasonography are the best tools a physician can employ to diagnose a heterotopic pregnancy.

References

1. Marcus SF, Dimitry ES, Dimitry M, et al. Heterotopic pregnancy and assisted reproduction. In Rizk B (Ed.) *Ultrasonography in Reproductive Medicine and Infertility*. Cambridge University Press; 2010: 271–275.

2. Serour GI. Complications of assisted reproductive technology. In: Rizk B, Garcia-Velasco J, Sallam H, Makrigiannakis (Eds.) *Infertility and Assisted Reproduction*. Cambridge University Press; 2008: 604–618.

3. Hubayter ZR, Muasher SJ. Ectopic and heterotopic pregnancies following in vitro fertilization. In: Rizk B, Garcia-Velasco J, Sallam H, Makrigiannakis (Eds.) *Infertility and Assisted Reproduction*. Cambridge University Press; 2008: 619–628.

4. Serour GI. Early and late pregnancy and psychological complications after assisted reproductive technology. In: Jauniaux ERM, Rizk B (Eds.) *Pregnancy after Assisted Reproductive Technology*. Cambridge University Press; 2012: 72–81.

5. Dicken D, Goldman G, Feldberg D, Ashkenazi J, Goldman JA. Heterotopic pregnancy after IVF-ET: report of a case and a review of the literature. *Hum Reprod* 1989; **4**: 335–336.

6. De Vroe RW, Pratt JH. Simultaneous intrauterine and extrauterine pregnancy. *Am J Obstet Gynecol* 1948; **56**: 1119–1123.

7. Seeber BE, Barnhart KT. Suspected ectopic pregnancy. *Obstet Gynecol* 2006; **107**: 399–413.

8. Dimitry ES, Subak-Sharpe R, Mills M, et al. Nine cases of heterotopic pregnancies in 4 years of in-vitro fertilization. *Fertil Steril* 1990; **53**: 107–110.

9. Rizk B, Tan SL, Morcos S, et al. Heterotopic pregnancies following in-vitro fertilization and embryo transfer. *Am J Obstet Gynecol* 1991; **164**(1): 161–164.

10. Marcus SF, Macnamee M, Brinsden P. Heterotopic pregnancies after in vitro fertilization and embryo transfer. *Hum Reprod* 1995; **10**(5): 1232–1236.

11. Finberg HJ. Ultrasound evaluation in multiple gestation. In: Callen PW (Ed.) *Ultrasonography in Obstetrics and Gynecology*. Philadelphia: W.B. Saunders Company; 1994: 124–125.

12. Dimitry ES, Soussis IS, Mastrominas M, Packham D, Margara R, Winston RML. Early diagnosis of asymptomatic heterotopic pregnancy after in vitro fertilization (IVF). *Assist Reprod Technol Androl J* 1991; (Suppl): 81–83.

13. BenNagi J, Helmy S, Ofili-Yebovi D, Yazbek J, Sawyer E, Jurkovic D. Reproductive outcome of women with a previous history of Caesarean scar ectopic pregnancies. *Hum Reprod* 2007; **22**(7): 2012–2015.

14. Rizk B, Dimitry ES, Marcus SF. A multi-centre study on combined intrauterine and extrauterine gestations after IVF. *Proceedings of the European Society of Human Reproduction and Embryology*, Milan, Italy, 1990; Abstract 43.

15. Rizk B, Marcus S, Fountain S, et al. The value of transvaginal sonography and hCG in the diagnosis of heterotopic pregnancy. 9th Annual meeting of the ESHRE, Thessaloniki, June. *Hum Reprod* 1993; Abstract No. 102.

16. Clayton HB, Schieve LA, Peterson HB, Jamieson DJ, Reynolds MA, Wright VC. A comparison of heterotopic and intrauterine-only pregnancy outcomes after assisted reproductive technologies in the United States from 1999 to 2002. *Fertil Steril* 2007; **87**(2): 303–309.

17. Goldstein JS, Ratts VS, Philpott T, Dahan MH. Risk of surgery after use of potassium chloride for treatment of tubal heterotopic pregnancy. *J Obstet Gynecol* 2006; **107**(2): 506–508.

18. Faschingbauer F, Mueller A, Voigt F, Beckmann MW, Goecke TW. Treatment of heterotopic cervical pregnancies. *Fertil Steril* 2011; **95**: 1787.e9–e13.

19. Tal J, Haddad S, Gordon N, Timor-Tritsch I. Heterotopic pregnancy after ovulation induction and assisted reproductive technologies: a literature review from 1971 to 1993. *Fertil Steril* 1996; **66**(1): 1–12.

20. Han SH, Jee BC, Suh CS, et al. Clinical outcomes of tubal heterotopic pregnancy: assisted vs. spontaneous conceptions. *Gynecol Obstet Invest* 2007; **64**(1): 49–54.

Ultrasound imaging in gestational trophoblastic neoplasia

Asim Kurjak and Kazuo Maeda

Introduction

Trophoblastic neoplasia is unique, i.e. it originates from fetal trophoblasts, and is classified into complete, partial, and invasive hydatidiform mole, choriocarcinoma, placental site trophoblastic tumor (PSTT), and epithelioid trophoblastic tumor (ETT). It is also divided into gestational and non-gestational. Gestational choriocarcinoma preceded by complete mole is the most significant, with systemic hematogenous metastases and fatal outcome unless treated with effective chemotherapy. Next most important are invasive mole, complete mole, and PSTT. Urinary hCG and serum β-hCG are clinical markers of trophoblastic neoplasia in their follow-up and chemotherapy. Choriocarcinoma was frequent in East Asia in the past, but is now infrequent following the introduction of effective chemotherapy. Medical ultrasound is indispensable for diagnosing trophoblastic neoplasia.

Classification, development, and pathology

Trophoblastic neoplasia is divided into hydatidiform mole, choriocarcinoma, and placental site trophoblastic tumor according to pathologic findings (Table 20.1) [1], because of well-defined differences in outcome between pathologically classified invasive hydatidiform mole and choriocarcinoma. There is also the clinical NCI (National Cancer Institute)/NIH (National Institutes of Health) classification and the FIGO (Federation Internationale Gynecologie et Obstetrique) staging.

Complete hydatidiform mole

Complete hydatidiform mole is an abnormal pregnancy where placental villi change into molar vesicles; there is no embryo, fetus, or umbilical cord (Figs 20.1–20.3). Amnion is, however, found in some cases [2]. No vessel is found in molar vesicles covered by trophoblasts. With an intravascular mole the vesicles spread into blood vessels. Metastasis rarely appears in distant organs. The chromosome is usually diploid 46,XX where the XX are both of male origin (androgenesis) and the mechanism is two X sperms fertilized in a vacant ovum without a nucleus [3]. The chromosome is rarely 46,XY, where X and

Table 20.1 Classification of trophoblastic neoplasia

1. Hydatidiform mole
Complete hydatidiform mole
Partial hydatidiform mole
Invasive hydatidiform mole
2. Choriocarcinoma
3. Persistent trophoblastic disease
4. Placental site trophoblastic tumor (PSTT) and epithelioid trophoblastic tumor (ETT)

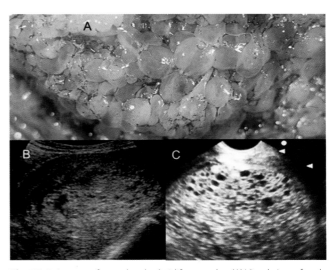

Fig. 20.1 Images of complete hydatidiform moles. (A) Visual view of molar vesicles. (B) B-mode image of complete hydatidiform mole at 11 weeks of pregnancy. Courtesy of Dr. M. Utsu. (C) B-mode image of established complete hydatidiform mole. Courtesy of Professor S. Kupesic.

Y are of male origin [4]. Complete mole can also develop in one of twins or triplets. Ovarian theca lutein cysts are frequent in developed complete and invasive moles, while their incidence is low in the first trimester. Since the lutein cyst is not a trophoblastic neoplasia and disappears after remission, surgical removal is not appropriate. Color and pulsed Doppler have

Ultrasonography in Gynecology, ed. Botros R. M. B. Rizk and Elizabeth E. Puscheck. Published by Cambridge University Press. © Cambridge University Press 2015.

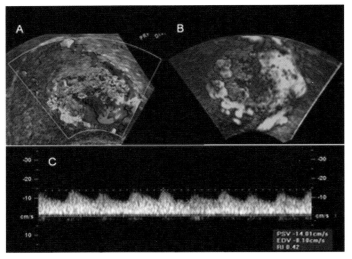

Fig. 20.2 Blood flow images of complete hydatidiform mole. Courtesy of Dr. G. Varga. (A) 2D color Doppler uterine blood flow in complete hydatidiform mole. (B) Molar vesicles are recognized by 2D power Doppler uterine blood flow in complete hydatidiform mole. (C) Pulsed Doppler flow wave in complete hydatidiform mole. Intervesicular maternal blood flow RI = 0.42.

been used to differentiate between normal and abnormal signs in early pregnancy [5,6]. Also the gene expression patterns of normal trophoblast and the choriocarcinoma cell line have been differentiated [7].

Partial hydatidiform mole

In a partial hydatidiform mole there is partial change of placental villi into molar vesicles, associated with embryo, fetus, or fetal parts (Fig. 20.4). Fetal anomalies are common. Chromosomes are usually triplets, 69,XXX, 69,XXY, or 69,XYY [8]. DNA analysis confirmed the androgenetic mechanism [9]. Capillary vessels are found in the interstitium of molar vesicles.

Invasive hydatidiform mole

Invasive hydatidiform mole involves the invasion of molar vesicles into the myometrium with destruction and hemorrhage. The lesion is found in either total or partial moles, usually after molar evacuation, although the invasion may develop before the termination. The change is visually noted in surgical specimens (Fig. 20.5) and microscopically confirmed, where the

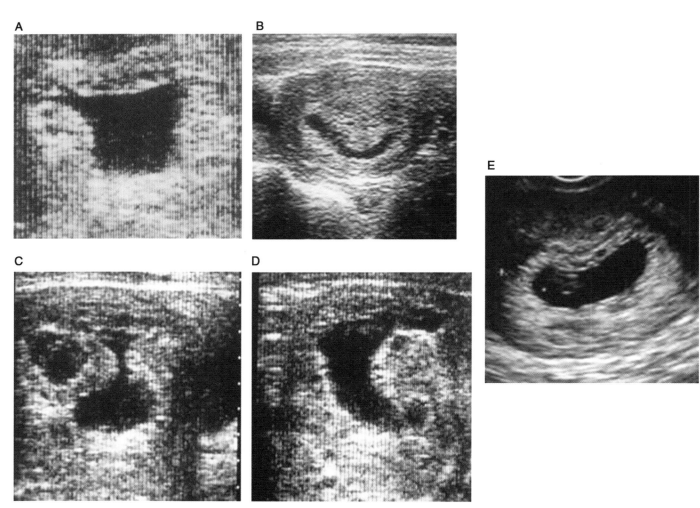

Fig. 20.3 2D images of complete hydatidiform moles in early pregnancy.

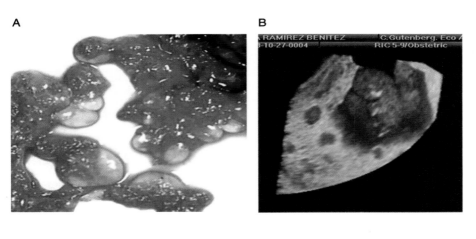

Fig. 20.4 Partial hydatidiform moles. (A) Partial hydatidiform mole developed in the placenta. (B) 3D ultrasound image of partial mole in early pregnancy. Courtesy of Dr. J. R. Benitez.

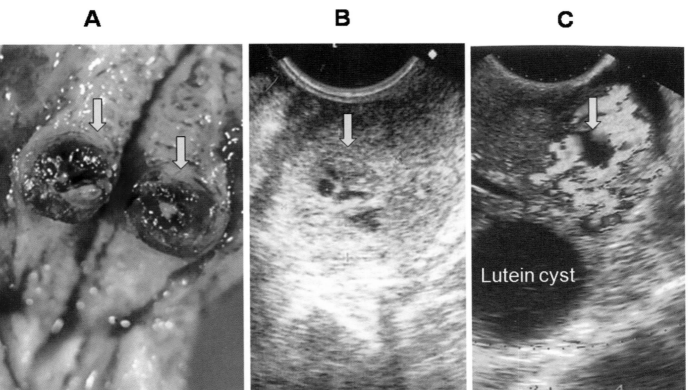

Fig. 20.5 Invasive hydatidiform moles (arrows). (A) Invasive moles developed in the myometrium. (B) B-mode image of villous pattern in the invasive mole. (C) Color Doppler image of blood flow around the villous pattern of an invasive mole.

trophoblasts proliferate, and hemorrhage and necrosis occur in the myometrium. An invasive mole rarely metastasizes and has low malignancy. The outcome is more favorable than for choriocarcinoma.

Choriocarcinoma

Choriocarcinoma is a solid trophoblastic tumor that develops primarily in the myometrium (Fig. 20.6), or in distant organs and tissues, usually after the removal of a complete or partial hydatidiform mole, and also infrequently after abortion or normal delivery. It is defined as gestational choriocarcinoma or trophoblastic neoplasia (Fig. 20.6). Non-gestational choriocarcinoma develops from germ cells or other cancer cells. Primary choriocarcinomas are also reported in both reproductive and non-reproductive organs, e.g. uterine cervix [10,11], lung, stomach, and pancreas [12].

Choriocarcinoma is composed of syncytio- and cyto-trophoblasts, and shows no villous pattern at all. Since the villous pattern is a characteristic sign of an invasive mole, and its outcome is less ominous than for choriocarcinoma, microscopic studies should be detailed on the whole specimen if the uterus is removed.

A

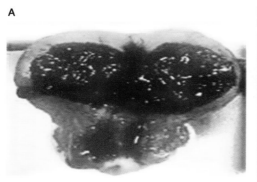

B

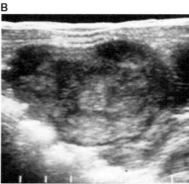

C

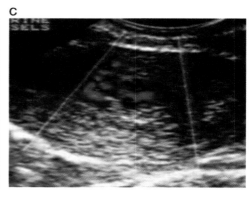

Fig. 20.6 Choriocarcinoma. (A) Choriocarcinoma in a uterus surgically removed before 1960. (B) B-mode image of choriocarcinoma. Courtesy of Dr. M. Terahara. (C) Color Doppler image of choriocarcinoma. Courtesy of Dr. S. Kondo.

Widespread distant metastases of choriocarcinoma were common before the introduction of effective chemotherapy. The interval between diagnosis and metastases was about six to 12 months. Early metastases were dark red tumors on the external genitalia and vaginal wall. Subsequent frequent spread was to the lung, where typical foci showed round shapes of various sizes, while a diffuse pulmonary shadow was found in multiple trophoblastic emboli in pulmonary arteries. Organs and/or tissues were affected after pulmonary metastasis, e.g. skin [13], subcutaneous tissue, intestine, liver, spleen, kidney, heart [14], and finally brain. Tumor cells were found also in blood vessels. Every organ was damaged by the trophoblasts and hemorrhage. Patients died from brain and multiple organ metastases due to damage and dysfunction occurring before effective chemotherapy. Choriocarcinoma is subdivided into three subtypes; gestational choriocarcinoma, non-gestational choriocarcinoma, and unclassified choriocarcinoma.

Gestational choriocarcinoma is related to pregnancy, and three categories are further classified:

(1) Uterine choriocarcinoma is the most common; it develops in the uterus after a hydatidiform mole, and rarely after abortion or normal delivery. Choriocarcinoma with an intact pregnancy has been reported [15].

(2) Extrauterine choriocarcinoma develops primarily at the site of ectopic pregnancy, where there is no tumor in the uterus.

(3) Intraplacental choriocarcinoma is found in the placenta mainly after delivery. These cases were reported to be associated with viable pregnancy [16].

Placental site trophoblastic tumor

Placental site trophoblastic tumor (PSTT) is a rare uterine tumor of proliferated intermediate trophoblasts [17]. It shows infiltrating growth penetrating between muscle fibers, while epithelioid trophoblastic tumor (ETT), another rare intermediate trophoblastic growth, has solitary nodules with a sharp tumor border growing in an expansive fashion [18].

The transvaginal sonography and color and pulsed Doppler are valuable in the diagnosis of PSTT [19,20].

The final diagnosis is made by histological study. There may have been gestational events in the past, e.g. mole, abortion, or delivery. PSTT produces less β-hCG and is less sensitive to chemotherapy than choriocarcinoma. More than half of patients present with disease confined to the uterus, and the remainder present with disease extension beyond the uterus. The outcome for patients with disease confined to the uterus is usually excellent, while most patients with extension beyond the uterus experience progression of disease and die despite surgery and intensive chemotherapy. Immunochemical and DNA analysis has been reported in metastasizing PSTT [21]. Adverse factors include interval from gestational events of more than 2 years, age older than 40 years, and mitotic count higher than 5 mitoses/10 HPF [22]. In another report on PSTT, statistically significant adverse survival factors were age over 35 years, interval since the last pregnancy of over 2 years, deep myometrial invasion, maximum hCG level >1000 mIU/mL, extensive coagulative necrosis, high mitotic rate, and the presence of cells with clear cytoplasm [23]. Simple hysterectomy is the mainstay of treatment, and multiagent chemotherapy with etoposide, methotrexate, actinomycin D, cyclophosphamide, and vinblastine appears to be the most effective [24].

Epithelioid trophoblastic tumor

Epithelioid trophoblastic tumor (ETT) appearing in the uterus is a discrete, hemorrhagic, solid and cystic lesion. Microscopically it is composed of intermediate trophoblastic cells forming nests and solid masses; typically islands of trophoblastic cells are surrounded by necrotic masses; mean mitosis is 2/10 HPF; and it is immunohistochemically positive for inhibin-alpha, cytokeratin, human placental lactogen (hPL), placental alkaline phosphatase, and Mel-CAM(CD-148) [18,25,26]. Its monomorphic growth pattern is closer to PSTT than to choriocarcinoma; ETT grows in a nodular fashion compared with the infiltrative pattern of PSTT; it appears to be less aggressive than choriocarcinoma, more closely resembling the behavior of PSTT where histological and immunohistochemical features are characteristic of ETT, although one report [25] included ETT in the category of PSTT. Two out of 14 ETT presented with extrauterine lesions. Serum hCG was elevated but lower than that of choriocarcinoma [25].

Persistent trophoblastic disease

Persistent trophoblastic tumor (PTD) is a postmolar persistent hCG, clinically invasive mole or metastatic mole, or clinical choriocarcinoma; no specimen has been obtained and the pathological status is unknown.

Postmolar persistent hCG is the most common PTD and shows an abnormal type II hCG regression pattern after the hydatidiform mole, i.e. urinary hCG is greater than 1000 mIU/mL after 5 weeks, serum hCG is greater than 100 mIU/mL after 8 weeks, or serum β-hCG is greater than 1.0 mIU/mL (β-hCG-cytidine 5′-triphosphate [CTP] 0.5 mIU/mL) after 20 weeks, where the focus is unknown.

Clinical invasive mole or metastatic mole is determined by either the symptoms or by the suspected focus.

Clinical choriocarcinoma is determined from the symptoms, suspected focus, or the postmolar state where hCG levels rise again after transient remission that is confirmed by lower than the cut-off hCG level, except for new pregnancies.

Symptoms of gestational trophoblastic neoplasia

Complete hydatidiform mole

Typical symptoms of well-developed complete hydatidiform moles are amenorrhea, hyperemesis, hypertension, no fetal movement, no fetal heartbeat with Doppler detector, larger uterus than in normal pregnancy, abdominal pain, hemorrhage, expelled molar vesicles, and urinary hCG levels usually higher than 100 000 mIU/mL. Typical symptoms are infrequently detected by ultrasonic screening in the first trimester of pregnancy; with transvaginal scan, an early stage hydatidiform mole can be detected and evacuated before its development. Ovarian theca lutein cysts are also detected by 2D real-time ultrasound. Twenty percent of complete moles are followed by sequelae and choriocarcinoma develops in 2%.

Partial hydatidiform mole

Symptoms of the mole associated with a living fetus are similar to normal pregnancy except for hyperemesis, enlarged uterus, and high-titer urinary hCG. Ultrasonic screening of pregnancy detects partial molar changes of the placenta with the embryo, fetus, or fetal particles being present. Partial moles are followed by sequelae in 5% of cases, and rarely progress to choriocarcinoma.

Invasive hydatidiform mole

An invasive mole is preceded by a molar pregnancy and presents with vaginal bleeding, enlarged uterus, bilaterally enlarged ovaries, and high urinary or serum hCG levels. The symptoms resemble those of choriocarcinoma, and differential diagnosis is needed. The interval from antecedent molar pregnancy is usually within six months and it is shorter than in choriocarcinoma. The hCG is continuously elevated after molar curettage, but the titer is lower than in choriocarcinoma. Ultrasonic study reveals the presence of molar vesicles in the myometrial mass.

Choriocarcinoma

Gestational choriocarcinoma is usually preceded by a molar pregnancy, and rarely by abortion or term delivery. The interval from antecedent pregnancy can be longer than one year and longer than with an invasive mole. There may be a period of partial remission, and it can exist for more than 10 years as an extrauterine choriocarcinoma. The symptoms are vaginal bleeding, enlarged uterus, high hCG titer, ovarian masses, and irregular basal body temperature (BBT). Choriocarcinoma is often diagnosed by the presence of metastasis. Multiple pulmonary foci show the progress of malignancy. The hCG titer should be checked even in non-gestational cases when round pulmonary foci are found in the female patient. The symptoms derived from distant metastases suggest choriocarcinoma, e.g. abdominal pain and hemorrhage in hepatic lesions, or persistent headache and vomiting followed by unconsciousness and apnea in brain metastasis.

PSTT and ETT

PSTT and ETT are rare trophoblastic neoplasia. Amenorrhea, vaginal bleeding, and enlarged uterus are their symptoms, and are preceded by gestational processes, e.g. molar pregnancy, abortion, or delivery. PSTT produces less β-hCG and is less sensitive to chemotherapy than choriocarcinoma. The hPL is higher than β-hCG in PSTT. Since metastasis and recurrence are commonplace [21,23,24], PSTT is malignant and can be fatal, while the prognosis is excellent when the disease is confined to the uterus without metastasis. In a report of 55 PSTT cases, statistically significant adverse survival factors were age greater age that 35 years, interval since the last pregnancy over 2 years, deep myometrial invasion, stage III or IV, maximum hCG level >1000 mIU/mL, extensive coagulative necrosis, high mitotic rate, and the presence of cells with clear cytoplasm [23]. A case of PSTT was reported in both mother and child [27]. ETT appears to be less aggressive than choriocarcinoma, more closely resembling the behavior of PSTT; metastatic extrauterine lesions were found in only 2 of 14 ETT cases.

Diagnosis of gestational trophoblastic neoplasia

Complete hydatidiform mole

Complete hydatidiform mole is diagnosed by symptoms such as high urinary and serum hCG titers, and particularly by ultrasonic B-mode, color Doppler, and Doppler flowmetry.

Transvaginal scan is useful in the first trimester. Ultrasonic B-mode detects molar vesicles in the uterine cavity without detecting a fetus or embryo or its particles (Figs 20.1, 20.2). Amniotic membrane and fluid are, however, occasionally detected by B-mode. Characteristic changes are found in complete hydatidiform moles by various ultrasonic imaging techniques.

Real-time B-mode

The complete hydatidiform mole is detected in its early stages by screening during the first trimester. An empty gestational sac, where the wall shows small cystic changes without an embryo, is ultrasonically detected before typical growth of the complete hydatidiform mole (Fig. 20.3). An early complete mole resembles a blighted ovum, whereas the vomiting and high urinary hCG titer of the molar case are contradictory to the presence of blighted ovum. The chorionic plate thickness increases, and typical molar cysts develop within 1–2 weeks in early pregnancy. A characteristic molar pattern is composed of multiple small cysts, but not a snowstorm pattern by ultrasonographic examination with a modern B-mode device (Fig. 20.1B and C). Complete hydatidiform mole develops in one of twins or triplets. It is diagnosed by ultrasound study where the molar tissue separated by the septum has originated from the fetus. A partial mole in a singleton pregnancy is differentiated from the complete mole of a multiple pregnancy by the partial molar change of the placental villi without separating the septum, or by the presence of a triploid chromosome.

Color Doppler flow mapping

A complete hydatidiform mole can be studied using 2D color and power Doppler flow mapping, pulsed Doppler flow wave with flow impedance, and by 3D power Doppler flow mapping. Color Doppler flow mapping discloses filling of the uterine cavity with color flow signals of various directions in the space between molar vesicles (Fig. 20.2).

2D and 3D power Doppler flow images

2D power Doppler of the complete mole reveals molar vesicles in the rich blood flow (Fig. 20.2B). The three sections of 3D power Doppler images also show rich blood flows and the surface image of 3D power Doppler displays blood streams that cover the molar vesicles (Fig. 20.2B). The blood flow stream ejected into the uterine cavity by an arterial aperture may flow through molar vesicles and return to the myometrial vein, because various blood flow directions are shown in 2D color Doppler; 3D power Doppler also shows intrauterine blood flow stream lines.

Pulsed Doppler flow wave and flow impedance

Diastolic flow is larger and the resistance index (RI) is lower in uterine, arcuate, radial, and spiral arteries in the mole than in normal pregnancy [5]. Also the RI is low in molar flow. In the present study [5], in the intervesicular space of the complete mole, peak systolic velocity of maternal arterial blood was as slow as 14 cm/s and the RI was also low at 0.42 (Fig. 20.2C).

Theoretically, fetal blood flow was not recorded, since there was no fetal capillary vessel in the complete mole vesicles. A complete mole was recognized by morphological and functional characters detected by ultrasound techniques.

hCG and other diagnostic methods

Complete hydatidiform mole is estimated when urinary or serum hCG levels are higher than 100 000 mIU/mL, which is within the higher normal range of early pregnancy. A complete mole can, however, be present with lower hCG levels. The postmolar state is monitored every 1–2 weeks by hCG levels, ultrasound, and local conditions after complete mole removal by repeated curettages until the hCG reaches a low cut-off level. Abnormal regression of hCG or persistent trophoblastic disease is treated with chemotherapy for the prophylaxis of choriocarcinoma. Chromosomal diploidy and DNA analysis report an androgenic origin of the complete mole [3,4].

Partial hydatidiform mole

Partial hydatidiform mole is diagnosed by symptoms such as high urinary hCG and ultrasound in the presence of the fetus, or the partial image of fetus and partial changes of the placenta into molar vesicles. 3D ultrasound shows the diagnosis of a partial mole in early pregnancy (Fig. 20.4B). Anomalies are frequent in the fetus with partial mole. Chromosomal examination discloses triploidy. Postmolar changes in urinary and serum hCG are the same as with a complete hydatidiform mole. Chemotherapy in the case of abnormal hCG regression and persistent trophoblastic disease is also the same as for a complete hydatidiform mole.

Invasive hydatidiform mole

Invasive hydatidiform moles are mainly found within six months of the termination of a complete or partial molar pregnancy, although the molar tissue can invade the myometrium during pregnancy. Myometrial invasion may be detected by detailed study with B-mode and color or power Doppler flow mapping of the uterine wall before the termination.

The symptoms of invasive mole are similar to those of choriocarcinoma, i.e. postmolar development, vaginal bleeding, enlarged uterus, and possible metastasis. Urinary or serum hCG is positive, but the levels are lower than with choriocarcinoma. Ultrasound B-mode shows a uterine mass. An invasive mole is usually diagnosed if molar cysts are imaged in the tumor (Fig. 20.5B and C). Rich blood flow is found by color/power Doppler flow mapping (Fig. 20.5). Pulsed Doppler flow impedance is low with an invasive mole. In contrast, flow impedance is high in the wall artery of a theca lutein cyst.

Gestational choriocarcinoma

Gestational choriocarcinoma develops after a hydatidiform mole, abortion, or normal delivery. Clinical symptoms are vaginal bleeding, enlarged uterus, ovarian masses, and high hCG titer, and are similar to those of an invasive mole before

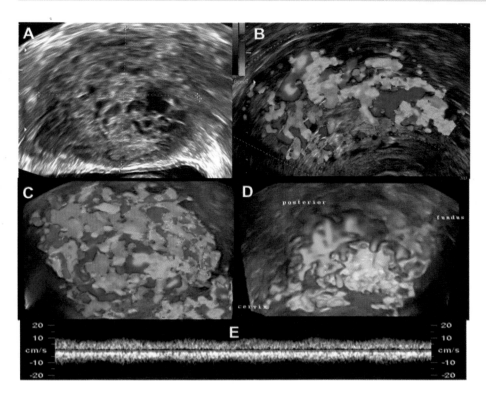

Fig. 20.7 Ultrasound images of a placental site trophoblastic tumor (PSTT). Courtesy of Dr. U. Honemeyer. (A) Lacunae of PSTT in B-mode images. (B) 2D color Doppler flow signs in the lacunae and surface of the neoplas. (C) Tumor covering color flow signs detected with 3D color Doppler. (D) 3D power Doppler. (E) Pulsed Doppler waves of tumor flow.

metastasis. The interval before its development is usually greater than that of an invasive mole, which is usually within six months. Metastases are found in external genitalia and the vaginal wall at an early stage, and then in the lung. An invasive mole rarely develops metastases.

Differential diagnosis of choriocarcinoma from an invasive mole is important, because the outcome is ominous in the former and less risky in the latter, despite the similarity of clinical symptoms. Ultrasonic detection of a cystic pattern in the focus is decisive evidence for an invasive mole (Fig. 20.5B and C), while a cystic villous pattern is not detected by various ultrasound imaging techniques in a choriocarcinoma (Fig. 20.6A and B). Color Doppler flow mapping shows a rich blood flow (Fig. 20.6C). Flow impedance is usually low in both diseases, but it is lower in choriocarcinoma than in an invasive mole. The RI of the uterine artery is significantly lower in a choriocarcinoma than in a hydatidiform mole [19]. A differential gene expression pattern is reported between normal trophoblast and choriocarcinoma cells [21]. Although the risk is clinically suspected by FIGO staging, NIC/NIH classification, and WHO scoring tables, it is important to examine the trophoblastic disease with objective imaging techniques, particularly with various ultrasound methods. Pelvic angiography was used in the past, but ultrasound is now an alternative to angiography.

PSTT and ETT

A long interval after antecedent gestation, and symptoms including vaginal bleeding, amenorrhea and enlarged uterus, and the lack of high hCG titer, suggest the presence of PSTT or ETT. Differential diagnosis from other malignant trophoblastic

diseases is required. In a case of PSTT shown in Fig. 20.7A, transvaginal ultrasound (TVS) disclosed intrauterine tumor with multiple lacunae and indistinct margins within the uterus. Color flow was remarkable surrounding the tumor and in the lacunae by color Doppler flow mapping (Fig.20.7B), and the flow signal covered the surface of the tumor with 3D color Doppler (Fig. 20.7C) and 3D power Doppler (Fig. 20.7D). Tumor malignancy was thought to be due to the very low resistance index of the pulsed Doppler flow velocity wave (Fig. 20.7E). In another PSTT case report [20], TVS showed a slightly enlarged uterus and the presence of an inhomogeneous lesion in the posterior myometrium, which had an ill-defined outer border and several blood vessels on power Doppler imaging.

A case of ETT [18] showed an enlarged uterus with irregular echolucent lacunae within the myometrium, where Doppler color flow image showed that some lacunae were filled with blood. Other than common gynecologic examinations and B-mode, color Doppler images indicated uterine vascularity characterized by low resistance to flow. Serial transvaginal color Doppler is useful for monitoring chemotherapy and residual tumor [19]. Final diagnosis is made by histology of the removed specimen. In one study, ETT was immunohistochemically positive for inhibin-alpha, cytokeratin, hPL, placental alkaline phosphatase, and Mel-CAM(CD-148) [25].

Therapy

Complete hydatidiform mole

Complete hydatidiform mole is treated primarily by curettage, where the massive, well-developed mole should be carefully treated, i.e. the cervix is slowly dilated and uterine contraction is induced by prostaglandin before expulsion and curettage to prevent excessive hemorrhage and uterine damage. Ultrasonically diagnosed early stage evacuation is easier than treating the developed mole at later stages. Curettage is repeated for complete evacuation. Ultrasound monitoring of the intra-uterine maneuver is useful for successful curettage and the prevention of uterine damage. No surgery is performed unless the disease is refractory to chemotherapy or massive hemorrhage occurs.

Partial hydatidiform mole

In the treatment of a partial hydatidiform mole, labor is induced by prostaglandin, followed by curettage for expulsion of the fetus and removal of the mole.

Postmolar monitoring

Postmolar monitoring is indispensable for the detection of any sequelae and prevention of malignant trophoblastic disease. After ultrasonically confirmed complete evacuation of the uterus, ultrasonic transvaginal scan and urinary or serum hCG are mandatory every 1–2 weeks until hCG decreases to normal cut-off levels, then every 1–2 months for a year. An X-ray image is studied when there is any suspicion of pulmonary change. The postmolar monitoring should be continued for 3 or more years, because 85% of choriocarcinomas develop within 3 years after treatment of the mole.

In type I post-molar hCG regression, the regression pattern is normal; urinary hCG decreases to 1000 mIU/mL or less after 5 weeks, serum hCG is 100 mIU/mL or less after 8 weeks, serum β-hCG is 1 mIU/mL or less, and β-hCG-CTP is 0.5 mIU/mL or less, which is the cut-off level 20 weeks after the mole. In the type II hCG regression pattern, hCG is re-elevated after transient remission, and should be treated by prophylactic chemotherapy for prevention of the development of choriocarcinoma, where the use of methotrexate (MTX) is common. Prophylactic chemotherapy was tried in a controlled study [28], where significantly less choriocarcinoma (actually zero) developed in the study group than in the control group.

Choriocarcinoma

Choriocarcinoma is treated by primary chemotherapy, which means the first choice of treatment for choriocarcinoma is chemotherapy. Hysterectomy was common in the past, but was frequently followed by metastases. Radiation was also a local therapy. MTX was the first primary chemotherapy in Kyushu University in the 1960s. It was systemic chemotherapy because choriocarcinoma was recognized as a systemic disease not a local one. The effect is further improved by combined chemotherapy, i.e. EMA (etoposide, MTX, and actinomycin-D) [28], or a further combination of CO (cyclophosphamide and vincristine), forming the EMA/CO regimen [29]. The most intensive therapy may be salvage chemotherapy including etoposide

or cisplatin [30]. Chemotherapy-resistant metastasis or recurrence is associated with surgery, e.g. pulmonary lobectomy or craniotomy [31], and if there is severe vaginal bleeding, the uterus and the focus are surgically removed. Active combination of hysterectomy or endoscopic surgery and chemotherapy may result in favorable remission [32].

Serum hCG level should be lower than the cut-off level for complete remission, that is, disappearance of primary and metastatic foci and lower hCG levels than the cut-off level. Since there is cross-sensitivity of hCG antibody to pituitary luteinizing hormone (LH), β-hCG or β-hCG-CTP antibody, which is more specific for hCG, are commonly used in trophoblastic diseases, particularly low-level hCG. However, some studies reported the presence of false-positive tests in some hCG antibodies including β-hCG and β-hCG-CTP [33,34]. The reports suggested repeated tests, urine instead of serum, serial serum dilution tests, or removal of interfering substances if there is any discrepancy between clinical conditions and the test results.

The systemic side effects of intensive chemotherapy include stomatitis, skin eruption, hair loss, fever, reduced granulocytes, bone marrow damage, hepatic lesions, and gastrointestinal damage. Bone marrow damage, manifested as leucopenia in peripheral blood, is life-threatening. Mild leucopenia is cured by steroids, while severe damage is treated by bone marrow transplantation and stem cell support [35].

Intra-arterial infusion chemotherapy has been used in the treatment of liver metastasis, which decreased by using this treatment. Internal iliac arterial infusion chemotherapy was tried in a uterine cervical choriocarcinoma, followed by tumor regression and necrotic change [11].

Pregnancy outcome after complete remission obtained by intensive chemotherapy is favorable and the treatment shows minimal impact. As for further long-term influence of chemotherapy, menopause was 3 years earlier than in control women [36].

The role of ultrasound in the chemotherapy of choriocarcinoma

Tumor size and blood flow are effectively monitored in chemotherapy by various ultrasound techniques. Primary or metastatic focus reduces the tumor size in the ultrasound image and the tumor blood flow reduces by color/power Doppler flow mapping when chemotherapy is effective (Fig. 20.8A). Early estimation of tumor sensitivity to the chemotherapy is recommended in the treatment of trophoblastic neoplasia.

Pulsed Doppler flow impedance for the early estimation of sensitivity to chemotherapy

Impedance to flow in the choriocarcinoma, e.g. RI and pulsatility index (PI), clearly rose immediately after initiation of chemotherapy in the first course, when the choriocarcinoma was sensitive to chemotherapy before later reduction of hCG, color Doppler flow mapping, and tumor size (Fig. 20.8B). The elevation of flow impedance may be caused by sudden shrinkage

A

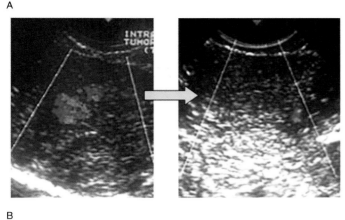

B

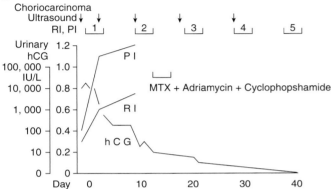

Fig. 20.8 The role of ultrasound in the chemotherapy of trophoblastic neoplasia. (A) Disappearance of color Doppler flow sign after choriocarcinoma chemotherapy. (B) Tumor vessel RI/PI rose immediately after the onset of chemotherapy on choriocarcinoma. Courtesy of Dr. S. Kondo.

of the tumor and the tumor vessels by the chemotherapy. In contrast, a chemotherapy-resistant invasive mole showed no change in RI or PI in tumor flow [33]. Another chemotherapy-resistant invasive mole also showed only mild increase of RI at the end of systemic chemotherapy. Therefore, tumor blood flow impedance can be the indicator of tumor sensitivity in the early period of chemotherapy. This method can also be tried in other chemotherapy treatments for malignancy.

Persistent trophoblastic disease

Post-molar hCG persistence is treated with prophylactic chemotherapy for the prevention of choriocarcinoma, usually with single MTX. The course is repeated until hCG reaches normal levels. Chemotherapy is given for clinical choriocarcinoma as described previously. Clinical invasive mole is also treated with chemotherapy, but with hysterectomy when it is refractory.

Invasive mole

Invasive moles are treated with systemic chemotherapy, although they tend to be refractory, because an invasive mole is a molar vesicle which is more differentiated than choriocarcinoma. A

higher local dose of agents may be needed for invasive moles than for choriocarcinoma. Local therapy before hysterectomy in the future may be tumor resection, laser evaporation etc., in the open uterus.

PSTT and ETT

PSTT is treated by hysterectomy when limited to the uterus, while chemotherapy is used when it has spread further than the uterus, although the clinical outcome has been reported to be poor when the preceding pregnancy was more than 2 years before the PSTT [37]. Janni et al. [38] recommended a cytostatic-surgical approach for metastatic PSTT. Furthermore, Tsuji et al. [39] reported that resection of the tumor and EMA/CO chemotherapy could achieve long-term remission. Other reports [40–42] obtained favorable results mainly by EMA/CO chemotherapy and further use of the etoposide-cisplatin cycle [43]. The outcome of FIGO stage I–II patients was excellent after hysterectomy, but for stage III–IV patients the survival rate was only for 30%. In the reports, PSTT responds to chemotherapy, and complete remission can be expected. ETT may be treated with a similar regimen.

As for other reported treatments, Watanabe et al. [44] reported a choriocarcinoma in the pulmonary artery which needed emergency pulmonary embolectomy under cardiopulmonary bypass. Kohyama et al. [45] reported the stereotactic radiation therapy of a choriocarcinoma in the cranium followed by conventional craniospinal irradiation. Bohlmann et al. [14] reported intracardiac resection of a metastatic choriocarcinoma. A combination of high-dose chemotherapy and bone marrow/blood stem cell transplantation was tried in the case of refractory choriocarcinoma [32].

Acknowledgments

The authors express sincere gratitude to Drs M. Utsu, S. Kupesic, G. Varga, J. R. Benitez, M. Terahara, S. Kondo, and U. Honemeyer for the very kind presentation of excellent sonograms and figures in this chapter.

References

1. Japan Society of Obstetrics and Gynecology and Japanese Pathological Society. *The General Rules for Clinical and Pathological Management of Trophoblastic Diseases*, 2nd edn. Tokyo: Kanehara Shuppan; 1995.

2. Weaver DT, Fisher RA, Newlands ES, Paradinas FJ. Amniotic tissue in complete hydatidiform moles can be androgenetic. *J Pathol* 2000; **191**: 67–70.

3. Kajii T, Ohama K. Androgenetic origin of hydatidiform mole. *Nature* 1977; **268**: 633–634.

4. Ohama K, Kajii T, Okamoto E, Fukuda Y, Imazumi K, Tsukahara M, Kobayashi K, Hagiwara K. Dispermic origin of XY hydatidiform mole. *Nature* 1981; **292**: 551–552.

5. Kurjak A, Zalud I, Predanic M, Kupesic S. Transvaginal color and pulsed Doppler study of uterine blood flow in the first and early

second trimesters of pregnancy: normal versus abnormal. *J Ultrasound Med* 1994; **13**: 43–47.

6. Gungor T, Ekin M, Dumanli H, Gokmen O. Color Doppler ultrasonography in the earlier differentiation of benign mole-hydatidiform from malignant gestational trophoblastic disease. *Acta Obstet Gynecol Scand* 1998; **77**: 860–862.

7. Vegan GI, Fulop V, Liu Y, et al. Differential gene expression pattern between normal human trophoblast and choriocarcinoma cell lines: down regulation of heat shock protein-27 in choriocarcinoma in vitro and in vivo. *Gynecol Oncol* 1999; **75**: 391–396.

8. Szulman AE, Philippe E, Boue JG, Boue A. Human triploidy. Association with partial hydatidiform moles and nonmolar conceptuses. *Human Pathol* 1981; **12**: 1016–1021.

9. Hirose M, Kimura T, Mitsuno N, Wakuda K, Fujita J, Noda Y. DNA flow cytometric quantification and DNA polymorphism analysis in the case of a complete mole with a coexisting fetus. *J Assist Reprod Genet* 1999; **16**: 263–267.

10. Yahata T, Kodama S, Kase H, et al. Primary choriocarcinoma of the uterine cervix: clinical MRI and color Doppler ultrasonographic study. *Gynecol Oncol* 1997; **64**: 274–278.

11. Koga K, Izuchi S, Maeda K, Noutomi Y. Treatment of chorionepithelioma of uterine cervix with hypogastric arterial infusion of amethopterin. *J Jpn Obstet Gynecol Soc* 1966; **13**: 245–249.

12. Coskun M, Agildere AM, Boyvart F, Tarhan C, Niron EA. Primary choriocarcinoma of the stomach and pancreas: CT findings. *Eur Radiol* 1998; **8**: 1425–1428.

13. Chama CM, Nggada HA, Nuhu A. Cutaneous metastasis of gestational choriocarcinoma. *Int J Gynecol Obstet* 2002; **77**: 249–250.

14. Bohlmann MK, Eckstein FS, Allemann Y, Stauffer E, Carrel TP. Intracardiac resection of a metastatic choriocarcinoma. *Gynecol Oncol* 2002; **84**: 157–160.

15. Steigrad SM, Cheung AP, Osborn RA. Choriocarcinoma coexistent with and intact pregnancy: case report and review of the literature. *J Obstet Gynecol Res* 1999; **25**: 197–203.

16. Jacque SM, Quershi F, Doss BJ, Munkarah A. Intraplacental choriocarcinoma associated with viable pregnancy: pathologic features and implications for the mother and infant. *Pediatr Dev Pathol* 1998; **1**: 380–387.

17. Feltmate CM, Genest DR, Goldstein DP, Berkowitz RS. Advances in the understanding of placental site trophoblastic tumor. *J Reprod Med* 2002; **47**: 337–341.

18. Okumura M, Fushida K, Rezende WW, Schultz R, Zugaib M. Sonographic appearance of gestational trophoblastic disease evolving into epithelioid trophoblastic tumor. *Ultrasound Obstet Gynecol* 2010; **36**: 249–251.

19. Bettencourt E, Pinto E, Abraul e, Dinis M, De Oliveira CF. Placental site trophoblastic tumor: the value of transvaginal colour and pulsed Doppler sonography (TV-CGS) in its diagnosis: case report. *Eur J Gynecol Oncol* 1997; **18**: 461–464.

20. Savelli L, Pollastri P, Mabrouk M, Seracchioli R, Ventuoli S. Placental site trophoblastic tumor diagnosed on transvaginal sonography ultrasound *Obstet Gynecol* 2009; **34**: 235–236.

21. Remadi S, Lifschita-Mercer B, Ben-Hur H, Dgani R, Czernobilsky B. Metastasizing placental site trophoblastic tumor: immunohistochemical and DNA analysis. 2 case reports and a review of the literature. *Arch Gynecol Obstet* 1997; **259**: 97–103.

22. Feltmate CM, Genest DR, Wise L, Bernstein MR, Goldstein CP. Berkowitz RS. Placental site trophoblastic tumor: a 17-year experience at the New England Trophoblastic Disease Center. *Gynecol Oncol* 2001; **82**: 415–419.

23. Baergen RN, Rutgers JL, Young RH, Osann K. Scully RE. Placental site trophoblastic tumor: a study of 55 cases and review of the literature emphasizing factors of prognostic significance. *Gynecol Oncol* 2006; **100**: 511–520.

24. Mangili G, Garavaglia E, De Marzi P, Zanetto F, Taccagni G. Metastatic placental site trophoblastic tumor. Report of a case with complete response to chemotherapy. *J Reprod Med* 2001; **46**: 259–262.

25. Shih IM, Kurman RJ. Epithelioid trophoblastic tumor: a neoplasm distinct from choriocarcinoma and placental site trophoblastic tumor simulating carcinoma. *Am J Surg Pathol* 1998; **22**: 1393–1403.

26. Allison KH, Love JE, Garcia RL. Epithelioid trophoblastic tumor; review of a rare neoplasma of the chorionic-type intermediate trophoblast. *Arch Pathol Lab Med* 2006; **130**: 1875–1877.

27. Monclair T, Abeler VM, Kren J, Salaas L, Zeller B. Placental site trophoblastic tumor (PSTT) in mother and child: first report of PSTT in infancy. *Med Pediatr Oncol* 2002; **38**: 187–191.

28. Soto-Wright V, Goldstein DP, Bernstein MR, Berkowitz RS. The management of gestational trophoblastic tumors with etoposide, methotrexate, and actinomycin D. *Gynecol Oncol* 1997; **64**: 156–159.

29. Nozue A, Ichikawa Y, Minami R, Tsunoda H, Nishida M, Kubo T. Postpartum choriocarcinoma complicated by brain and lung metastases treated successfully with EMA/CO regimen. *BJOG* 2000; **107**: 1171–1172.

30. Okamoto T, Goto S. Resistance to multiple agent chemotherapy including cisplatin after chronic low-dose oral etoposide administration in gestational choriocarcinoma. *Gynecol Obstet Invest* 2001; **52**: 139–141.

31. Kang SB, Lee CM, Kim JW, Park NH, Lee HP. Chemoresistant choriocarcinoma cured by pulmonary lobectomy and craniotomy. *Int J Gynecol Cancer* 2000; **10**: 165–169.

32. Chou HH, Lai CH, Wang PN, Tsai KT, Liu HP, Hsueh S. Combination of high-dose chemotherapy, autologous bone marrow/peripheral blood stem cell transplantation, and thoracoscopic surgery in refractory nongestational choriocarcinoma of a 45XO/46XY female: a case report. *Gynecol Oncol* 1997; **64**: 521–525.

33. Cole LA, Butler S. Detection of hCG in trophoblastic disease. The USA hCG reference service experience. *J Reprod Med* 2002; **47**: 433–444.

34. ACOG Committee opinion. Avoiding inappropriate clinical decisions based on false-positive human chorionic gonadotropin test results. *Am J Obstet Gynecol* 2002; **100**: 1057–1059.

35. Knox S, Brooks SE, Wog-You-Cheong J, Ioffe O, Meisenberg B, Goldstein DP. Choriocarcinoma and epithelial trophoblastic tumor: successful treatment of relapse with hysterectomy and high dose chemotherapy with peripheral stem cell support. A case report. *Gynecol Oncol* 2002; **85**: 204–208.

36. Bower M, Rustin GJ, Newlands ES, et al. Chemotherapy for gestational trophoblastic tumours hastens menopause by 3 years. *Eur J Cancer* 1998; **34**: 1204–1207.

37. Newlands ES, Bower M, Fisher RA, Paradinas FJ. Management of placental site trophoblastic tumors. *J Reprod Med* 1995; **3**: 53–59.

38. Janni W, Hantschmann P, Rehbock J, Braun S, Lochmueller E, Kindermann G. Successful treatment of malignant placental site trophoblastic tumor with combined cytostatic-surgical approach, case report and review of literature. *Gynecol Oncol* 1999; **75**: 164–169.

39. Tsuji Y, Tsubamoto H, Hori M, Ogasawara T, Koyama K. Case of PSTT treated with chemotherapy followed by open uterine tumor resection to preserve fertility. *Gynecol Oncol* 2002; **87**: 303–307.

40. Twigs LB, Hartenbach E, Saltzman AK, King LA. Metastatic placental site trophoblastic tumor. *Int J Gynecol Obstet* 1998; **60**(Suppl 1): S51–S55.

41. Swisher E, Drescher CW. Metastatic placental site trophoblastic tumor: long-term remission in a patient treated with EMA/CO chemotherapy. *Gynecol Oncol* 1998; **58**: 62–65.

42. Chang YL, Chang TC, Hsuen KG, Wand PN, Liu HP, Soong YK. Prognostic factors and treatment for placental site trophoblastic tumor – report of 3 cases and analysis of 88 cases. *Gynecol Oncol* 1999; **73**: 216–222.

43. Randall TC, Coukos G, Wheeler JE, Rubin SC. Prolonged remission of recurrent, metastatic placental site trophoblastic tumor after chemotherapy. *Gynecol Oncol* 2000; **76**: 115–117.

44. Watanabe S, Shimokawa K, Masuda H, Sakata R, Higashi M. Choriocarcinoma in the pulmonary artery treated with emergency pulmonary embolectomy. *Chest* 2002; **121**: 654–656.

45. Kohyama S, Uematsu M, Ishihara S, Shima K, Tamai S, Kusano A. An experience of stereotactic radiation therapy for primary intracranial choriocarcinoma. *Tumori* 2001; **87**: 162–165.

Chapter

21

Ultrasound imaging in ovarian masses: benign or malignant?

Elizabeth E. Puscheck and Jashoman Banerjee

Introduction

Ultrasonography should be the first imaging modality utilized to evaluate pelvic masses. Most ovarian masses are asymptomatic. Occasionally, patients may present with abdominal pain secondary to torsion, rupture, or bleeding within ovarian cysts [1,2]. Asymptomatic ovarian masses are often detected during the annual pelvic exam and an ultrasound should be ordered for the initial assessment. Ovarian masses may be incidentally identified when doing a pelvic ultrasound or other imaging test. Pelvic ultrasound may be ordered to evaluate the pelvis when an inadequate exam is noted (often due to obesity). A clinical exam has a low sensitivity to detect adnexal masses [3], so there should be a low threshold to do a baseline pelvic ultrasound. Of course, ultrasound should be the first modality to evaluate the pelvis if the ovarian mass presents with pelvic pain.

Ultrasound imaging to rule out ovarian malignancy has not been accepted as a standard screening tool. In fact, there is no diagnostic imaging test or screening test to rule out ovarian malignancy. Patients typically remain asymptomatic until an advanced stage and even then, the most common presenting symptoms are nonspecific abdominal symptoms. However, there are pelvic ultrasound characteristics that we can group into the following categories: (1) normal appearance, (2) benign characteristics, (3) indeterminate, but probably benign, and (4) suspicious for malignancy. Recent advances in ultrasound technology including improved resolution, color or power Doppler, three-dimensional ultrasound (3D-US), and contrast-enhanced techniques have made diagnosis of pelvic masses better.

Recently, the Society of Radiology in Ultrasound convened a consensus conference to discuss the management of asymptomatic ovarian masses. The panel included experts in gynecology, reproductive endocrinology and infertility, gynecologic oncology, radiology, pathology, and epidemiology. The result of this conference is a white paper of recommendations published in *Radiology* [4]. The recommendations were made after analyzing the current literature as well as discussing common practice and expert experience. Within this paper are four tables categorizing ovarian masses into normal appearance, cysts with benign characteristics, cysts with indeterminate but probably benign characteristics, and cysts with characteristics worrisome for malignancy. These tables are very helpful for clinical guidance in distinguishing benign from malignant masses and in determining when and how to follow up (Figs 21.1 and 21.2).

The International Ovarian Tumor Assessment (IOTA) group is another group of experts who have also come up with a classification system to distinguish benign from malignant masses (Figs 21.3 and 21.4). The IOTA group consists of gynecologic oncologists with extensive ultrasound experience. They have identified a set of 10 rules to follow when evaluating ovarian masses by ultrasound. Their goal was to develop a set of rules for any sonographer (regardless of experience) to use to distinguish benign from malignant masses. They also did a prospective, multicenter study to evaluate the effectiveness of these rules compared to expert sonographer/sonologist assessment. These results show that there are masses that are characteristically benign and remain benign. Masses that are suspicious for malignancy require surgical intervention. Both groups identified masses that would be indeterminate. The IOTA group used expert sonographers to give input in such cases. The other group took into consideration the hormonal status of the woman in such cases. Both recommend considering surgical evaluation in many of these cases. Neither system is perfect but both provide assistance in making this distinction.

There are several other classification systems that have been attempted. We have found the white paper and the IOTA classification the most useful. In the following sections we review some of the more classic ultrasound characteristics in benign and malignant masses.

Benign ovarian masses

Most ovarian masses in reproductive age women are benign. They range from normal physiologic findings (i.e. follicular cysts, corpora lutea) to hemorrhagic corpora lutea, serous cystadenomas, endometriomas, dermoid cysts, and fibroadenomas [5]. Functional ovarian cysts (which should not really be called cysts since they are normal physiologic findings) rarely

Normal Appearance		Follow-up*	Comments
Normal ovary appearance: Reproductive age Follicles • Thin and smooth walls • Round or oval • Anechoic • Size ≤3 cm • No blood flow	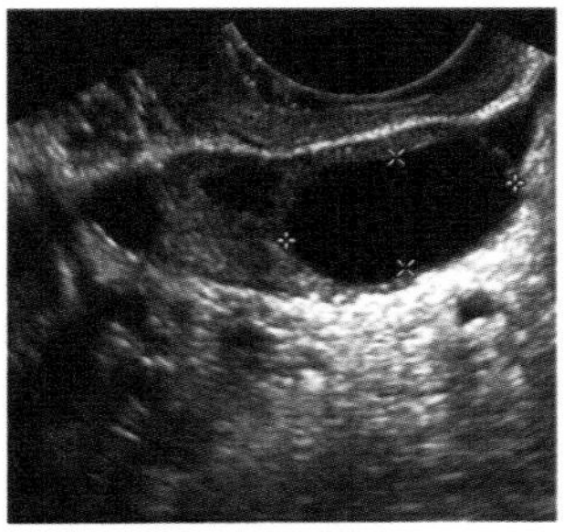	Not needed	Developing follicles and dominant follicle ≤3 cm are normal findings
Normal ovary appearance: Reproductive age Corpus luteum • Diffusely thick well • Peripheral blood flow • Size ≤3 cm • +/− internal echoes • +/− crenulated appearance	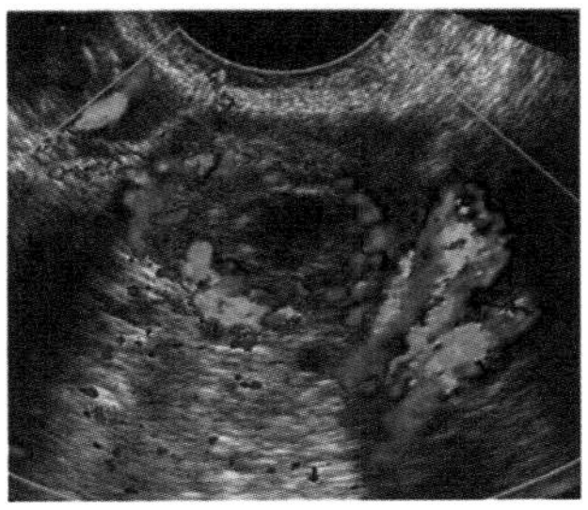	Not needed	Corpus luteum ≤3 cm is a normal findings
Normal ovary appearance: Postmenopausal • Small • Homogenous	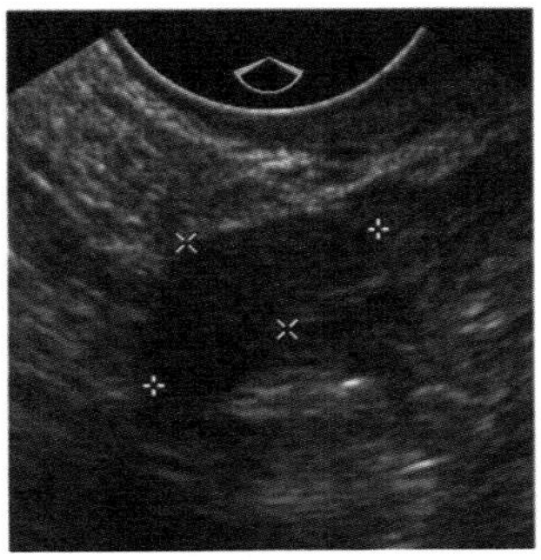	Not needed	Normal postmenopausal ovary is atrophic without follicles
Clinically inconsequential: Postmenopausal Simple cyst ≤1 cm • Thin wall • Anechoic • No flow	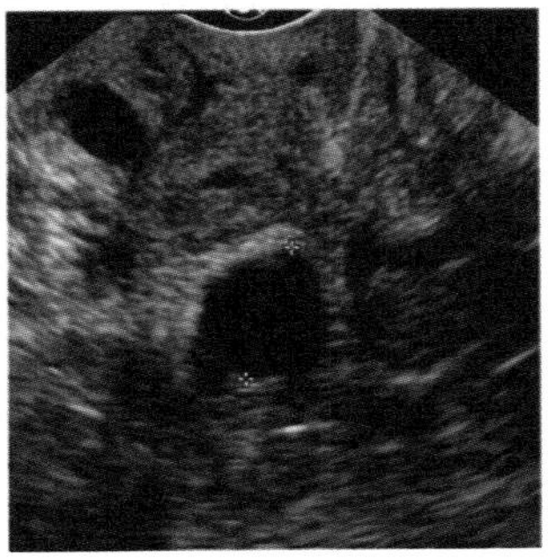	Not needed	Small simple cysts are common; cyst ≤1 cm are considered clinically unimportant

Fig. 21.1 Summary of recommendations for management of asymptomatic ovarian and other adnexal cysts. * Follow-up recommendations are for US, unless otherwise indicated. ** Some practices may choose a threshold size slightly higher than 1 cm before recommending yearly follow-up. Practices may choose to decrease the frequency of follow-up once stability or decrease in size has been confirmed. *(Figure continues.)* Reproduced with permission from *Radiology* (Levine D. et al. Management of asymptomatic ovarian and other adnexal cysts imaged at US: Society of Radiologists in Ultrasound Consensus Conference Statement. *Radiology* 256(3): 949–951, 2010).

measure above 8 cm. However, 20% of postmenopausal women will present with small functional neoplasms [3,6]. Most common ovarian masses in reproductive-age women are follicular cysts and corpus luteal cysts. So correlating the findings with the stage of the menstrual cycle is also critical. These follicles may enlarge up to 2–3 cm and larger when the patient is undergoing controlled ovarian stimulation for in vitro fertilization, where they can be multiple and bilateral. These cysts have a thin wall and homogeneous, hypoechoic pattern [7]. Corpus luteal cysts are commonly unilateral in natural cycles. Bilateral follicular cysts are also commonly seen in ovulation induction cycles. Presence of free fluid in the luteal phase with presence

Cysts with indeterminate, but probably benign, characteristics		Follow-up*	Comments
Findings suggestive of, but not classic for, hemorrhagic cyst, endometrioma, or dermoid	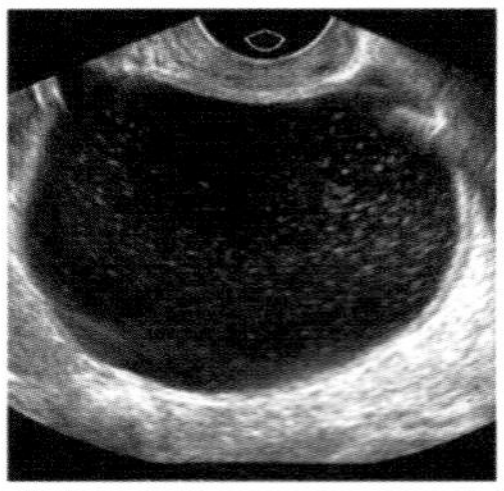	Reproductive age: 6–12 weeks follow-up to ensure resolution. If the lesion is unchanged, then hemorrhagic cyst is unlikely, and continued follow-up with either ultrasound or MRI should then be considered. If these studies do not confirm an endometrioma or dermoid, then surgical evaluation should be considered. Postmenopausal: Consider surgical valuation	
Thin-walled cyst with single thin septation or focal calcification in the wall of a cyst	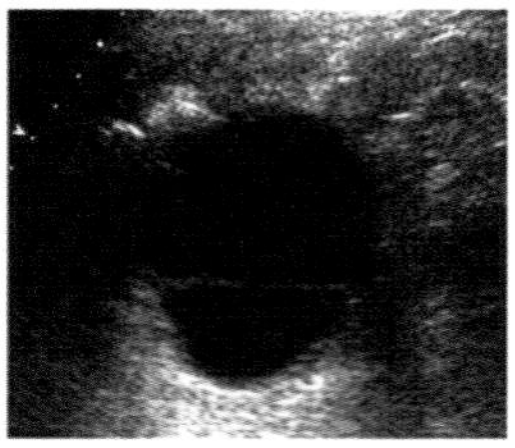	Follow-up based on size and menopausal status, same as simple cyst described above	
Multiple thin septations (<3 mm)	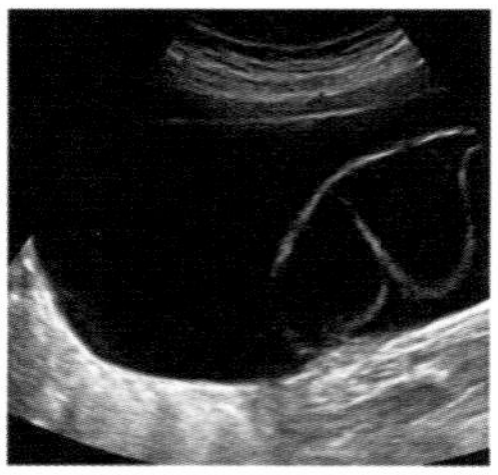	Consider surgical evaluation	Multiple septations suggest a neoplasm, but if thin, the neoplasm is likely benign
Nodule (non-hyperechoic) without flow	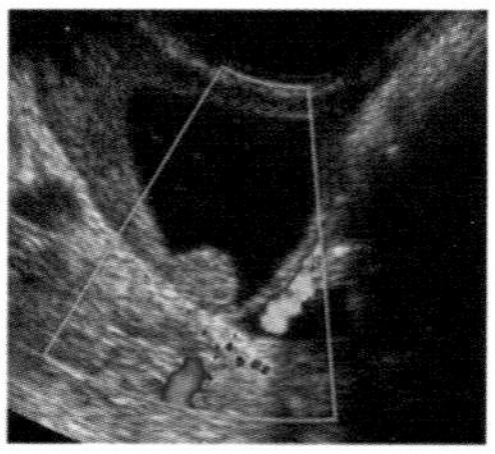	Consider surgical evaluation or MRI	Solid nodule suggests neoplasm, but if no flow (and not echogenic as would be seen in a dermoid) this is likely a benign lesion such as a cystadenofibroma
Cysts with characteristics worrisome for malignancy		Follow-up*	Comments
Thick (>3mm) irregular septations	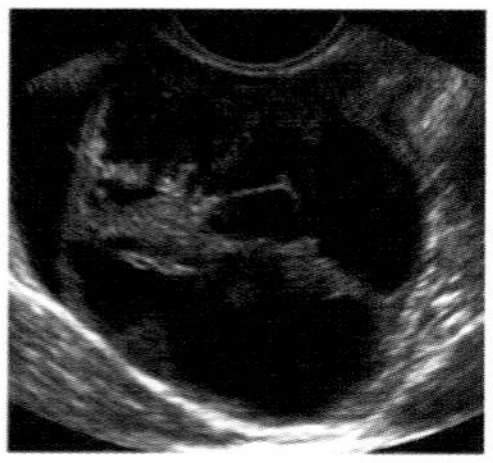	Any age: Consider surgical evaluation	
Nodule with blood flow	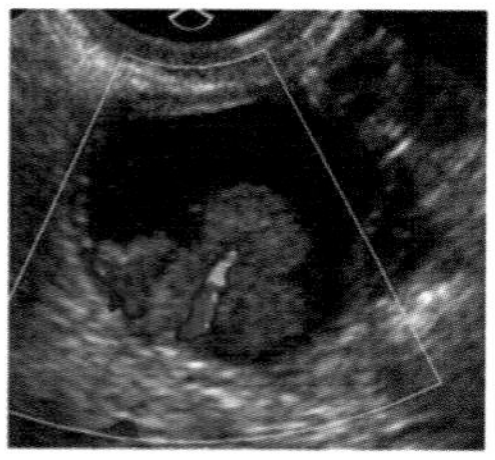	Any age: Consider surgical evaluation	

Fig. 21.2 Benign and malignant cyst: ultrasonographic appearances and fallow up. Reproduced with permission from *Radiology* (Levine D et al. Management of asymptomatic ovarian and other adnexal cysts imaged at US: Society of Radiologists in Ultrasound Consensus Conference Statement. *Radiology* 256(3): 949–951, 2010).

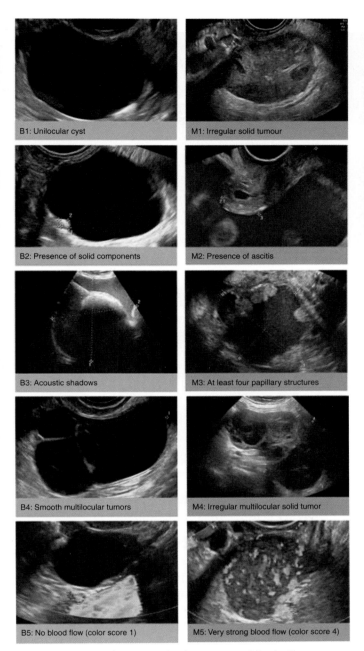

Fig. 21.3 Ultrasound features used in the International Ovarian Tumor Analysis (IOTA) simple rules, illustrated by ultrasound images. B1–B5, benign features; M1–M5, malignant features. Reproduced with permission from Kaijser J et al. Improving strategies for diagnosing ovarian cancer: a summary of the International Ovarian Tumor Analysis (IOTA) studies. *Ultrasound Obstet Gynecol* 41: 9–20, 2013.

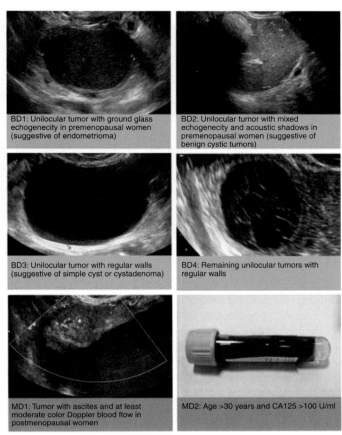

Fig. 21.4 International Ovarian Tumor Analysis (IOTA) "easy descriptors" illustrated by ultrasound images. BDI-BD4, benign descriptors; MDI-MDI, malignant descriptors. Reproduced with permission from Kaijser J et al. Improving strategies for diagnosing ovarian cancer: a summary of the International Ovarian Tumor Analysis (IOTA) studies. *Ultrasound Obstet Gynecol* 41: 9–20, 2013.

of a cyst may indicate ovulation. Benign serous cysts, which are common in the reproductive-age group, demonstrate an anechoic pattern without vegetations [7].

When an adnexal mass is noted on pelvic ultrasound, each mass should be evaluated by grayscale 2D ultrasound with measurements and its origin determined (ovarian, paraovarian, tubal, uterine, or extrapelvic in origin). Then color or power Doppler is very helpful in distinguishing between benign masses and masses suspicious for malignancy [5,8–12]. Although some of the literature recommends a resistivity index less than 0.4 and pulsatility index less than 1.0 as being suspicious for malignancy, there is much overlap in this data and obtaining accurate reproducible results is difficult when looking at ovarian masses (not ovarian vessels). Instead of the specific Doppler measurements (i.e. resistivity index or pulsatility index or maximum velocity), Doppler flow into the mass indicates vascular flow into the mass and this is more reliable and concerning for malignancy. A hallmark of malignancy is neovascularization. There are benign conditions, such as corpus luteum, in which there is markedly increased vascularity but this vascularity remains in the tissue surrounding the ovarian cyst for most benign conditions and not into the mass as in malignancy or suspected malignancy.

Ovarian simple cyst

An ovarian mass is more likely to be benign if it is a simple cyst with a thin wall (Figure 21.5) [2]. It is important to carefully evaluate the entire cyst wall to make sure that there are no nodules, papillations, or septa. If the entire cyst wall cannot be

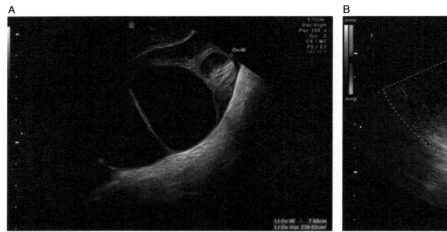

Fig. 21.5 (A and B) Simple cysts. Simple cysts are hypoechoic and have smooth borders with no separations, papillary projections, or color flow into the cyst.

visualized, then this limitation should be noted in the report and this ovarian cyst cannot be called a simple cyst since it is not completely evaluated. So the size limitation is dependent on the penetration of the vaginal probe and we put this limit at 7–10 cm. Masses larger than this cannot reliably be evaluated. Occasionally, a simple cyst may have a very small nodule (<3 mm in size) with no color Doppler flow into this nodule and this can be accepted as an atypical finding that is benign. Similarly, a thin septation (<3 mm) without vascularity may occasionally be seen in benign masses. Simple cysts may represent an enlarged follicle, hemorrhagic follicle, serous cystadenoma, mucinous cystadenoma, or adenofibroma. These are all benign tumors and they may have ultrasound characteristics that overlap with those of a simple cyst. Some may be unilocular or bilocular. The mucinous cystadenoma does tend to be larger and multilocular with regular wall and septa (no papillary vegetations or nodules). Septations thicker than 3 mm are concerning [5]. Ovarian masses that have solid components are more suspicious for malignancy. Color and power Doppler should be utilized to determine whether there is any color flow noted in the nodule, vegetation, papillation, septum, or solid area. This finding is much more worrisome for neovascularization, which one expects with malignancy. However, even suspicious masses on ultrasound may actually be benign upon surgical evaluation.

Paraovarian and paratubal cysts

These cysts are typically unilocular and move separately from the ovary and the uterus. There is no Doppler flow into the cyst. These cysts do tend to persist.

Corpus luteum and hemorrhagic corpus luteum

Reproductive-age women have cyclic changes in their ovary due to ovulation. An ovulatory follicle may reach 3–4 cm and be a normal physiologic follicular development. After ovulation these follicles become corpora lutea and these corpora lutea have increased vascularity surrounding them. The corpus luteum typically is involuting and decreasing in size, but

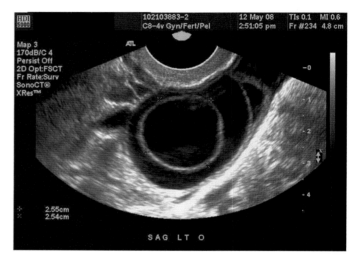

Fig. 21.6 Functional cyst. (Courtesy of Leeber Cohen MD.)

occasionally there is a bleed into the corpus luteum and it increases in size. The hemorrhagic corpus luteum has Doppler flow around the cyst but no blood flow into the cyst, which consists mainly of a blood clot. The blood clot may have a variety of ultrasound appearances from solid, low-level echoes, hypoechoic areas to a combination of these. The ultrasound findings may note low-level echoes consistent with fibrin which have small, thin hyperechoic areas. Others have been described as spiderweb-like in appearance. Some have solid components without Doppler flow consistent with the clot. And others have a combination consistent with a retracting clot. Some may even look like a simple cyst as the clot liquefies. These benign masses have a variety of appearances and have been confused on occasion with a malignancy. Typically, the hemorrhagic corpus luteum will resolve in 6–8 weeks.

Endometrioma

The endometrioma is a benign ovarian tumor. The endometrioma is usually a single cyst with the cyst wall composed

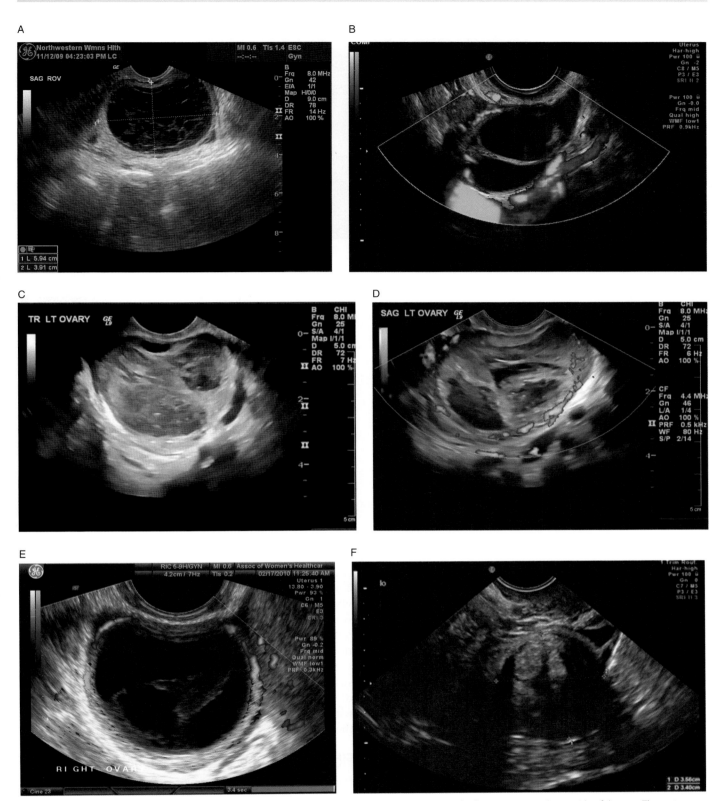

Fig. 21.7 Hemorrhagic corpus luteum cysts. These have a wide range of appearances. Again, the Doppler flow remains on the outside of the cyst. The cyst may appear hypoechoic or it may be a mix of low-level echoes or even a solid mass (clot) without Doppler flow within it. (A) Classic hemorrhagic corpus luteum (courtesy of Leeber Cohen MD) – see the lines consistent with fibrin within the clot. (B) Hemorrhagic corpus luteum with hypoechoic and low-level echoes layered along with a strong Doppler signal around the corpus luteum. (C) Hemorrhagic corpus luteum. (D) Hemorrhagic corpus luteum with ring of fire, power Doppler. (E) Hemorrhagic corpus luteum with cystic and solid areas, power Doppler. (F) Hemorrhagic corpus luteum with solid parts and shadowing.

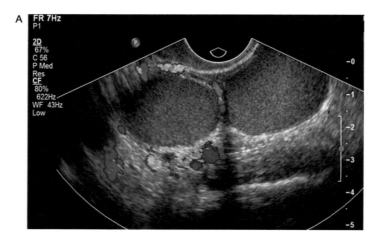

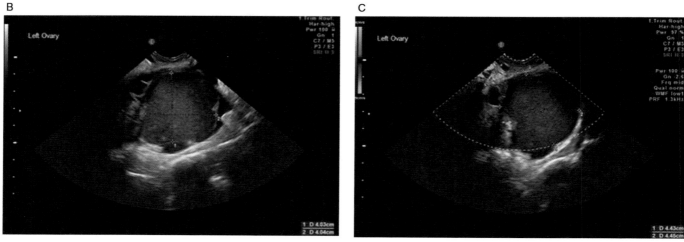

Fig. 21.8 (A) Endometrioma with color Doppler. (B) Endometrioma. (C) Endometrioma showing no Doppler within the cyst.

of endometrium and the contents of the cyst are typically blood or hemolytic components of blood giving a chocolate appearance when entered surgically. Consequently, the typical ultrasound findings are homogeneous low-level echoes. Some describe the findings as having a "ground-glass" appearance. These masses can often be confused with a hemorrhagic corpus luteum for obvious reasons. However, an endometrioma will not resolve and more often enlarges in size over time.

Dermoid

The dermoid cyst or mature cystic teratomas are the commonest ovarian tumors removed in surgery [13]. This cyst is of embryonal origin and can have structures within it of any tissue. Most commonly these cysts are made up of sebaceous material, hair, and calcified components (consistent with teeth). Consequently, these masses may have a variety of appearances. Occasionally, the dermoid may look like an endometrioma with low-level echoes and some fine reticular echoes [14]. Thin echogenic bands may represent hair [13]. Some have cystic and solid components which may be

described as complex. The solid components may be due to the calcifications or teeth. Some have a nodule or tubercle (Rokitansky nodule) with acoustic shadowing below it [13]. Teratomas less than 5–6 cm are amenable to close follow-up whereas larger ones need surgery because of the risk of torsion [13]. Though most ovarian dermoid cysts are mature teratomas and may demonstrate imaging features as mentioned, immature and malignant teratomas may present with mixed echo patterns [13]. When the ultrasound of a mass is suspicious for a dermoid but there is uncertainty, then an MRI of this mass may be helpful since MRI easily detects the fat within the mass, which is common in dermoids and clinches the diagnosis.

Fibroma, fibrothecoma, fibroadenoma, thecofibroma, and thecoma

These ovarian cysts typically are solid benign neoplasms. The echogenicity is more like a leiomyoma. To determine the origin of the mass, one looks to see whether it is attached to the uterus as a myoma or a pedunculated myoma. It may be confused with an exophytic myoma. The fibromas tend to be more regular in

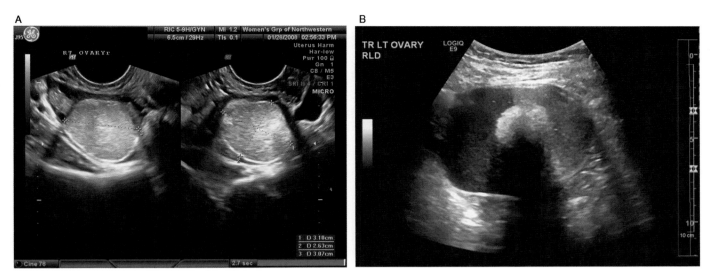

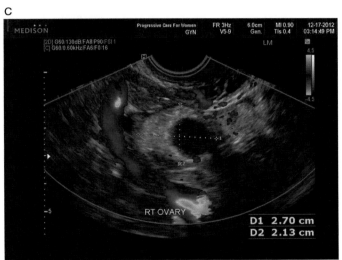

Fig. 21.9 Dermoid. (A) Hyperechoic with extenuated posterior border with shadowing. (Courtesy of Leeber Cohen MD.) (B) Dermoid with Rokitansky nodule. (C) Dermoid. (Courtesy of Leeber Cohen MD.)

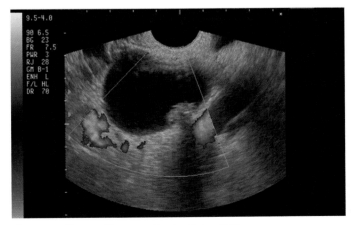

Fig. 21.10 Fibroma. (Courtesy of Leeber Cohen MD.)

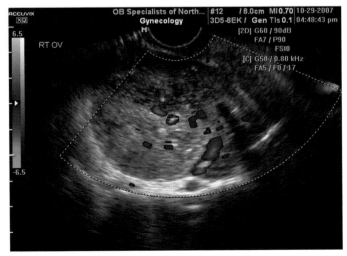

Fig. 21.11 Thecoma. (Courtesy of Leeber Cohen MD.)

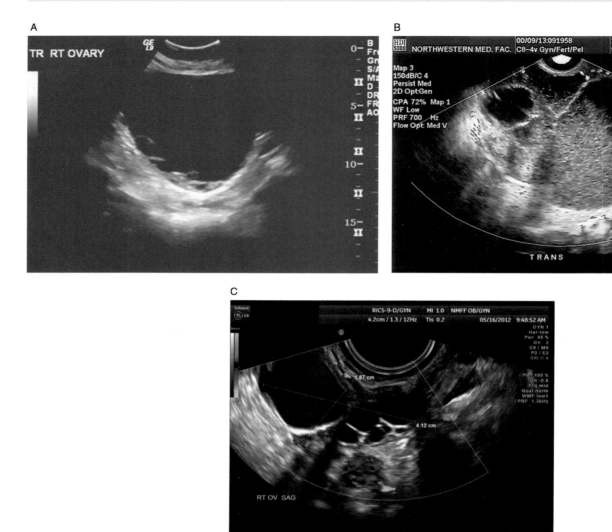

Fig. 21.12 (A–C) Mucinous cystadenoma. (B and C courtesy of Leeber Cohen MD.)

comparison with the thecomas or thecofibromas, which tend to be more lobular and irregular in echogenicity. Brenner tumors also fall within this category.

Malignant neoplasms

In the United states almost 3% of all cancers are ovarian cancers and to date no proper screening tool has been standardized [8]. Pelvic ultrasonography has a very important role to play since it is the first line in imaging to diagnose an ovarian mass. Malignant ovarian tumors consist of borderline tumors (or ovarian tumors of low malignant potential), epithelial tumors, germ cell tumors, sex cord/stromal tumors, granulosa cell tumors, and metastatic cancer to the ovary. Most common ovarian malignancies are of epithelial origin, namely cystadenocarcinoma with tumors of low malignant potential comprising 20% and less than 5% being germ cell tumors. Transvaginal ultrasound characteristics of unilateral or bilateral

masses, along with the clinical context such as age, menopausal status, clinical exam, and tumor markers, have improved the diagnosis and management of adnexal masses[15]. Grayscale transvaginal ultrasonography combined with color and power Doppler techniques have improved sensitivity for detecting malignant neoplasms [6,8], with a sensitivity of 87.5% and specificity of 91.2% [16]. Ultrasound characteristics suspicious for malignancy include: color/power Doppler within the ovarian mass indicating angiogenesis and increased vascularity [9,17], the presence of septations (particularly thick septations or multiple septations), papillations or vegetations within the cysts with Doppler flow, irregular papillations, and solid components or solid mass [6]. Localizing increased blood flow has been helpful in differentiating benign and malignant ovarian masses. Peripheral vascularization is detected in benign masses whereas central localization within the mass is suspicious for a malignant lesion [9]. Color Doppler ultrasound characterizes the hemodynamics of the neoplasm. It demonstrates

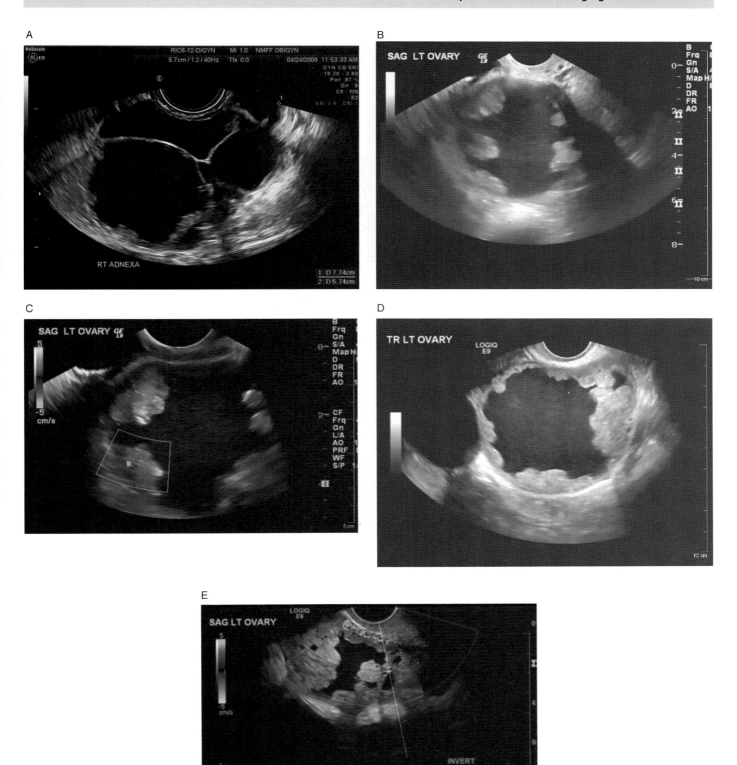

Fig. 21.13 Carcinomas. (A) Borderline. (Courtesy of Leeber Cohen MD.) (B) Serous borderline. (C) Serous borderline with Doppler. (D) Mixed serous endometrioid. (E) Mixed serous endometrioid with Doppler.

A
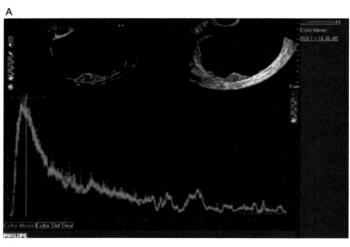

B
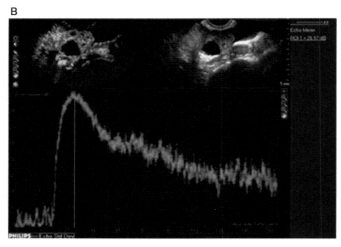

Fig. 21.14 Contrast-enhanced imaging of ovarian masses. (Reproduced with permission from Art Fleischer MD.) (A) Quick wash-in and wash-out of contrast consistent with a benign mass. Diagnosis: serous cystadenoma. (B) Quick wash-in and slow wash-out is consistent with malignancy. Diagnosis: Stage 1 papillary serous cystadenocarcinoma.

impedance in the vasculature surrounding the neoplasms, and low impedance in these vessels indicates malignancy compared with high impedance in benign masses [3]. Some cut-off values of less than 1.0 for pulsatility index and less than 0.6 for resistivity index have been suggested [3].

3D ultrasound, power Doppler, and contrast-enhanced ultrasonography are also helpful but contrast is an expensive tool to aid in diagnosis and not individually superior to color Doppler ultrasound at this time [6,18].

Contrast agents and ovarian masses

In contrast-enhanced ultrasound studies, 2D or 3D power Doppler is utilized after injecting contrast medium and the pattern of blood flow is observed over time [19,20]. Other than morphology of blood flow patterns, the kinetics of wash-out and peak flow of contrast material have been studied. It was found that malignant ovarian neoplasms have slower wash-out of contrast compared with benign lesions [21–23]. It is controversial whether this technique adds to diagnostic accuracy and hence it is not recommended for screening of ovarian masses [8,24].

Utilizing other imaging modalities like MRI or PET scans has added to the sensitivity in detecting malignant ovarian neoplasms when combined with transvaginal ultrasonography [25].

Conclusion

Ultrasonography has been utilized extensively in gynecological diseases. Though its sensitivity in diagnosing benign conditions like teratomas and functional cysts is very high, the main outcome and modality of treatment depends on repeat imaging in 1–2 months in reproductive-age women. The advances in this noninvasive technology utilizing color or power Doppler, 3D or contrast-enhanced tools have aided in characterizing ovarian malignant neoplasms, but none of these tools has proven

to be superior to the others. Combination of ultrasound findings with clinical and laboratory evaluations may differentiate benign and malignant ovarian masses, but no single ultrasound technique has been standardized as a screening tool for ovarian cancer. Color Doppler is often utilized to diagnose torsion of ovarian cysts and also to characterize masses that are suspicious of malignancy.

References

1. Bottomley C, Bourne T. Diagnosis and management of ovarian cyst accidents. *Best Pract Res Clin Obstet Gynaecol* 2009; **23**(5): 711–724.

2. Osmers R. Sonographic evaluation of ovarian masses and its therapeutic implications. *Ultrasound Obstet Gynecol* 1996; **8**(4): 217–222.

3. Murta EF, Nomelini RS. Early diagnosis and predictors of malignancy of adnexal masses. *Curr Opin Obstet Gynecol* 2006; **18**(1): 14–19.

4. Levine D, Brown DL, Andreotti RF, et al. Management of asymptomatic ovarian and other adnexal cysts imaged at US: Society of Radiologists in Ultrasound consensus conference statement. *Radiology* 2010; **256**(3): 943–954.

5. Brown DL, Dudiak KM, Laing FC. Adnexal masses: US characterization and reporting. *Radiology*. 2010; **254**(2): 342–354.

6. Bell DJ, Pannu HK. Radiological assessment of gynecologic malignancies. *Obstet Gynecol Clin North Am* 2011; **38**(1): 45–68, vii.

7. Guerriero S, Alcazar JL, Pascual MA, et al. Diagnosis of the most frequent benign ovarian cysts: is ultrasonography accurate and reproducible? *J Womens Health* (Larchmt) 2009; **18**(4): 519–527.

8. Rao A, Carter J. Ultrasound and ovarian cancer screening: is there a future? *J Minim Invasive Gynecol* 2011; **18**(1): 24–30.

9. Kurjak A, Predanic M, Kupesic-Urek S, Jukic S. Transvaginal color and pulsed Doppler assessment of adnexal tumor vascularity. *Gynecol Oncol* 1993; **50**(1): 3–9.

10. Hassen K, Ghossain MA, Rousset P, et al. Characterization of papillary projections in benign versus borderline and malignant ovarian masses on conventional and color Doppler ultrasound. *AJR Am J Roentgenol* 2011; **196**(6): 1444–1449.

11. Murta EF, da Silva CS, Gomes RA, Tavares-Murta BM, Melo AL. Ultrasonographic criteria and tumor marker assay are good procedures for the diagnosis of ovarian neoplasia in preselected outpatients. *Eur J Gynaecol Oncol* 2004; **25**(6): 707–712.

12. van Nagell JR, Jr., DePriest PD, et al. The efficacy of transvaginal sonographic screening in asymptomatic women at risk for ovarian cancer. *Gynecol Oncol* 2000; **77**(3): 350–356.

13. Outwater EK, Siegelman ES, Hunt JL. Ovarian teratomas: tumor types and imaging characteristics. *Radiographics* 2001; **21**(2): 475–490.

14. Patel MD, Feldstein VA, Chen DC, Lipson SD, Filly RA. Endometriomas: diagnostic performance of US. *Radiology* 1999; **210**(3): 739–745.

15. Knudsen UB, Tabor A, Mosgaard B, et al. Management of ovarian cysts. *Acta Obstet Gynecol Scand* 2004; **83**(11): 1012–1021.

16. Daskalakis G, Kalmantis K, Skartados N, Thomakos N, Hatziioannou L, Antsaklis A. Assessment of ovarian tumors using transvaginal color Doppler ultrasonography. *Eur J Gynaecol Oncol* 2004; **25**(5): 594–596.

17. Kinkel K, Hricak H, Lu Y, Tsuda K, Filly RA. US characterization of ovarian masses: a meta-analysis. *Radiology* 2000; **217**(3): 803–811.

18. Alcazar JL, Castillo G. Comparison of 2-dimensional and 3-dimensional power-Doppler imaging in complex adnexal masses for the prediction of ovarian cancer. *Am J Obstet Gynecol* 2005; **192**(3): 807–812.

19. Kohzuki M, Kanzaki T, Murata Y. Contrast-enhanced power Doppler sonography of malignant ovarian tumors using harmonic flash-echo imaging: preliminary experience. *J Clin Ultrasound* 2005; **33**(5): 237–242.

20. Kupesic S, Kurjak A. Contrast-enhanced, three-dimensional power Doppler sonography for differentiation of adnexal masses. *Obstet Gynecol* 2000; **96**(3): 452–458.

21. Orden MR, Jurvelin JS, Kirkinen PP. Kinetics of a US contrast agent in benign and malignant adnexal tumors. *Radiology* 2003; **226**(2): 405–410.

22. Fleischer AC, Lyshchik A, Jones HW, 3rd, et al. Diagnostic parameters to differentiate benign from malignant ovarian masses with contrast-enhanced transvaginal sonography. *J Ultrasound Med* 2009; **28**(10): 1273–1280.

23. Marret H, Sauget S, Giraudeau B, et al. Contrast-enhanced sonography helps in discrimination of benign from malignant adnexal masses. *J Ultrasound Med* 2004; **23**(12): 1629–1639.

24. Fleischer AC, Lyshchik A, Jones HW, Jr., et al. Contrast-enhanced transvaginal sonography of benign versus malignant ovarian masses: preliminary findings. *J Ultrasound Med* 2008; **27**(7): 1011–1018.

25. Grab D, Flock F, Stohr I, et al. Classification of asymptomatic adnexal masses by ultrasound, magnetic resonance imaging, and positron emission tomography. *Gynecol Oncol* 2000; **77**(3): 454–459.

Ultrasound imaging of ovarian cancer

Osama M. Azmy and Amr Abbasy

Ovarian cancer is a silent killer, its management remains a common clinical problem in the practice of gynecology, and it continues to be a formidable challenge and elusive task. Ovarian cancer varies widely in frequency among different geographic regions and ethnic groups, with a high incidence in northern Europe and the United States and a low incidence in Japan [1]. It accounts for approximately 3% of all cancers in women and is the fifth leading cause of cancer-related death among women in the United States because ovarian cancer is often diagnosed at an advanced stage, after the cancer has spread beyond the ovary [2].

The incidence rate for ovarian cancer has been declining since the mid-1980s in the United States. Nevertheless, it has the highest mortality of all cancers of the female reproductive system. This reflects, in part, a lack of early symptoms and effective ovarian cancer screening tests. Furthermore, the majority of cases are sporadic, and only 5–10% of ovarian cancers are familial. White women have higher incidence and mortality rates than women of other racial and ethnic groups and it is estimated that approximately $4.4 billion is spent in the United States each year on ovarian cancer treatment [3].

Since the ultrasound evaluation of the female pelvis has been extensively studied, the normal and abnormal characteristics have been clarified. Thus, pelvic ultrasonography is the examination of choice and the most common scenario for investigating malignant ovarian tumors [4,5]. Although tumor markers, such as CA-125, have an important role in clinical evaluation of ovarian cancer, multiple recent studies have explored the superiority of ultrasound in both diagnosis and outcome in these women [6].

Ultrasound of ovarian cancer

Transvaginal ultrasonographic assessment has improved the visualization of the ovary and its morphology. Thus, normal ovarian anatomy and ovarian abnormality can be distinguished. Many studies have been done to define and standardize ovarian characteristics, which can be used as criteria to diagnose and evaluate ovarian cancer [7].

Ovarian size

Non-neoplastic ovarian and adnexal masses, such as functional cysts, tubal inflammatory diseases, and endometriosis, are usually smaller in size than reported in ovarian neoplasms. However, each of these non-neoplastic masses may have a sonographic appearance that mimics neoplastic appearance. Thus, other sonographic ovarian characteristics should be included, with ovarian size, during evaluation of ovarian masses [8,9].

The size of a normal ovary varies throughout a woman's life. Normal ovary measurements are $3.5 \times 2 \times 1.5$ cm in the premenopausal woman and $1.5 \times 0.7 \times 0.5$ cm 2–5 years after menopause [10]. Large ovarian mass, with other characteristics, has been proposed as significant in predicting ovarian cancer. Koonings et al. performed a study in 1989 on postmenopausal women and they concluded that ovarian masses exceeding 10 cm were significantly more likely to be associated with malignancy [11]. Many later studies have confirmed that the larger ovarian masses are significantly associated with an increased likelihood of ovarian cancer [6]. However, the incorporation of tumor size does not improve the accuracy of the morphologic criteria and is, therefore, not included in most of the more recent studies of ovarian masses. Ovarian lesions greater than 10 cm are difficult to assess morphologically. For ovarian masses less than 5 cm, sono-morphology and Doppler assessment are most efficacious [12]. With masses between 5 cm and 10 cm, determining a course of action should be individualized. The patient's age, history, symptoms, adequacy of the ultrasound examination, and possibly observation over 6–8 weeks should be considered.

Ovarian morphology

Many studies of ovarian cancer recognized neoplastic sonographic features to predict and diagnose ovarian neoplasms and to distinguish neoplastic ovarian masses from non-neoplastic masses.

Once an ovarian neoplasm is predicted, it is important to determine whether it is a benign or malignant neoplasm. A dermoid tumor of the ovary, or teratoma, is the most common

A

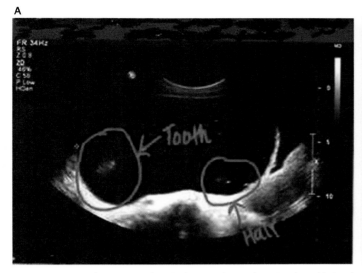

B

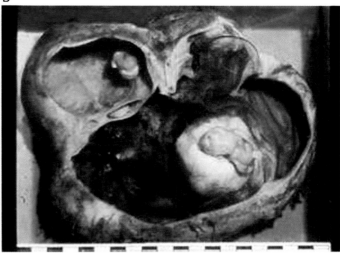

Fig. 22.1 Dermoid cyst as seen by 2D ultrasound; note that a tooth and hair tuft were suspected (A). This was confirmed by the postoperative findings (B).

benign ovarian neoplasm and it has several classic appearances. In most studies, dermoid tumors appear in ultrasound as a hyperechoic mass with acoustic attention, with/without hyperechoic fat-fluid level, with/without hyperechoic Rokitansky nodules, and with/without hyperechoic lines and punctate dots representing hair tufts (Fig. 22.1). However, dermoid tumors, due to their solid and echogenic appearance, may be misdiagnosed as malignant neoplasm [13].

Ovarian cancer can be predicted by its morphology. Sassone et al. proposed a scale for morphological ovarian characteristics, including inner wall structure, wall thickness, the presence of septa, and echogenicity of the mass (Table 22.1) [14,15].

Evaluation of the regularity of the ovarian cyst wall is valuable in studying ovarian mass (Fig. 22.2). Evaluating whether or not the ovarian cyst contains solid mass is important in suspecting ovarian malignancy, although this is a subjective method [16].

The risk of malignancy index (RMI) was developed to increase the predictive accuracy of diagnosing ovarian malignancy. It includes incorporating ultrasound impression, CA-125 level, and the menopausal state of the woman [17]. In 1999 a prospective study was done in nine centers from five countries (Belgium, Sweden, Italy, France, and the United Kingdom). The International Ovarian Tumor Analysis (IOTA) study has used quantitative and qualitative recognition algorithms to categorize the adnexal mass [7]. The masses are categorized into four subgroups according to their sonographic appearance: (1) unilocular cyst; (2) multilocular cyst; (3) presence of a solid component but not papillation; and (4) presence of papillation (Table 22.2).

Although sonographic characteristics of an ovarian mass can help clinicians diagnose ovarian cancer, it is not possible to recommend clinical management of an ovarian malignancy on the basis of the sonographic study only. Management of an ovarian malignancy depends on many other factors along with

ultrasound examination, such as symptoms, tumor marker levels, operative risk, and the patient's anxiety (Table 22.3). The Risk of Ovarian Malignancy Algorithm (ROMA) was devised to increase the sensitivity of diagnosing ovarian cancer [18]. The ROMA model utilizes the combination of human epididymis protein 4 (HE4) and CA-125 values to assess the risk of epithelial ovarian cancer in women with a pelvic mass. One hundred and four women were diagnosed with a pelvic mass (55 with epithelial ovarian cancer and 49 benign cases scheduled to have surgery were enrolled), along with 49 healthy females [18].

Separate logistic regression algorithms (ROMA) for premenopausal and postmenopausal women were used to categorize patients into low-risk and high-risk groups for epithelial ovarian cancer. The area under the curve, sensitivity, and specificity were calculated for HE4, CA-125, and ROMA for the diagnosis of ovarian cancer using receiver operating characteristic analysis. The study showed that the median CA-125 and HE4 serum concentrations were significantly higher in epithelial ovarian cancer women than in healthy females (both $P < 0.05$) and those with a benign mass (both $P < 0.05$). The premenopausal group included 36 benign cases (29 of which were classified by ROMA as low risk with a specificity of 80.6%) [18].

However, more recent studies have questioned these findings. A Dutch study compared the diagnostic accuracy of ROMA to the diagnostic accuracy of the two most widely used ultrasound methods: RMI and subjective assessment by ultrasound [19]. Four hundred and thirty-two women with a pelvic mass who were scheduled to have surgery were enrolled in a prospective cohort study. The diagnostic accuracy and performance indices of ROMA, RMI, and subjective assessment were calculated after surgery. Subjective assessment had the highest area under the receiver operator characteristic curve (0.968, 95% CI 0.945–0.984), followed by RMI (0.931, 95% CI 0.901–0.955). Subjective assessment and RMI both had significantly higher area under the curve than ROMA (0.893, 95% CI

Table 22.1 Variables considered for association with the type of ovarian mass (benign, malignant)

1. Continuous demographic characteristics

· Age	· Number of years postmenopause
· Parity	

2. Continuous grayscale ultrasound findings

· Maximal diameter of the lesion (mm)	· Volume of lesion (mL)
· Fluid in the anteroposterior plane of the pouch of Douglas (mm)	· Thickness of the thickest septum where it appeared to be at its thickest (mm)
· Height of largest papillary projection (mm)	· Maximal diameter of papillary projection (mm)
· Ratio between the volume of the largest papillary projection and the volume of the lesion	· Number of separate papillary projections (1, 2, 3, or >3)
· Number of locules (0, 1, 2, 3, 4, 5–10, or >10)	· Maximum diameter of the largest solid component (mm)
· Volume of the largest solid component (mL)	· Ratio between the volume of the largest solid component and the volume of the lesion

3. Continuous blood flow indices

· Pulsatility index	· Resistance index
· Peak systolic velocity (cm/s)	· Time-averaged maximum velocity (cm/s)

4. Categorical characteristics

· Tumor type (unilocular, unilocular-solid, multilocular, multilocular-solid, solid, not classifiable)	· Echogenicity of cyst fluid (anechoic, low-level, ground-glass, hemorrhagic, mixed echogenicity, no cyst fluid)
· Color score (no flow, minimal flow, moderately strong flow, very strong flow according to subjective evaluation of the color content of the tumor scan at color Doppler examination)	

5. Tumor markers

· CA-125	· HE4

6. Binary variables

· First-degree relatives with ovarian cancer	· First-degree relatives with breast cancer
· Personal history of ovarian cancer	· Personal history of breast cancer
· Nulliparous	· Hysterectomy
· Postmenopausal	· Hormone therapy
· Postmenopausal bleeding within 1 year before the ultrasound examination	· Bilateral lesions
· Pain during the ultrasound examination	· Ascites
· Incomplete septum	· Papillation
· Flow within at least one of the papillary projections	· Irregular papillary projection
· Irregular cyst walls	· Acoustic shadows
· Venous blood flow only	

0.857–0.922; $P < 0.0001$ and $P = 0.0030$, respectively). The pre- and postmenopausal populations generated similar results. Therefore, although new tumor marker models are promising, they do not contribute significantly to the diagnosis of ovarian cancer.

Ultrasound, especially subjective assessment by ultrasound, remains superior in discriminating malignant from benign ovarian masses and clinicians should consider ultrasound examination as the primary tool in their work to diagnose ovarian cancer along with other clinical, laboratory, and radiology studies. Another study from Italy showed that lesion size can affect the diagnostic performance of the IOTA logistic regression models, the IOTA simple rules, and RMI to estimate the risk of malignancy in adnexal masses [20]. A moderate amount of cul-de-sac fluid in a postmenopausal patient should increase the index of suspicion for an ovarian malignancy. Unfortunately, this sign is usually only present with advanced ovarian carcinoma [21]. The presence of normal ovarian tissue adjacent to an adnexal mass has been described as the ovarian crescent sign (Fig. 22.3). In one observational study of 100 women with adnexal masses, the absence of an ovarian crescent sign had a sensitivity of 96% and a specificity of 76% for the diagnosis of ovarian carcinoma [22]. However, this sign cannot differentiate between benign and borderline tumors. In addition, it is more difficult to document this sign in the postmenopausal age group.

Doppler study

Doppler study to examine ovarian vascularity can evaluate neovascularity of ovarian neoplasms. Doppler study, in

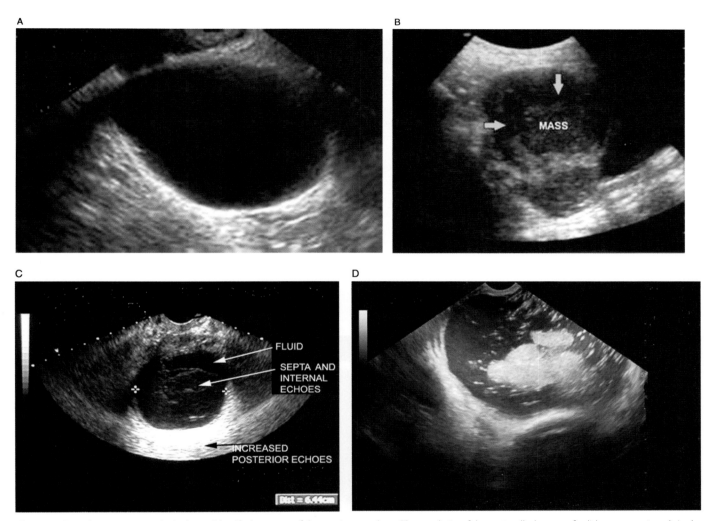

Fig. 22.2 Several parameters are looked at to identify the nature of the ovarian neoplasm. The regularity of the cyst wall, absence of solid component, and single cyst is in favor of a benign nature as seen in (A), while the presence of complex structure with septa, internal solid elements, and multilocular character is in support of malignant behavior (B, C, D).

Table 22.2 Selected historical comparisons of ultrasound and clinical criteria for cancer prediction

Study	No. of patients	Characteristics	Accuracy
Sassone et al. [14]	143	Grayscale characteristics score	Sensitivity, 100%; specificity, 83%; PPV, 37%; NPV, 100%
Fleischer et al. [23]	43	Pulsatility index	Pulsatility index; sensitivity, 100%; specificity, 82%; PPV, 73%; NPV, 100%
Fleischer et al. [24]	50	Color and spectral Doppler characteristics	Other variables significant
UKCTOCS [5]	50 640	Multi-technique screening (ultrasound and serum CA-125)	Sensitivity, 89%; specificity, 99%; PPV, 35%; NPV, 99%
IOTA [7]	1 573	Combined grayscale and color mapping, age, and other clinical variables	AUC = 0 0.96; pattern recognition: sensitivity, 90%; specificity, 88%; logistic regression: sensitivity, 95%; specificity, 74%; and subgroup category: sensitivity, 88%, specificity, 90%

UKCTOCS = United Kingdom Collaborative Trial of Ovarian Cancer Screening; IOTA = International Ovarian Tumor Analysis Group; PPV = positive predictive value; NPV = negative predictive value; AUC = area under the receiver operating characteristic curve.

Table 22.3 Differential diagnosis of selected causes of adnexal masses

Diagnosis	Possible symptoms	Examination findings	Suggested laboratory testing	Suggested imaging
Ectopic pregnancy	Lower abdominal (usually unilateral and severe) or pelvic pain	Adnexal mass or tenderness; hypotension; tachycardia	Blood type and Rh; CBC; quantitative β-hCG	Transvaginal ultrasonography
Endometrioma	Abnormal uterine bleeding; dyspareunia; worsening pain with menses	Adnexal mass or tenderness; tenderness over uterosacral ligaments	–	Transvaginal ultrasonography
Leiomyoma	Dysmenorrhea; menorrhagia	Abdominal mass; uterine enlargement	–	Transabdominal or transvaginal ultrasonography
Ovarian cancer	Abdominal fullness and pressure; back pain; bloating; constipation; difficulty eating; early satiety; fatigue; increased abdominal size; indigestion; lack of energy; pelvic or abdominal pain; urinary urgency, frequency, or incontinence; weight loss	Abdominal or adnexal mass; ascites; lymphadenopathy; nodularity of uterosacral ligaments; pleural effusion	Cancer antigen 125; inhibin A and B (if granulosa cell tumor); serum α-fetoprotein (if germ cell tumor); quantitative β-hCG (if germ cell tumor)	Transabdominal or transvaginal ultrasonography; computed tomography of the head, chest, and abdomen (to rule out metastasis

A B

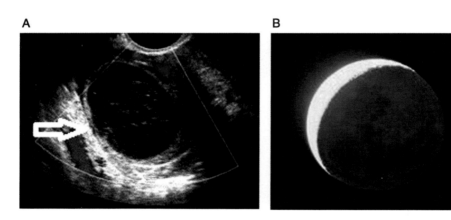

Fig. 22.3 The presence of the ovarian crescent sign is confirmatory of the origin of the adnexal cyst. It can be seen with ordinary 2D ultrasound (white arrow in A) and it becomes more obvious with CT scanning (B).

combination with other ultrasound markers, often has a role in the management of ovarian cancer.

The vascular characteristics of a malignant neoplasm often differ from those of a benign neoplasm. Malignant lesions usually show angiogenesis that produces an increase in neovascularization, causing a significant increase in color Doppler flow signals. The color content of the tumor reflects the vascularity better than any other parameters of Doppler. The number, size, and functional capacity of the tumor vessels are concluded from overall evaluation of tumor vascularity [23,24].

One hundred and twenty-one women with adnexal masses were examined over a period of 2 years in India, out of which 60 women with neoplastic ovarian tumors were retained as study subjects. Color Doppler showed blood flow in 92.59% of malignant tumors in contrast to only 42.24% of benign tumors [25]. Absent blood flow in a solid tumor almost always ruled out the possibility of malignancy. Spectral Doppler helped to assess the nature of the blood vessels picked up on color Doppler. More than 95% of the malignant tumors had a pulsatility index (PI) less than 0.8 in contrast to only 6.06% of benign tumors. Similarly, 92.59% of the malignant tumors showed a

resistance index (RI) less than 0.6 in contrast to only 9.09% of the benign tumors. Thus, color Doppler and spectral Doppler markedly increased the reliability in diagnosing a malignant ovarian tumor.

The IOTA study has described a color score for the assessment of the blood flow in ovarian masses. This color score evaluates the tumor as a whole: color score 1, no detectable blood flow; score 2, minimal flow; score 3, moderate flow; and score 4, highly vascular tumor [7].

While benign lesions often exhibit their increased flow signals only at the periphery of the mass, malignancies often exhibit their increased flow signals at both the periphery and central regions of the mass, including within septations and solid tumor areas (Fig. 22.4). The neovascularity within malignancy is formed by multiple abnormal small blood vessels that lack smooth muscle within their wall and contain multiple arteriovenous shunts [26]. Therefore, Doppler study of malignant neoplasms reveals low-impedance flow with PI below 1.0 and RI below 0.4. The blood flow in malignant neovascularity shows high time-averaged maximum velocity, higher than 15 cm/s, and an absence of a diastolic notch (Fig. 22.5).

A

B

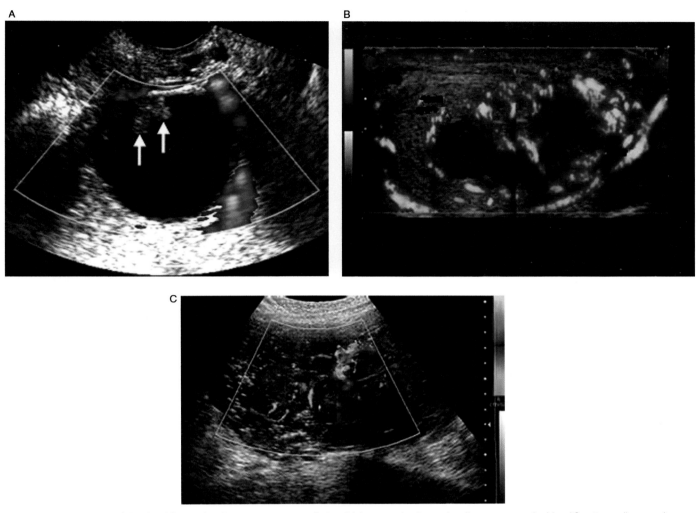

C

Fig. 22.4 Doppler study of the blood flow within the ovarian mass can distinguish between benign and malignant nature; the blood flow is usually around the periphery in benign cysts even if it contains a solid component (A) where the arrows point to a solid part lacking flow within. However, due to increased neoangiogenesis, blood flow tends to be around and inside the mass in malignant neoplasms (B and C).

Nevertheless, there is an overlap of vascular parameters between benign and malignant neoplasms. Thus, it is not possible to differentiate with high accuracy between benign and malignant neoplasms based on spectral Doppler evaluation alone [27].

Three-dimensional ultrasound and power Doppler

Three-D ultrasound is a new imaging technique that has become available in clinical practice. It is being increasingly used in women with gynecologic cancer. A systematic review [28] critically examined the current evidence on the role of this technique in this clinical setting. The authors included 46 studies using 3D ultrasound in women with gynecological cancer (28 studies involving ovarian cancer, 15 studies involving endometrial cancer, and 6 studies involving cervical cancer). Most studies were prospective and observational. Moreover, the series were small in most of them. Ten studies addressed the

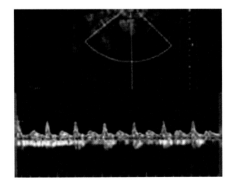

Fig. 22.5 Estimating the blood flow characteristics in ovarian malignancies shows low-impedance flow that is reflected in both a low pulsatility index and resistance index.

technical and reproducibility issues. All of them demonstrated that 3D ultrasound is a reproducible technique among examiners. Studies involving ovarian cancer showed that grayscale 3D ultrasound is not superior to conventional 2D ultrasound for

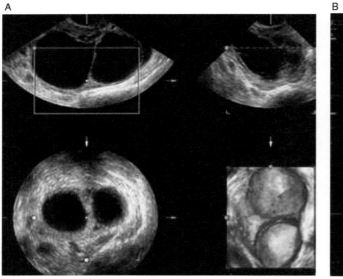
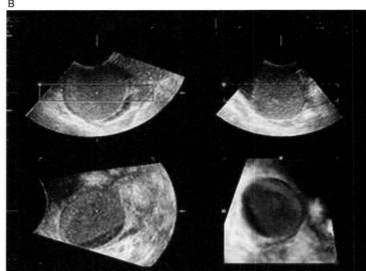
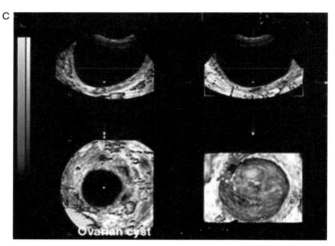

Fig. 22.6 3D ultrasound can show more detailed anatomy of the ovary. This may have an impact on the differentiation between benign and malignant neoplasms. This is obvious in A and B, where the inside of the cyst can be seen with great precision and any solid component is seen clearly. Adding Doppler to 3D can also help in delineating benign from malignant masses, as seen in part C.

predicting ovarian cancer. Tumor vascular assessment by 3D power Doppler showed that this method might be useful in a selected subset of adnexal masses.

The application of 3D ultrasound and power Doppler imaging facilities, as a secondary screening test preceded by transvaginal ultrasound and transvaginal color Doppler as a primary screening test for ovarian malignancy, was set up to represent a new approach for the early and accurate detection of ovarian cancer through screening [29]. 3D power Doppler imaging better defines the morphological and vascular characteristics of ovarian lesions. Although both 2D and 3D imaging can identify ovarian malignancies, the specificity was significantly improved with the addition of 3D power Doppler [30]. This improved diagnostic accuracy may promote differentiation between benign and malignant ovarian masses and might be useful in some clinical circumstances (Fig. 22.6).

Conclusion

Subjective assessment of grayscale and Doppler ultrasound features by an experienced sonographer is an excellent method for discriminating between benign and malignant adnexal masses. Ultrasound study is superior to serum CA-125 in the diagnosis of benign and malignant ovarian masses. However, it is recommended to use ultrasound examination in conjunction with other clinical and laboratory studies to increase the diagnostic accuracy of differentiating between the benign and malignant potential of an adnexal mass.

References

1. Holschneider CH, Berek JS. Ovarian cancer: epidemiology, biology, and prognostic factors. *Semin Surg Oncol* 2000; **19**(1): 3–10.

2. Cancer Statistics Working Group. United States Cancer Statistics: 1999–2008 Incidence and Mortality Web-based Report. Atlanta (GA): Department of Health and Human Services, Centers for Disease Control and Prevention, and National Cancer Institute; 2012.

3. Cancer Trends Progress Report (http://progressreport.cancer. gov).

4. Granberg S, Wikland M, Jansson I. Macroscopic characterization of ovarian tumors and the relation to the histological diagnosis: criteria to be used for ultrasound evaluation. *Gynecol Oncol* 1989; **35**: 139–144.

5. Menon U, Gentry-Maharaj A, Hallett R, et al. Sensitivity and specificity of multimodal and ultrasound screening for ovarian cancer, and stage distribution of detected cancers: results of the prevalence screen of the UK Collaborative Trial of Ovarian Cancer Screening (UKCTOCS). *Lancet Oncol* 2009; **10**(4): 327–340.

6. Van Calster B, Timmerman D, Bourne T, et al. Discrimination between benign and malignant adnexal masses by specialist ultrasound examination versus serum CA-125. *J Natl Cancer Inst* 2007; **99**: 1706–1714.

7. Timmerman D, Valentin L, Bourne TH, et al. Terms, definitions and measurements to describe the sonographic features of adnexal tumors: a consensus opinion from the International Ovarian Tumor Analysis (IOTA) group. *Ultrasound Obstet Gynecol* 2000; **16**: 500–505.

8. Twickler DM, Moschos E. Ultrasound and assessment of ovarian cancer risk. *AJR Am J Roentgenol* 2010; **194**: 322–329.

9. Twickler DM, Forte TB, Santos-Ramos R, et al. The ovarian tumor index predicts risk for malignancy. *Cancer* 1999; **86**: 2280–2290.

10. Herrmann UJ. Sonographic patterns of ovarian tumors. *Clin Obstet Gynecol* 1993; **36**: 375–383.

11. Koonings PP, Campbell K, Mischell DR Jr, Grimes DA. Relative frequency of primary ovarian neoplasm: a 10-year review. *Obstet Gynecol* 1989; **74**: 921–926.

12. Kinkel K, Hricak H, Lu Y, et al. US characterization of ovarian masses: a meta-analysis. *Radiology* 2000; **217**: 803–811.

13. Timmerman D. Lack of standardization in gynecological ultrasonography. *Ultrasound Obstet Gynecol* 2000; **16**: 395–398.

14. Sassone AM, Timor-Trish IE, Artner A, et al. Transvaginal sonographic characterization of ovarian disease: evaluation of a new scoring system to predict ovarian malignancy. *Obstet Gynecol* 1991; **78**: 70–76.

15. Timmerman D, Testa AC, Bourne T, et al. Logistic regression model to distinguish between the benign and malignant adnexal mass before surgery: a multicenter study by the International Ovarian Tumor Analysis Group. *J Clin Oncol* 2005; **23**: 8794–8801.

16. Ameye L, Valentin L, Testa AC, et al. A scoring system to differentiate malignant from benign masses in specific ultrasound-based subgroups of adnexal tumors. *Ultrasound Obstet Gynecol* 2009; **33**: 92–101.

17. van den Akker PA, Aalders AL, Snijders MP, et al. Evaluation of the Risk of Malignancy Index in daily clinical management of adnexal masses. *Gynecol Oncol* 2010; **116**(3): 384–388.

18. Bandiera E, Romani C, Specchia C, et al. Serum human epididymis protein 4 and risk for ovarian malignancy algorithm as new diagnostic and prognostic tools for epithelial ovarian cancer management. *Cancer Epidemiol Biomarkers Prev* 2011; **20**(12): 2496–2506.

19. Van Gorp T, Veldman J, Van Calster B, et al. Subjective assessment by ultrasound is superior to the risk of malignancy index (RMI) or the risk of ovarian malignancy algorithm (ROMA) in discriminating benign from malignant adnexal masses. *Eur J Cancer* 2012; **5**: 163–169.

20. Di Legge A, Testa A, Ameye L, et al. Lesion size affects the diagnostic performance of the International Ovarian Tumor Analysis logistic regression models, the IOTA simple rules and the Risk of Malignancy Index to estimate the risk of malignancy in adnexal masses. *Ultrasound Obstet Gynecol* 2012; **18**: 298–305.

21. Osmers RGW, Osmers M, Von Maydell B, et al. Preoperative evaluation of ovarian tumors in the premenopausal by transvaginosonography. *Am J Obstet Gynecol* 1996; **175**: 428–434.

22. Hillaby K, Aslam N, Salim R, et al. The value of detection of normal ovarian tissue (the "ovarian crescent sign") in the differential diagnosis of adnexal masses. *Ultrasound Obstet Gynecol* 2004; **23**: 63–67.

23. Fleischer AC, Rodgers WH, Kepple DM, et al. Color Doppler sonography of ovarian masses: a multi-parameter analysis. *J Ultrasound Med* 1993; **12**: 41–48.

24. Fleischer AC, Cullinan JA, Peery CV, Jones HW III. Early detection of ovarian carcinoma with transvaginal color Doppler ultrasonography. *Am J Obstet Gynecol* 1996; **174**: 101–106.

25. Taori KB, Mitra KR, Ghonge NP, Ghonge SN. Doppler determinants of ovarian malignancy: experience with 60 patients. *Ind J Radiol Imaging* 2002; **12**(2): 245–249.

26. Guerriero S, Alcazar JL, Ajossa S, et al. Transvaginal color Doppler imaging in the detection of ovarian cancer in a large study population. *Int J Gynecol Cancer* 2010; **20**(5): 781–786.

27. Valentin L. Gray scale sonography, subjective evaluation of the color Doppler image and measurement of blood flow velocity for distinguishing benign and malignant tumors of suspected adnexal origin. *Eur J Obstet Gynecol Reprod Biol* 1997; **72**: 63–72.

28. Alcázar JL, Jurado M. Three-dimensional ultrasound for assessing women with gynecological cancer: a systematic review. *Gynecol Oncol* 2011; **120**(3): 340–346.

29. Kurjak A, Prka M, Arenas JM, et al. Three-dimensional ultrasonography and power Doppler in ovarian cancer screening of asymptomatic peri- and postmenopausal women. *Croat Med J* 2005; **46**(5): 757–764.

30. Cohen LS, Escobar PF, Scharm C, et al. Three-dimensional power Doppler ultrasound improves the diagnostic accuracy for ovarian cancer prediction. *Gynecol Oncol* 2001; **82**(1): 40–48.

Ultrasound imaging of endometrial cancer

Osama M. Azmy and Haitham Badran

Introduction

There is a worldwide trend for increasing endometrial cancer as it is the fourth most common malignancy in women in the United States, with more than 23 000 new cases each year and 6300 deaths occurring annually [1]. The incidence has increased by almost 38% (from 120 per 100 000 in 1994 to 163 per 100 000 in 2006) in the United Kingdom over the past two decades [2]. In New Zealand and some Asian countries this incidence is even higher – 1.5–2.5 times higher than European rates [3]. This increase in the rate of endometrial cancer relates to rising obesity [4], falling fertility, and the aging of the population. Most women with endometrial cancer are postmenopausal and present with vaginal bleeding [5,6]. Therefore, the majority of them will have endometrial sampling with an endometrial biopsy or dilatation and curettage performed. Endometrial cancer is detected in between 5% and 60% of these postmenopausal women with vaginal bleeding, depending on age and other risk factors (Table 23.1).

Normal ultrasonographic endometrial pattern

In most women, transvaginal sonography (TVS) of the endometrium and uterine cavity should be the preferred method of scanning the uterus in order to obtain valuable data. Nonetheless, a transabdominal scan may be required in the presence of large fibroids, a globally enlarged uterus, or when a transvaginal scan is considered inappropriate (e.g. declined, virgins, vaginismus, or secondary vaginal stenosis). If the transabdominal scan is inconclusive, a transrectal ultrasound examination should be considered. The use of transabdominal sonography in the detection of endometrial pathology is well documented. Limited spatial resolution, obesity, retroflection, and multiple leiomyomas of the uterus, however, can occasionally make assessment of the endometrial stripe using the transabdominal route technically difficult. With the advent of endovaginal sonography, these technical limitations have largely been overcome. Moreover, the greater resolution afforded with the higher-frequency endovaginal probe can improve the detection of endometrial carcinoma and other endometrial abnormalities.

A prospective study of TVS and transabdominal sonography by Tsuda et al. in 1995 compared transabdominal ultrasound to TVS for endometrial cancer screening among 91 postmenopausal women [7]. The mean endometrial thickness estimated by the vaginal route was larger than that obtained by the transabdominal method. Furthermore, the sensitivity and specificity of transabdominal sonography were 83.3% and 58.8%, respectively, compared with 100% and 54.1%, respectively, for TVS [7]. Moreover, they reported that endovaginal scans yielded new information in 60% of cases and allowed better visualization of pelvic structures in 22% of cases. The clinical diagnosis was altered on the basis of endovaginal sonographic findings in 24% of women and confirmed with certainty in 72% of them.

Technique of TVS

It is recommended that a relatively strict scanning routine should be followed and an empty bladder is needed. Overfilling of the bladder will cause cephalad displacement or retroversion of the uterus, pushing it out of the imaging plane. Higher frequency transducers (5–7.5 MHz) are used, allowing better resolution of structures in close proximity of the probe. The disadvantage of TVS is the limited field of view. Therefore, a quick scan of the pelvis using the abdominal probe with a full bladder may be advisable to detect big masses that are too far from the tip of the transducer, and hence out of the view. The transducer is covered with a condom containing a transducer gel. Then, the probe is introduced into the vagina and placed close to the cervix for optimal visualization of the uterus and ovaries. In the beginning, as the vaginal probe advances, the cervix is scanned and the uterus evaluated. This is followed by scanning of the ovaries, tubes, and cul-de-sac. Finally, other planes and structures can be studied. Coronal and sagittal planes are examined by moving the probe from side to side. Variations in depth of the probe insertion optimize visualization of the uterus, as does having the woman tilt her pelvis up to facilitate scanning of the uterine fundus (Fig. 23.1).

Ultrasonography in Gynecology, ed. Botros R. M. B. Rizk and Elizabeth E. Puscheck. Published by Cambridge University Press. © Cambridge University Press 2015.

Table 23.1 Risk factors for endometrial cancer and their associated relative risk

Factor	Relative risk
Long-term use of high-dosage and/or unopposed menopausal estrogens	10–20
High cumulative doses of tamoxifen	3–7
Estrogen-producing tumor	>5
Obesity	
BMI 30–34 kg/m²	1.7[a]
BMI 35–39 kg/m²	4.3[a]
BMI ≥40 kg/m²	6.4[a]
Nulliparity	3
Diabetes, hypertension, thyroid or gallbladder disease	1.3–3
Older age	2–3
History of infertility	2–3
Late age at natural menopause (older than 52 years)	2–3
Early age at menarche (younger than 12 years)	1.5–2
Menstrual irregularities	1.5
White race	2
Long-term use of high dosages of combination oral contraceptives	0.3–0.5 (decreased risk)
Cigarette smoking	0.5 (decreased risk)

BMI, body mass index.

[a] Compared with women who have a BMI of 20–24 kg/m².

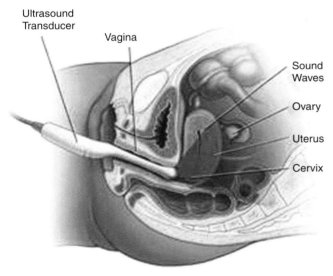

Fig. 23.1 Schematic representation of transvaginal sonography. Note the close proximity of the probe to the pelvic organs but with limited view.

Orientation of vaginal images

On the sagittal longitudinal plane, the bladder appears on the upper left side of the screen, with the cervix to the right of the picture, while on the cross-sectional plane, the patient's right side will appear on the left side of the screen. Images obtained by TVS do not usually correspond to the normal anatomical planes, since the vagina runs superiorly and posteriorly and the pelvis itself is tilted at an angle of 30 degrees to the longitudinal axis of the body. Therefore, instead of referring to coronal and sagittal planes, the terminology of trans-pelvic and anteroposterior planes is more appropriately used. Another orientation approach is to focus on target organs rather than anatomic planes: "organ-oriented scanning." An evaluation of endometrial morphology includes an assessment of endometrial echogenicity, the endometrial midline, and the endometrial–myometrial junction.

The echogenicity of the endometrium is described as hyperechogenic, isoechogenic, or hypoechogenic compared with the echogenicity of the myometrium. The endometrial echogenicity is usually defined as "uniform" if the endometrium is homogeneous, with symmetrical anterior and posterior sides. This definition includes the different appearances seen throughout the menstrual cycle and the monolayer pattern found in most postmenopausal patients. A uniform endometrium includes the three-layer pattern, as well as the homogeneous hyperechogenic, hypoechogenic, and isoechogenic endometrium (Fig. 23.2).

The echogenicity is defined as "non-uniform" if the endometrium appears heterogeneous, asymmetrical, or cystic. Also, the endometrial midline is defined as "linear, non-linear, or irregular." A linear endometrial line is seen when a straight hyperechogenic interface within the endometrium is visualized. A non-linear endometrial line is seen when a waved hyperechogenic interface is observed. An irregular or undefined endometrial line is seen when there is an absence of a distinct interface (Fig. 23.3).

The "bright edge" is the echo formed by the interface between an intracavitary lesion and the endometrium. In some women, the endometrial interface is better detected by gently pushing the transvaginal probe against the uterine corpus, which makes the two endometrial surfaces slide against each other ("the sliding sign"). This technique may help characterize pathology, as also small amounts of fluid in the cavity may help delineate structures in the cavity (Fig. 23.4). The endometrial–myometrial junction is described as "regular," "irregular," "interrupted," or "not defined." Intracavitary fluid is described as "anechogenic or of low-level echogenicity," "ground glass," or of "mixed" echogenicity.

Endometrial thickness is measured from the highly reflective interface of the junction of the endometrium and myometrium. This measurement represents two layers of the endometrium. The measurement should not include the surrounding low-amplitude echo layer, as this represents the inner layer of the compact and vascular myometrium. If fluid appears to separate the endometrial cavity, a single wall thickness should be taken. It is recommended that the endometrial thickness be measured on the longitudinal axis image of the uterus rather than on the axial scan because of more reliable and reproducible plane selection (Fig. 23.5). On the other hand, endometrium of

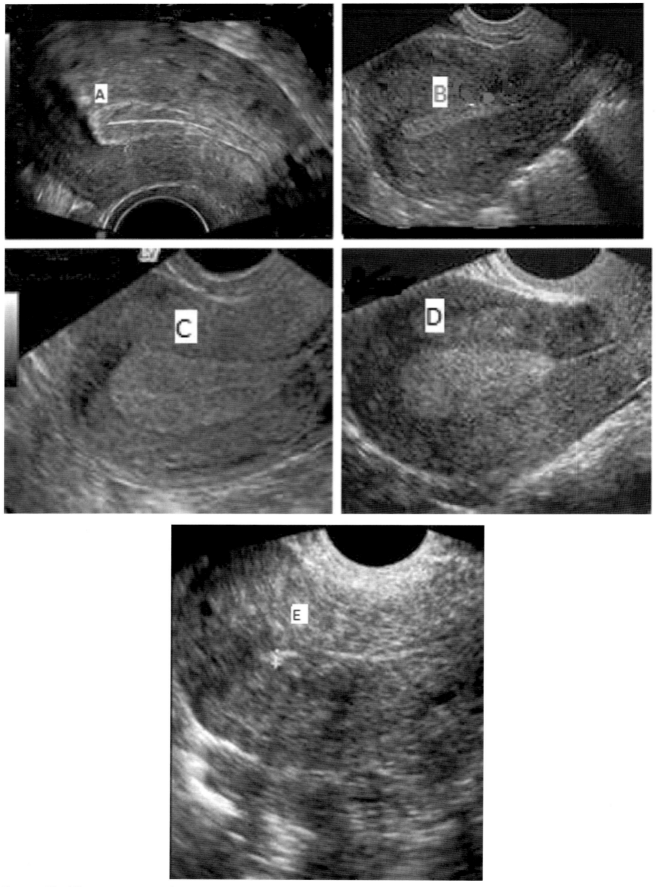

Fig. 23.2 The different presentations of a normal endometrium during the menstrual cycle. (A) The triple line appearance during the follicular phase; (B) the endometrium during the immediate postmenstrual days; (C) the endometrium during the luteal phase; (D) ultrasound image of the endometrium just premenstrual (note the change in endometrial thickness and echogenicity); (E) the thin normal monolayer state of the endometrium during the menopause.

normal thickness may appear falsely thickened if oblique slices are taken, or if there is a mass in the endometrial cavity that is isoechoic with the endometrium.

Grayscale ultrasound and endometrial cancer

Over recent years TVS has significantly improved our ability to accurately diagnose and manage intrauterine abnormalities. TVS scanning is an excellent tool for the determination of whether further investigation with curettage or some form of endometrial biopsy is necessary. Before menopause, a sonographic examination should preferably be performed in the early proliferative phase (cycle days 4–6), while in postmenopausal women on cyclic hormonal replacement therapy it should be performed 5–10 days after the last progestin tablet [8,9].

The chief goal of TVS examination of the endometrium is to exclude pathological conditions and thereby make endometrial sampling unnecessary. Many published studies have assessed the accuracy of TVS in evaluating the endometrium for malignancy. Thin endometrium generally is considered normal, whereas thickened endometrium may represent cancer, hyperplasia, or polyps. In a study by Goldstein [10], it was reported that a thin, distinct endometrial echo on TVS has a risk of malignancy of 1 in 917 and does not require an endometrial biopsy. If the endometrial echo is poorly visualized, then in such women, saline infusion sonohysterography is an appropriate next step. The prevalence of asymptomatic endometrial thickening (mostly due to inactive polyps) is

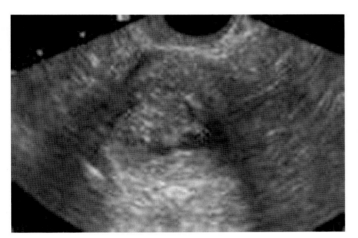

Fig. 23.3 Irregular endometrium with no clear demarcation between the myometrium and the endometrium (isoechoic appearance).

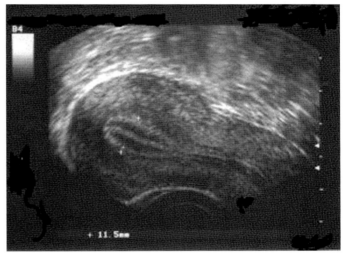

Fig. 23.5 Sagittal view of the uterus showing endometrial thickness of 11.5 mm. The measurement is taken between the highly reflective interface of the junction between the endometrium and myometrium on both sides.

A   B

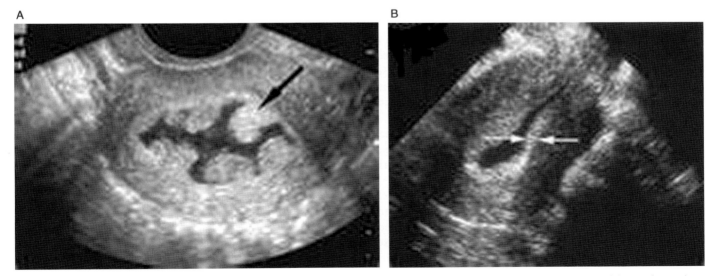

Fig. 23.4 (A) shows the bright edge echo between an intracavitary polyp and the myometrium (black arrow), while the white arrows in (B) delineate the regular endometrial line. Note that a minimal amount of fluid in the uterine cavity allows better visualization and differentiation between different uterine layers and intracavitary pathology.

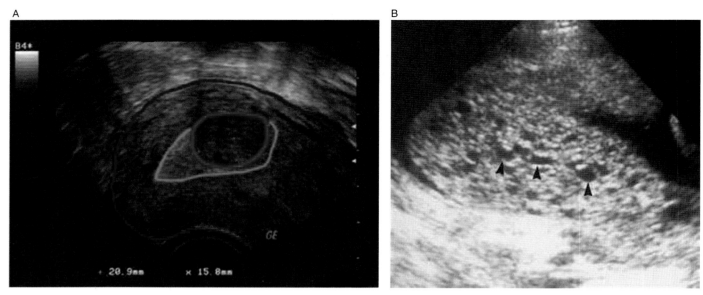

Fig. 23.6 Endometrial cancer appearances on transvaginal ultrasonography as hyperechoic thickened endometrium (green line) or hypoechoic (red color) in a postmenopausal woman are highly suggestive of endometrial cancer (A); also areas of degeneration and bleeding can be seen (black arrowheads, B).

approximately 10–17% of postmenopausal women. The risk of malignancy in such polyps is low (approximately 0.1%), as well as in structures that mimic polyps (0.3%). Thus, automatic intervention in such women, without any high-risk status, is not warranted.

Moreover, the Nordic multicenter study evaluated the predictive value of endometrial thickness to exclude endometrial abnormalities in postmenopausal women. Endometrial thickness of less than 4 mm had a negative predictive value of 100% for endometrial cancer [11]. The ACOG Committee Opinion [12] reviewed the use of TVS in the evaluation of postmenopausal bleeding. The opinion clarified that an endometrial biopsy or TVS may be used in the initial evaluation of postmenopausal bleeding, but both tests may not be necessary. It further concluded that "when an endometrial thickness less than or equal to 4 mm is found, endometrial sampling is not required." However, when the endometrium cannot be reliably assessed by ultrasonography in women with postmenopausal bleeding because of marked obesity, myomas, or other anatomic limitations, an alternative method of evaluation is necessary.

In women with postmenopausal bleeding, a simple measurement of endometrial thickness can reliably discriminate between women who are at low or high risk of endometrial cancer (Fig. 23.6).

Endometrial thickness of 4 mm or less decreases the likelihood of endometrial cancer by a factor of ten in both users and non-users of hormone replacement therapy. In a retrospective observational study in Belgium on 187 women diagnosed with endometrial malignancy with endometrial thickness <5 mm in which an ultrasound evaluation of the endometrium had been performed before the diagnosis [13], it was shown that the median endometrial thickness was 15 mm. In

13 women (6.9%), the endometrial thickness was <5 mm. The characteristics of those patients presenting with an endometrial thickness <5 mm were analyzed. In 12 of these patients, the measurement was compromised in some way. Nine of these patients had undergone endometrial sampling before the ultrasound examination. In two cases, focal malignant lesions were not included in the recorded endometrial thickness. Then, in one case, the endometrial thickness was visualized poorly due to myometrial distortion. Finally, in only one case was the endometrium correctly measured to be <5 mm; this woman had diffuse uterine and endometrial metastases of a breast cancer.

In another retrospective study at the University of Göteborg, Gull and his colleagues evaluated 394 women with postmenopausal bleeding and TVS measurement of endometrial thickness as predictors of endometrial cancer and atypical hyperplasia [14]. These women were followed for at least 10 years after referral for postmenopausal bleeding. In their study, it was possible to assess the medical records in 86% of women. Thirty-nine of the 339 women (11.5%) had endometrial cancer and five women (1.5%) had atypical hyperplasia. The relative risk of endometrial cancer in women who were referred for postmenopausal bleeding was 63.9 (95% CI 46.0–88.8); the corresponding relative risk for endometrial cancer and atypical hyperplasia together was 72.1 (95% CI 52.8–98.5), as compared with women of the same age from the general population of the same region of Sweden. No woman with an endometrial thickness of ≤4 mm was diagnosed as having endometrial cancer. The relative risk of the development of endometrial cancer in women with an endometrial thickness of >4 mm was 44.5 (95% CI 6.5–320.1) compared with women with an endometrial thickness of ≤4 mm [14].

The reliability of endometrial thickness (cut-off value, ≤4 mm) as a diagnostic test for endometrial cancer was assessed with a sensitivity of 100%, specificity of 60%, positive predictive value of 25%, and negative predictive value of 100%. Furthermore, the incidence of endometrial cancer or atypical hyperplasia in women with an intact uterus whose cases had been followed for ≥10 years was 5.8% (15/257 women) as compared with 22.7% (15/66 women) of women who had only one episode of recurrent bleeding [14]. No endometrial cancer was diagnosed in women with recurrent postmenopausal bleeding who had an endometrial thickness of ≤4 mm at the initial scan. Thus, in the high-risk group of women, i.e. those with an endometrial thickness of 5 mm or more, an evaluation of endometrial morphology and vascularization using gray-scale and Doppler ultrasound imaging [15] with or without the added use of sonohysterography [16] can be used to further refine the estimation of risk of pathology and in particular the risk of endometrial cancer.

The usefulness of an ultrasound examination of the endometrium in premenopausal women with bleeding problems is much less obvious. A prospective Danish study [17] recruited 355 premenopausal women with abnormal uterine bleeding and indications for endometrial sampling or surgery from two centers. The thickness of the endometrium was measured, and the midline echoes were evaluated using TVS. The findings from the endometrial sampling were combined with the evaluation of the uterine cavity using operative hysteroscopy in 115 women, hysterectomy in 74 women, and hysterosonographic examination in 166 women for use as the true values. The mean endometrial thickness was significantly different in women with hyperplasia 11.5±5 mm, polyps 11.8±5.1 mm, submucous myomas 7.1±3.4 mm, and in women without these abnormalities 8.37±3.9 mm. Hyperplasia and/or polyps were present in 20% of all women, and in 8% of 143 women with an endometrial thickness of ≤7 mm. This proportion did not decrease with lower cut-off levels for endometrial thickness. Receiver operating characteristic curves were not optimal for excluding hyperplasia or polyps by endometrial thickness. In 173 women with a distinct, regular midline echo without echo-dense foci in TVS, the proportion of women with abnormalities was 16%. This proportion did not decrease with cut-off levels for endometrial thickness. Accordingly, the use of TVS with low levels of endometrial thickness reduced the possibility of abnormalities such as polyps and hyperplasia, but did not exclude them and low cut-off levels for endometrial thickness did not increase the diagnostic performance in cases with normal sonograms.

Saline infusion sonography

In saline infusion sonography (also known as sonohysterography), sterile saline is instilled into the uterine cavity before ultrasound evaluation to allow for more precise visualization of the endometrial structures. Saline infusion sonography is often used as a second step in the evaluation of abnormal bleeding. It is particularly useful when ultrasonography suggests a focal

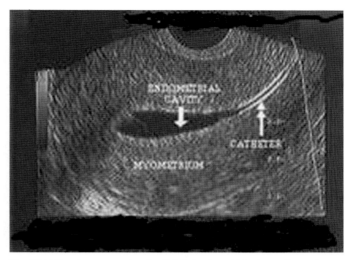

Fig. 23.7 Sonohysterography after fluid injection within the uterine cavity. This technique is helpful to delineate intracavitary lesions but with the risk of disseminating cancer cells into the peritoneal cavity.

lesion, when endometrial biopsy is non-diagnostic, or when abnormal bleeding persists despite normal initial workup (Fig. 23.7). If a focal lesion is noted on saline infusion sonography, hysteroscopy with directed biopsy is traditionally indicated. However, newer techniques are being developed that combine saline infusion hysterography with endometrial sampling under direct visualization, with highly accurate results [18]. Saline infusion sonography should not be performed if endometrial biopsy detects malignant cells or when ultrasonography suggests endometrial cancer because of concerns of peritoneal spread [19].

Doppler and endometrial cancer

Color Doppler has an important role in evaluating the endometrial cavity at risk of cancer. It is considered a reliable method for assessing endometrial angiogenesis. The color and power Doppler box should include the endometrium with the surrounding myometrium. Magnification and settings should be adjusted to ensure maximal sensitivity for blood flow (ultrasound frequency of at least 5.0 MHz, pulse repetition frequency of 0.3–0.9 kHz, wall filter of 30–50 Hz, and color power Doppler gain should be reduced until all color artifacts disappear). The vascular pattern within the endometrium is reported with respect to the presence or absence of "dominant vessels" or of other specific patterns. Dominant vessels are defined as one or more distinct vessels (arterial and/or venous) traversing the endometrial–myometrial junction. This dominant vessel may show branching within the endometrium, which may be described as either orderly or disorderly/chaotic. Furthermore, the dominant vessel may present as a single vessel (formerly referred to as the "pedicle artery sign") with or without branching. Multiple dominant vessels may have a "focal origin" at the endometrial–myometrial junction or may have a "multifocal origin." Other vascular patterns within the

A

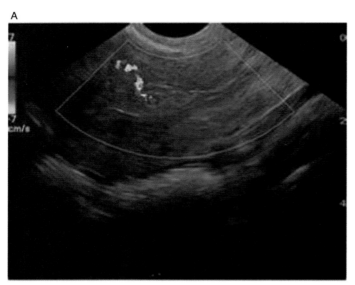

B

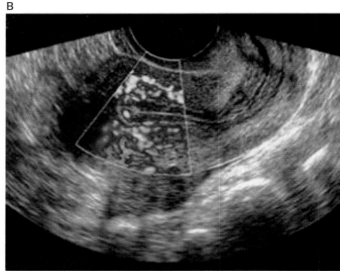

Fig. 23.8 Doppler blood flow study of the endometrium. A. Normal blood flow within the endometrium in a premenopausal woman. B. Increased blood flow in a woman who had proven endometrial cancer after surgery.

endometrium include scattered vessels (dispersed color signals within the endometrium but without visible origin at the myometrial–endometrial junction) and circular flow (Fig. 23.8).

Studies indicate that blood flow rates correspond with increased angiogenesis in endometrial cancers and might potentially be used as a good prediction factor for tumor progression and metastasis in affected women. To investigate the diagnostic value of blood flow measurements in endometrial, myometrial, and uterine vasculature by transvaginal Doppler ultrasonography in the differentiation of the neoplastic endometrial pathologies in women with postmenopausal bleeding, Bezircioglu and colleagues [20] enrolled 106 women who presented with postmenopausal bleeding in a prospective cohort study. Endometrial thickness, pulsatility index (PI), and resistance index (RI) of the uterine, myometrial, and endometrial vasculature and endometrial histopathology were measured by transvaginal Doppler sonography. Dilatation and curettage were performed for all women. Endometrial malignancy was diagnosed in 24 of the patients (22.7%). Endometrial thickness was found to be higher in women with malignant histopathology compared with women who had benign histopathology. Statistically, uterine artery PI, RI, radial artery PI, spiral artery PI, and RI were also significantly lower in patients with malignant histopathology. According to ROC curve analysis, endometrial thickness of 5 mm, uterine artery PI of 1.45, uterine artery RI of 0.72, radial artery PI of 1.06, and radial artery RI of 0.65 were defined as the cut-off points. The multivariate regression model showed only that uterine artery PI is an independent determinant of malignant endometrium. The authors concluded that uterine artery blood flow and also vasculature displayed lower impedance in patients with malignant indices and are not yet adequate for use as diagnostic tests.

Transvaginal color and pulsed Doppler ultrasound was carried out by Sawicki et al. [21] on 90 women with uterine

cancer in order to determine the location and intensity of angiogenesis as well as selected flow parameters, and to evaluate the relation of myometrial invasion, histological grading, lymph nodes, and omental and adnexal metastasis to blood flow characteristics in endometrial cancer. The degree of invasion as well as adnexal, omental, and pelvic lymph node metastasis were assessed. Location of the blood vessels (peripheral, central, mixed) and vascular density, as well as selected Doppler blood flow indices, peak systolic velocity (PSV), and RI of neoplastic infiltration were assessed. The median age of the women was 63.3 ± 12.3 years; of these women, 92.2% were postmenopausal. Cancer concerned only the endometrium in 14.4%, with superficial and deep infiltration established in 45.6%, and 40%, respectively. The histological maturity was as follows: grade 1 (17.6% of cases), grade 2 (66.7% of cases), and grade 3 (16.6% of cases). Adnexal, omental, and lymph node metastasis was found in 12.2%, 3.3%, and 16.6%, respectively. Abnormal low impedance and high velocity flow (mean RI 0.38 ± 0.09, PSV 20.45 ± 9.6 cm/s) were found in 88.9% of women. Peripheral and mixed vascularity were found more frequently in all women and a positive significant correlation was found between vascular density increase and the surgical-pathological stage of cancer. There were significant differences in vascular density, Doppler blood flow indices, and vascular location in each type of histological malignancy. Also, there were significant differences in vascular density in lymph node-positive women whereas there were no significant differences in each flow parameter in hematogenous-adnexal/omental metastatic and non-metastatic women.

Color Doppler also may distinguish between different intracavitary pathologies by the pedicle artery test and may replace more invasive established second-stage tests, such as saline contrast sonohysterography and office hysteroscopy. Furthermore, advanced tumors often have higher color score and multiple globally entering vessels, whereas less advanced tumors are more often hyperechoic and have no or a low color score.

A prospective observational study involving 3099 consecutive women referred for assessment of the endometrium and myometrium was carried out by Timmerman et al. in 2003. The uterus was assessed in sagittal and coronal planes using color Doppler sonography. Women with suspected endometrial pathology on sonography were noted and the volume of the focal lesion was calculated [22]. Women with a clearly visible pedicle artery reaching the central part of the endometrium were regarded as test-positive. The gold standard was defined as the presence or absence of an endometrial polyp at hysterectomy, hysteroscopy, and/or endometrial histology on dilatation and curettage within 1 year of sonography. Of the 3099 women, 2230 did not meet the gold standard. Only 28 of the 199 women who were test-positive did not meet the gold standard. In the 869 women in whom a gold standard was met, 182 had one or more endometrial polyps. The pedicle artery test had an apparent sensitivity for detection of endometrial polyps of 76.4%, specificity of 95.3%, positive predictive value of 81.3%, and negative predictive value of 93.8%. When extending the test to the prediction of any focal intracavitary pathology, the positive predictive value was 94.2%.

Another prospective multicenter study was performed in Sweden to describe the grayscale and vascular characteristics of endometrial cancer in relation to stage, grade, and size using two-dimensional and three-dimensional TVS [23]. The study included 144 women with endometrial cancer who were undergoing TVS before surgery. The sonographic characteristics assessed were echogenicity, endometrial/myometrial border, fibroids, vascular pattern, color score, and tumor/uterus anteroposterior ratio. Histological assessment of tumor stage, grade, type, and growth pattern was performed. Hyperechoic or isoechoic tumors were more often seen in stage IA cancer, whereas mixed or hypoechoic tumors were more often found in cancers of stage IB or greater. Hyperechogenicity was more common in grade 1–2 tumors (well or moderately differentiated) and in tumors with a tumor/uterine anteroposterior ratio of <50%. A non-hyperechoic appearance was more commonly found in grade 3 tumors (poorly differentiated) and in tumors with a tumor/uterine anteroposterior ratio of ≥50%. Multiple global vessels were more often seen in tumors of stage IB or greater (rather than in stage IA tumors), in grade 3 tumors (rather than in grade 1 and 2 tumors), and in tumors with a tumor/uterine anteroposterior ratio of ≥50%. A moderate/high color score was significantly more common in tumors of higher stage and larger size.

Three-dimensional ultrasound and endometrial cancer

Three-D ultrasound is an imaging technique that has become widely available in clinical practice. It is increasingly being used in women with gynecological cancer and current evidence demonstrates that it is a reproducible technique among examiners and might be useful in some clinical circumstances. Three-D ultrasound is even useful to determine myometrial infiltration in women with endometrial cancer. However, the role of 3D power Doppler in endometrial cancer is controversial and further studies are still needed to establish its role in clinical practice in gynecologic oncology.

A meta-analysis from Spain looking at 15 prospective and observational studies involving endometrial cancer showed that endometrial volume estimation is more specific than endometrial thickness measurement for predicting endometrial cancer. Moreover, it concluded that this method is useful for determining myometrial infiltration in women with endometrial cancer [24].

Combining 3D ultrasound with Doppler analysis of tumor vascularization in endometrial cancer may correlate with some prognostic histological characteristics. In order to assess the correlation between intra-tumor vascularization using 3D power Doppler angiography (3D-PDA) and several histological tumor characteristics, a cohort of 99 women with endometrial carcinoma were assessed [25]. The mean age of the women was 61.7 years. The women were diagnosed as having endometrial cancer and assessed by transvaginal 3D-PDA before surgical staging. Endometrial volume and 3D-PDA vascular indices (vascularization index, flow index, and vascularization flow index) were calculated using the virtual organ computer-aided analysis method and all women were surgically staged. Individual tumor features such as histological type, tumor grade, myometrial infiltration depth, lymph-vascular space involvement, cervical involvement, lymph node metastases, and tumor stage were considered for analysis. Multivariate logistic regression analysis was used to determine which 3D-PDA parameters were independently associated with each histological characteristic. The multi-variant logistic regression analysis showed that only endometrial volume and vascularization index were independently associated with myometrial infiltration and tumor stage (OR 1.119 [95% CI 1.025–1.221]; 1.127 [95% CI 1.063–1.195]), respectively. Only vascularization index was independently associated with tumor grade (OR 1.056 [95% CI 1.023–1.091]), while endometrial volume was independently associated with lymph node metastases (OR 1.086 [95% CI 1.017–1.161]).

Tips for clinical practice

- Most women with endometrial cancer are postmenopausal.
- They usually present with recurrent attacks of postmenopausal bleeding.
- Simple measurement of endometrial thickness by TVS is the first line of investigation.
- Postmenopausal bleeding and endometrial thickness <5 mm are unlikely to be of malignant origin.
- Color Doppler may also distinguish between different intracavitary pathology using the pedicle artery test.

- Endometrial volume by 3D ultrasound may have better predictive value than endometrial thickness.
- The role of 3D power Doppler in endometrial cancer is still controversial.

References

1. Duong LM, Wilson RJ, Ajani UA, et al. Trends in endometrial cancer incidence rates in the United States, 1999–2006. *J Womens Health* 2011; **20**(8): 1157–1163.

2. Evans T, Sany O, Pearmain P, et al. Differential trends in the rising incidence of endometrial cancer by type: data from a UK population-based registry from 1994 to 2006. *Br J Cancer* 2011; **104**(9): 1505–1510.

3. Blakely T, Shaw C, Atkinson J, et al. Social inequalities or inequities in cancer incidence? Repeated census-cancer cohort studies, New Zealand 1981–1986 to 2001–2004. *Cancer Causes Control* 2011; **22**(9): 1307–1318.

4. Lambe M, Wigertz A, Garmo H, et al. Impaired glucose metabolism and diabetes and the risk of breast, endometrial, and ovarian cancer. *Cancer Causes Control* 2011; **22**(8): 1163–1171.

5. Jillani K, Khero RB, Maqsood S, Siddiqui MA. Prevalence of malignant disorders in 50 cases of postmenopausal bleeding. *J Pak Med Assoc.* 2010; **60**(7): 540–543.

6. Burbos N, Musonda P, Crocker SG, et al. Outcome of investigations for postmenopausal vaginal bleeding in women under the age of 50 years. *Gynecol Oncol* 2012; **125**(1): 120–123.

7. Tsuda H, Kawabata M, Kawabata K, Yamamoto K, Hidaka A, Umesaki N. Comparison between transabdominal and transvaginal ultrasonography for identifying endometrial malignancies. *Gynecol Obstet Invest* 1995; **40**(4): 271–273.

8. Dijkhuizen FP, Brölman HA, Potters AE, Bongers MY, Heinz AP. The accuracy of transvaginal ultrasonography in the diagnosis of endometrial abnormalities. *Obstet Gynecol* 1996; **87**: 345–349.

9. Omodei U, Ferrazzi E, Ramazzotto F, et al. Endometrial evaluation with transvaginal ultrasound during hormone therapy: a prospective multicenter study. *Fertil Steril* 2004; **81**: 1632–1637.

10. Goldstein SR. Significance of incidentally thick endometrial echo on transvaginal ultrasound in postmenopausal women. *Menopause* 2011; **18**(4): 440–442.

11. Karlsson B, Granberg S, Wikland M, et al. Transvaginal ultrasonography of the endometrium in women with postmenopausal bleeding – a Nordic multicenter study. *Am J Obstet Gynecol* 1995; **172**: 1488–1494.

12. ACOG Committee Opinion No. 426: the role of transvaginal ultrasonography in the evaluation of postmenopausal bleeding. *Obstet Gynecol* 2009; **113**: 462–464.

13. Van den Bosch T, Van Schoubroeck D, Domali E, et al. A thin and regular endometrium on ultrasound is very unlikely in patients with endometrial malignancy. *Ultrasound Obstet Gynecol* 2007; **29**: 674–679.

14. Gull B, Karlsson B, Milsom I, Granberg S. Can ultrasound replace dilation and curettage? A longitudinal evaluation of postmenopausal bleeding and transvaginal sonographic measurement of the endometrium as predictors of endometrial cancer. *Am J Obstet Gynecol* 2003; **188**: 401–408.

15. Epstein E, Skoog L, Isberg PE, et al. An algorithm including results of gray-scale and power Doppler ultrasound examination to predict endometrial malignancy in women with postmenopausal bleeding. *Ultrasound Obstet Gynecol* 2002; **20**: 370–376.

16. Epstein E, Valentin L. Gray-scale ultrasound morphology in the presence or absence of intrauterine fluid and vascularity as assessed by color Doppler for discrimination between benign and malignant endometrium in women with postmenopausal bleeding. *Ultrasound Obstet Gynecol* 2006; **28**: 89–95.

17. Dueholm M, Jensen ML, Laursen H, Kracht P. Can the endometrial thickness as measured by trans-vaginal sonography be used to exclude polyps or hyperplasia in pre-menopausal patients with abnormal uterine bleeding? *Acta Obstet Gynecol Scand* 2001; **80**: 645–651.

18. Moschos E, Ashfaq R, McIntire DD, Liriano B, Twickler DM. Saline-infusion sonography endometrial sampling compared with endometrial biopsy in diagnosing endometrial pathology. *Obstet Gynecol* 2009; **113**(4): 881–887.

19. Amant F, Moerman P, Neven P, et al. Endometrial cancer. *Lancet* 2005; **366**: 491–505.

20. Bezircioglu I, Baloglu A, Cetinkaya B, Yigit S, Oziz E. The diagnostic value of the Doppler ultrasonography in distinguishing the endometrial malignancies in women with postmenopausal bleeding. *Arch Gynecol Obstet* 2012; **285**(5): 1369–1374.

21. Sawicki V, Spiewankiewicz B, Stelmachów J, Cendrowski K. Color Doppler assessment of blood flow in endometrial cancer. *Eur J Gynaecol Oncol* 2005; **26**(3): 279–284.

22. Timmerman D, Verguts J, Konstantinovic ML, et al. The pedicle artery sign based on sonography with color Doppler imaging can replace second-stage tests in women with abnormal vaginal bleeding. *Ultrasound Obstet Gynecol* 2003; **22**(2): 166–171.

23. Epstein E, Van Holsbeke C, Mascilini F, et al. Gray-scale and color Doppler ultrasound characteristics of endometrial cancer in relation to stage, grade and tumor size. *Ultrasound Obstet Gynecol* 2011; **38**(5): 586–593.

24. Alcázar JL, Jurado M. Three-dimensional ultrasound for assessing women with gynecological cancer: a systematic review. *Gynecol Oncol.* 2011; **20**(3): 340–346.

25. Galván R, Mercé L, Jurado M, Mínguez JA, López-García G, Alcázar JL. Three-dimensional power Doppler angiography in endometrial cancer: correlation with tumor characteristics. *Ultrasound Obstet Gynecol* 2010; **35**(6): 723–729.

Use of ultrasound imaging in "one-stop" fertility diagnosis

Geeta Nargund

The first advertisement using the term "one-stop shop" was in a local newspaper in Lincoln, Nebraska in 1930 with the strapline: "Have it all done in one place. Save your time. Save your money." This ideal is essentially what is offered by one-stop fertility treatment. For the infertile couple "save your time" has even greater significance, for it essentially implies "save your fertility potential" because age is the greatest adverse prognostic factor contributing to female infertility. Another adverse factor is stress and there is nothing more stressful than uncertainty and delay. Unfortunately, infertility investigations are frequently strung out over many months and the process is not only lengthy, but frequently repetitive. For the older woman especially, this delay significantly reduces her chances of successful treatment. One-stop fertility testing is therefore rational and desirable, because it can provide valuable information about fertility potential within one hour during one visit.

The aim is to complete investigations within one hour, providing time for discussions with a fertility expert who will discuss management options with the couple. Investigation of the woman is based upon the availability of high-quality ultrasound equipment with Doppler and (preferably) 3D facilities, and usually involves assessment of tubal patency. Investigations on the male partner are run in parallel, and semen analysis results should be available for the post-test discussions.

The fertility scan

The ultrasound scan performed for the one-stop fertility investigation should be called the "fertility scan" (as opposed to the gynecological scan or the early pregnancy scan), as this is targeted to address specific questions concerning the fertility potential of the woman. The scan should be performed at a time which maximizes the amount and quality of information provided, and should therefore be between days 10 and 12 of a 28-day menstrual cycle. Clearly some compromise has to be made as to the timing of this scan, for most studies on ovarian reserve assessment are performed on days 2–3. However, in our experience, the advantages of determining whether a "good" dominant follicle is present, the improved ability to diagnose polycystic ovaries, and the ability to assess the endometrial response to follicular development all favor performing the scan on days 10 to 12.

The scan must be performed transvaginally and the equipment should be of high resolution with sensitive color and spectral Doppler modalities. A three-dimensional (3D) facility, while not essential, can provide additional valuable information, and in future 3D color power angiography (3D-CPA) may become an essential prerequisite.

A summary of the checklist for the fertility scan is given below:

Fertility scan (days 10 to 12 of a 28-day menstrual cycle)

• Uterus:
    position, mobility
    dimensions
    congenital anomaly (3D)
    fibroids/adenomyosis
    uterine cavity investigation by hydrosonography
    uterine blood flow; uterine artery pulsatility index (PI); peak systolic velocity (PSV)
• Endometrium:
    thickness
    morphology
    color or power Doppler assessment
• Ovary:
    morphology: normal, polycystic, or multicystic
    position and mobility
    volume/antral follicle count (AFC)
    stromal blood flow (PSV)
    identification of cysts, endometrioma, dermoid, etc.
    Doppler assessment of cyst
    dominant follicle; mean diameter
    perifollicular blood flow
    fallopian tube; hysterosalpingo-contrast-sonography (HyCoSy)
    presence of hydrosalpinx
• Pouch of Douglas:
    free fluid
    masses

Ultrasonography in Gynecology, ed. Botros R. M. B. Rizk and Elizabeth E. Puscheck. Published by Cambridge University Press. © Cambridge University Press 2015.

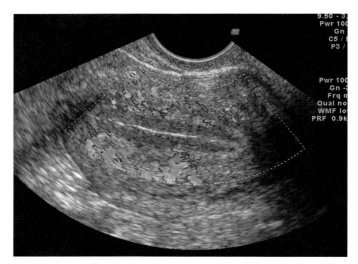

Fig. 24.1 Pre-ovulatory, triple-layer endometrium with good spiral artery flow.

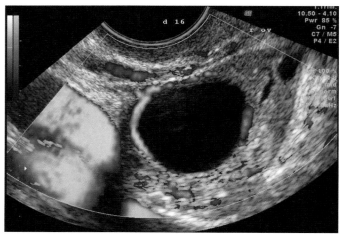

Fig. 24.2 Pre-ovulatory follicle with good perifollicular vascularity.

Ideally the scan should show an anteverted uterus of approximately 75 mm in length (from fundus to cervix), with normal myometrium and a triple-layer endometrium of greater than 7 mm thickness. A clear layer of mucus in the cervical canal is a favorable sign. Blood flow in the uterine arteries should show good diastolic velocities with a mean PI of less than 3. Endometrial color Doppler should demonstrate vessels (spiral arteries) extending into the triple layer (Fig. 24.1).

There should be a dominant follicle in one of the ovaries of about 16–18 mm in diameter with a circle of blood vessels around the follicle demonstrated on color or power Doppler (Fig. 24.2), with a peak systolic velocity of 5–10 cm/s. The stroma of each ovary should contain four or five late antral follicles (mean diameter greater than 5 mm) and the stromal blood flow velocity should be around 6–12 cm/s. Mobility of the pelvic organs is an important feature and movement of the ovaries in relation to the uterus in response to abdominal palpation should be clearly demonstrated.

Unfavorable features would be large fibroids close to the endometrium, evidence of adenomyosis, an echogenic or thin endometrium, an endometrial polyp greater than 5 mm in diameter, high-resistance uterine artery blood flow, polycystic ovaries or ovaries with no dominant follicle, few late antral follicles (combined total less than 5), low ovarian volume (nondominant ovary less than 3 mL), and low-velocity stromal blood flow (PSV less than 6 cm/s). A poorly mobile uterus or ovary is another unfavorable sign. These ultrasound results are considered together with the woman's follicle-stimulating hormone (FSH) and anti-müllerian hormone (AMH) levels, which for women over 35 years are routinely estimated on days 1 to 3 of the cycle by the patient's general practitioner.

Immediately following the fertility scan, HyCoSy is performed using initially negative contrast (saline) to outline the endometrium, which is followed by positive contrast (Echovist, Schering AG, Berlin, Germany) to demonstrate the medium in the fallopian tubes and the spill of medium into the peritoneal cavity. This is carried out under antibiotic prophylaxis. It is now our policy to routinely perform a 3D scan to obtain a coronal plane of the uterus to identify congenital defects such as subseptate uterus or uterus didelphys and also to demonstrate the precise position of submucous fibroids (Fig. 24.3A and B). All patients have *Chlamydia* screening and those with irregular cycles have prolactin and thyroid function assays performed.

Rationale

The importance of excluding gross abnormalities of the uterus and ovaries, such as large fibroids or complex ovarian cysts, is self-evident. Large fibroids that grossly distort the endometrial cavity, or endometrial polyps greater than 5 mm, require removal before fertility treatment begins. Similarly, large complex ovarian cysts will require removal prior to treatment. However, for endometriotic cysts less than 5 cm, previous surgery to the ovaries or the patient's age may indicate a need to proceed with treatment without delay. These gross abnormalities would of course be detected by a standard gynecological scan performed at any time during the menstrual cycle. Nevertheless, the fertility scans described above have a greater agenda: the evaluation of the fertility potential of the woman. That analysis together with the partner's semen results will have a bearing on which type of treatment should be offered or indeed whether treatment should be offered at all.

Polycystic ovaries

Ovarian morphology can be accurately assessed by ultrasound. On days 10 to 12 of the cycle, normal ovaries can easily be differentiated from those that are polycystic, which by definition have more than 12 small antral follicles in each ovary. Even without evidence of polycystic ovarian syndrome (PCOS), polycystic ovaries (PCO) are an important diagnosis as this also has significant implications for treatment. First, the fertility scan should be able to differentiate ovulatory from anovulatory PCO. Second, patients with PCO who may require ovarian

A   B

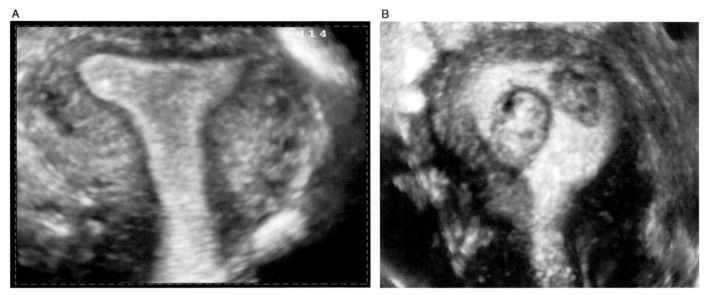

Fig. 24.3 3D transverse coronal view of the cavity of a normal uterus (A) and one containing submucous fibroids (B).

stimulation are more likely to develop ovarian hyperstimulation syndrome (OHSS). The use of Doppler to assess ovarian stromal flow in women with PCO may have a useful predictive role for the future development of OHSS. Patients with PCO who have a high ovarian stromal flow are more likely to be at risk of ovarian hyperstimulation during treatment.

Ovarian reserve

The role of ultrasound in the assessment of ovarian reserve is becoming more widely recognized [1]. This assessment is based principally on the measurement of ovarian volume and counting the number of late antral follicles in each ovary. When the ovarian volume is less than 3 mL or there are fewer than five antral follicles between the two ovaries, ovarian reserve is diminished. Ovarian volume is more precisely measured by 3D ultrasound, but the standard technique of measuring three orthogonal diameters in centimeters and multiplying this by the constant 0.5233 provides acceptable results. There have been a number of papers extolling the value of 3D automatic calculations [2,3] for the number of antral follicles. However, the standard 2D measurement is accurate, especially (and very importantly) when the AFC is low and when the 3D method may be less efficient.

Another parameter in estimating ovarian reserve is the Doppler measurement of peak systolic velocity in stromal vessels [4]. This is a simple technique and it only takes a few seconds to gate out one or two stromal vessels to measure the peak systolic velocity. Difficulty in visualizing stromal vessels [5] or vessels with velocities of less than 6 cm/s indicates reduced ovarian reserve. One of the questions to be addressed is whether hormonal ovarian reserve testing performed on days 2 to 3 of the cycle provides better (or different) information on ovarian reserve than the ultrasound parameters described above. There

is no clear answer at the present time for there are advocates for both methods [6,7], with some recommending a cumulative score of hormonal and ultrasound parameters [8,9]. It is possible that those who favor hormonal assessment have no advanced ultrasound facilities in their service with which to make a fair comparison. Certainly in our practice we have found ultrasound parameters predictive of an ovarian response during treatment. However, for women more than 35 years of age, it is advisable to obtain a days 2 to 3 FSH or AMH level prior to the one-stop visit so that all the results can be discussed with the couple after the fertility scan.

Dysfunctional ovulation

Failure to demonstrate a dominant follicle or the presence of a functional cyst indicates ovarian dysfunction and requires further investigation. Even the presence of a dominant follicle of an appropriate size does not guarantee that it contains an oocyte of good quality. Demonstration of perifollicular flow on color or power Doppler is a depiction of angiogenesis in the theca interna [10], which is itself essential for the production of a good-quality oocyte. It has been shown that there is a positive correlation between peak systolic velocity in the perifollicular vessels and the production of a good-quality embryo during in vitro fertilization (IVF) cycles [11]. Even the demonstration of power Doppler signals around more than 50% of the follicular perimeter is associated with a good-quality oocyte [12]. It is, therefore, an important part of the fertility scan to demonstrate perifollicular vascularity as an indicator of a normal ovulatory process.

Endometrial receptivity

An important aspect of the fertility scan is examination of the endometrium in the assessment of endometrial receptivity. In this regard, ultrasound is unique for there is no other practical method of making this evaluation. Previous methods of analyzing endometrial receptivity have revolved around obtaining endometrial tissue for histology and its correlation with various biochemical and molecular markers. However, this process lacked both specificity and practicality. The assessment of endometrial receptivity at the fertility scan is based on endometrial thickness and the morphological appearance of the endometrium in conjunction with an estimation of uterine artery blood flow velocities using Doppler ultrasound.

A trilaminar appearance with a minimum thickness of 7 mm and a uterine artery pulsatility index of less than 3 are regarded as reliable markers of good endometrial receptivity. More recently, the visualization of spiral arteries "pallisading" into the endometrium has been shown to correlate with good receptivity. Most of the evidence for this comes from studies performed during IVF cycles, but it is likely that the same inferences can be drawn from the finding of poor endometrial blood flow during a fertility scan. The latest 3D studies where endometrial and subendometrial vascularity is assessed using semi-quantitative indices (vascularization index [VI], flow index [FI], and vascularization-flow index [VFI]) demonstrate reduced endometrial vascularity and flow in women with unexplained infertility [13]. In the future, improved understanding of the inter-relation between specific hormonal, angiogenic, and molecular factors and morphological and vascular parameters on ultrasound imaging will allow us to formulate reliable ultrasonographic criteria to determine receptivity [14,15].

Tubal patency assessment

Normal tubes are not visible with ultrasound imaging unless there is fluid within the pouch of Douglas. However, hydrosalpinges are generally visible and can be clearly delineated by operators with moderate experience. The gold standard for confirmation of tubal patency has historically been either X-ray hysterosalpingography (HSG) or laparoscopy with chromopertubation. There is a growing body of opinion against performing routine laparoscopy for tubal evaluation due to its expense and increased morbidity. The old argument that the pelvic organs could be examined at the same time has little support now, because although laparoscopy is better able to identify extra ovarian endometriosis and adhesions, ultrasound provides more comprehensive information without morbidity.

The development of HyCoSy offers an alternative to HSG as it appears to provide similar information with respect to both the uterine cavity and tubal patency [16,17]. It has the additional patient benefit of being combined with the fertility scan and is carried out by the same team who will be responsible for her fertility management. In other words, there is a seamless progression from the fertility scan to tubal evaluation. Furthermore, hydrosonography is part of the HyCoSy test so endometrial evaluation is improved. Recent evidence suggests, at least from the patient's perspective, that HyCoSy is a more acceptable investigation than HSG [18]. Total pain scores for HyCoSy are reported to be significantly less than for HSG in

the majority of patients. The instigation of a HyCoSy-based tubal investigation service reduces the number of laparoscopies and allows patients to proceed to corrective surgery without resorting to a second planned operative procedure [19]. The original HyCoSy technique recommended injecting 10 mL of Echovist into each fallopian tube through a balloon catheter. We have adapted the original HyCoSy technique to even further reduce any side effects by:

1. Injecting only 2–5 mL of Echovist very slowly into each tube.
2. Dispensing with the balloon catheter and using a fine, intrauterine insemination catheter instead.

These modifications do not reduce the effectiveness of the technique and our patients have had very little pain or other side effects since we adopted this policy. A further refinement, which has been shown to reduce pelvic discomfort, is warming the Echovist to room temperature before the procedure [20].

Although HyCoSy is a standard part of the one-stop fertility assessment, there are circumstances when it should not be performed. For example, when there is a severe male factor problem, ovarian reserve is low, or there are bilateral hydrosalpinges, IVF is the only treatment option, so there is no need to carry out an unnecessary invasive procedure. Also, if there is any evidence of a low-grade pelvic infection it would be unwise to proceed to HyCoSy for this could precipitate an acute infection.

Evidence

It is extremely difficult, if not impossible, to perform a randomized study comparing the diagnostic information obtained in a conventional, multi-visit infertility workup to a one-stop clinic. Our group has been practicing an ultrasound-based one-stop assessment for 10 years [10,21], and we would not contemplate returning to the prolonged, rather unfocused workup which previously existed. The concept of a focused one-hour diagnostic workup with a management plan at the end seems to us to be ideal. We have analyzed 154 sequential one-stop assessments performed in our clinic between March 2005 and July 2006 to provide a yardstick as to what findings might be obtained in other clinics if they set up a similar program. It is unlikely that the percentage distribution of the diagnoses would be the same in each clinic, because infertility populations differ. Our program deals with couples referred on a tertiary referral basis with almost 50% of women over the age of 36.

Surprisingly only about a quarter of the women were found to have normal ovaries with a dominant follicle. Low ovarian reserve was found in 30% (11% in women less than 38 years of age and 19% in women 38 years or older). As expected, PCO was found in 21% of the population and dysfunctional ovulation in a further 11%. Endometriomas were found in 9%. It is important to realize that only 30% of women required IVF as the first line of treatment because of ovarian problems.

Only half of the women had absolutely normal uterine findings. Over 44% had abnormalities that could affect implantation, such as poor uterine vascularity, submucous fibroids, adenom–yosis, large endometrial polyps, intrauterine adhesions, and asynchronous thin endometrium. Less than 15% of women required a surgical procedure before commencing treatment.

Normal tubes with spill were found in 71% of the population following HyCoSy. Hydrosalpinges were found in 12.5% of women and they required surgical removal of these before commencing. Ten percent of women had tubal blockage, but in 6% this was confined to one tube. However, it was reasonable to offer IVF to all these women. In 6% of cases, tubal patency could not be confirmed as there were technical problems associated with the procedure. Severe male factor problems were found in 28% of male partners, with mild to moderate problems in a further 16%.

Comparative costs

We have compared the cost of a conventional multiple visit workup with that of a one-stop clinic. The average costs of the conventional workup were three times higher (£964 versus £316), mainly due to the cost of laparoscopy and repeat visits. The average duration of the complete conventional workup was 62 weeks, principally due to delays in arranging for HSG, ultrasound scans, and laparoscopy.

Conclusions

One-stop fertility assessment adheres strictly to the principles of the one-stop shop, i.e. it is carried out in one place, it saves the couple vital time, and is much less expensive. It offers a quick, one-hour diagnosis and a management plan at the end. It is comprehensive, cost effective, and minimally invasive. In our experience, it has demonstrated a high patient satisfaction rate. One-stop fertility diagnosis requires that the clinic is more organized, that the ultrasound equipment is of high quality, and that the team is skilled in ultrasound diagnosis.

References

1. Sharara F, Scott RJ, Seifer D. The detection of diminished ovarian reserve in infertile women. *Am J Obstet Gynecol* 1998; **179**: 804–812.

2. Raine-Fenning NJ, Lamb PM. Assessment of ovarian reserve using the inversion mode. *Ultrasound Obstet Gynecol* 2006; **27**(1): 104–106.

3. Jayapraksan K, Hilwah N, Kendall NR, et al. Does 3D ultrasound offer any advantage in the pre treatment assessment of ovarian reserve and prediction of outcome after assisted reproduction treatment? *Hum Reprod* 2007; **22**(7): 1932–1941.

4. Engmann L, Sladkevicius P, Agrawal R, et al. Value of ovarian stromal blood flow velocity measurement after pituitary suppression in the prediction of ovarian responsiveness and outcome of in vitro fertilization treatment. *Fertil Steril* 1999; **71**(1): 22–29.

5. Younis JS, Haddad S, Matilsky M, et al. Undetectable basal ovarian stromal blood flow in infertile women is related to low ovarian reserve. *Gynecol Endocrinol* 2007; **23**(5): 284–289.

6. Hendricks DJ, Mol EW, Banksi LF, et al. Antral follicle count in the prediction of poor ovarian response and pregnancy after invitro fertilisation; a meta analysis and comparison with basal follicle stimulating hormone level. *Fertil Steril* 2005; **83** 2): 291–301.

7. McIlveen M, Skull JE, Ledger WL. Evaluation of the utility of multiple endocrine and ultrasound measures of ovarian reserve in the prediction of cycle cancellation in a high risk IVF population. *Hum Reprod* 2007; **22**(3): 778–785.

8. Muttukrishna S, McGarrigle H, Wakim R, et al. Antral follicle count, anti-mullerian hormone and inhibin B; predictors of ovarian response in assisted reproductive technology? *BJOG* 2005; **112**(10): 1384–1390.

9. Coctia ME, Rizzello F. Ovarian reserve. *Ann NY Acad Sci* 2008; **1127**: 27–30.

10. Nargund G. Time for an ultrasound revolution in reproductive medicine. *Ultrasound Obstet Gynecol* 2002; **20**: 107–111.

11. Nargund G, Bourne T, Doyle P, et al. Ultrasound derived indices of follicular blood flow before HCG administration and the prediction of oocyte recovery and pre-implantation embryo quality. *Hum Reprod* 1996; **11**: 2512–2517.

12. Bhal P. Pugh N, Chui DK, et al. The use of transvaginal power Doppler ultrasonography to evaluate the relationship between perifollicular vascularity and outcome of in-vitro fertilisation treatment cycles. *Hum Reprod* 1999; **14**(4): 919–945.

13. Raine-Fenning NJ, Campbell BK, Kendall NR, et al. Endometrial and subendometrial perfusions are impaired in women with unexplained subfertility. *Hum Reprod* 2004; **19**(11): 2605–2614.

14. Lédéé N, Chaouat G, Serazin V, et al. Endometrial vascularity by three dimensional power Doppler ultrasound and cytokines: a complementary approach to assess uterine receptivity. *J Reprod Immunol* 2008; **77**(1): 57–62.

15. Mona R, Carine M, Valerie S, et al. Study of uterine spiral arteries during implantation window in women with normal fertility or implantation failure. *Am J Reprod Immunol* 2008; **60**(1): 87–88.

16. Campbell S, Bourne TH, Tan SL, Collins WP. Hysterosalpingo-contrast sonography (HyCoSy) and its future role within the investigation of infertility in Europe. *Ultrasound Obstet Gynecol* 1994 May 1; **4** (3); 245–253.

17. Strandell A, Bourne T, Berg C, et al. The assessment of endometrial pathology and tubal patency; a comparison between the use of ultrasonography and X-ray hysterosalpingography for the investigation of infertile patients. *Ultrasound Obstet Gynecol* 1999; **14** (3): 200–204.

18. Ghazeeri G, Kutteh W, Ke R. Sonohysterography (SHG); a prospective study to determine patient acceptability of SHG over hysterosalpingography (HSG) in the assessment of uterine structural abnormalities and tubal patency. *Fertil Steril* 1974; **1**(Suppl): 234–235.

19. Killick S. Hysterosalpingo-contrast sonography as a screening test for tubal patency in infertile women. *J R Soc Med* 1999; **92**: 628–631.

20. Nirmal B, Griffiths AN, Jose G, Evans J. Warming Echovist contrast medium for hystero-contrast sonography and the effect on the incidence of pelvic pain. A randomized controlled study. *Hum Reprod* 2006; **21**(4): 1052–1054.

21. Kelly SM, Sladkevicius P, Campbell S, Nargund G. Investigation of the infertile couple; a one stop ultrasound based approach. *Hum Reprod* 2001; **16**(12): 2481–2484.

Chapter

25

Ultrasound assessment prior to infertility treatment

Valerie Shavell and Elizabeth E. Puscheck

Imaging has become a critical component of the diagnostic workup for female infertility. Preceding the development of advanced imaging modalities, laparoscopy served as the primary method to assess pelvic organ structure and function. Fortunately, the development of transvaginal sonography (TVS) and saline infusion sonohysterography (SIS) has enabled less invasive evaluation of the female reproductive tract prior to infertility treatment. Over the past several decades, these imaging modalities have been refined. The introduction of color Doppler and three-dimensional (3D) imaging technologies has further improved assessment of the female reproductive tract.

Transvaginal sonography

In women undergoing evaluation for infertility, baseline TVS provides valuable information regarding the pelvic anatomy and ovarian reserve. Evaluation should be performed in a systematic fashion to ensure assessment of all reproductive structures, including the uterus, adnexa, and cervix. Transvaginal scans should utilize frequencies of 5 MHz or greater, recognizing that there is an inverse relationship between resolution and penetration [1]. The urinary bladder should preferably be empty. When all necessary information cannot be obtained via TVS, a transabdominal scan should be performed.

Uterus

The size, shape, and orientation of the uterus should be determined during TVS. Three measurements of the uterus are obtained: uterine length (measured as the distance from the cervix to the uterine fundus on a long-axis view), the anteroposterior diameter (measured perpendicular to uterine length), and transverse diameter (measured perpendicular to the long axis on a coronal view) (Fig. 25.1) [1]. Uterine length dramatically increases after puberty. The shape and contour of the uterus should also be assessed to determine if a congenital malformation is present. For a comprehensive review of congenital malformations of the uterus, please refer to **Chapter 6**.

The uterine cervix may be visualized on TVS, and the cervical canal will appear as either a hyperechoic line or a sonotranslucent canal when cervical mucus is present. Cervical length may be determined by measuring the length of the cervix along the cervical canal from the external to the inner os. The inner os of the cervix is delineated from the uterine corpus by the absence of endometrium.

Endometrial lining

The endometrial lining should be assessed for thickness, abnormalities, and the presence of fluid during TVS. The endometrial lining is measured in the sagittal plane approximately 1 cm from the uterine fundus, and the maximal thickness is recorded (Fig. 25.2) [2]. Fluid within the endometrial cavity should be excluded from the measurement. It is important to note the last menstrual period for the patient at the time of the ultrasound so that the ultrasound can be interpreted in the context of the menstrual cycle. Following menstruation, the endometrial lining appears as a thin, well-defined line. As the menstrual cycle progresses, the endometrial lining becomes characteristically hypoechoic and multilayered and typically proliferates to 4–10 mm in thickness (Fig. 25.2). Subsequent to ovulation, the lining becomes homogeneous and echogenic. Thus, knowing the timing in the menstrual cycle when the ultrasound is performed really helps understand whether the findings are normal or pathological. Endometrial polyps or submucosal fibroids may give the false appearance of a thickened endometrial lining on TVS. A dilated, fluid-filled endometrial cavity may suggest hematometra due to cervical stenosis.

Although there is no consensus in the literature as to whether or not there should be a lower limit for endometrial lining thickness prior to embryo transfer in women undergoing assisted reproductive techniques (ART), a lining less than 6 mm has a high negative predictive value for successful pregnancy [3]. The impact of a thickened endometrial lining on pregnancy outcome in women undergoing ART is also debatable. While several studies have found decreased pregnancy rates with an endometrial lining greater than 14 mm on the day of human chorionic gonadotropin (hCG) administration, greater than 15 mm on the day of embryo transfer, and greater than 16 mm on the day of oocyte retrieval, others have published conflicting results [2].

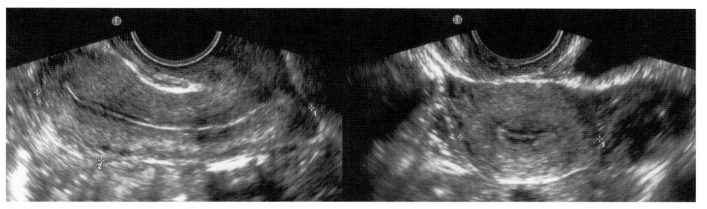

Fig. 25.1 Sagittal and horizontal views of the uterus demonstrating normal appearance of the endometrium and the myometrium.

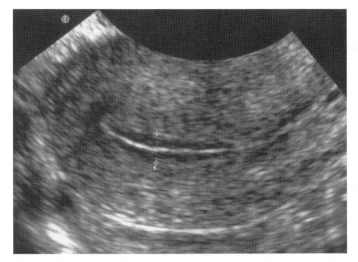

Fig. 25.2 Sagittal view of the uterus demonstrating normal appearance of the uterus and its measurements.

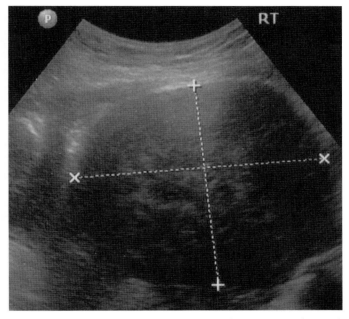

Fig. 25.3 Uterine lieomyoma demonstrating typical appearance outlines and the measurements.

The pattern of the endometrial lining, defined as the relative echogenicity of the endometrium contrasted with the adjacent myometrium, may be classified using several different grading systems [3]. Gonen and Casper [4] described a three-category grading system: an entirely homogeneous, hyperechogenic pattern without a central echogenic line (type A); intermediate (type B); and a multilayered "triple-line" endometrium consisting of a prominent outer and central hyperechogenic line and inner hypoechogenic region (type C). This grading system has been further simplified into either "non-multilayered" (grade I) or "multilayered" (grade II) by Sher and colleagues [5]. Although a hyperechogenic solid pattern has a relatively high negative predictive value for pregnancy, the appearance of this pattern does not necessitate cancellation of embryo transfer in women undergoing ART [2].

Fibroids

Uterine fibroids, also known as leiomyomas, are the most common benign tumor of the female reproductive tract, affecting 30–70% of reproductive age women [6]. Uterine enlargement or distortion is suggestive of uterine fibroids, and discrete

fibroids typically appear as spherical hypoechoic masses with well-defined borders on TVS (Fig. 25.3). Depending on the degree of calcification, however, fibroids may appear heterogeneous or hyperechoic [7]. High-resolution TVS may detect fibroids as small as 4 to 5 mm in diameter [8]. Depending on location, fibroids may be classified as intramural, submucosal, subserosal, pedunculated, or cervical. Large pedunculated fibroids may be missed during TVS because they may be out of the field of view of the transducer; thus, transabdominal ultrasound should also be performed if the serosal border is not complete or when clinically indicated [8].

Although approximately 5–10% of women have infertility associated with fibroids, fibroids are thought to be the isolated factor associated with infertility in only 1–3% of cases [9]. Fibroids may interfere with fertility by obstructing sperm transport or by impeding implantation. For a detailed discussion of the relationship between fibroids and infertility, please refer to Chapter 31.

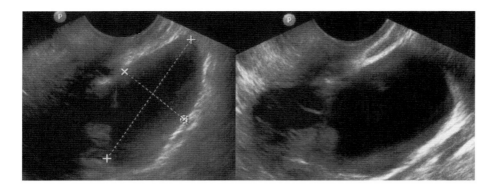

Fig. 25.4 Transvaginal ultrasound image of Hydorsalpinx and measurements in two plains.

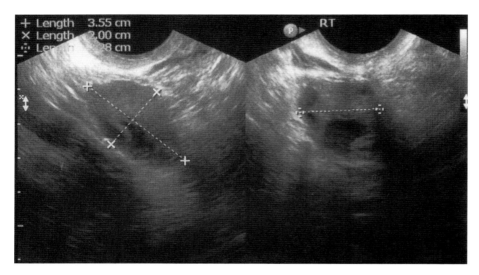

Fig. 25.5 Tranvaginal ultrasound image of normal ovary image.

Adenomyosis

Fibroids may be mistaken for adenomyosis, which is defined as ectopic endometrial glands and stroma within the smooth muscle of the uterus. Adenomyosis may be diffuse or focal. An enlarged uterus, poor definition of the endomyometrial interface, heterogeneous myometrial echogenicity, asymmetric thickening of the myometrium, subendometrial echogenic linear striations, and visualization of myometrial cysts on TVS suggest the presence of adenomyosis [2,10]. A globular, enlarged uterus, myometrial cysts, and subendometrial linear striations were found to have the greatest accuracy in the detection of adenomyosis [11]. In contrast with fibroids, the borders of the lesions are often poorly defined, and the blood supply, as depicted on Doppler imaging, is more penetrating than peripheral. In a recent meta-analysis, TVS had a pooled sensitivity of 72% and specificity of 81% for the accurate diagnosis of adenomyosis [10]. Magnetic resonance imaging (MRI) may further assist in the diagnosis of adenomyosis, particularly if fibroids are also present [12]. Adenomyosis may potentially impair uterine contractility; however, the association between adenomyosis and infertility remains unclear.

Fallopian tubes

During evaluation of the adnexa, fallopian tubes are typically not seen unless there is a pathologic finding, such as hydrosalpinges which may be detected on TVS. Hydrosalpinges represent fluid-filled fallopian tubes resulting from distal tubal obstruction [13]. In addition to impairing natural conception, hydrosalpinges have a significant affect on ART outcomes. The presence of hydrosalpinx is associated with a reduction in pregnancy rate by half and a doubling of the rate of spontaneous abortion in women undergoing in vitro fertilization (IVF) [13]. The fluid within the dilated tubes is thought to have a detrimental effect on endometrial receptivity by altering the intrauterine environment.

On TVS, the characteristic cogwheel or beads-on-a-string sign represent inflammation present in acute disease, while chronic hydrosalpinges will appear serpiginous with incomplete septa (Fig. 25.4) [2,14]. In women with an adnexal mass, hydrosalpinx may be detected during TVS with an accuracy of 98% [15]. Furthermore, 3D ultrasound inversion rendering may be utilized to confirm the diagnosis of hydrosalpinx [16]. If the hydrosalpinx is visible on ultrasound, surgical treatment

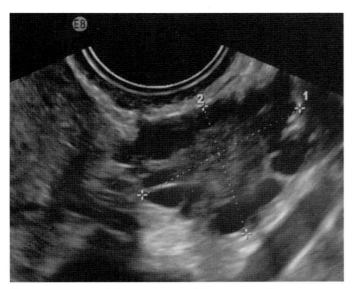

Fig. 25.6 Transvaginal ultrasound image of classic pearl necklace appearance of PCOS.

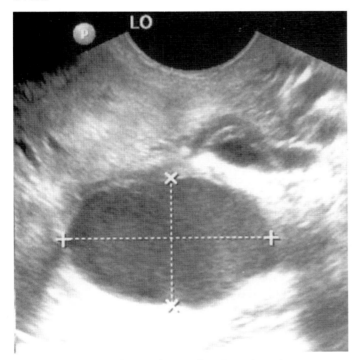

Fig. 25.7 Transvaginal ultrasound image of ovarian endometrioma.

prior to IVF is recommended in order to improve IVF success. In a recent Cochrane review, the odds of clinical pregnancy were shown to be increased in women who underwent laparoscopic salpingectomy or tubal occlusion prior to IVF [17].

Ovaries

The ovaries should be identified during TVS. The ovaries are typically located anterior to the internal iliac vessels and lateral to the uterus [1]. The size of each ovary should be measured in

three dimensions (Fig. 25.5). The volume of each ovary may be very helpful in the infertility evaluation and can be calculated with minimal inter-observer and intra-observer variability using the formula for an ellipsoid ($0.52 \times$ length $\times$ height $\times$ width) [18] or 3D ultrasound volumes. Ovarian cysts may falsely elevate ovarian volume, and women on oral contraceptives have smaller ovarian volumes [18]. Ovarian volume is known to decline significantly with each decade of life from 30 to 70 years of age [19], and reduced ovarian volume is associated with decreased ovarian responsiveness and a lower pregnancy rate in IVF [20]. For a comprehensive review of the use of ultrasound to predict ovarian reserve, please refer to Chapter 27.

During TVS, antral follicle count (AFC) may be determined. Each ovary should be scanned systematically in a sweeping motion, and the total number of follicles measuring between 2 and 10 mm in diameter should be determined [18]. As with ovarian volume, AFC declines with age and is associated with ovarian responsiveness in ART [21]. An AFC less than 10 has been associated with a higher IVF cancellation rate, and the presence of 12 or more follicles between 2 and 9 mm in one ovary or combined with both ovaries is suggestive of polycystic ovarian syndrome (PCOS) or a multifollicular ovary [18]. Women with PCOS often have enlarged ovaries and increased echogenicity of the ovarian stoma as well (Fig. 25.6). Please refer to Chapter 22 for a detailed discussion of AFC.

In addition to determining ovarian size and AFC, the ovaries should be assessed for pathologic findings during TVS. For example, ovarian endometriomas, often referred to as "chocolate cysts," have the characteristic appearance of cysts with diffuse, low-level internal echoes (Fig. 25.7). Hyperechoic foci may be visualized within the cyst wall, and peripheral blood flow may be noted on color Doppler imaging [18]. An endometrioma may be mistaken for hemorrhagic corpus luteum cyst; however, endometriomas tend to persist over time. The ovaries should also be evaluated for the presence of other benign and malignant findings, which are discussed in detail in Chapter 21.

Saline infusion sonohysterography

Saline infusion sonohysterography has become an attractive alternative to hysterosalpingography (HSG) in the evaluation of the uterine cavity and saline infusion salpingography for tubal patency. The procedure, which involves transcervical injection of sterile saline into the uterine cavity under real-time ultrasonographic imaging, is noninvasive, well tolerated, and does not require exposure to ionizing radiation [22,23]. This imaging technique allows for excellent visualization of the uterine cavity (Fig. 25.8), including the detection of intrauterine pathology such as endometrial polyps, submucosal fibroids, intrauterine adhesions, and foreign objects within the uterine cavity. Of importance, SIS should not be performed if a woman has an ongoing pelvic infection or is possibly pregnant [22]. Therefore, SIS is typically performed in the follicular phase of

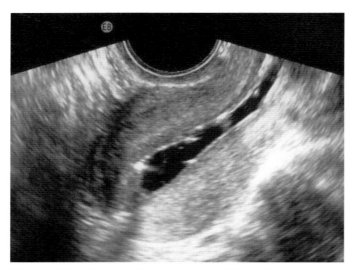

Fig. 25.8 Saline infusion sonohystrogram image of the endometrium cavity.

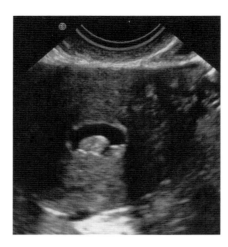

Fig. 25.9 Saline infusion sonohystrogram image defenestrating posterior wall endometrial polyp.

the menstrual cycle after menstrual bleeding has ended and prior to ovulation (approximately cycle days 5–12). The ideal time is right after the period is over when the endometrial lining is thinnest. Furthermore, the endometrium appears more heterogeneous and irregular during the proliferative phase, which may obscure visualization and lead to false-positive or false-negative diagnoses [24]. Routine use of prophylactic antibiotics prior to SIS is not advised and should be individualized based on the patient's risk for pelvic infection [25].

Intrauterine pathology is frequently encountered in the setting of infertility. In 600 infertile women who underwent evaluation with SIS, 16.2% were found to have an intracavitary abnormality, of which 13% were endometrial polyps and 2.8% were submucosal fibroids [26]. In a recent study evaluating the diagnostic accuracy of SIS as compared to hysteroscopy with directed biopsy, SIS had an overall sensitivity of 98% and positive predictive value (PPV) of 96% in the detection of polypoid lesions and endometrial hyperplasia and a sensitivity of 99% and PPV of 96% in the detection of submucosal fibroids [23]. Therefore, the technique of SIS has been shown to offer excellent detection of intrauterine pathology.

Polyps

Intrauterine polyps are localized areas of hyperplasia consisting of benign glands and stroma that have an estimated prevalence ranging from 1.4% to 41% in the subfertile female population [27]. Although polyps may be recognized as irregularities within the endometrial echo on TVS, SIS is able to deliver a much more definitive diagnosis given real-time ultrasonographic imaging during distension of the uterine cavity. During SIS, endometrial polyps will typically appear as homogeneous, echogenic, smooth intracavitary masses that are attached to the underlying endometrium by a narrow base (Fig. 25.9) [7]. Less commonly, polyps may have a broad base, contain cystic foci, or appear heterogeneous [24]. A single central vascular stalk

may be observed on color Doppler imaging with a sensitivity of 81% and a specificity of 88% [28].

Polyps have been shown to have an adverse effect on fertility, and the removal of intrauterine polyps via operative hysteroscopy has been shown to confer a higher pregnancy rate in women undergoing intrauterine insemination [29]. In a retrospective study, hysteroscopic polypectomy was associated with an improvement in pregnancy rates in infertile women, irrespective of the size or number of intrauterine polyps removed [23]. The location of the polyps may impact fertility, as removal of polyps from the uterotubal junction significantly improved pregnancy rates compared with removal from other locations within the uterus [31]. The mechanism by which endometrial polyps interfere with implantation is not entirely clear; however, inflammatory changes or distortion of the uterine cavity at the site of the polyp may result in defective implantation or embryogenesis.

Fibroids

As with endometrial polyps, submucosal fibroids alter the uterine cavity and may interfere with implantation. Submucosal fibroids may be clearly visualized during SIS as broad-based hypoechoic solid masses that distort the endometrium (Fig. 25.10). At times, endometrium lining the protruding submucosal fibroid may be visualized [24]. Opposed to a single-vessel pattern seen with polyps, submucosal fibroids tend to have a rim-like vessel pattern on power Doppler sonography with a sensitivity of 70.6% and specificity of 100% [28].

As SIS is performed under real-time ultrasonographic imaging, a more accurate determination of fibroid location is possible. Typically, hysteroscopic resection of submucosal fibroids may be successfully performed when greater than 50% of the fibroid is projecting into the endometrial cavity [24]. As with submucosal fibroids, intramural fibroids that distort the endometrium appear to have a detrimental effect on pregnancy rates with in vitro fertilization (IVF). The impact of fibroids that do not distort the uterine cavity remains controversial [32]. For

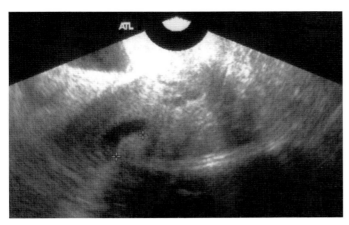

Fig. 25.10 Saline infusion sonohystrogram image demonstrating submucosal fibroid.

a thorough discussion of the relationship between fibroids and infertility, please refer to **Chapter 12**.

Intrauterine adhesions

Intrauterine adhesions, also referred to as Asherman's syndrome or intrauterine synechiae, are frequently associated with infertility. Intrauterine adhesions originate from injury to the pars basalis of the endometrium, typically related to a pregnancy [33]. These adhesions are fibrous connective tissue bands that range from minimal involvement to complete obliteration of the uterine cavity.

The presence of an echogenic area or an asymmetric thickness of the endometrium on transverse view of the uterus during TVS may suggest the presence of intrauterine adhesions, but with limited sensitivity [34]. Saline infusion sonohysterography, however, may be utilized to detect intrauterine adhesions, which may appear as an echogenic area between the anterior and posterior walls of the uterine cavity. In a small case series of women suspected to have intrauterine adhesions, SIS had a sensitivity of 100% in the detection of intrauterine adhesions [34]. In cases of complete obliteration of the uterine cavity, injection of saline during SIS may not be feasible.

Fallopian tubes

In addition to detection of hydrosalpinges as described above, SIS may be utilized to determine tubal patency. Prior to the introduction of sterile saline into the uterine cavity, the cul-de-sac should be assessed for the presence of free fluid. If free fluid is absent prior to instillation of saline but present subsequently, at least one fallopian tube must be patent [1]. Contrast material or air bubbles may also be visualized traversing through and exiting the fallopian tubes as a means of determining individual tubal patency. In a study of 115 women undergoing evaluation for infertility, air-contrast sonohysterography demonstrated agreement with laparoscopy and chromopertubation for the investigation of tubal patency in 79.4% with a sensitivity of 85.7% and specificity of 77.2% [35]. Therefore, air-contrast

sonohysterography during SIS may be utilized to assess tubal patency with high accuracy.

Summary

The improvements in ultrasound and particularly transvaginal ultrasound have transformed our infertility evaluation. A baseline transvaginal ultrasound can not only confirm normal anatomy of the uterus and ovaries, but also alert us to common pathologies in reproductive-aged women (fibroids, polyps, adenomyosis, uterine anomalies, synechiae, and ovarian masses) which may impact their fertility. In addition, transvaginal ultrasound can give us an indication of the patient's ovarian reserve and, combined with an agitated saline sonohysterogram, we can confirm tubal patency with a high degree of accuracy. These advances allow us to do the entire infertility evaluation within the office. This approach decreases anxiety for patients since they do not have to go to a radiology suite for a hysterosalpingogram and decreases their exposure and the physician's exposure to radiation, which is safer. Of course, it saves the physician time as well by allowing the entire evaluation to be done in the office without needing the physician to leave the office to transit to a radiology suite and back. There are limits to ultrasound, and radiology can be very helpful, for example when fibroids are too large or calcifications interfere with the full visualization of the uterus, or when tubal patency could not be confirmed by the agitated saline SIS approach. However, these cases that require further assessment in radiology account for less than 10% of all cases when one is serious about the ultrasound assessment.

References

1. American Institute of Ultrasound in Medicine; Society for Reproductive Endocrinology and Infertility; American Society of Reproductive Medicine. AIUM practice guideline for ultrasonography in reproductive medicine. *J Ultrasound Med* 2009; **28**: 128–137.

2. Van Voorhis BJ. Ultrasound assessment of the uterus and fallopian tube in infertile women. *Semin Reprod Med* 2008; **26**: 232–240.

3. Friedler S, Schenker JG, Herman A, Lewin A. The role of ultrasonography in the evaluation of endometrial receptivity following assisted reproductive treatments: a critical review. *Hum Reprod Update* 1996; **2**: 323–335.

4. Gonen, Y, Casper RF. Prediction of implantation by the sonographic appearance of the endometrium during controlled ovarian stimulation for in vitro fertilization (IVF). *J In Vitro Fertil Embryo Transf* 1990; **7**: 146–152.

5. Sher G, Herbert C, Maassarani G, Jacobs MH. Assessment of the late proliferative phase endometrium by ultrasonography in patients undergoing in-vitro fertilization and embryo transfer (IVF/ET). *Hum Reprod* 1991; **6**: 232–237.

6. Okolo S. Incidence, aetiology and epidemiology of uterine fibroids. *Best Pract Res Clin Obstet Gynaecol* 2008; **22**: 571–588.

7. Nalaboff KM, Pellerito JS, Ben-Levi E. Imaging the endometrium: disease and normal variants. *Radiographics* 2001; **21**: 1409–1424.

8. Hurley V. Imaging techniques for fibroid detection. *Baillieres Clin Obstet Gynaecol* 1998; **12**: 213–224.

9. Kolankaya A, Arici A. Myomas and assisted reproductive technologies: when and how to act? *Obstet Gynecol Clin North Am* 2006; **33**: 145–152.

10. Champaneria R, Abedin P, Daniels J, Balogun M, Khan KS. Ultrasound scan and magnetic resonance imaging for the diagnosis of adenomyosis: systematic review comparing test accuracy. *Acta Obstet Gynecol Scand* 2010; **89**: 1374–1384.

11. Kepkep K, Tuncay YA, Göynümer G, Tutal E. Transvaginal sonography in the diagnosis of adenomyosis: which findings are most accurate? *Ultrasound Obstet Gynecol* 2007; **30**: 341–345.

12. Bazot M, Cortez A, Darai E, et al. Ultrasonography compared with magnetic resonance imaging for the diagnosis of adenomyosis: correlation with histopathology. *Hum Reprod* 2001; **16**: 2427–3243.

13. Strandell A. The influence of hydrosalpinx on IVF and embryo transfer: a review. *Hum Reprod Update* 2000; **6**: 387–395.

14. Patel MD, Acord DL, Young SW. Likelihood ratio of sonographic findings in discriminating hydrosalpinx from other adnexal masses. *AJR Am J Roentgenol* 2006; **186**(4): 1033–1038.

15. Sokalska A, Timmerman D, Testa AC, et al. Diagnostic accuracy of transvaginal ultrasound examination for assigning a specific diagnosis to adnexal masses. *Ultrasound Obstet Gynecol* 2009; **34**: 462–470.

16. Timor-Tritsch IE, Monteagudo A, Tsymbal T. Three-dimensional ultrasound inversion rendering technique facilitates the diagnosis of hydrosalpinx. *J Clin Ultrasound* 2010; **38**: 372–376.

17. Johnson N, van Voorst S, Sowter MC, Strandell A, Mol BW. Surgical treatment for tubal disease in women due to undergo in vitro fertilisation. *Cochrane Database Syst Rev* 2010; **1**: CD002125.

18. Van Voorhis BJ. Ultrasound assessment of the ovary in the infertile woman. *Semin Reprod Med* 2008; **26**: 217–222.

19. Pavlik EJ, DePriest PD, Gallion HH, et al. Ovarian volume related to age. *Gynecol Oncol* 2000; **77**: 410–412.

20. Syrop CH, Willhoite A, Van Voorhis BJ. Ovarian volume: a novel outcome predictor for assisted reproduction. *Fertil Steril* 1995; **64**: 1167–1171.

21. Frattarelli JL, Lauria-Costab DF, Miller BT, Bergh PA, Scott RT. Basal antral follicle number and mean ovarian diameter predict cycle cancellation and ovarian responsiveness in assisted reproductive technology cycles. *Fertil Steril* 2000; **74**: 512–517.

22. American College of Obstetricians and Gynecologists. ACOG Technology Assessment in Obstetrics and Gynecology No. 5: sonohysterography. *Obstet Gynecol* 2008; **112**: 1467–1469.

23. Bingol B, Gunenc Z, Gedikbasi A, Guner H, Tasdemir S, Tiras B. Comparison of diagnostic accuracy of saline infusion sonohysterography, transvaginal sonography and hysteroscopy. *J Obstet Gynaecol* 2011; **31**: 54–58.

24. O'Neill MJ. Sonohysterography. *Radiol Clin North Am* 2003; **41**: 781–797.

25. ACOG Committee on Practice Bulletins – Gynecology. ACOG practice bulletin No. 104: antibiotic prophylaxis for gynecologic procedures. *Obstet Gynecol* 2009; **113**: 1180–1189.

26. Tur-Kaspa I, Gal M, Hartman M, Hartman J, Hartman A. A prospective evaluation of uterine abnormalities by saline infusion sonohysterography in 1,009 women with infertility or abnormal uterine bleeding. *Fertil Steril* 2006; **86**: 1731–1735.

27. Afifi K, Anand S, Nallapeta S, Gelbaya TA. Management of endometrial polyps in subfertile women: a systematic review. *Eur J Obstet Gynecol Reprod Biol* 2010; **151**: 117–121.

28. Cil AP, Tulunay G, Kose MF, Haberal A. Power Doppler properties of endometrial polyps and submucosal fibroids: a preliminary observational study in women with known intracavitary lesions. *Ultrasound Obstet Gynecol* 2010; **35**: 233–237.

29. Pérez-Medina T, Bajo-Arenas J, Salazar F, et al. Endometrial polyps and their implication in the pregnancy rates of patients undergoing intrauterine insemination: a prospective, randomized study. *Hum Reprod* 2005; **20**: 1632–1635.

30. Stamatellos I, Apostolides A, Stamatopoulos P, Bontis J. Pregnancy rates after hysteroscopic polypectomy depending on the size or number of the polyps. *Arch Gynecol Obstet* 2008; **277**: 395–399.

31. Yanaihara A, Yorimitsu T, Motoyama H, Iwasaki S, Kawamura T. Location of endometrial polyp and pregnancy rate in infertility patients. *Fertil Steril* 2008; **90**: 180–182.

32. Surrey ES. Impact of intramural leiomyomata on in-vitro fertilization-embryo transfer cycle outcome. *Curr Opin Obstet Gynecol* 2003; **15**: 239–242.

33. Berman JM. Intrauterine adhesions. *Semin Reprod Med* 2008; **26**: 349–355.

34. Salle B, Gaucherand P, de Saint Hilaire P, Rudigoz RC. Transvaginal sonohysterographic evaluation of intrauterine adhesions. *J Clin Ultrasound* 1999; **27**: 131–134.

35. Jeanty P, Besnard S, Arnold A, Turner C, Crum P. Air-contrast sonohysterography as a first step assessment of tubal patency. *J Ultrasound Med* 2000; **19**: 519–527.

Doppler ultrasonography in infertility

L. T. Polanski, M. N. Baumgarten, Nicholas J. Raine-Fenning and
Kannamannadiar Jayaprakasan

Introduction and overview

Pelvic ultrasound has become an essential investigation for assessing subfertile women during the last two to three decades. While grayscale B-mode ultrasonography of the female pelvis provides anatomical information, Doppler ultrasonography may allow a more detailed insight into the vascularity and functional components of the female pelvis. Doppler ultrasonography is based on the concept of the "Doppler principle." When a signal with a known frequency is emitted by the transducer and is reflected by a moving object (blood cells in the blood vessels), the return frequency is altered proportionally to the velocity of the object. This frequency change as perceived by a static observer allows for the assessment of the direction and velocity of blood flow within a selected vessel.

Pulse-wave Doppler uses the signals from a specific, or gated, area of a blood vessel to display a velocity waveform (Fig. 26.1) that can be measured to produce indices of velocity of blood flow (PSV: peak systolic velocity; and S/D: systole to diastole ratio) and of resistance to flow (the pulsatility and resistance indices). However, pulse-wave Doppler ultrasonography may have certain limitations as the information regarding vascularity and blood flow is obtained from a single artery, which may not be truly representative of the surrounding vasculature or total organ blood flow. Development of three-dimensional (3D) power Doppler allows for global assessment of total vascularity and blood flow within an acquired volume, and the results are expressed by volumetric vascularity indices: vascularization index (VI), flow index (FI), and the vascularization–flow index (VFI) [1–4] (Fig. 26.2). The VI represents the ratio of power Doppler information within the total dataset relative to both color and gray information, the FI is proportional to the power Doppler signal intensity, and the VFI reflects a combination of the two. While these vascularity indices are reproducible in both in vitro and in vivo settings [2–6] and may be reflective of the concentration of blood vessels and, therefore, the volume of blood and vascularity within the region of interest, the exact relationship of these indices to true blood flow remains to be explored further. Although both pulse-wave and power Doppler ultrasound may have some clinical application in

subfertile women, these are not universally practiced and their use is generally restricted to the advanced user and research setting.

In this chapter, we will describe the technique and clinical application of Doppler sonography within an infertility clinic and the evidence base for its clinical use. We will outline the physiological changes depicted by Doppler sonography during the menstrual cycle within the female reproductive tract, as well as its usefulness in supplementing the diagnosis of various pathologies that may have adverse effects on fertility and treatment outcome. Future trends and new developments, as well as pitfalls, are also discussed.

Doppler assessment of the uterus

Anatomy and physiology

The blood supply to the uterus comes mainly from the uterine arteries, branches of the anterior division of internal iliac arteries, located on both sides of the organ between the two layers of the broad ligament. Once in the broad ligament, the uterine arteries divide into the ascending and descending branches supplying the cervix, and uterus and cervix and vagina, respectively. Within the uterus, uterine arteries give off further branches: the arcuate arteries and spiral arteriolar plexus [7–9]. A small proportion of the blood supply to the uterus comes from the ovarian arteries, originating from the abdominal aorta and anastomosing with the superior branches of the uterine arteries within the broad ligaments.

The majority of studies assessing uterine and endometrial blood flow have utilized pulse-wave Doppler of the easily accessible uterine arteries and not their smaller branches. During a normal menstrual cycle, pulse-wave Doppler studies have shown a rise in the pulsatility index (PI) values and blood flow velocity of the uterine arteries around the time of menses and ovulation, with decline in PI approximately 1 week prior to and 1 week after ovulation; however, few studies have found a statistically significant difference [10–14]. The assessment of uterine arteries might not necessarily give accurate information on the actual blood supply within the endometrium.

Ultrasonography in Gynecology, ed. Botros R. M. B. Rizk and Elizabeth E. Puscheck. Published by Cambridge University Press. © Cambridge University Press 2015.

A

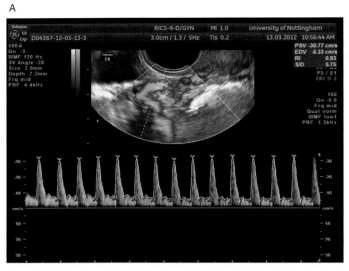

B

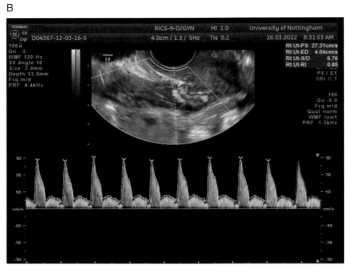

Fig. 26.1 Normal spectral Doppler images of the uterine arteries.

A

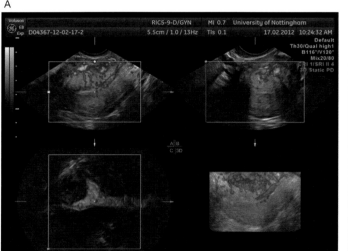

B

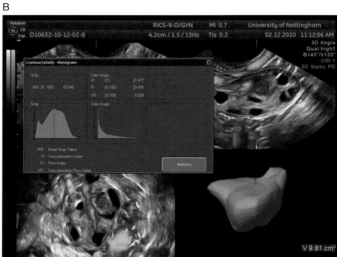

Fig. 26.2 3D static Doppler acquisition of the uterus (A) and ovary (B). The ovarian volume is calculated and the vascularity indices are displayed within the histogram window (B).

Studies assessing the blood flow within spiral arteries of the sub-endometrium (single vessel assessment) suggest the same pattern of blood flow as described for the uterine arteries during the menstrual cycle [10,13,15]. However, this is still a subjective method and relies on selection of a single, visible vessel for analysis. An overall assessment of the whole endometrium and sub-endometrium is possible with the use of 3D Doppler sonography [16,17]. A study performed by Raine-Fenning et al. using 3D power Doppler sonography of the endometrium and sub-endometrium has shown a gradual increase in all three vascularity indices (VI, FI, and VFI) in the follicular phase, reaching a peak around 3 days prior to ovulation [18,19]. This was followed by decrease in these indices, reaching a trough 5 days after ovulation and a subsequent rise until the mid-luteal phase

of the cycle. Emerging histological and embryological data suggest that a relatively low pO_2 environment may be necessary for successful implantation of the human blastocyst [6]. Variations in the vascularity indices during a normal menstrual cycle seem to indicate that such a low-oxygen environment is created during the window of implantation, as demonstrated by a fall in vascular indices approximately on day 5 post-ovulation [18,19].

Doppler sonography of the uterus

Technique

The use of up-to-date sonographic equipment allows for the most detailed assessment of the pelvic organs and permits detailed evaluation of blood flow. Pulse-wave (PW) Doppler is

A

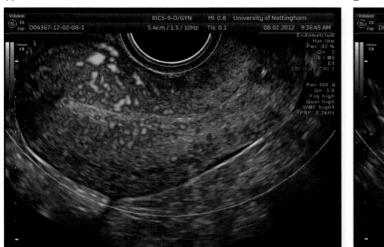

B

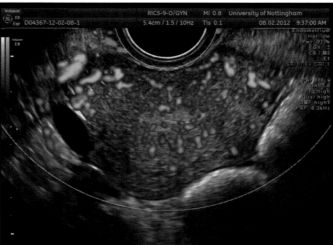

Fig. 26.3 Longitudinal (A) and transverse views (B) of a normal uterus on day 4 of the menstrual cycle. Power Doppler acquisition.

Table 26.1 3D Doppler sonography ultrasound machine settings providing optimal definition of small vessels without artifact induction

Machine settings	Value
Color gain	−2.0
Power	100%
Wall motion filter	low1
PRF (pulse repetition frequency)	0.6 kHz
Frequency	mid
Flow resolution	mid1
Balance	G >225
Smooth (rise/ fall)	2/2
Ensemble	12
Line density	7
Power Doppler map	5
Gently color	On
Artifact suppression	On
Line filter	2

potentially the quickest of the Doppler modalities, as it does not require time-consuming off-machine computer analysis of the acquired data. Following introduction of the transvaginal transducer (working frequencies typically 6–9 MHz) into the vagina and identification of the uterus, the probe should be directed towards the vaginal fornix. Using power Doppler, the ascending branch of the uterine artery is identified. The angle of insonation should be as small as possible to maximize the accuracy of the gathered information and not exceed 30 degrees [18]. The Doppler gate should be placed in the middle of the artery and data recorded. The size of the Doppler gate should be adjusted to the inner diameter of each vessel, in order to avoid the distortions caused by the movement of the vascular walls and errors resulting from lower blood flow velocities in the proximity of the vascular wall [20,21]. Automated analysis of the selected fragment will produce vascularity indices.

Three-dimensional Doppler sonography relies on an initial optimal two-dimensional (2D) image; hence every effort should be made to enhance the standard 2D view before proceeding to volume acquisition. Modern transvaginal transducers have multiple piezoelectric crystals that are capable of performing the sweep automatically without the need for movement of the probe. Following visualization of the midline-sagittal section of the uterus, 3D power Doppler mode should be activated (Fig. 26.3). The angle of acquisition should be increased to cover the entire uterus during the automated sweep. It is advisable to ask the patient to lie as still as possible in order to prevent movement artifacts. Used settings differ from machine to machine and the patient's body habitus might necessitate adjustment of the settings used in order to improve the quality of the image. However it is advisable, especially in a research setting, to adhere strictly to selected settings in order to obtain true and reproducible results (Table 26.1). Offline analysis of the acquired dataset using computer software (4D view, GE Medical Systems, Zipf, Austria) will produce volumetric vascularity indices (VI, FI, and VFI).

Uterine Doppler

All investigations prior to infertility treatment aim to identify treatable causes, predict successful treatment, and improve outcome. Many studies have undertaken to correlate the Doppler vascularity indices of the uterus and endometrium with treatment outcome in an IVF setting, with the day of Doppler assessment varying in different studies: on the day of hCG injection, on the day of oocyte retrieval, or on the day of embryo transfer [22–26]. The conflicting results in different studies suggest that the ability of Doppler ultrasonography to predict fertility treatment outcome in a day-to-day clinical practice is limited.

Doppler sonography can be a useful tool to assess uterine pathology that is commonly associated with infertility.

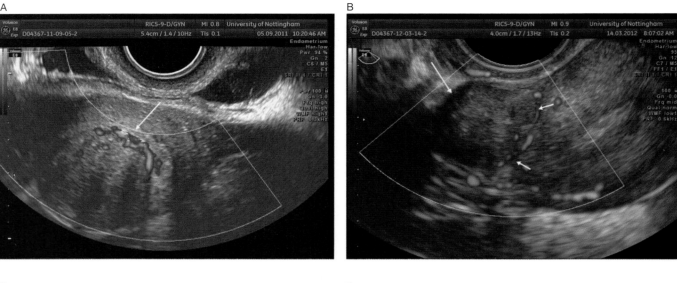

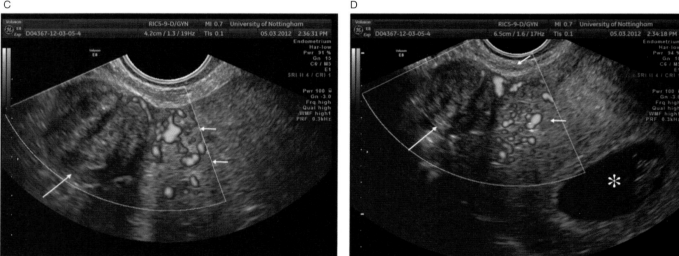

Fig. 26.4 Leiomyomas. (A) A submucosal fibroid (large arrow) indenting the endometrial cavity. A typical "rim-like" pattern of blood vessels is noted (small arrow) (B, C, and D). A subserosal fibroid protruding from the lateral aspect of the uterus (large arrow) (B, C and D). On image D a gestational sac is noted (asterisk).

Leiomyomas

Uterine leiomyomas are the most common benign tumors of the female genital tract and are known to cause various gynecologic symptoms including subfertility. Current evidence suggests that submucosal fibroids and intramural fibroids have a negative impact on implantation rates [27,28]. The majority of fibroids are easily diagnosed by conventional ultrasound during either an opportunistic scan or a targeted infertility workup. Within an infertility clinic setting, the frequency of uterine fibroids is in the range of 25%, possibly even higher [29]. Transvaginal ultrasound is highly accurate in detecting intramural and subserosal fibroids, with a sensitivity of 99% and a specificity of 91%, and can be used to categorize the number, size, and position of each. The sensitivity and specificity of standard ultrasound for detection of submucous myomas varies, and has been reported to be as low as 21% and 53%, respectively [30]. Adding Doppler sonography to standard 2D ultrasound improves the sensitivity significantly [31]. Fibroids are generally low-vascularity lesions with the majority of the blood flow demonstrated in the periphery, within the capsule. The typical blood flow pattern seen when assessing fibroids using power Doppler is that of a ring or rim of Doppler signal with a relatively avascular lesion in the center (Fig. 26.4). This "rim-like pattern" has been reported to have a sensitivity and positive predictive value of 70.6% and 100%, respectively, for detection of submucosal leiomyomas [31].

Endometrial polyps

The prevalence of endometrial polyps in women undergoing hysteroscopy for investigation of infertility is quoted to be as high as 25% [32–34]. Polyps can vary in size from millimeters to a few centimeters and they can be single or multiple. While its effect on fertility is less clear, the prevalence of endometrial polyp is increased in subfertile populations. The adverse

A

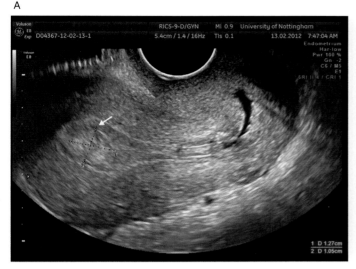

B

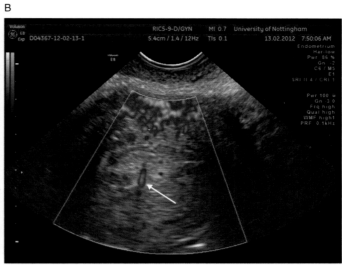

Fig. 26.5 Endometrial polyp as demonstrated by two-dimensional ultrasound (small arrow, image A). Application of the Doppler modality allows for identification of the feeding vessel to the polyp (large arrow).

influence of polyps on conception and implantation may possibly be related to formation of a mechanical barrier for gamete migration as well as alteration of receptivity of the endometrium, which prevents implantation [35]. Vascular patterns observed in endometrial polyps using Doppler sonography usually comprise a single feeding vessel running from the base and branching within the polyp (Fig. 26.5). With broad-base polyps, there can be few feeding vessels, however the vascular pattern does not resemble that of a submucosal leiomyoma [31]. The addition of Doppler sonography when assessing intrauterine lesions increases diagnostic accuracy and adds useful information prior to surgical planning (Fig. 26.6). When compared to the diagnostic gold standard, which is hysteroscopy, transvaginal ultrasound for diagnosis of endometrial pathology has been shown to have a sensitivity ranging from 23% to 57%, and specificity of 69% to 93% [36,37]. Addition of color Doppler and the presence of single-vessel pedicle increases the sensitivity and specificity to values between 80% and 90% [31,38].

Adenomyosis

These ectopic endometrial implants within the uterine muscle have been linked to infertility, although there is no convincing evidence to support this cause–effect relationship [39]. The confounding factor is that adenomyosis often coexists with endometriosis, which has a confirmed link with failure to conceive. The true prevalence of adenomyosis within the infertile population is thought to be as high as 50%; however, that figure was derived from studies reporting the disruption of the myometrial junctional zone (JZ), which is a feature of adenomyosis [40]. The presence of myometrial cysts and distorted or irregular endomyometrial JZ have been reported to be the best diagnostic features on 2D and 3D sonography with diagnostic accuracy, as compared to histopathology, in the range of 83% and 89% for 2D and 3D sonography, respectively [41] (Fig. 26.7). Doppler sonography often allows distinction of

adenomyosis from intramural fibroids. As the blood vessels within the area affected by adenomyosis course uninterrupted by, the pattern of the Doppler signal is similar to that of the normal myometrium (Fig. 26.2). The diameter of vessels within the lesion is often large compared with vessels within the normal myometrium [42].

Uterine and endometrial blood flow: prediction of pregnancy

Early studies of endometrial blood flow using color Doppler on the day of hCG administration have demonstrated that lack of color Doppler signals within the sub-endometrium of women undergoing ovarian stimulation predicts a non-conception cycle [43,44]. A more recent study using pulse-wave Doppler to assess the endometrium and sub-endometrium has demonstrated that the presence of blood flow within the inner hypoechogenic zone of the endometrium on the day of hCG administration is correlated with a successful pregnancy [45]. However, the authors gave no Doppler index values. Color Doppler assessment of the endometrial blood flow has been positively correlated in another study with viable intrauterine pregnancy. The S/D ratio and PI and RI indices of the endometrial spiral artery blood flow on the day of hCG administration [46] or on the day of embryo transfer [47] have been found to be significantly lower in patients with a successful pregnancy [46,47].

Assessment of the uterine arteries has been so far the "gold standard" of analysis of the blood flow to the uterus during or preceding IVF treatment. This technique has its limitations as it assesses the big vessels and not the vasculature of the actual site of implantation. Studies differ in conclusions as to the usefulness of Doppler indices as markers of implantation. Some seem to support the predictive value, while others refute it [15,46,48]. Analysis of the waveform obtained during pulse-wave Doppler sonography suggests that the presence of end-diastolic flow within the vessel is a good prognostic factor for successful

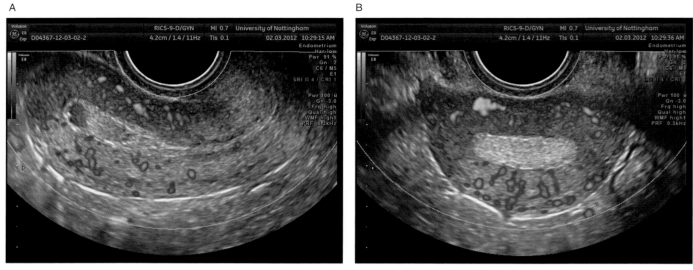

Fig. 26.6 Intracavitary fluid (menstrual blood) around the time of menstruation. Lack of Doppler signal within the uterine cavity helps to differentiate between a polyp and coagulated blood.

pregnancy [49,50]. A combination of this feature with endometrial thickness and appearance was reported to have a sensitivity and specificity in the range of 81%, with positive and negative predictive values for pregnancy of 68.2% and 89.7%, respectively [22]. End-diastolic flow has also been reported to be predictive of pregnancy and term birth by other authors [49,50]. Assessment of the uterine artery (UA) by Wang et al. did not reveal any predictive values correlated with successful pregnancy; the PI values were in the range of 2.0 ± 1.1 [46]. Serial assessment of uterine artery indices in patients undergoing IVF-stimulated cycles did not yield a predictive cut-off for vascular indices in a group of 83 patients, with PI values ranging from 1.72 to 2.32 across the pregnant and non-pregnant subjects [51]. Some studies, however, have found significant correlations between the vascular indices in a successful cycle versus an unsuccessful one. The most often quoted cut-off values for PI are in the range of 3.0 to 3.3, with lower values being deemed normal [17,52,53]. Using PI of 3.0 in the uterine artery, the estimated chance of implantation failure is in the range of 35% [52].

With the increasing availability of 3D Doppler sonography, it is being evaluated as a possibly useful tool for prediction of pregnancy outcome in fresh or frozen IVF cycles. Studies using 3D uterine Doppler in prediction of outcome of frozen embryo transfer cycles during a natural and clomiphene-stimulated cycle did not show any significant difference in endometrial and subendometrial vascularity indices between patients that conceived and those that did not [54,55]. It is, however, interesting and worth highlighting that some differences have been found between natural and stimulated IVF cycles with regard to vascular indices as assessed by 3D Doppler sonography. Endometrial and subendometrial vascular indices were found to be lower in stimulated cycles compared with non-stimulated cycles, which might be due to the effects of the supraphysiological levels of estrogen during stimulated cycles [56,57]. Patient age, smoking habits, and type and cause of infertility did not have a profound impact on the vascular indices [57]. Subfertile women having anovulatory PCOS associated with hyperandrogenemia have been shown to have an impaired endometrial blood flow as expressed by VI and VFI values [58]. A large study conducted by Ng et al. [59] on 293 patients undergoing their first IVF cycle has failed to identify values of endometrial vascularity indices predictive of conception when 3D Doppler was applied. Other data are also ambiguous as to the usefulness of 3D Doppler indices as predictors of successful IVF outcome, as VI, FI, and VFI differ between studies not just in numeric value but also in terms of being higher or lower than controls [17,24,47,60]. However, correlation between Doppler indices and pregnancy outcome has been demonstrated when a non-grade 1 embryo is transferred, as shown by an analysis of 43 cycles [61]. Other studies have not found any statistically significant relationship between the endometrial vascularity as assessed by 3D Doppler sonography and pregnancy outcome in the IVF setting [62,63]. A cut-off value for prediction of pregnancy was suggested by Wu et al. in a study of 54 patients undergoing stimulated IVF cycles. The VFI of the subendometrium above 0.24 on day of the hCG administration gave a positive predictive value and negative predictive value of 93.8% and 72.7%, respectively [60]. However, other studies have failed to establish similar values for prediction of outcome. Therefore no single values of 3D power Doppler vascularity indices exist that could be reliably used in IVF setting.

Doppler sonography is potentially a useful tool to assess the endometrium during IVF treatment as demonstrated by the large numbers of studies present in the literature. However, the conclusions that are drawn from these studies are conflicting and these discrepancies are possibly related to different study design, populations, timings of assessment,

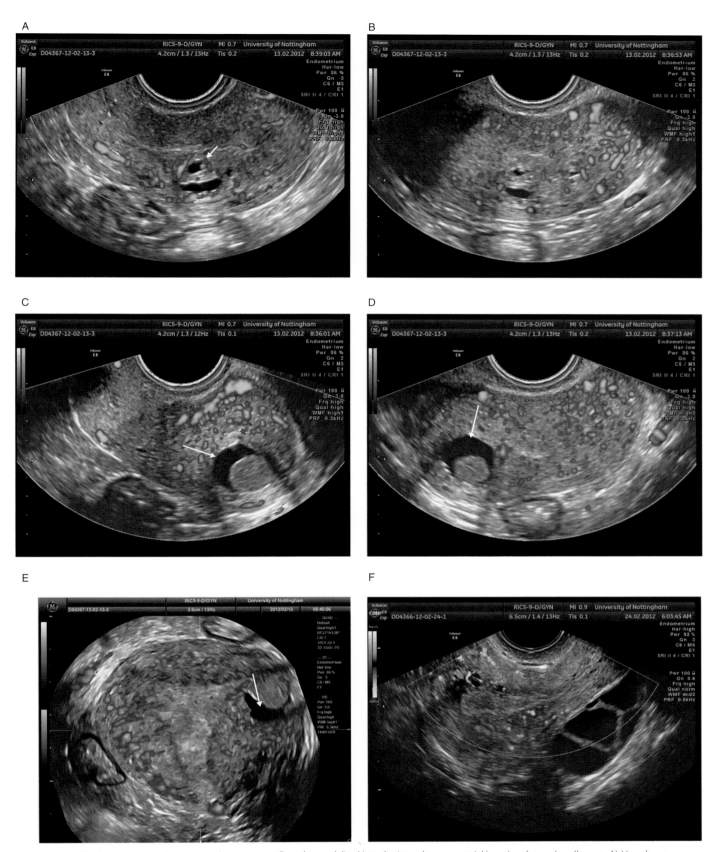

Fig. 26.7 (A–D) Adenomyosis as demonstrated using power Doppler modality. Note the irregular myometrial junctional zone (small arrow, A). Vessels are traversing the affected myometrium without interruption (A and B), except for a large intramyometrial cyst that is completely distorting the structure of the myometrium (arrow, C and D). (E) A coronal reconstruction of the endometrial cavity. The inclusion cyst (large arrow) is clearly located beyond the cavity and is not distorting it. (F) Adenomyosis during ovarian stimulation protocol using high-definition Doppler imaging.

and varying experience of sonographers. With the rapid technological advancement in improving the resolution and sensitivity of the Doppler signal, these discrepancies may be ameliorated in order to draw a single conclusion in the future.

Doppler assessment of the ovaries

Anatomy and physiology

An oval-shaped ovary normally measures 4 cm in length, 1.5–2 cm in width, and 1 cm in depth. There are two distinguishable layers: cortex and medulla. Blood flow to the ovary is via the ovarian artery, which arises from the abdominal aorta below the origin of the renal artery. Ovarian arteries pass downward and laterally, entering the pelvis through the infundibulopelvic ligament, and reach the ovary via the mesovarium and pass through the hilus of the ovary to give rise to numerous spiral branches. Blood flow to the ovary is also derived from the ovarian branch of the uterine artery, which anastomoses with the ovarian artery near the ovary [64].

Doppler sonography of the ovaries in the infertility setting

Technique

As previously described in the section dealing with Doppler assessment of the uterus, optimal acquisition commences with localization of the ovary using a 2D scan. The biggest diameter is most likely to correspond with the middle of the ovary. Following identification of the middle portion of the ovary, the same principles as when assessing the uterus should be applied. When the volume of one ovary is obtained, the same should be done for the opposite side. When Doppler acquisition is part of the desired examination, transvaginal ultrasound is preferred to abdominal, to minimize the distance between the probe and the ovary, minimizing the attenuation.

Pulse-wave Doppler and 3D power Doppler ultrasonography or angiography can be used to assess both ovarian and stromal blood flow. Pulse-wave Doppler is used for assessment of blood flow through the individual ovarian stromal arteries, providing information about the direction and velocity of blood going through the specified vessel. Volume acquisition using 3D power Doppler is relatively slow, making it sensitive to movement artifacts, by movement of the sonographer or patient [65]. Once an ovarian volume dataset is obtained, Virtual Organ Computer-aided AnaLysis (VOCAL) software is utilized to measure ovarian volume and semi-quantify the blood flow within the whole ovary [66].

Conventional B-mode ultrasonography is adequate to confirm normal ovarian morphology and to diagnose ovarian pathologies. However, application of Doppler sonography can sometimes aid the diagnosis of certain ovarian pathologies that are commonly associated with infertility.

Polycystic ovary syndrome

The most common cause of medically treatable infertility is polycystic ovarian syndrome (PCOS), which is the cause of anovulatory infertility in 70% of cases [67] and, therefore, is an important condition to diagnose in the assessment of infertile couples. The diagnosis of PCOS not only carries important long-term health implications, such as increased metabolic risks, but also helps to guide the assisted reproduction treatment. In the Rotterdam criteria, PCOS is defined as either 12 or more follicles measuring 2–9 mm in diameter or an increased ovarian volume greater than 10 cm³, while the distribution of follicles, a description of the stroma, and blood flow indices are not included. However, the evaluation of ovarian stroma by ultrasound could be too subjective or too difficult to apply in routine daily practice.

Ovarian vascularity is generally assumed to be higher in PCOS than in normal ovaries owing to hypertrophy of ovarian stroma. Ovarian vascularity can be assessed subjectively through the application of color or power Doppler maps to a single plane to examine the flow pattern, or can be assessed objectively by measuring flow velocity and the resistance to flow through pulse-wave Doppler on a single vessel. It has been observed that the pulsatility index and resistance index of both ovarian artery and stromal artery were significantly lower in women with PCOS [68], but this was not supported by other investigators [69]. Quantitative 3D power Doppler angiography facilitates the assessment of total blood flow within the defined volume of interest, allowing the objective assessment of total vascular flow within an organ or a specified volume of tissue. The data on ovarian blood flow quantified using 3D power Doppler in a polycystic ovary are conflicting, with some groups reported higher values of ovarian Doppler vascularity indices (VI, FI, VFI) in PCOS patients on day 3 of menses, compared with non-PCOS patients [70] while others reported no apparent difference in ovarian blood flow [71,72].

Endometriosis

Endometriosis is a diagnosis frequently made in subfertile women. The disease and targeted therapy can influence the response to fertility treatment. Wu et al. [73] found all 3D power Doppler ovarian indices to be lower in women with ovarian endometriosis. However, it remains unclear whether the observed changes are due to the disease or the fact that studied patients underwent cystectomies. Their control group consisted of patients with tubal factor infertility also undergoing IVF treatment. The outcome in terms of number of oocytes collected and pregnancy rates was lower in the endometriosis group. Interestingly, if the vascularity indices were compared between the operated and not-operated-on ovary, no difference in the values was noted.

Ovarian cysts

In the population having IVF treatment, ovarian cysts are a common ultrasound finding. Although the likelihood of having a malignant ovarian mass in the fertile age group is small,

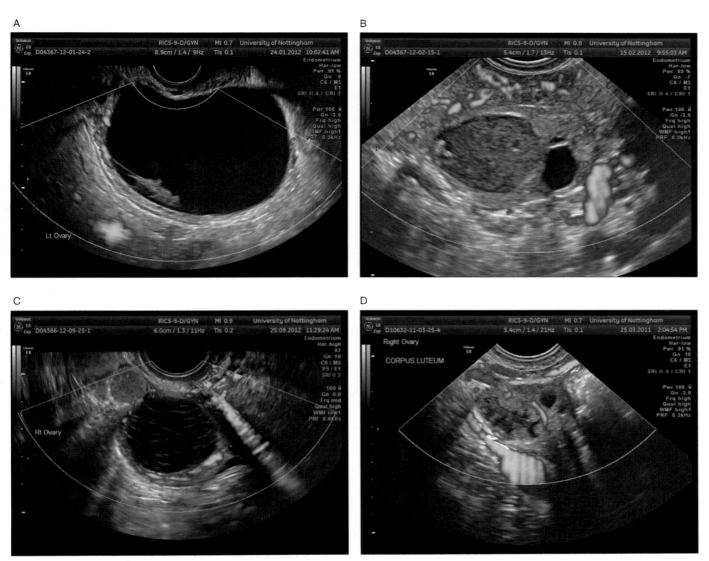

Fig. 26.8 Various ovarian masses assessed by Doppler sonography in patients undergoing IVF treatment. (A and C) Hemorrhagic cysts. (B) A dermoid cyst. Note lack of blood flow within the content of the dermoid cysts, as well as within the "papillary" projections that are formed by coagulated blood (A and C). (D) A physiological corpus luteum within the right ovary.

imaging using Doppler can help adequate assessment. Low or no blood flow in the mass is most likely to be benign [74] (Fig. 26.8). Other chance findings in this population are mature cystic teratomas (dermoid cysts). The ultrasound appearances are nonspecific, although the tumors are typically mixed lesions, usually with scattered calcifications [75]. During ovarian stimulation protocols, formation of simple cysts may occur. Follow-up remains necessary, especially when a high vascularity is present.

Intrauterine insemination (IUI)

While there are many studies [76–78] evaluating the relationship between follicular and perifollicular blood flow of the leading ovarian follicle and IUI outcome, the clinical application of Doppler indices to improve the treatment success is limited. During IUI treatment, timing in relation to predicting

maturation of the follicle, administration of hCG ovulation trigger, and insemination is possibly one of the most crucial steps in achieving a pregnancy. In a recent study of 79 IUI cycles [79], there was no statistically significant difference in the values of vascularity indices of the dominant follicle as measured by 3D power Doppler in patients who achieved ovulation and those who did not, and between pregnant and non-pregnant women.

Prediction of IVF outcome

An adequate ovarian blood supply is essential to its normal function and may influence the endocrine and paracrine signals that effect the growth and development of follicles. It has been suggested that an increased ovarian blood flow may lead to a higher delivery of gonadotropins and other growth factors to the granulosa–theca cell complex of the developing follicles, resulting in a multifollicular response to ovarian stimulation during IVF. Ultrasound assessment of ovarian blood flow may be helpful in predicting the response to controlled ovarian stimulation during assisted reproduction treatment. There are various studies which have evaluated ovarian and follicular blood flow to predict embryo quality and implantation.

Zaidi et al. were the first group to evaluate the correlation between ovarian stromal blood flow and follicular response in an IVF program [80]. They measured the ovarian stromal PSV and PI in 105 women in the early follicular phase and found that poor responders, defined as those who developed six or fewer follicles at the time of oocyte retrieval, had a significantly lower mean ovarian PSV, but no difference in PI, when compared with normal responders. The adjusted odds of a poor response increased significantly by an estimated 22% per 1 cm/s decrease in velocity. Most subsequent work based on 2D pulse-wave Doppler assessment of individual ovarian stromal vessels showed a significant correlation between the absolute velocity and impedance to blood flow and ovarian response in terms of the number of oocytes retrieved [81,82], although recent studies utilizing larger populations did not reveal an association between blood flow indices and ovarian response during IVF [83].

More recently, work has been done utilizing 3D ultrasound and power Doppler angiography, allowing the demonstration and quantification of the total blood flow within ovaries. Kupesic et al. used 3D power Doppler angiography to evaluate ultrasound-derived ovarian predictors of ovarian response and outcome in 56 women with normal basal serum follicle-stimulating hormone (FSH) concentrations (<10 mIU/mL) undergoing their first cycle of IVF [84]. Multiple regression analysis of the six most predictive variables – including the peak estradiol on the day of human chorionic gonadotropin (hCG) administration, total ovarian volume, total ovarian stromal area, age, and total antral follicle count (AFC) – revealed ovarian flow index to be the second best predictor of the number of mature oocytes collected and pregnancy, followed by the ovarian stromal flow index (FI) after AFC. However, most subsequent larger studies did not find a strong relationship between 3D power Doppler indices and poor ovarian response or exaggerated ovarian response or pregnancy during IVF [85–88]. It seems that the use of ovarian 3D vascular indices as an independent predictor of ovarian response is limited and should be restricted to use as a research tool until convincing evidence for routine clinical use is reported.

Doppler assessment of the testes

While ultrasound seems to be the most frequent investigation that women undergo in an infertility setting, imaging modality is rarely used in male infertility. Ultrasound and Doppler imaging can be a useful diagnostic tool in cases of male-factor infertility.

Anatomy and physiology

Adult male testes are ovoid organs measuring 2–3 cm in width and 3–5 cm in length. The testicles are supplied with blood via the testicular artery arising from the aorta and entering the scrotum via the inguinal canal. After passing the tunica albuginea, the artery forms capsular arteries located beneath the tunica. These give off centripetal arteries heading towards the mediastinum and divide into recurrent rami heading away from the mediastinum. Additional blood supply to the testes comes from the cremasteric (external spermatic) artery and deferential artery (artery to the ductus deferens), branches of inferior epigastric artery and superior vesical artery, respectively. In approximately 50% of patients, a large mediastinal artery (branch of testicular artery) with accompanying vein courses through the testicle from the mediastinum to the capsular arteries [89,90]. The venous drainage is by the pampiniform plexus emptying into the testicular veins, of which the right empties into the inferior vena cava and the left into the left renal vein [91].

Technique

The patient is assessed in a supine position with scrotal support if necessary. Linear array transducers with scan frequency range 7–10 MHz are used in order to obtain best results. Assessment of the testicle is carried out in at least two planes: longitudinal and transverse. The texture and dimensions are then assessed and comparison between the two sides is made. Valsalva maneuver or upright position might be used to evaluate venous blood flow characteristics [92].

Doppler ultrasound of testes

Simple color Doppler sonography is useful to demonstrate blood flow within the testicular tissue [93]. Power Doppler has the advantage of being almost angle independent and has the ability to detect lower velocities of blood flow; hence this modality may be more appropriate in assessing testes [94]. Pulse-wave Doppler sonography is also used and assesses single vessel blood flow parameters. In gonads of at least 4 cm³ in volume, blood flow within intra-testicular arteries is usually a low-resistance one with RI ranging from 0.48 to 0.75 and PI values from 0.7 to 2.3 [93,95]. Some authors suggest the cut-off for normal vasculature of the testicle to have an RI of below 0.6 [96]. In gonads smaller than 4 cm³, the diastolic flow may not be detectable, as is often the case in the pre-pubertal state [97]. The RI of the epididymis is reported to be similar to that found in the testicle and ranges from 0.46 to 0.68 [98]. In general, Doppler sonography is a useful tool to assess the testicular anatomy and assess its pathology.

Presence and quality of sperm often dictate the artificial reproductive technique used, starting with IUI and ending with donor sperm. Within the IVF setting the common conditions requiring Doppler assessment of the testicle are azoospermia and palpable varicocele. Other conditions potentially associated with male infertility such as testicular microlithiasis, hydrocele, and infections usually do not require the use of Doppler sonography; however, in cases of orchitis slight hyperemia might be present [92]. Testicular malignancies generally have an increased blood flow as demonstrated by Doppler sonography [92,99].

Testicular perfusion may be related to sperm quality, as Herwig et al. have demonstrated an inverse relationship between testicular RI and sperm parameters [100]. While correlation of FSH with testicular volume has revealed an inverse association, a positive correlation exists between testicular vascularization and serum FSH levels [101]. Doppler sonography may be a supplementary investigation to differentiate between obstructive and non-obstructive azoospermia. In obstructive azoospermia, testicular vasculature is usually intact and can be easily demonstrated by normal distribution of the Doppler signal. Absent or significantly reduced blood flow might suggest a non-obstructive cause of azoospermia [96]. Some authors have suggested targeted surgical sperm retrieval at areas of visible perfusion, as biopsies from vascular regions are more likely to produce viable spermatozoa because residual active spermatogenic regions might still be present in perfused regions of the testicle [102].

Varicocele is a pathological dilatation of the veins surrounding the vas deferens. It affects approximately 15% of adult males, but can be as common as a third of patients presenting for primary infertility investigations, and even 80% in the secondary infertility [103–105]. Diagnosis is important, as presence of palpable varicocele may have an impact on semen quality and a possible benefit of surgical intervention in oligozoospermic men with varicocele has been observed [92,106]. While clinical evaluation is usually adequate to make a diagnosis, ultrasound and Doppler assessment might be beneficial in occult cases. Ultrasound examination reveals multiple, dilated, tortuous tubular structures most commonly located superior and to the side of the testicle; however, in extreme cases they might also occupy the space posteriorly and inferiorly to the affected testicle. Doppler assessment optimized for low-velocity blood flow demonstrates venous flow pattern with retrograde flow and phasic variation. These findings are best visible during Valsalva maneuver [92]. In addition, decreased blood flow within the testicular artery [96,107] is a coexistent finding. The sensitivity and specificity of detection of varicocele during Doppler evaluation reaches 100% [92].

Procedure-related application of Doppler in infertility

Doppler sonography has been evaluated in certain other procedure-related applications such as hysterosalpingo-contrast-sonography (HyCoSy) and vascular Doppler during testicular surgery. Tubal patency can be assessed using HyCoSy, by injecting a contrast medium through the cervix and demonstrating its spill through the fimbrial end of the fallopian tubes on transvaginal ultrasound. Doppler imaging may be helpful to increase the diagnostic accuracy by limiting false-negative test results. Identification of the flow of contrast in the tube from the uterus towards the peritoneal cavity improves the diagnostic accuracy, and the appearance of color in the abdominal cavity confirms tubal patency. Limitations of Doppler application in HyCoSy are associated with the presence of significant

Doppler motion artifacts generated by the small bowel, making interpretation of the test often unreliable [108,109].

Research suggests that routine use of intraoperative vascular Doppler during varicocele surgery is helpful to identify and spare as many testicular and spermatic arteries as possible [110]. Inadvertent ligation of arterial blood supply to the testicle during surgery has been related to slow return to normal of semen parameters, damage to seminiferous tubules, and even testicular atrophy [111–113]. Doppler sonography used in this setting may also be beneficial to achieve successful obliteration of venous vessels and consequent improvement in semen parameters [110,114].

Conclusion

Doppler ultrasound has a role in the field of fertility in both clinical and research settings. Clinically it can be used to help in confirming and differentiating certain pathological diagnoses made on grayscale imaging and may provide additional diagnostic information for adequate surgical planning. However, its use is generally restricted to subjective impression of color flow rather than a quantitative analysis of blood flow velocity or volume vascularity. Although many studies have reported evaluating the role of quantitative analysis of blood flow within the uterus and ovaries in predicting pregnancy and fertility treatment outcome in subfertile population, the conclusions were conflicting. This may relate to the limitation of Doppler ultrasound in that the measurable vascularity indices may not be reflective of endometrial or follicular microcirculation, which is possibly below the resolution limit of the currently available Doppler ultrasound both in terms of the vessel size and flow velocity. Technology is fast advancing with emerging new techniques including spatio-temporal image correlation (STIC) sonography, which assesses the blood flow within a volume during systole and diastole in real time. This technology needs to be assessed in a research setting before its application in day-to-day clinical practice can be implemented. Rapid improvement of the sensitivity of the Doppler software and hardware will allow for even more detailed assessment of the microvasculature of the endometrium and ovary. Hopefully, this will allow fertility specialists to obtain true and reproducible results, which in turn will translate into predictive models for use in tailoring the treatment protocols and improving the treatment outcomes.

References

1. Jones N, Hutchinson ES, Brownbill P, et al. In vitro dual perfusion of human placental lobules as a flow phantom to investigate the relationship between fetoplacental flow and quantitative 3D power Doppler angiography. *Placenta* 2009; **30**(2): 130–135.

2. Martins W. Three-dimensional power Doppler: validity and reliability. *Ultrasound Obstet Gynecol* 2010; **36**(5): 530–533.

3. Raine-Fenning N, Nordin NM, Ramnarine KV, et al. Evaluation of the effect of machine settings on quantitative three-dimensional power Doppler angiography: an in-vitro flow phantom experiment. *Ultrasound Obstet Gynecol* 2008; **32**(4): 551–559.

4. Raine-Fenning N, Nordin NM, Ramnarine KV, et al. Determining the relationship between three-dimensional power Doppler data and true blood flow characteristics: an in-vitro flow phantom experiment. *Ultrasound Obstet Gynecol* 2008. **32**(4): 540–550.

5. Raine-Fenning N, Campbell BK, Clewes JS, Kendall NR, Johnson IR. The interobserver reliability of three-dimensional power Doppler data acquisition within the female pelvis. *Ultrasound Obstet Gynecol* 2004; **23**(5): 501–508.

6. Graham C, Postovit LM, Park H, Canning MT, Fitzpatrick TE. Adriana and Luisa Castellucci award lecture 1999: role of oxygen in the regulation of trophoblast gene expression and invasion. *Placenta* 2000; **21**(5–6): 443–450.

7. Farrer-Brown G, Beilby JO, Tarbit MH. The blood supply of the uterus. 1. Arterial vasculature. *J Obstet Gynaecol Br Commonw* 1970; **77**(8): 673–681.

8. Farrer-Brown, G, Beilby JO, Tarbit MH. The blood supply of the uterus. 2. Venous pattern. *J Obstet Gynaecol Br Commonw* 1970; **77**(8): 682–689.

9. Farrer-Brown, G, Beilby JO, Rowles PM. Microvasculature of the uterus. An injection method of study. *Obstet Gynecol* 1970; **35**(1): 21–30.

10. Bourne TH, Hagström HG, Granberg S, et al. Ultrasound studies of vascular and morphological changes in the human uterus after a positive self-test for the urinary luteinizing hormone surge. *Hum Reprod* 1996; **11**(2): 369–375.

11. Tan SL, Zaidi J, Campbell S, Doyle P, Collins W. Blood flow changes in the ovarian and uterine arteries during the normal menstrual cycle. *Am J Obstet Gynecol* 1996; **175**(3 Pt 1): 625–631.

12. Zaidi J, Collins W, Campbell S, Pittrof R, Tan SL. Blood flow changes in the intraovarian arteries during the periovulatory period: relationship to the time of day. *Ultrasound Obstet Gynecol* 1996; **7**(2): 135–140.

13. Sladkevicius P, Valentin L, Marsal K. Blood flow velocity in the uterine and ovarian arteries during the normal menstrual cycle. *Ultrasound Obstet Gynecol* 1993; **3**(3): 199–208.

14. Steer C, Campbell S, Pampiglione JS, Kingsland CR, Mason BA, Collins WP. Transvaginal colour flow imaging of the uterine arteries during the ovarian and menstrual cycles. *Hum Reprod* 1990; **5**(4): 391–395.

15. Achiron R, Levran D, Sivan E, Lipitz S, Dor J, Mashiach S. Endometrial blood flow response to hormone replacement therapy in women with premature ovarian failure: A transvaginal Doppler study. *Fertil Steril* 1995; **63**(3): 550–554.

16. Ng E, Chan CC, Tang OS, Yeung WS, Ho PC. Relationship between uterine blood flow and endometrial and subendometrial blood flows during stimulated and natural cycles. *Fertil Steril* 2006; **85**(3): 721–727.

17. Ng, E, Chan CC, Tang OS, Yeung WS, Ho PC. The role of endometrial blood flow measured by three-dimensional power Doppler ultrasound in the prediction of pregnancy during in vitro fertilization treatment. *Eur J Obstet Gynecol Reprod Biol* 2007; **135**(1): 8–16.

18. Raine-Fenning N, Campbell BK, Kendall NR, Clewes JS, Johnson IR. Endometrial and subendometrial perfusion are impaired in women with unexplained subfertility. *Hum Reprod* 2004; **19**(11): 2605–2614.

19. Raine-Fenning N, Campbell BK, Kendall NR, Clewes JS, Johnson IR. Quantifying the changes in endometrial vascularity throughout the normal menstrual cycle with three-dimensional power Doppler angiography. *Hum Reprod* 2004.;**19**(2): 330–338.

20. Gill RW. Measurement of blood flow by ultrasound: accuracy and sources of error. *Ultrasound Med Biol* 1985; **11**(4): 625–641.

21. Ranke C, Hendrickx P, Roth U, Brassel F, Creutzig A, Alexander K. Color and conventional image-directed Doppler ultrasonography: accuracy and sources of error in quantitative blood flow measurements. *J Clin Ultrasound* 1992; **20**(3): 187–193.

22. Dechaud H, Bessueille E, Bousquet PJ, Reyftmann L, Hamamah S, Hedon B. Optimal timing of ultrasonographic and Doppler evaluation of uterine receptivity to implantation. *Reprod BioMed Online* 2008; **16**(3): 368–375.

23. Salle B, Bied-Damon V, Benchaib M, Desperes S, Gaucherand P, Rudigoz RC. Preliminary report of an ultrasonography and colour Doppler uterine score to predict uterine receptivity in an in-vitro fertilization programme. *Hum Reprod* 1998; **13**(6): 1669–1673.

24. Schild R, Holthaus S, d'Alquen J, et al. Quantitative assessment of subendometrial blood flow by three-dimensional-ultrasound is an important predictive factor of implantation in an in-vitro fertilization programme. *Hum Reprod* 2000; **15**(1): 89–94.

25. Dietterich C, Check JH, Choe JK, Nazari A, Lurie D. Increased endometrial thickness on the day of human chorionic gonadotropin injection does not adversely affect pregnancy or implantation rates following in vitro fertilization-embryo transfer. *Fertil Steril* 2002; **77**(4): 781–786.

26. Chien L, Lee WS, Au HK, Tzeng CR. Assessment of changes in utero-ovarian arterial impedance during the peri-implantation period by Doppler sonography in women undergoing assisted reproduction. *Ultrasound Obstet Gynecol* 2004; **23**(5): 496–500.

27. Pritts EA, Parker WH, Olive DL. Fibroids and infertility: an updated systematic review of the evidence. *Fertil Steril* 2009; **91**(4): 1215–1223.

28. Klatsky PC, Tran ND, Caughey AB, Fujimoto VY. Fibroids and reproductive outcomes: a systematic literature review from conception to delivery. *Am J Obstet Gynecol* 2008; **198**(4): 357–366.

29. Bulletti C, De Ziegler D, Polli V, Flamigni C. The role of leiomyomas in infertility. *J Am Assoc Gynecol Laparosc* 1999; **6**(4): 441–445.

30. Farquhar C, Ekeroma A, Furness S, Arroll B. A systematic review of transvaginal ultrasonography, sonohysterography and hysteroscopy for the investigation of abnormal uterine bleeding in premenopausal women. *Acta Obstet Gynecol Scand* 2003; **82**(6): 493–504.

31. Cil A, Tulunay G, Kose MF, Haberal A. Power Doppler properties of endometrial polyps and submucosal fibroids: a preliminary observational study in women with known intracavitary lesions. *Ultrasound Obstet Gynecol* 2010; **35**(2): 233–237.

32. de Sá Rosa e de Silva AC, Rosa e Silva JC, Cândido dos Reis FJ, Nogueira AA, Ferriani RA. Routine office hysteroscopy in the investigation of infertile couples before assisted reproduction. *J Reprod Med* 2005; **50**(7): 501–506.

33. Kim M, Kim YA, Jo MY, Hwang KJ, Ryu HS. High frequency of endometrial polyps in endometriosis. *J Am Assoc Gynecol Laparosc* 2003; **10**(1): 46–48.

34. Shokeir T, Shalan H, El-Shafei M. Significance of endometrial polyps detected hysteroscopically in eumenorrheic infertile women. *J Obstet Gynaecol Res* 2004; **30**(2): 84–89.

35. Rackow B, Jorgensen E, Taylor H. Endometrial polyps affect uterine receptivity. *Fertil Steril* 2011; **95**(8): 2690–2692.

36. Krampl E, Bourne T, Hurlen-Solbakken H, Istre O. Transvaginal ultrasonography sonohysterography and operative hysteroscopy for the evaluation of abnormal uterine bleeding. *Acta Obstet Gynecol Scand* 2001; **80**(7): 616–622.

37. Bonnamy L, Marret H, Perrotin F, Body G, Berger C, Lansac J. Sonohysterography: a prospective survey of results and complications in 81 patients. *Eur J Obstet Gynecol Reprod Biol* 2002; **102**(1): 42–47.

38. Hosny I, Elghawabit H, Mosaad M. The role of 2D, 3D ultrasound and color Doppler in the diagnosis of benign and malignant endometrial lesions. *J Egypt Natl Cancer Inst* 2007; **19**(4): 275–281.

39. Tremellen K, Russell P. Adenomyosis is a potential cause of recurrent implantation failure during IVF treatment. *Aust N Z J Obstet Gynaecol* 2011; **51**: 280–283.

40. de Souza NM, Brosens JJ, Schwieso JE, Paraschos T, Winston RM. The potential value of magnetic resonance imaging in infertility. *Clin Radiol* 1995; **50**(2): 75–79.

41. Exacoustos C, Brienza L, Di Giovanni A, et al. Adenomyosis: three-dimensional sonographic findings of the junctional zone and correlation with histology. *Ultrasound Obstet Gynecol* 2011; **37**(4): 471–479.

42. Perrot N, Frey I, Mergui JL, Bazot M, Uzan M, Uzan S. Picture of the month. Adenomyosis: power Doppler findings. *Ultrasound Obstet Gynecol* 2001; **17**(2): 177–178.

43. Zaidi J, Campbell S, Pittrof R, Tan SL. Endometrial thickness, morphology, vascular penetration and velocimetry in predicting implantation in an in vitro fertilization program. *Ultrasound Obstet Gynecol* 1995; **6**(3): 191–198.

44. Applebaum M. The uterine biophysical profile. *Ultrasound Obstet Gynecol* 1995; **5**(1): 67–68.

45. Singh N. Bahadur A, Mittal S, Malhotra N, Bhatt A. Predictive value of endometrial thickness, pattern and sub-endometrial blood flows on the day of hCG by 2D doppler in in-vitro fertilization cycles: a prospective clinical study from a tertiary care unit. *J Hum Reprod Sci* 2011; **4**(1): 29–33.

46. Wang L, Qiao J, Li R, Zhen X, Liu Z. Role of endometrial blood flow assessment with color Doppler energy in predicting pregnancy outcome of IVF-ET cycles. *Reprod Biol Endocrinol* 2010; **8**: 122.

47. Kupesic S, Bekavac I, Bjelos D, Kurjak A. Assessment of endometrial receptivity by transvaginal color Doppler and three-dimensional power Doppler ultrasonography in patients undergoing in vitro fertilization procedures. *J Ultrasound Med* 2001; **20**(2): 125–134.

48. Engmann L, Sladkevicius P, Agrawal R, Bekir J, Campbell S, Tan S. The pattern of changes in ovarian stromal and uterine artery blood flow velocities during in vitro fertilization treatment and its relationship with outcome of the cycle. *Ultrasound Obstet Gynecol* 1999; **13**(1): 26–33.

49. Sterzik K, Grab D, Sasse V, Hütter W, Rosenbusch B, Terinde R. Doppler sonographic findings and their correlation with implantation in an in vitro fertilization program. *Fertil Steril* 1989; **52**(5): 825–828.

50. Serafini P, Batzofin J, Nelson J, Olive D. Sonographic uterine predictors of pregnancy in women undergoing ovulation induction for assisted reproductive treatments. *Fertil Steril* 1994; **62**(4): 815–822.

51. Hoozemans DA, Schats R, Lambalk NB, Homburg R, Hompes PG. Serial uterine artery Doppler velocity parameters and human uterine receptivity in IVF/ICSI cycles. *Ultrasound Obstet Gynecol* 2008; **31**: 432–438.

52. Steer CV, Campbell S, Tan SL, et al. The use of transvaginal color flow imaging after in vitro fertilization to identify optimum uterine conditions before embryo transfer. *Fertil Steril* 1992; **57**(2): 372–376.

53. Coulam CB, Bustillo M, Soenksen DM, Britten S. Ultrasonographic predictors of implantation after assisted reproduction. *Fertil Steril* 1994; **62**(5): 1004–1010.

54. Zackova T, Järvelä IY, Tapanainen JS, Feyereisl J. Assessment of endometrial and ovarian characteristics using three dimensional power Doppler ultrasound to predict response in frozen embryo transfer cycles. *Reprod Biol Endocrinol* 2009; **7**: 151.

55. Ng EH, Chan CC, Tang OS, Yeung WS, Ho PC. The role of endometrial and subendometrial vascularity measured by three-dimensional power Doppler ultrasound in the prediction of pregnancy during frozen-thawed embryo transfer cycles. *Hum Reprod* 2006; **21**(6): 1612–1617.

56. Ng EH, Chan CC, Tang OS, Yeung WS, Ho PC. Comparison of endometrial and subendometrial blood flow measured by three-dimensional power Doppler ultrasound between stimulated and natural cycles in the same patients. *Hum Reprod* 2004; **19**(10): 2385–2390.

57. Ng EH, Chan CC, Tang OS, Yeung WS, Ho PC. Factors affecting endometrial and subendometrial blood flow measured by three-dimensional power Doppler ultrasound during IVF treatment. *Hum Reprod* 2006; **21**(4): 1062–1069.

58. Lam P, Johnson I, Raine-Fenning N. Endometrial blood flow is impaired in women with polycystic ovarian syndrome who are clinically hyperandrogenic. *Ultrasound Obstet Gynecol* 2009; **34**(3): 326–334.

59. Ng E, Chan CC, Tang OS, Yeung WS, Ho PC. Changes in endometrial and subendometrial blood flow in IVF. *Reprod BioMed Online* 2009; **18**(2): 269–275.

60. Wu HM, Chiang CH, Huang HY, Chao AS, Wang HS, Soong YK. Detection of the subendometrial vascularization flow index by three-dimensional ultrasound may be useful for predicting the pregnancy rate for patients undergoing in vitro fertilization-embryo transfer. *Fertil Steril* 2003; **79**(3): 507–511.

61. Merce L, Barco MJ, Bau S, Troyano J. Are endometrial parameters by three-dimensional ultrasound and power Doppler angiography related to in vitro fertilization/embryo transfer outcome? *Fertil Steril* 2008; **89**(1): 111–117.

62. Dorn C, Reinsberg J, Willeke C, Wendt A, van der Ven H, Schild RL. Three-dimensional power Doppler ultrasound of the subendometrial blood flow under the administration of a contrast agent (Levovist). *Arch Gynecol Obstet* 2004; **270**(2): 94–98.

63. Jarvela I, Sladkevicius P, Kelly S, Ojha K, Campbell S, Nargund G. Evaluation of endometrial receptivity during in-vitro fertilization using three-dimensional power Doppler ultrasound. *Ultrasound Obstet Gynecol* 2005; **26**(7): 765–769.

64. Hackeloer BJ, Nitschke-Dabelstein S. Ovarian imaging by ultrasound: an attempt to define a reference plane. *J Clin Ultrasound* 1980; **8**(6): 497–500.

65. Raine-Fenning NJ, Nordin NM, Ramnarine KV, et al. Evaluation of the effect of machine settings on quantitative three-dimensional power Doppler angiography: an in-vitro flow phantom experiment. *Ultrasound Obstet Gynecol* 2008; **32**(4): 551–559.

66. Raine-Fenning N, Campbell B, Collier J, Brincat M, Johnson I. The reproducibility of endometrial volume acquisition and measurement with the VOCAL-imaging program. *Ultrasound Obstet Gynecol* 2002; **19**(1): 69–75.

67. Revised 2003 consensus on diagnostic criteria and long-term health risks related to polycystic ovary syndrome (PCOS). *Hum Reprod* 2004; **19**(1): 41–47.

68. Ozkan S, Vural B, Caliṣkan E, Bodur H, Türköz E, Vural F. Color Doppler sonographic analysis of uterine and ovarian artery blood flow in women with polycystic ovary syndrome. *J Clin Ultrasound* 2007; **35**(6): 305–313.

69. Tugrul S, Oral O, Güçlü M, Kutlu T, Uslu H, Pekin O. Significance of Doppler ultrasonography in the diagnosis of polycystic ovary syndrome. *Clin Exp Obstet Gynecol* 2006; **33**(3): 154–158.

70. Pan HA, Wu MH, Cheng YC, Li CH, Chang FM. Quantification of Doppler signal in polycystic ovary syndrome using three-dimensional power Doppler ultrasonography: a possible new marker for diagnosis. *Hum Reprod* 2002; **17**(1): 201–206.

71. Jarvela IY, Mason HD, Sladkevicius P, et al. Characterization of normal and polycystic ovaries using three-dimensional power Doppler ultrasonography. *J Assist Reprod Genet* 2002; **19**(12): 582–590.

72. Ng EH, Chan CC, Yeung WS, Ho PC. Comparison of ovarian stromal blood flow between fertile women with normal ovaries and infertile women with polycystic ovary syndrome. *Hum Reprod* 2005; **20**(7): 1881–1886.

73. Wu M, Tsai SJ, Pan HA, Hsiao KY, Chang FM. Three-dimensional power Doppler imaging of ovarian stromal blood flow in women with endometriosis undergoing in vitro fertilization. *Ultrasound Obstet Gynecol* 2003; **21**(5): 480–485.

74. Timmerman D, Testa AC, Bourne T, et al. Simple ultrasound-based rules for the diagnosis of ovarian cancer. *Ultrasound Obstet Gynecol* 2008; **31**(6): 681–690.

75. Sokalska A, Timmerman D, Testa AC, et al. Diagnostic accuracy of transvaginal ultrasound examination for assigning a specific diagnosis to adnexal masses. *Ultrasound Obstet Gynecol* 2009; **34**(4): 462–470.

76. Freiesleben N, Lossl K, Bogstad J, et al. Predictors of ovarian response in intrauterine insemination patients and development of a dosage nomogram. *Reprod BioMed Online* 2008; **17**(5): 632–641.

77. Ragni G, Anselmino M, Nicolosi AE, Brambilla ME, Calanna G, Somigliana E. Follicular vascularity is not predictive of pregnancy outcome in mild controlled ovarian stimulation and IUI cycles. *Hum Reprod* 2007; **22**(1): 210–214.

78. Bhal PS, Pugh ND, Gregory L, O'Brien S, Shaw RW. Perifollicular vascularity as a potential variable affecting outcome in stimulated intrauterine insemination treatment cycles: a study using transvaginal power Doppler. *Hum Reprod* 2001; **16**(8): 1682–1689.

79. Engels V, Sanfrutos L, Perez-Medina T, et al. Periovulatory follicular volume and vascularization determined by 3D and power Doppler sonography as pregnancy predictors in intrauterine insemination cycles. *J Clin Ultrasound* 2011; **39**(5): 243–247.

80. Zaidi J, Barber J, Kyei-Mensah A, Bekir J, Campbell S, Tan SL. Relationship of ovarian stromal blood flow at the baseline ultrasound scan to subsequent follicular response in an in vitro fertilization program. *Obstet Gynecol* 1996; **88**(5): 779–784.

81. Engmann L, Sladkevicius P, Agrawal R, Bekir JS, Campbell S, Tan S. Value of ovarian stromal blood flow velocity measurement after pituitary suppression in the prediction of ovarian responsiveness and outcome of in vitro fertilization treatment. *Fertil Steril* 1999; **71**(1): 22–29.

82. Bassil S, Wyns C, Toussaint-Demylle D, Nisolle M, Gordts S, Donnez J. The relationship between ovarian vascularity and the duration of stimulation in in-vitro fertilization. *Hum Reprod* 1997; **12**(6): 1240–1245.

83. Ng EH, Tang OS, Chan CC, Ho PC. Ovarian stromal blood flow in the prediction of ovarian response during in vitro fertilization treatment. *Hum Reprod* 2005; **20**(11): 3147–3151.

84. Kupesic S, Kurjak A. Predictors of IVF outcome by three-dimensional ultrasound. *Hum Reprod* 2002; **17**(4): 950–955.

85. Mercé LT, Barco MJ, Bau S, Troyano JM. Prediction of ovarian response and IVF/ICSI outcome by three-dimensional ultrasonography and power Doppler angiography. *Eur J Obstet Gynecol Reprod Biol* 2007; **132**(1): 93–100.

86. Ng EH, Tang OS, Chan CC, Ho PC. Ovarian stromal vascularity is not predictive of ovarian response and pregnancy. *Reprod Biomed Online* 2006; **12**(1): 43–49.

87. Jayaprakasan K, Jayaprakasan R, Al-Hasie HA, et al. Can quantitative three-dimensional power Doppler angiography be used to predict ovarian hyperstimulation syndrome? *Ultrasound Obstet Gynecol* 2009; **33**(5): 583–591.

88. Jayaprakasan K, Al-Hasie H, Jayaprakasan R, et al. The three-dimensional ultrasonographic ovarian vascularity of women developing poor ovarian response during assisted reproduction treatment and its predictive value. *Fertil Steril* 2009; **92**(6): 1862–1869.

89. Middleton W, Bell M. Analysis of intratesticular arterial anatomy with emphasis on transmediastinal arteries. *Radiology* 1993; **189**(1): 157–160.

90. Siegel BA (Ed.) *Diagnostic Ultrasonography Test and Syllabus (Second Series)*. Reston, VA: American College of Radiology; 1994.

91. Cardiovascular (inferior vena cava). In: Williams PL, Bannister LH (Eds.) *Gray's Anatomy: The Anatomical Basis of Medicine and Surgery*. New York: Churchill Livingstone; 1995: 1600–1601.

92. Dogra V, Gottlieb RH, Oka M, Rubens DJ. Sonography of the scrotum. *Radiology* 2003; **227**(1): 18–36.

93. Middleton W, Thorne D, Melson G. Color Doppler ultrasound of the normal testis. *AJR Am J Roentgenol* 1989; **152**(2): 293–297.

94. Rubin J, Bude RO, Carson PL, Bree RL, Adler RS. Power Doppler US: a potentially useful alternative to mean frequency- based color Doppler US. *Radiology* 1994; **190**(3): 853–856.

95. Siegel M. The acute scrotum. *Radiol Clin North Am* 1997; **35**(4): 959–976.

96. Schurich M, Aigner F, Frauscher F, Pallwein L. The role of ultrasound in assessment of male fertility. *Eur J Obstet Gynecol Reprod Biol* 2009; **144**(Suppl 1): S192–198.

97. Paltiel HJ, Rupich RC, Babcock DS. Maturational changes in arterial impedance of the normal testis in boys: Doppler sonographic study. *AJR Am J Roentgenol* 1994; **163**(5): 1189–1193.

98. Keener TS, Winter TC, Nghiem HV, Schmiedl UP. Normal adult epididymis: evaluation with color Doppler US. *Radiology* 1997; **202**(3): 712–714.

99. Horstman WG, Melson GL, Middleton WD, Andriole GL. Testicular tumors: findings with color Doppler US. *Radiology* 1992; **185**(3): 733–737.

100. Herwig R, Tosun K, Schuster A, et al. Tissue perfusion-controlled guided biopsies are essential for the outcome of testicular sperm extraction. *Fertil Steril* 2007; **87**(5): 1071–1076.

101. Battaglia C, Pasini A, Mancini F, Burnelli R, Cicognani A, de Aloysio D. Role of intratesticular ultrasonographic and Doppler flow analyses in evaluating gonadal status in male survivors of childhood malignancy. *Fertil Steril* 2005; **83**(6): 1867–1870.

102. Foresta C, Garolla A, Bettella A, Ferlin A, Rossato M, Candiani F. Doppler ultrasound of the testis in azoospermic subjects as a parameter of testicular function. *Hum Reprod* 1998; **13**(11): 3090–3093.

103. Meacham RB, Townsend RR, Rademacher D, Drose JA. The incidence of varicoceles in the general population when evaluated by physical examination, gray scale sonography and color Doppler sonography. *J Urol* 1994; **151**(6): 1535–1538.

104. Pierik FH, Dohle GR, van Muiswinkel JM, Vreeburg JT, Weber RF. Is routine scrotal ultrasound advantageous in infertile men? *J Urol* 1999; **162**(5): 1618–1620.

105. Gorelick JI, Goldstein M. Loss of fertility in men with varicocele. *Fertil Steril* 1993; **59**(3): 613–616.

106. Mehta AL, Dogra VS. Intratesticular varicocele. *J Clin Ultrasound* 1998; **26**(1): 49–51.

107. Tarhan S, Gümüs B, Gündüz I, Ayyildiz V, Göktan C. Effect of varicocele on testicular artery blood flow in men – color Doppler investigation. *Scand J Urol Nephrol* 2003; **37**(1): 38–42.

108. Boudghene FP, Bazot M, Robert Y, et al. Assessment of Fallopian tube patency by HyCoSy: comparison of a positive contrast agent with saline solution. *Ultrasound Obstet Gynecol* 2001; **18**(5): 525–530.

109. Kleinkauf-Houcken A, Hüneke B, Lindner C, Braendle W. Combining B-mode ultrasound with pulsed wave Doppler for the assessment of tubal patency. *Hum Reprod* 1997; **12**(11): 2457–2460.

110. Cocuzza M, Pagani R, Coelho R, Srougi M, Hallak J. The systematic use of intraoperative vascular Doppler ultrasound during microsurgical subinguinal varicocelectomy improves precise identification and preservation of testicular blood supply. *Fertil Steril* 2010; **93**(7): 2396–2399.

111. Silber SJ. Microsurgical aspects of varicocele. *Fertil Steril* 1979; **31**(2): 230–232.

112. Steinberger E, Tjioe DY. Spermatogenesis in rat testes after experimental ischemia. *Fertil Steril* 1969; **20**(4): 639–649.

113. Penn I, Mackie G, Halgrimson CG, Starzl TE. Testicular complications following renal transplantation. *Ann Surg* 1972; **176**(6): 697–699.

114. Pasqualotto FF, Lucon AM, de Góes PM, et al. Relationship between the number of veins ligated in a varicocelectomy with testicular volume, hormonal levels and semen parameters outcome. *J Assist Reprod Genet* 2005; **22**(6): 245–249.

Chapter

27

Ultrasound assessment of ovarian reserve

Bradley J. Van Voorhis

Societal trends towards delayed childbearing mean that more women will be faced with the unexpected problem of infertility due to reduced ovarian reserve. The rate of decline in ovarian reserve greatly varies in individuals, so having an accurate assessment of ovarian reserve may be useful in counseling women about the cause of infertility and the prognosis for treatment. Transvaginal ultrasound (TVUS) has revolutionized the practice of assisted reproduction. TVUS has been utilized for many years to diagnose reproductive tract abnormalities and to monitor follicular development. It has also allowed for transvaginal oocyte retrieval in IVF procedures. One of the newer uses is to assess ovarian reserve in women with infertility. In this chapter, I will review ultrasound assessment of ovarian reserve and compare this test with other available tests of ovarian reserve.

Assessment of ovarian reserve

The aim of ovarian reserve testing is to estimate the number of eggs remaining in the ovaries of women. Since this number cannot be determined without removing the ovaries, various tests of ovarian reserve have been developed which reflect the size of the pool of the primordial follicles and thus eggs remaining in the ovary. Serum tests include follicle-stimulating hormone (FSH), estradiol, inhibin B, and anti-müllerian hormone (AMH) levels which reflect, either directly or indirectly, granulosa cell production of hormones in ovarian follicles and, therefore, estimate the ovarian follicular pool. TVUS can also be utilized to directly estimate ovarian reserve, either by measuring ovarian volume or by determining the antral follicle count (AFC). A key point to be made is that all tests to date measure the quantity of ovarian follicles and eggs and do not measure the quality of those eggs. This is important since all measures of ovarian reserve are better at predicting ovarian responsiveness to gonadotropin stimulation than they are at predicting pregnancy, which is very dependent on egg quality.

An individual's ovarian reserve can have important clinical consequences. If there is a high ovarian reserve, women can be expected to have a more robust response to gonadotropin stimulation and may be at increased risk for ovarian hyperstimulation syndrome. In contrast, women with reduced ovarian reserve are at increased risk of cycle cancellation due to inadequate follicle development to gonadotropin stimulation. In an IVF cycle, women with reduced ovarian reserve will have fewer oocytes retrieved, fewer embryos, and because IVF success is somewhat dependent on embryo number, possibly a reduced chance for pregnancy. Theoretically, ovarian stimulation protocols could be selected and gonadotropin doses adjusted to optimize ovarian responsiveness based on ovarian reserve. However, at least in the case of reduced ovarian reserve, increasing doses of gonadotropins do not necessarily lead to increases in the number of retrieved eggs at IVF [1]. At the very least, couples can be counseled about expected outcomes of ovarian stimulation prior to deciding to pursue a given treatment.

All tests of ovarian reserve should accurately estimate the primordial follicular pool and thus the number of remaining eggs, which in turn is most often determined by measuring the ovarian response to gonadotropins in an infertility treatment cycle. An ideal test would not only be accurate but would inform the clinician beyond what is already known from the woman's age—that the chances for a poor ovarian stimulation rise and the chances for pregnancy drop as women age is well known. An ovarian reserve test becomes most useful when it can predict prognosis when controlling for age. Can the test differentiate the 38-year-old who will conceive easily from the one who will have a cycle cancelled for poor ovarian response and who will never conceive a pregnancy?

In the following sections, I will review ultrasound-based measures of ovarian reserve and compare these tests with other serum-based measures.

Ovarian reserve and ovarian volume

The first studies of ultrasound-based determination of ovarian reserve looked at ovarian volumes. The volume of the ovary is easily measured by TVUS and is commonly calculated by the formula of an ellipsoid (0.52 × the length × height × width of the ovary in centimeters) (Fig. 27.1). To make these measurements, the ovary is imaged in a plane that captures the long axis of the

Ultrasonography in Gynecology, ed. Botros R. M. B. Rizk and Elizabeth E. Puscheck. Published by Cambridge University Press. © Cambridge University Press 2015.

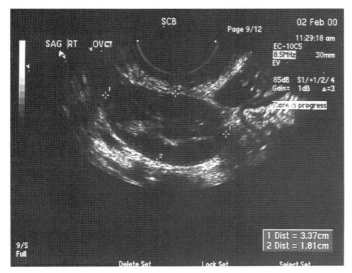

Fig. 27.1 Ultrasound determination of ovarian volume. The ovary is measured in three dimensions for this purpose.

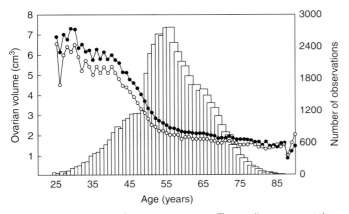

Fig. 27.2 Mean ovarian volumes as women age. The two lines represent the right and left ovary. ([2]: Reprinted with permission from Pavlik et al., *Gynecol Oncol* 2000; **77**: 410–412.)

ovary. Perpendicular measurements (length and width) are made in this plane and then the ultrasound transducer is turned to create a plane perpendicular to the first plane and the final measurement (height) is determined. The inter- and intra-observer variability of ovarian volume determinations is small (both under 7%) and cycle-to-cycle variation in a given woman is also low. Recently, ovarian volumes have been determined by 3D ultrasonography and these measures have been shown to correlate quite closely with estimates of volume calculated from 2D measurements.

Ovarian volume declines in women as they age. Pavlik et al. [2] studied nearly 14 000 women, aged 25–91 years, as part of an ovarian cancer-screening program and found that ovarian volume declined, particularly after ages 35–37 (Fig. 27.2). Indeed, the mean ovarian volume for women <30 (6.6 cm³ ± 0.19) was significantly greater than for women aged 30–39 (6.1 cm³ ± 0.06) or women aged 40–49 (4.8 cm³ ± 0.03). Although women over 68 inches tall had larger mean volumes, the authors found no relation between ovarian volume and weight or parity [2].

When controlling for a woman's age, reduced ovarian volume has been shown to predict reduced ovarian responsiveness and a lower pregnancy rate following IVF [3]. In this study, ultrasound measurement of the ovary was made on day 21 of a natural cycle. Because there was often the presence of a corpus luteum or an ovarian cyst which inflated the true ovarian volume in one ovary, the volume of the smallest ovary was studied. The median volume of the smallest ovary was 6.4 cm³ with the 10th percentile at 3.2 c m³ in this population of women presenting for IVF treatment. When the volume of the smallest ovary was <3 cm³, patients had a higher cycle cancellation rate, fewer eggs retrieved, and a lower clinical pregnancy rate. Specifically, a volume reduction in the smallest ovary from 12 cm³ to 3 cm³ increased the odds of obtaining <8 mature oocytes (25th percentile performance for numbers of retrieved mature oocytes) by 380% and decreased the odds of pregnancy by 50%. In contrast, when the volume of the smallest ovary was >9 cm³, cycle cancellations were very rare, more eggs were retrieved, and clinical pregnancy rates were improved. In a direct comparison, ovarian volume was found to be superior to cycle day 3 FSH as a measure of ovarian reserve [4]. Thus, ovarian volume can be a useful prognostic test prior to an IVF cycle.

High ovarian volumes have also been shown to predict increased ovarian reserve and a higher risk of ovarian hyperstimulation syndrome (OHSS) [5]. Following pre-treatment with an oral contraceptive, the pre-stimulation "pooled" ovarian volume on 3D ultrasound was significantly greater in patients who developed OHSS than in those who did not (11.3 ± 4.9 cm³ vs. 8.9 ± 3.7 cm³, $P < 0.035$). In women with a pooled ovarian volume <10 cm³ ($n = 65$), the risk of OHSS was 10% compared with 23.5% if the volume was >10 cm³ ($n = 34$). It has been suggested that baseline ovarian volume assessment prior to stimulation may help prevent OHSS by early adjustment of gonadotropin dosage or careful monitoring [5].

In addition to age, other factors that affect ovarian volume include past cigarette smoking (smokers have a decreased ovarian volume), polycystic ovarian syndrome, and the presence of larger ovarian cysts, functional or otherwise. Because ovarian cysts are common and may falsely inflate the basal ovarian volume, it is best to use the smallest ovarian volume to estimate ovarian reserve. Due to suppression of gonadotropins, women on birth control pills have small ovarian volumes and these measurements cannot be used to estimate reserve in this circumstance.

Ovarian reserve and antral follicle counts

Although there is a direct correlation between ovarian volume and antral follicle count (AFC), AFC has been found to be superior to ovarian volume as a predictor of reduced ovarian reserve [6]. For this test, both ovaries are scanned systematically with a sweeping motion while counting the number of ovarian follicles present in both ovaries (Fig. 27.3). In the literature, studies have used different size criteria for determining AFC. Some studies have counted follicles between 2 and 5 mm

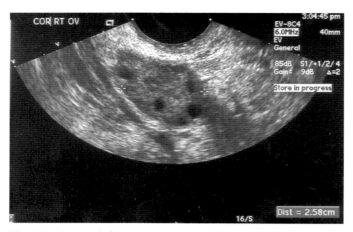

Fig. 27.3 Ultrasound of the ovary showing several antral follicles in this section.

whereas others have counted follicles between 2 and 10 mm. The variability of AFC measurements depends, in part, on the size of the follicles being counted. There is less cycle variability when counting all follicles between 2 and 10 mm as compared with counting follicles between 2 and 5 mm [7]. Due to its better test characteristics, AFC between 2 and 10 mm may be the preferred measure of ovarian reserve using ultrasonography, and this seems to be the method that is most commonly used at this time [7].

Based on autopsy studies, depletion of ovarian follicles from the ovary has been described as a biphasic phenomenon with a more rapid loss of follicles occurring after approximately 37 years of age [8]. A recent cross-sectional study of 252 white women suggests that this may not be the case, at least based on AFC [9]. In this study, AFC (2–10 mm) was determined in a cross-sectional study of regularly cycling women from 25 to 45 years of age. When graphing the average AFC versus age, the line was best described as a gradual acceleration in decline with age. This finding was recently confirmed by a large Italian study, evaluating 362 patients with AFC measurements, that also found the decline to be essentially linear with mean AFC, decreasing by about 0.4 follicles for every year of age [10]. The mean AFC was 16.6 in women 16 years of age and reduced to 3.3 by age 49. At age 35, the mean AFC was 9.0. Both studies only included women with regular menstrual cycles who were not infertile and who were not taking hormonal medications. Thus women with PCOS were excluded. Therefore, these findings reflect AFC in normal women and it remains possible that AFC counts and declines could differ in an infertile population.

Many studies have now demonstrated that a reduced AFC in infertile women is associated with a higher cycle cancellation rate and a reduced number of eggs retrieved in an IVF cycle. For example, Tomas et al. [11] found that AFC correlated more strongly with numbers of oocytes recovered during IVF than age alone. Although ovarian volume was linearly related with AFC preceding stimulation, AFC was a better predictor of oocytes retrieved. Frattarelli et al. [12] studied 278 IVF patients and found that AFC (2–10 mm follicles) was correlated with

numbers of recovered eggs and negatively correlated with patient age and day 3 FSH. An AFC of ≤10 increased the risk of cancellation significantly (OR 4.71, CI 1.28–20.47). Bancsi et al. [13] studied day 3 total ovarian volume, AFC, basal FSH, estradiol, and inhibin B levels. AFC was the single best predictor of poor ovarian response (ROC = 0.87).

Although there is general agreement in the literature that a lower AFC predicts reduced ovarian reserve leading to fewer eggs being recovered with IVF, the exact cut-off has varied in published studies. A reduced AFC has been defined anywhere from ≤3 follicles to <10 follicles. Test characteristics (sensitivity, specificity, positive and negative predictive values) will change depending on the cut-off used. The positive and negative predictive values are generally improved by using lower cut-offs (<4 follicles) although this naturally reduces the sensitivity of AFC [14].

A recent systematic review of ultrasound-based tests of ovarian reserve (AFC, ovarian volume, and Doppler studies of ovarian stromal blood flow) concluded that all are better predictors of ovarian response to gonadotropins than to pregnancy after treatment [15]. This study found that an AFC (2–10 mm) <4 has high specificity in predicting cycle cancellation. Women with an AFC <4 were 37 times more likely to have their cycle cancelled than were women with an AFC of 4 or more. Likewise, ovarian volume measurements of less than 3 cm^3 had specificity for predicting cycle cancellation of 92%. AFC and ovarian volume are useful in predicting poor response at extreme cut-offs, which are rarely found in regularly cycling young women. However, these values are found more frequently in older reproductive-age women and are moderately useful for planning ovarian stimulation and counseling women about the likelihood of cycle cancellation. Although some have reported that ovarian vascular flow by Doppler studies may be predictive of outcomes, this systematic review found conflicting data in the literature and did not find sufficient evidence to justify its use as a measure of ovarian reserve. More studies are warranted regarding this technology.

AFC versus day 3 FSH for ovarian reserve

A meta-analysis concluded that AFC is a better test than a cycle day 3 FSH level for predicting poor response and it was determined to be a moderately useful test for this purpose [14]. Neither test performs very well for predicting pregnancy.

AFC versus serum AMH for ovarian reserve

Recently, AMH levels have emerged as an important predictor of ovarian reserve. AMH is made by the granulosa cells of secondary, preantral, and small antral follicles up to 6 mm in diameter and therefore serum levels directly correlate with ovarian reserve. This test is easily measured by serum immunoassay and it requires less skill to perform than an ultrasound of the ovary.

A meta-analysis comparing AFC to AMH concluded that these two tests had equal accuracy and clinical value for predicting poor response in an IVF cycle [16]. Both tests performed poorly for predicting the occurrence of pregnancy after treatment.

The ideal ovarian reserve test would change little over the course of the reproductive cycle and would be relatively stable from cycle to cycle, allowing the test to be performed virtually any time. The inter- and intra-cycle variability of both AMH levels and AFC was recently investigated [7]. The inter-cycle variability was assessed in 77 regularly cycling infertile women between the ages of 24 and 40 on cycle day 3 for up to four cycles. The intra-cycle variation was assessed by taking measurements from 44 regularly cycling women every 1–3 days in a cycle. When comparing the two tests, mean AMH and AFC levels were not statistically different over four consecutive cycles; however, the variability was less with AMH levels than with AFC. Likewise, the intra-cycle variability was less for AMH than for AFC. Better consistency favors AMH levels, especially when ovarian reserve testing is done at random times in the reproductive cycle.

Not only can ovarian reserve tests predict reduced ovarian reserve and, therefore, poor responsiveness to gonadotropins, they also can predict excessive response. Several studies have evaluated the ability of AMH and AFC to predict excessive response (variably defined as anywhere from 14 to greater than 21 eggs retrieved in a cycle) or by the occurrence of ovarian hyperstimulation syndrome. A recent meta-analysis of these studies concluded that AMH and AFC counts were both clinically useful, and equally accurate in predicting this outcome [17]. Thus, if excessive response is predicted, perhaps strategies can be implemented, including use of lower doses of gonadotropins, in an effort to reduce this complication.

Summary

Ultrasound measures of ovarian reserve are clinically useful in counseling patients about expected response to gonadotropins and, perhaps, in adjusting doses of gonadotropins to either increase or decrease the ovarian response. AFC appears to be the best ultrasound measure of ovarian reserve and is better than all serum measures except AMH. AMH measures appear to be equal to AFC for predicting ovarian response and AMH may have advantages since it requires less skill and may have improved consistency over the reproductive cycle. No tests of ovarian reserve can measure egg quality and they are poor tests for predicting who will and will not conceive a pregnancy. Therefore these tests should not routinely be used to exclude patients from treatment.

References

1. Klinkert ER, Broekmans FJ, Looman CW, et al. Expected poor responders on the basis of an antral follicle count do not benefit from a higher starting dose of gonadotrophins in IVF treatment; a randomized controlled trial. *Hum Reprod* 2005; **20**: 611–615.

2. Pavlik EJ, DePriest PD, Gallion HH, et al. Ovarian volume related to age. *Gynecol Oncol* 2000; **77**: 410–412.

3. Syrop CH, Willhoite A, Van Voorhis BJ. Ovarian volume: a novel outcome predictor for assisted reproduction. *Fertil Steril* 1995; **64**: 1167–1171.

4. Syrop CH, Dawson JD, Husman KJ, Sparks, et al. Ovarian volume may predict assisted reproductive outcomes better than follicle stimulating hormone concentration on day 3. *Hum Reprod* 1999; **14**: 1752–1756.

5. Danniger B, Brunner M, Obruca A, et al. Prediction of ovarian hyperstimulation syndrome of baseline ovarian volume prior to stimulation. *Hum Reprod* 1996; **11**: 1597–1599.

6. Hendricks DJ, Kwee J, Mol, et al. Ultrasonography as a tool for the prediction of outcome in IVF patients: a comparative meta-analysis of ovarian volume and antral follicle count. *Fertil Steril* 2007; **87**(4): 764–775.

7. van Disseldorp J, Lambalk CB, Kwee J, et al. Comparison of inter- and intra-cycle variability of anti-Mullerian hormone and antral follicle counts. *Hum Reprod* 2010; **25**(1): 221–227.

8. Faddy MJ, Gosden RG, Gougeon A, et al. Accelerated disappearance of ovarian follicles in mid-life: implications for forecasting menopause. *Hum Reprod* 1992; **7**: 1342–1346.

9. Rosen MP, Sternfeld B, Schuh-Huerta SM, et al. Antral follicle count: absence of significant midlife decline. *Fertil Steril* 2010; **94**: 2182–2185.

10. La Marca A, Spada E, Sighinolfi G, et al. Age-specific nomogram for the decline in antral follicle count throughout the reproductive period. *Fertil Steril* 2011; **95**: 684–688.

11. Tomas C, Nuojua-Huttunen S, Martikainen H. Pretreatment transvaginal ultrasound examination predicts ovarian responsiveness to gonadotrophins in in-vitro fertilization. *Hum Reprod* 1997; **12**: 220–223.

12. Frattarelli JL, Lauria-Costa DF, Miller BT, et al. Basal antral follicle number and mean ovarian diameter predict cycle cancellation and ovarian responsiveness in assisted reproductive technology cycles. *Fertil Steril* 2000; **74**: 512–517.

13. Bancsi LFJMM, Broekmans FJM, Eijkemans MJC, et al. Predictors of poor ovarian response in in vitro fertilization: a prospective study comparing basal markers of ovarian reserve. *Fertil Steril* 2002; **77**: 328–336.

14. Hendriks DJ, Mol B-WJ, Bancsi LFHMM, et al. Antral follicle count in the prediction of poor ovarian response and pregnancy after in vitro fertilization: a meta-analysis and comparison with basal follicle-stimulating hormone level. *Fertil Steril* 2005; **83**: 291–301.

15. Gibreel A, Maheshwari A, Bhattacharya S, et al. Ultrasound tests of ovarian reserve: a systematic review of accuracy in predicting fertility outcomes. *Hum Fertil* 2009; **12**(2): 95–106.

16. Broer SL, Mol BWJ, Hendriks D, et al. The role of antimüllerian hormone in prediction of outcome after IVF: comparison with the antral follicle count. *Fertil Steril* 2009; **91**(3): 705–714.

17. Broer SL, Dolleman M, Opmeer BC, et al. AMH and AFC as predictors of excessive response in controlled ovarian hyperstimulation: a meta-analysis. *Hum Reprod Update* 2011; **17**(1): 46–54.

Ultrasound assessment of antral follicle count

Kannamannadiar Jayaprakasan and Nicholas J. Raine-Fenning

Introduction

Ovarian reserve, a measure of ovarian aging, is defined by the quantity and quality of the remaining primordial follicular pool within the ovaries at any given time [1]. Ovarian reserve diminishes with age [2,3] and the gradual decline dictates the onset of several age-related reproductive events including shortening of the length of the menstrual cycle, menstrual irregularity [4,5], and, finally, the menopause [6]. The associated and well-known age-related decrease in fecundity [7,8] is also primarily related to declining ovarian reserve rather than uterine aging, as evident by the equivalent pregnancy rates seen in women of all ages undergoing assisted reproduction treatment (ART) with oocyte donation from younger women [9,10]. Ovarian reserve, therefore, clearly reflects the fertility potential of a woman and strongly influences the possibility of conception either spontaneously or in conjunction with fertility treatment. Women with decreased ovarian reserve may also be at an increased risk of experiencing adverse obstetric events such as miscarriage [11], aneuploidy [12], multiple pregnancy [13], and pre-eclampsia [14].

Careful evaluation of subfertile women for signs of reduced ovarian reserve by reliable tests at the outset will help the clinician provide appropriate counseling of the couple about their realistic chances of conception, both spontaneously and after treatment, and may facilitate the choice of treatment for that individual couple. The evaluation of ovarian reserve is now an integral part of the pre-treatment assessment of a woman about to undergo ART, and is generally recommended for all women planning in vitro fertilization (IVF). The aim is to identify those women likely to respond poorly, who have a low chance of success and are more likely to have their treatment cycle cancelled, and those prone to ovarian hyperstimulation syndrome (OHSS), which is associated with significant morbidity and potential mortality. An accurate assessment of ovarian reserve and a prediction of ovarian response is important as it allows the treatment protocol to be tailored to the individual, thus potentially increasing the number of oocytes retrieved without risking an exaggerated response. Furthermore, ovarian reserve assessment is increasingly being requested and performed in

young patients with cancer prior to and following adjuvant treatment in order to predict the degree of potential impact of chemotherapy and radiotherapy on their reproductive life span. Girls and young women affected with cancer who wish to have children in the future could be advised on their fertility options, which include a rapid cycle prior to cancer treatment, fertility preservation, or no action dependent on their ovarian reserve, which can be used to guide them and the treating physicians.

Ovarian reserve tests

While chronological age is a marker of ovarian reserve, there is a considerable inter-individual variation in quantitative and qualitative ovarian reserve as indicated by histological studies demonstrating a variable number of primordial follicle cohort within the ovaries at any given age [15,16] and in the clinically evident variability in response to gonadotropin stimulation and live birth rates following IVF in women of the same age group [17]. Several ultrasound and endocrine markers of ovarian reserve based on the mechanism of ovarian aging have been identified and proposed for the prediction of fertility. Primarily, all of these tests aim to estimate the number of gonadotropin-responsive or "selectable follicles," which are assumed to be reflective of primordial follicle population. Two key challenges in assessing these markers are the population in whom the predictive evaluation should be performed and the outcome against which the markers need to be evaluated [18,19]. While the ideal population to be assessed would be the general population of woman wishing to delay conception, studies are invariably conducted on those women attending the infertility clinic and those undergoing IVF. The IVF population offers an ideal clinical group in which a defined clinical outcome directly relating to ovarian reserve, but not influenced by male factor, can be evaluated as it provides a quantitative assessment of the number of eggs retrieved and poor ovarian response to gonadotropin stimulation or cycle cancellation due to inadequate follicle development, both of which are closely linked to the likelihood of the desired outcome, namely live birth [18].

Ultrasonography in Gynecology, ed. Botros R. M. B. Rizk and Elizabeth E. Puscheck. Published by Cambridge University Press. © Cambridge University Press 2015.

The reported endocrine markers of ovarian reserve include factors produced by the developing follicles, such as estradiol, inhibin B, and anti-müllerian hormone (AMH), or the hormones under the inhibitory control of these factors, predominantly follicle-stimulating hormone (FSH). The ultrasound markers include the total antral follicle count, ovarian volume, and ovarian vascularity. The sensitivities, specificities, and predictive values of these tests have been evaluated in many studies by correlating the test results with the number of oocytes retrieved, the poor or exaggerated ovarian response to controlled ovarian stimulation and pregnancy, or live birth rates following IVF [1].

Ultrasound markers

Over the past two decades, various ultrasound markers have been investigated to evaluate their role in the prediction of ovarian reserve. The three most common markers that have been specifically addressed are ovarian volume, antral follicle count (AFC), and ovarian stromal blood flow. Most investigators have used conventional two-dimensional (2D) ultrasound to assess ovarian morphology and quantify these ovarian reserve variables. The introduction of three-dimensional (3D) ultrasound, quantitative 3D power Doppler angiography (3D-PDA), and automated volume measurements (sonography-based automatic volume count: SonoAVC: GE Healthcare) has enabled clinicians and researchers to use these advanced ultrasound modalities with a view to improving the predictive accuracy of ultrasound assessment of ovarian reserve.

Ovarian volume

The first ultrasound marker of ovarian reserve to be evaluated was ovarian volume [20]. It can easily be measured from 2D ultrasound images, using the principle of the volume of an ellipsoid using the formula: length × width × depth × π/6 (Fig. 28.1) or with 3D ultrasound. The commonly used method to calculate ovarian volume from 3D ultrasound ovarian volume dataset is the "rotational" method possible through Virtual Organ Computer-aided AnaLysis (VOCAL: GE Healthcare), which also generates a 3D model of the ovary (Fig. 28.2). The technique involves manual delineation of the ovary in the multiplanar display that shows the three perpendicular planes characteristic of 3D ultrasound. VOCAL allows rotation of the 3D dataset about a central axis through a number of pre-defined rotation steps [21]. The most appropriate rotation step for its use in a clinical or research setting is 9° as it provides the best compromise between reliability, validity, and time taken for measurement. Whilst the volume measurements using 3D technique have been shown to be statistically more reproducible than 2D measurements, the degree of reproducibility between observers is extremely high [21].

The role of ovarian volume as a marker of reserve has been evaluated in many studies, with conflicting results. The rationale of using ovarian volume as an ovarian reserve marker is that the volume reflects the size of the total follicle population

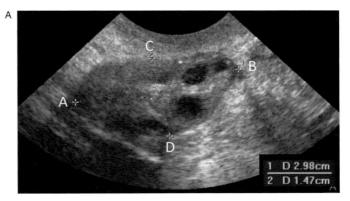

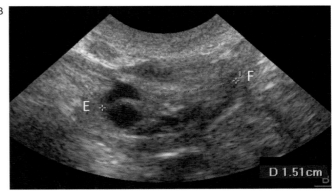

Fig. 28.1 2D method of volume calculation. Volume is measured using an ellipsoid formula: length × width × depth × π/6. (A) Longitudinal and anteroposterior diameters are measured in the longitudinal plane. (B) Transverse diameter is measured in the transverse plane.

remaining within the ovary, which was confirmed in a histological study [22]. Syrop et al. that found a reduction in estradiol levels, the number of oocytes collected, and pregnancy rates correlated with decreasing ovary volume in women undergoing assisted reproduction cycles [20], while Bowen et al. found a significant correlation between reduced ovarian volume, increasing age, and FSH levels [23]. Schild et al. examined the role of ovarian volume measurements made using pretreatment 3D datasets in 152 IVF cycles and found no relation to IVF outcome other than a nonsignificant trend of smaller ovarian measurements in the conception group [24]. Subgroup analysis comparing absolute ovarian size revealed a pregnancy rate of only 6.7% in patients with a minimum unilateral ovarian volume of no more than 3 cm³, which represented a single standard deviation below the mean, compared with 21.9% in patients with a minimum ovarian volume of more than 3 cm³. However, other studies have not seen such significant differences in ovarian volume between normal and poor responders in women aged less than 37 years [25], or in women at high risk for cancellation of assisted reproduction cycles [26]. While the value of ovarian volume on its own in predicting poor ovarian response is limited, ovarian volume measurement in women with or without polycystic ovaries may be a useful tool for predicting excessive response to ovarian stimulation [27]. An ovarian volume of more than 10 cm³ in the absence of a

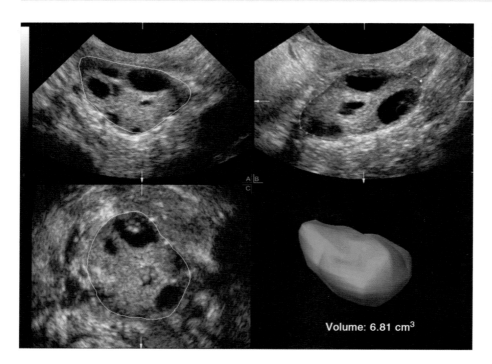

Fig. 28.2 3D method of volume calculation: the Virtual Organ Computer-aided AnaLysis (VOCAL). The measurement is performed in the B-plane by outlining the ovarian cortex manually. The ovarian dataset has been rotated 180° through twenty 9° rotation steps about a central vertical axis denoted by the blue arrow in the B-plane. The resultant three-dimensional model of the ovary is shown in the lower right image.

Volume: 6.81 cm³

dominant follicle or cyst of more than 10 mm is diagnostic of a polycystic ovary [28], which itself is a risk factor for excessive ovarian response and OHSS.

The data on the predictive ability of ovarian volume as an individual marker of ovarian reserve are conflicting therefore. A systematic review of all the relevant high-quality studies concluded that ovarian volume, as an individual marker of ovarian reserve and predictor of response to stimulation, has minimal clinical application [1]. Further, the use of ovarian volume as a marker in routine clinical practice is limited if there is a cyst or a large follicle in the ovary as it will falsely increase the baseline ovarian volume. The value of ovarian volume as a prognosticator of ovarian response is limited in certain other clinical situations such as in women with polycystic ovary syndrome who have an increased ovarian volume due to a possible increase in the ovarian stroma and in women who had ovarian surgery, which may decrease ovarian volume without reducing the follicular pool [29] although recent evidence suggests surgery may have a detrimental effect on ovarian reserve and the number of follicles.

Antral follicle count

The three different types of follicle seen within the ovaries, depending on the stages of development, include primordial follicles, early growing follicles, and antral follicles. While the ovarian reserve is principally composed of primordial or resting follicles, early growing follicles, which measure <1–2 mm in diameter, are composed of large primary, secondary, and pre-antral follicles, which grow at a slow rate in response to local regulatory factors, with endogenous FSH playing a permissive role. A small proportion of follicles develop into antral follicles that measure 2 mm or more in diameter, which are

highly sensitive and responsive to FSH and are commonly termed "selectable follicles" therefore. Larger antral follicles measuring 5–10 mm are gonadotropin-dependent. The number of "selectable" gonadotropin-responsive (2–5 mm) and gonadotropin-dependent (5–10 mm) follicles present in the ovaries is believed to reflect the number of remaining primordial follicles and, thus, the ovarian reserve. Further, the number of selectable follicles that are available to recruit determines the ovarian response to controlled ovarian stimulation during IVF. Antral follicles of at least 2 mm will be readily seen on transvaginal ultrasound and the antral follicle count measured using ultrasound is considered a good predictor of ovarian reserve and ovarian response to gonadotropin stimulation during IVF treatment [1].

The number of gonadotropin-responsive antral follicles detected by transvaginal ultrasound has been evaluated in the general subfertility population and in women undergoing ART, as a measure of ovarian aging. The correlation between the number of antral follicles with a diameter of up to 10 mm measured during the early follicular phase and reproductive aging has been investigated in a cohort of 162 regularly cycling women of 25–46 years of age with proven fertility [30]. The AFC ($r = -0.67$) showed a higher correlation with chronological age than the total ovarian volume ($r = -0.29$) and there was a decline in the mean number of antral follicles of 8.2% (95% CI 5.2–11.2%) per chronological year. This was evident when the range of follicles across different age groups was evaluated, with the number of follicles ranging from 7 to 22 at the age of 30 and from 2 to 7 by 40 years of age. There was a biphasic pattern of decline in AFCs, with a mean yearly decline of 4.8% before the age of 37 years compared with 11.7% thereafter. This finding was concordant with the age-related decline in primordial follicles as noted in a classic histological study of the ovaries obtained during autopsy or surgery in premenopausal women [6]. When the histological data were restricted to women of the same age group in this study, as in the study by Scheffer et al. [30], the disappearance rate of primordial follicles was similar before 37 years at 4.0% per year but higher at 23% after this age. Even though this study is limited by its cross-sectional study design, the data indicate that AFC, which is thought to be reflective of the primordial follicle population, is a marker of ovarian aging.

Tomas et al. were the first to report the role of AFC in predicting the ovarian response during IVF treatment [31]. The number of antral follicles measuring 2–5 mm was measured using conventional 2D transvaginal ultrasound, performed after pituitary down-regulation in 166 women undergoing their first cycle of IVF treatment. Based on the total number of antral follicles, the women were divided into those with inactive ovaries that contained less than 5 follicles, those with normal ovaries containing 5–15 follicles, and those with polycystic-like ovaries (PCO) with more than 15 follicles. Despite a similar total gonadotropin dose for ovarian stimulation in all three groups, there was a significant difference in the mean number of oocytes retrieved (5.4 ± 2.5, 7.4 ± 4.5, and 10.5 ± 5.1, respectively; $P = 0.006$), which was directly related to the number of antral follicles ($r^2 = 0.131$; $P < 0.001$). Although the ovarian volume was correlated with the AFC ($r^2 = 0.097$; $P < 0.001$), it had no relationship to the number of oocytes retrieved. The authors concluded that the number of small follicles observed before the ovarian stimulation was a better predictor of IVF outcome than ovarian volume or age alone.

Subsequently many studies have evaluated the predictive ability of AFC in assessing ovarian response and conception following IVF treatment. A significant correlation between the number of antral follicles with diameters measuring between 2 and 10 mm [32] or 2 and 6 mm [33] or 2 and 8 mm [34] or 2 and 5 mm [35,36], as assessed by both conventional 2D [37,38] and 3D [39,40] transvaginal ultrasound, and the number of oocytes retrieved has been observed. However, the relationship between AFC and conception following IVF has been poor in most of these studies. This has been confirmed in a recent meta-analysis [1], which concluded that the performance of AFC in the prediction of poor response in IVF was adequate and better than the widely used "ovarian reserve" marker, the basal FSH level, although its performance for predicting conception is poor. The optimum cut-off level of AFC (2–10 mm in diameter) with the maximum sum of sensitivity and specificity for the prediction of poor ovarian response is reported as 10 [32]. Further reports indicated that AFC is equal to AMH, the best endocrine marker of ovarian reserve, in predicting poor ovarian response, but both AFC and AMH are poor predictors of pregnancy rates following IVF treatment [32,41]. This suggests that the AFC is able to quantify the quantity but not the quality of the remaining follicle pool.

AFC has also been considered the most significant predictor of the development of OHSS and ovarian hyper-response in women undergoing IVF treatment. The optimum cut-off level with the maximum sum of sensitivity and specificity for the prediction of exaggerated response is 22 [42], which seems more in keeping with the normal ranges defined by the Rotterdam consensus on the ultrasonographic diagnostic criteria for the PCO, which by definition represents the upper extreme of normality. A recent meta-analysis by Broer et al. confirmed that the predictive ability of AFC for exaggerated ovarian response is equivalent to AMH, which is the best endocrine marker in predicting exaggerated ovarian response [43].

While the AFC is confirmed to be the best available predictor of ovarian reserve, there is wide variation in terms of measurement techniques, the timing of AFC measurement in relation to menstrual cycle and phase of IVF treatment (pretreatment or after down-regulation), and the size of antral follicle cohorts that are included in the total AFC. The AFC can be measured using conventional 2D or 3D ultrasound (Fig. 28.3) with an acceptably high level of clinical agreement [44,45]. Recent developments have seen the introduction of a 3D automated technique, Sonography-based Automated Volume Count (SonoAVC) (Fig. 28.4), which allows a semi-automated analysis of the antral follicle population [46]. Although 3D ultrasound and SonoAVC have been shown to offer a significant advantage over 2D imaging in terms of measurement reliability of AFC, the predictive ability of AFC for ovarian response during IVF has been similar with all the measurement methods. Further, there are limitations to routine use of 3D ultrasound and SonoAVC with its relatively higher cost limiting widespread uptake, particularly if its use is limited to the field of reproductive medicine. It has therefore generally been agreed that the use of real-time 2D ultrasound imaging is adequate for measurement and counting of antral follicles in routine clinical practice [47]. AFC is best performed in the early follicular phase of the menstrual cycle (days 2 to 4) to minimize the effect of intracycle fluctuations and reduce the likelihood of incorrectly including coexisting ovarian cysts or the corpus luteum in the AFC. Further, this helps to schedule all pre-treatment assessment concurrently as it is widespread clinical practice to perform standard baseline endocrine assays such as basal FSH and luteinizing hormone levels in the early follicular phase. Use of GnRH agonist therapy as part of the conventional "long" down-regulation protocol does not influence the AFC, which has a similar accuracy for the prediction of ovarian response regardless of whether the assessment is performed before treatment is commenced or after down-regulation [48]. However, assessment prior to treatment has an additional advantage in that it provides an opportunity for a pre-treatment evaluation of the pelvis to screen for pathology such as a hydrosalpinx, endometrial polyp, uterine anomaly, submucosal fibroid, or an endometriotic cyst, all of which have been shown to have an adverse effect on IVF outcome and are amenable to surgery.

As discussed before, there is limited consensus on which follicles should be included in the total AFC, and the current evidence base includes studies using follicles measuring 2–5 mm, 2–6 mm, 2–8 mm, or 2–10 mm in diameter. Manual

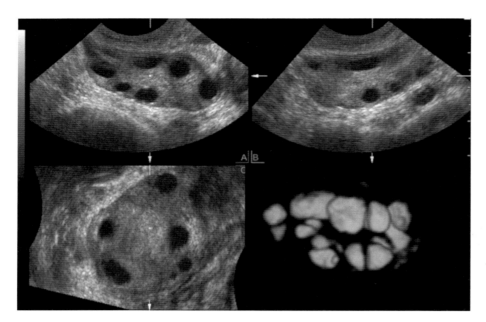

Fig. 28.3 3D multiplanar display of the ovary displaying antral follicles. Three mutually related orthogonal image planes at 90° to one another are shown – (upper left) longitudinal view or A-plane, (upper right) transverse view or B-plane, and (lower left) coronal view or C-plane. Antral follicles are clearly visualized with the application of "inversion mode" to a three-dimensional ultrasonographic dataset that allows immediate demonstration of antral follicles within an ovary (lower right).

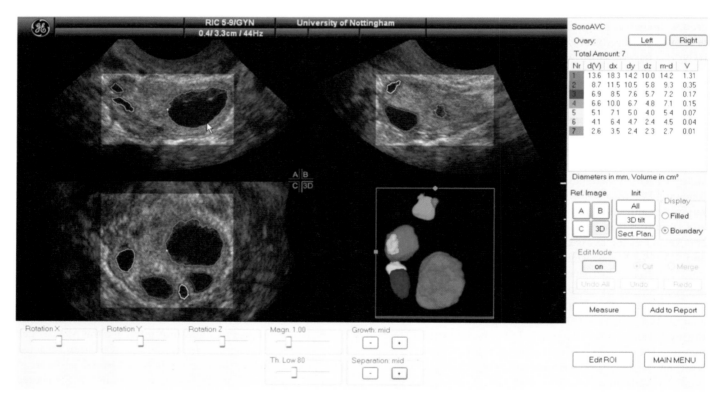

Fig. 28.4 Semi-automated antral follicle counts made using SonoAVC. It identifies the follicles and color codes each follicle differently. It also provides an automated assessment of the number of follicles with their size and volume. This ovary has one follicle above 10 mm, which needs to be excluded from the total antral follicle count.

measurement of the number and diameter of each and every antral follicle, especially the smaller ones, is labor intensive and not straightforward. A recent study utilizing SonoAVC for automated antral follicle measurements reported that the number of antral follicles measuring 2–6 mm is most reflective of the quantitative status of ovarian reserve, as this follicular cohort is most closely related to serum AMH levels and is the best predictor of ovarian response as assessed by the number of mature oocytes retrieved at egg collection [49]. However, the predictive ability of this cohort of antral follicles is equivalent to that of total follicle counts made using cohorts of 2–5 mm, 2–8 mm, and 2–10 mm for the prediction of poor ovarian response, the most clinically useful information required prior to enrolling a woman into an IVF treatment program. This is possibly because of the fact that the total follicle count is largely defined by the number of smaller antral follicles measuring 2–6 mm anyway, as these follicles accounted for 76% and 70% of the total number of antral follicles measuring 2–8 mm and 2–10 mm, respectively, in one study [49]. In order to avoid the time-consuming process of measuring each every follicle, it is recommended that counting all identifiable antral follicles of 2–10 mm in diameter would provide the most practical method for assessment of AFC in day-to-day clinical practice.

While the biological variation in the number of antral follicles between cycles has been reported [50], the predictive value of AFCs demonstrated minimal inter-cycle variation [51]. The inter-cycle variability was greater [50], as was the inter-observer variability [52] at higher AFCs, and this indicates that the cycle variability may partly be due to the variation in the reproducibility between observers. When the impact of inter-cycle variability on the response to gonadotropin stimulation in two consecutive IVF cycle was evaluated, there was no difference in ovarian response or cycle cancellation rates between the low and high AFC cycles in an individual [50]. The variability was relatively low in older women and women with a low AFC. This finding is clinically valuable as little difference in AFCs between cycles is expected once a woman is predicted to have low ovarian reserve due to a reduced AFC [53]. A study utilizing 3D ultrasound to limit the observer variation in measurement reproducibility reported minimal variation in AFC between cycles, with a mean interval of 5.4 ± 1.2 months. This observation obviates the need for repeating follicle count to predict ovarian response in women undergoing repeated IVF cycles, if the subsequent treatment cycle is performed within 6 months of the initial assessment.

In summary, AFC can be performed in the early follicular phase using conventional 2D ultrasound using a high-resolution transvaginal ultrasound transducer of a minimum frequency of 7 MHz, which allows clear visualization of 2 mm follicles. Antral follicle cohorts of 2–10 mm in diameter can be included in the total AFC. A systematic approach should be adopted for AFC assessment, which should ideally be performed by an appropriately trained person. A practical approach to measuring the number antral follicles in the ovary is described in Table 28.1.

Ovarian stromal blood flow

Various endocrine and paracrine factors are involved in the complex process of ovarian folliculogenesis [54]. An adequate ovarian blood supply is essential to its normal function and may influence the endocrine and paracrine signals that effect the growth and development of follicles [55]. It has been suggested that an increased ovarian blood flow may lead to a higher delivery of gonadotropins and other growth factors to the granulosa–theca cell complex of the developing follicles, resulting in a multifollicular response to ovarian stimulation during ART [56,57]. Other studies, although cross-sectional in

Table 28.1 A systematic approach to counting antral follicles

Should say TV scan/empty bladder

1. Transvaginal ultrasound scan using high-resolution transducer of at least 7 MHz frequency
2. Women should empty their bladder prior to ultrasound assessment
3. Identify the ovary
4. Perform a sweep through the ovary in longitudinal and transverse planes to identify the follicles and to rule out any pathologies
5. Keep the ovary in its longitudinal plane and decide on the direction of the sweep to measure and count follicles
6. Measure the largest follicle in two dimensions

If the largest follicle is ≤10 mm in diameter:

- Start to count from outer ovarian margin of the sweep to the opposite margin
- Consider every round or oval transonic structure within the ovarian margins to be a follicle
- Repeat the procedure in the contralateral ovary
- Combine the number of follicles in each ovary to obtain the total AFC

If the largest follicle is >10 mm in diameter:

- Measure all the other larger follicles sequentially in order of reducing size until a follicle with a diameter of 10 mm is identified
- Perform a total count (as described) regardless of follicle diameter
- Subtract the number of follicles of >10 mm from the total follicle count

nature, have reported an age-related decline in ovarian stromal vascularity in both fertile and subfertile populations [40,58,59]. Ultrasound assessment of ovarian blood flow may be helpful in predicting the response to controlled ovarian stimulation during assisted reproduction treatment. Due to the anatomical difficulty in visualizing the infundibulo-ovarian vessels, and in order to standardize measurements, a main artery in the ovarian stroma is generally examined to elicit flow velocity waveforms, which are assumed to be representative of the total ovarian vascular dynamics [60].

With the conventional 2D pulse-wave Doppler technique, the arteries within the ovarian stroma are visualized with the color Doppler technique, ensuring that no artery near the surface is measured. The blood flow velocity waveforms (Fig. 28.5) are obtained by placing the Doppler gate over the colored areas and activating the pulsed Doppler function. No correction is usually made for the angle of insonation in the vessels of the ovarian stroma because it cannot be detected for smaller vessels. However, the highest achievable signals are sought. Blood flow velocity waveforms illustrating the frequency and intensity of the shifted Doppler frequencies are demonstrated. Optimal flow velocity waveforms with maximum Doppler shift are selected for analysis. Peak systolic velocity (PSV) and measures of impedance to blood flow (pulsatility index [PI] and resistance index [RI]) are measured.

With 3D power Doppler angiography, a 3D ovarian volume dataset with power Doppler signals can be obtained. The power Doppler setting should be kept optimum so as to offer the best compromise between small ovarian vessel detection and artifact, and these are kept constant for each and every patient for

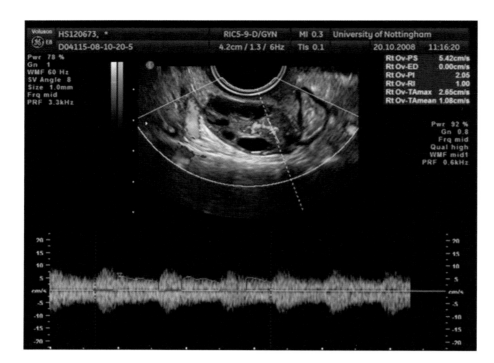

Fig. 28.5 2D pulse-wave Doppler of ovary: the Doppler gate is applied to the prominent ovarian stromal vessel to obtain blood flow velocity waveform, which is used to analyze blood flow velocity and resistance indices.

a meaningful comparison to be possible. As discussed before, ovarian volume is measured from the 3D power Doppler dataset of the ovary by using VOCAL through the manual delineation of the ovarian cortex in the transverse or longitudinal plane as the volume is rotated about a central axis through a number of rotation steps. Quantification of power Doppler information within the resultant 3D ovarian model (Fig. 28.6) can be performed using the "histogram facility." Three indices of vascularity are generated: the vascularization index (VI), which represents the ratio of power Doppler information within the total dataset relative to both color and gray information; the flow index (FI), which is proportional to the power Doppler signal intensity; and the vascularization flow index (VFI), which reflects a combination of the two (Fig. 28.7). These indices are generally thought to indicate the degree of vascularity and the volume flow rate within the ovaries.

Zaidi et al. were the first group to evaluate the correlation between ovarian stromal blood flow and follicular response in an IVF program [56]. They measured the ovarian stromal PSV and PI in 105 women in the early follicular phase and found that poor responders, defined as those who developed six or fewer follicles at the time of oocyte retrieval, had a significantly lower mean ovarian PSV, but no difference in PI, when compared with normal responders. The adjusted odds of a poor response increased significantly by an estimated 22% per cm/s decrease in velocity. While most subsequent work based on 2D pulse-wave Doppler assessment of individual ovarian stromal vessels showed a significant correlation between the absolute velocity and impedance to blood flow and ovarian response in terms of the number of oocytes retrieved [60,61], recent studies utilizing larger populations did not reveal an

association between blood flow indices and ovarian response during IVF [62].

More recently, work has been done utilizing 3D ultrasound and power Doppler angiography allowing the demonstration and quantification of the total blood flow within ovaries. Kupesic and Kurjak used 3D power Doppler angiography to evaluate ultrasound-derived ovarian predictors of ovarian response and outcome in 56 women with normal basal serum FSH concentrations (<10 mIU/mL) undergoing their first cycle of IVF [63]. Multiple regression analysis of the six most predictive variables – including the peak estradiol on the day of human chorionic gonadotropin (hCG) administration, total ovarian volume, total ovarian stromal area, age, and total AFC – revealed ovarian flow index to be the second best predictor of the number of mature oocytes collected and pregnancy, followed by the ovarian stromal flow index (FI) after AFC. However, most subsequent larger studies did not find a strong relationship between 3D power Doppler indices and poor ovarian response or exaggerated ovarian response or pregnancy during IVF [39,42,64,65]. It appears that the value of ovarian 3D vascular indices as an independent predictor of ovarian reserve is limited and their use should be restricted as a research tool until convincing evidence for routine clinical use is reported.

Conclusions

Antral follicle count is the most significant predictor of ovarian reserve and ovarian response among the ultrasound markers, although decreased ovarian volume (<3 cm³) and stromal blood flow are also implicated for poor treatment outcome during IVF treatment. While the antral follicle cohort of 2–6 mm reflects the most "functional quantitative ovarian reserve," it is

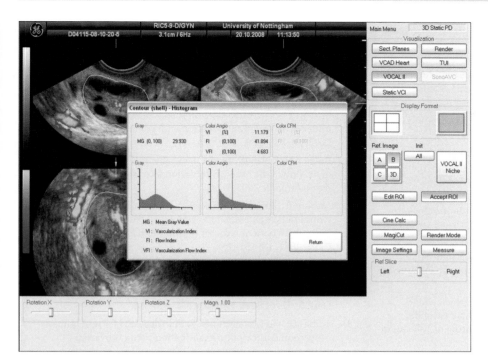

Fig. 28.6 3D power Doppler assessment of ovarian vascularity: The power Doppler information within the defined 3D model of the ovary (using VOCAL) is quantified using the histogram facility. Three vascular indices – vascularization index, flow index, and vascularization flow index – are demonstrated.

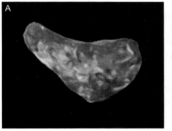 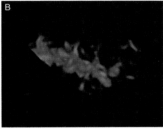

Fig. 28.7 (A) Both grayscale and Doppler information are shown in the three-dimensional "glass body" model of an ovary. The vascularization index (VI) represents the proportion of power Doppler information within this defined volume relative to both color and gray information, providing an indication of the degree of vascularity. (B) The same ovary is shown but with the grayscale information removed. The flow index (FI) represents the mean power Doppler signal intensity within the dataset and reflects the volume flow rate.

recommended to include follicles of 2–10 mm in the total AFC as it is practically easier to count this follicle pool, the majority of which are 2–6 mm follicles anyway, without compromising the predictive accuracy. The total AFC can be measured using 2D or 3D ultrasound with an acceptably high level of agreement both between and within observers. Total follicle counts of 10 and 22 are generally considered as the optimum cut-off levels for the prediction of poor and exaggerated ovarian response, respectively. The AFC measurement can be performed either in the early follicular phase of the cycle before treatment begins or after down-regulation with similar predictive accuracy. However, assessment prior to treatment has an additional advantage in that it provides an opportunity for a pre-treatment evaluation of the pelvis to screen for pathology. AFC and AMH are currently the best two predictors of ovarian reserve among all the endocrine and ultrasound markers

and are equally predictive of poor ovarian response during IVF treatment. AFC is currently considered the ovarian reserve test of choice in routine clinical practice, as it is easy to perform while there is limited availability of AMH assays. The new development in automated assessment of follicle count using SonoAVC is promising and has the potential to improve the reproducibility and accuracy of AFC measurements.

References

1. Broekmans FJ, Kwee J, Hendriks DJ, Mol BW, Lambalk CB. A systematic review of tests predicting ovarian reserve and IVF outcome. *Hum Reprod Update* 2006; **12**: 685–718.

2. Gougeon A. Ovarian follicular growth in humans: ovarian ageing and population of growing follicles. *Maturitas* 1998; **30**: 137–142.

3. Baird DT, Collins J, Egozcue J, et al. Fertility and ageing. *Hum Reprod Update* 2005; **11**: 261–276.

4. Treloar AE, Boynton RE, Behn BG, Brown BW. Variation of the human menstrual cycle through reproductive life. *Int J Fertil* 1967; **12**: 77–126.

5. Treloar AE. Menstrual cyclicity and the pre-menopause. *Maturitas* 1981; **3**: 249–264.

6. Faddy MJ, Gosden RG, Gougeon A, Richardson SJ, Nelson JF. Accelerated disappearance of ovarian follicles in mid-life: implications for forecasting menopause. *Hum Reprod* 1992; **7**: 1342–1346.

7. van Noord-Zaadstra BM, Looman CW, Alsbach H, Habbema JD, te Velde ER, Karbaat J. Delaying childbearing: effect of age on fecundity and outcome of pregnancy. *Br Med J* 1991; **302**: 1361–1365.

8. Menken J, Trussell J, Larsen U. Age and infertility. *Science* 1986; **233**: 1389–1394.

9. Van Voorhis BJ. Clinical practice. In vitro fertilization. *N Engl J Med* 2007; **356**: 379–386.

10. Navot D, Drews MR, Bergh PA, et al. Age-related decline in female fertility is not due to diminished capacity of the uterus to sustain embryo implantation. *Fertil Steril* 1994; **61**: 97–101.

11. Trout SW, Seifer DB. Do women with unexplained recurrent pregnancy loss have higher day 3 serum FSH and estradiol values? *Fertil Steril* 2000; **74**: 335–337.

12. Freeman SB, Yang Q, Allran K, Taft LF, Sherman SL. Women with a reduced ovarian complement may have an increased risk for a child with Down syndrome. *Am J Hum Genet* 2000; **66**: 1680–1683.

13. Lambalk CB, De Koning CH, Braat DD. The endocrinology of dizygotic twinning in the human. *Mol Cell Endocrinol* 1998; **145**: 97–102.

14. Woldringh GH, Frunt MH, Kremer JA, Spaanderman ME. Decreased ovarian reserve relates to pre-eclampsia in IVF/ICSI pregnancies. *Hum Reprod* 2006; **21**: 2948–2954.

15. Gougeon A, Ecochard R, Thalabard JC. Age-related changes of the population of human ovarian follicles: increase in the disappearance rate of non-growing and early-growing follicles in aging women. *Biol Reprod* 1994; **50**: 653–663.

16. Hansen KR, Knowlton NS, Thyer AC, Charleston JS, Soules MR, Klein NA. A new model of reproductive aging: the decline in ovarian non-growing follicle number from birth to menopause. *Hum Reprod* 2008; **23**: 699–708.

17. Arslan M, Bocca S, Mirkin S, Barroso G, Stadtmauer L, Oehninger S. Controlled ovarian hyperstimulation protocols for in vitro fertilization: two decades of experience after the birth of Elizabeth Carr. *Fertil Steril* 2005; **84**: 555–569.

18. Maheshwari A, Bhattacharya S, Johnson NP. Predicting fertility. *Hum Fertil* (Camb) 2008; **11**: 109–117.

19. Sunkara SK, Rittenberg V, Raine-Fenning N, Bhattacharya S, Zamora J, Coomarasamy A. Association between the number of eggs and live birth in IVF treatment: an analysis of 400 135 treatment cycles. *Hum Reprod* 2011; **26**: 1768–1774.

20. Syrop CH, Willhoite A, Van Voorhis BJ. Ovarian volume: a novel outcome predictor for assisted reproduction. *Fertil Steril* 1995; **64**: 1167–1171.

21. Raine-Fenning NJ, Campbell BK, Clewes JS, Johnson IR. The interobserver reliability of ovarian volume measurement is improved with three-dimensional ultrasound, but dependent upon technique. *Ultrasound Med Biol* 2003; **29**: 1685–1690.

22. Lass A, Silye R, Abrams DC, et al. Follicular density in ovarian biopsy of infertile women: a novel method to assess ovarian reserve. *Hum Reprod* 1997; **12**: 1028–1031.

23. Bowen S, Norian J, Santoro N, Pal L. Simple tools for assessment of ovarian reserve (OR): individual ovarian dimensions are reliable predictors of OR. *Fertil Steril* 2007; **88**: 390–935.

24. Schild RL, Knobloch C, Dorn C, Fimmers R, van der Ven H, Hansmann M. The role of ovarian volume in an in vitro fertilization programme as assessed by 3D ultrasound. *Arch Gynecol Obstet* 2001; **265**: 67–72.

25. Elgindy EA, El-Haieg DO, El-Sebaey A. Anti-Mullerian hormone: correlation of early follicular, ovulatory and midluteal levels with ovarian response and cycle outcome in intracytoplasmic sperm injection patients. *Fertil Steril* 2008; **89**: 1670–1676.

26. McIlveen M, Skull JD, Ledger WL. Evaluation of the utility of multiple endocrine and ultrasound measures of ovarian reserve in the prediction of cycle cancellation in a high-risk IVF population. *Hum Reprod* 2007; **22**: 778–785.

27. Lass A, Vassiliev A, Decosterd G, Warne D, Loumaye E. Relationship of baseline ovarian volume to ovarian response in World Health Organization II anovulatory patients who underwent ovulation induction with gonadotropins. *Fertil Steril* 2002; **78**: 265–269.

28. Balen AH, Laven JS, Tan SL, Dewailly D. Ultrasound assessment of the polycystic ovary: international consensus definitions. *Hum Reprod Update* 2003; **9**: 505–514.

29. Nahum R, Shifren JL, Chang Y, Leykin L, Isaacson K, Toth TL. Antral follicle assessment as a tool for predicting outcome in IVF – is it a better predictor than age and FSH? *J Assist Reprod Genet* 2001; **18**: 151–155.

30. Scheffer GJ, Broekmans FJ, Dorland M, Habbema JD, Looman CW, te Velde ER. Antral follicle counts by transvaginal ultrasonography are related to age in women with proven natural fertility. *Fertil Steril* 1999; **72**: 845–851.

31. Tomas C, Nuojua-Huttunen S, Martikainen H. Pretreatment transvaginal ultrasound examination predicts ovarian responsiveness to gonadotrophins in in-vitro fertilization. *Hum Reprod* 1997; **12**: 220–223.

32. Jayaprakasan K, Campbell B, Hopkisson J, Johnson I, Raine-Fenning N. A prospective, comparative analysis of anti-Mullerian hormone, inhibin-B, and three-dimensional ultrasound determinants of ovarian reserve in the prediction of poor response to controlled ovarian stimulation. *Fertil Steril* 2010; **93**: 855–864.

33. Haadsma ML, Bukman A, Groen H, et al. The number of small antral follicles (2–6 mm) determines the outcome of endocrine ovarian reserve tests in a subfertile population. *Hum Reprod* 2007; **22**: 1925–1931.

34. Sharara FI, McClamrock HD. Antral follicle count and ovarian volume predict IVF outcome. *Fertil Steril* 2000; **74**: S176.

35. Bancsi LF, Broekmans FJ, Eijkemans MJ, de Jong FH, Habbema JD, te Velde ER. Predictors of poor ovarian response in in vitro fertilization: a prospective study comparing basal markers of ovarian reserve. *Fertil Steril* 2002; **77**: 328–336.

36. Chang MY, Chiang CH, Hsieh TT, Soong YK, Hsu KH. Use of the antral follicle count to predict the outcome of assisted reproductive technologies. *Fertil Steril* 1998; **69**: 505–510.

37. Hsieh YY, Chang CC, Tsai HD. Antral follicle counting in predicting the retrieved oocyte number after ovarian hyperstimulation. *J Assist Reprod Genet* 2001; **18**: 320–324.

38. Ng EH, Yeung WS, Ho PC. The significance of antral follicle count in controlled ovarian stimulation and intrauterine insemination. *J Assist Reprod Genet* 2005; **22**: 323–328.

39. Ng EH, Tang OS, Chan CC, Ho PC. Ovarian stromal vascularity is not predictive of ovarian response and pregnancy. *Reprod Biomed Online* 2006; **12**: 43–49.

40. Kupesic S, Kurjak A, Bjelos D, Vujisic S. Three-dimensional ultrasonographic ovarian measurements and in vitro fertilization outcome are related to age. *Fertil Steril* 2003; **79**: 190–197.

41. Broer SL, Mol BW, Hendriks D, Broekmans FJ. The role of antimullerian hormone in prediction of outcome after IVF:

comparison with the antral follicle count. *Fertil Steril* 2009; **91**: 705–714.

42. Jayaprakasan K, Jayaprakasan R, Al-Hasie HA, et al. Can quantitative three-dimensional power Doppler angiography be used to predict ovarian hyperstimulation syndrome? *Ultrasound Obstet Gynecol* 2009; **33**: 583–591.

43. Broer SL, Dolleman M, Opmeer BC, Fauser BC, Mol BW, Broekmans FJ. AMH and AFC as predictors of excessive response in controlled ovarian hyperstimulation: a meta-analysis. *Hum Reprod Update* 2011; **17**: 46–54.

44. Jayaprakasan K, Walker KF, Clewes JS, Johnson IR, Raine-Fenning NJ. The interobserver reliability of off-line antral follicle counts made from stored three-dimensional ultrasound data: a comparative study of different measurement techniques. *Ultrasound Obstet Gynecol* 2007; **29**: 335–341.

45. Deb S, Jayaprakasan K, Campbell BK, Clewes JS, Johnson IR, Raine-Fenning NJ. Intraobserver and interobserver reliability of automated antral follicle counts made using three-dimensional ultrasound and SonoAVC. *Ultrasound Obstet Gynecol* 2009; **33**: 477–483.

46. Raine-Fenning N, Jayaprakasan K, Clewes J, et al. SonoAVC: a novel method of automatic volume calculation. *Ultrasound Obstet Gynecol* 2008; **31**: 691–696.

47. Broekmans FJ, de Ziegler D, Howles CM, Gougeon A, Trew G, Olivennes F. The antral follicle count: practical recommendations for better standardization. *Fertil Steril* 2010; **94**(3): 1044–1051.

48. Jayaprakasan K, Hopkisson JF, Campbell BK, Clewes J, Johnson IR, Raine-Fenning NJ. Quantification of the effect of pituitary down-regulation on 3D ultrasound predictors of ovarian response. *Hum Reprod* 2008; **23**: 1538–1544.

49. Jayaprakasan K, Deb S, Batcha M, et al. The cohort of antral follicles measuring 2–6 mm reflects the quantitative status of ovarian reserve as assessed by serum levels of anti-Mullerian hormone and response to controlled ovarian stimulation. *Fertil Steril* 2010; **94**(5): 1775–1781.

50. Hansen KR, Morris JL, Thyer AC, Soules MR. Reproductive aging and variability in the ovarian antral follicle count: application in the clinical setting. *Fertil Steril* 2003; **80**: 577–583.

51. Bancsi LF, Broekmans FJ, Looman CW, Habbema JD, te Velde ER. Impact of repeated antral follicle counts on the prediction of poor ovarian response in women undergoing in vitro fertilization. *Fertil Steril* 2004; **81**: 35–41.

52. Scheffer GJ, Broekmans FJ, Bancsi LF, Habbema JD, Looman CW, Te Velde ER. Quantitative transvaginal two- and three-dimensional sonography of the ovaries: reproducibility of antral follicle counts. *Ultrasound Obstet Gynecol* 2002; **20**: 270–275.

53. Elter K, Sismanoglu A, Durmusoglu F. Intercycle variabilities of basal antral follicle count and ovarian volume in subfertile women and their relationship to reproductive aging: a prospective study. *Gynecol Endocrinol* 2005; **20**: 137–143.

54. McGee EA, Hsueh AJ. Initial and cyclic recruitment of ovarian follicles. *Endocr Rev* 2000; **21**: 200–2014.

55. Redmer DA, Reynolds LP. Angiogenesis in the ovary. *Rev Reprod* 1996; **1**: 182–192.

56. Zaidi J, Barber J, Kyei-Mensah A, Bekir J, Campbell S, Tan SL. Relationship of ovarian stromal blood flow at the baseline ultrasound scan to subsequent follicular response in an in vitro fertilization program. *Obstet Gynecol* 1996; **88**: 779–784.

57. Zaidi J, Campbell S, Pittrof R, et al. Ovarian stromal blood flow in women with polycystic ovaries – a possible new marker for diagnosis? *Hum Reprod* 1995; **10**: 1992–1996.

58. Pan HA, Cheng YC, Li CH, Wu MH, Chang FM. Ovarian stroma flow intensity decreases by age: a three-dimensional power doppler ultrasonographic study. *Ultrasound Med Biol* 2002; **28**: 425–430.

59. Ng EH, Chan CC, Yeung WS, Ho PC. Effect of age on ovarian stromal flow measured by three-dimensional ultrasound with power Doppler in Chinese women with proven fertility. *Hum Reprod* 2004; **19**: 2132–2137.

60. Bassil S, Wyns C, Toussaint-Demylle D, Nisolle M, Gordts S, Donnez J. The relationship between ovarian vascularity and the duration of stimulation in in-vitro fertilization. *Hum Reprod* 1997; **12**: 1240–1245.

61. Engmann L, Sladkevicius P, Agrawal R, Bekir JS, Campbell S, Tan SL. Value of ovarian stromal blood flow velocity measurement after pituitary suppression in the prediction of ovarian responsiveness and outcome of in vitro fertilization treatment. *Fertil Steril* 1999; **71**: 22–29.

62. Ng EH, Tang OS, Chan CC, Ho PC. Ovarian stromal blood flow in the prediction of ovarian response during in vitro fertilization treatment. *Hum Reprod* 2005; **20**: 3147–3151.

63. Kupesic S, Kurjak A. Predictors of IVF outcome by three-dimensional ultrasound. *Hum Reprod* 2002; **17**: 950–955.

64. Merce LT, Barco MJ, Bau S, Troyano JM. Prediction of ovarian response and IVF/ICSI outcome by three-dimensional ultrasonography and power Doppler angiography. *Eur J Obstet Gynecol Reprod Biol* 2007; **132**: 93–100.

65. Jayaprakasan K, Al-Hasie H, Jayaprakasan R, et al. The three-dimensional ultrasonographic ovarian vascularity of women developing poor ovarian response during assisted reproduction treatment and its predictive value. *Fertil Steril* 2009; **92**: 1862–1869.

Ultrasound monitoring of ovulation induction

Josef Blankstein, Sarika Arora and Joel Brasch

The ultimate goal of the female reproductive process is the periodic maturation and discharge of a fertilizable egg. Recent advances in reproductive endocrinology have led to greater understanding of the basic regulatory mechanisms governing the reproductive process. It is fitting to introduce our topic by outlining the major morphological changes of the menstrual cycle that can be visualized by ultrasound.

The physiological concept of follicular selection

In the beginning of each ovarian or menstrual cycle a few primordial follicles (cohort) begin to grow; one is selected to continue development while the remainders undergo atresia. While oocyte recruitment and development is predominately dependent upon genetic endowment, follicular growth, in contrast is a gonadotropin- and sex steroid-regulated phenomenon.

The early follicular phase of the ovarian cycle is characterized by relatively elevated levels of follicle stimulating hormone (FSH) and low levels of luteinizing hormone (LH), estrogens, and progesterone. During this early cycle phase, the growth of a number of follicles is initiated. It has been demonstrated that this oocyte selection process involves two main processes. First, a number of follicles are recruited, and secondly a number of growing follicles are selected out of the recruited group to continue toward maturation. Studies supporting the "dominant follicle theory" suggest that new follicular growth is arrested in the presence of a single dominant follicle (Fig. 29.1). Moreover, the responsiveness of other follicles to human menopausal gonadotropin (hMG) therapy was found to be suppressed in the presence of the overt dominant follicle, while the same dose of hMG early in the follicular cycle increased the number of follicles recruited and/or selected for maturation.

In the normal ovulatory cycle the dominant follicle steadily increases in size, while the accompanying smaller follicles are not observed to show a similar increase. Thus, while one or more follicles will grow to full maturity and ovulate, others are destined for atresia and degeneration.

Ovarian secretion of estradiol (E_2) and estrone, from the granulosa cells, promotes follicular maturation by increasing follicular sensitivity to gonadotropin stimulation. This is accepted to be a gonadotropin receptor-mediated process.

The dominant follicle is selected due to its responsiveness to elevated circulatory FSH levels. It is not uncommon to observe two follicles developing to approximately 10 mm, with one achieving dominance and growing while the others regress. LH reinitiates meiosis of the oocyte, and typically, ovulation occurs within 36 hours of its "surge."

Small follicles can be visualized easily as echo-free structures and usually lie towards the periphery of the more echogenic ovarian tissue. As the follicle matures, more fluid is released and accumulates into its center. The granulosa cell mass, lining the inner wall of the follicle, increases. Microscopically the oocyte itself, which is less than one-tenth of 1 mm, is surrounded by a cluster of granulosa cells. This complex surrounding the oocyte is termed the cumulus oophorus. It measures approximately 1 mm and can occasionally be depicted by transvaginal scan (TVS) adjacent to the wall of a mature follicle. Immediately prior to ovulation the cumulus separates from the wall and floats freely within the follicle's center. Today, even with the enhanced resolution afforded by TVS, the attached or floating cumulus is only rarely seen. However, new technological developments, mainly high-resolution probes (40 MHz), have enabled clinical researchers to clearly visualize clearly the cumulus–oocyte complex (Fig. 29.2).

Mature follicles, those containing a mature oocyte, typically measure from 17 to 25 mm in average inner dimension. Intrafollicular echoes may be observed with mature follicles, probably arising from clusters of granulosa cells that shear off the wall near the time of ovulation. After ovulation, the follicular wall becomes irregular as the follicle becomes "deflated." The fresh corpus luteum usually appears as a hypoechoic structure with an irregular internal wall and may contain some internal free-floating or fixed echoes that correspond to hemorrhage. As the corpus luteum develops 4–8 days after ovulation, it appears as an echogenic structure of approximately 15 mm in size. Its wall is thickened due to the process of luteinization. TVS shows the neovascularity within the wall that is associated with formation of the corpus luteum. In addition to delineation of changes in follicle size and structure, TVS can

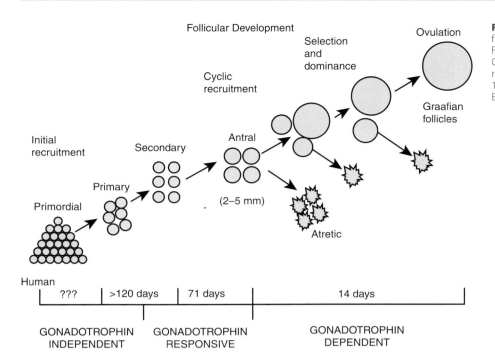

Fig. 29.1 Follicular development. Reprinted from *Fertility and Sterility*, Vol. 94, Broekmans FJM, Ziegler DD, Howles CM, Gougeon A, Trew G, Olivennes F. The antral follicle count: practical recommendations for better standardization, 1044–1051, Copyright 2010, with permission from Elsevier.

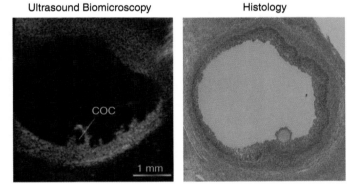

Fig. 29.2 Cumulus–oocyte complex (COC). Reprinted from *Fertility and Sterility*, Vol. 91, Pallares P, Letelier C, Gonzalez-Bulnes A. Progress toward "in vitro virtual histology" of ovarian follicles and corpora lutea by ultrasound biomicroscopy, 624–626, Copyright 2009, with permission from Elsevier.

depict the presence of intraperitoneal fluid. It is normal to have approximately 1–3 mL of intraperitoneal fluid in the cul-de-sac throughout the cycle. When ovulation occurs, there typically is between 4 and 5 mL within the cul-de-sac. The intraperitoneal fluid resulting from ovulation may be located outside of the posterior cul-de-sac, surrounding bowel loops in the lower abdomen, and in the upper pelvis or in the anterior cul-de-sac superior to the uterine fundus.

The role of Doppler in ovulation induction

It was recognized as early as in 1926 that neovascularization may be of prime importance in the growth and selection of ovulatory follicles, in addition to the subsequent development and function of the corpus luteum [1]. Studies of ovarian vascular morphology showed that the capillary network of pre-ovulatory follicles was more extensive than that of other follicles [2], consequently proposing that initiation and maintenance of follicular growth depends on development of the follicular microvasculature.

A study done by Shrestha et al. [3], to determine whether ovarian perifollicular blood flow (PFBF) in the early follicular phase (EFP) is associated with treatment outcome of in vitro fertilization (IVF), showed high-grade ovarian PFBF in the EFP during IVF to be associated with a higher clinical pregnancy rate. Coulam et al. [4] correlated peak systolic velocity (PSV) of individual follicles with oocyte recovery, fertilization rate, and embryo quality in women undergoing IVF and embryo transfer. They assessed the role of quantitative and qualitative indices of follicular vascularity in predicting pregnancy after IVF and embryo transfer. Women who had PSV ≥10 cm/s in at least one follicle on the day of hCG administration more often became pregnant than those with PSV <10 cm/s (*P* = 0.05). Nargund et al. [5] demonstrated that there was a 70% chance of producing a grade I or II embryo if the follicular blood velocity was >10 cm/s, compared with 14% if the PSV was <10 cm/s. This study concluded that there is a physiological relationship between follicular blood velocity, oocyte recovery, and the production of a high-grade preimplantation embryo, which may form the basis of a useful clinical test. Jayaprakasan et al. [6], on the other hand, concluded that ovarian vascularity as measured by 3D ultrasound is not decreased in women who demonstrate poor ovarian response to controlled ovarian stimulation as part of assisted reproduction treatment.

Perifollicular vascular perfusion appears to be an important factor in determining the outcome of stimulated cycles, and may have clinical implications in assisted reproduction

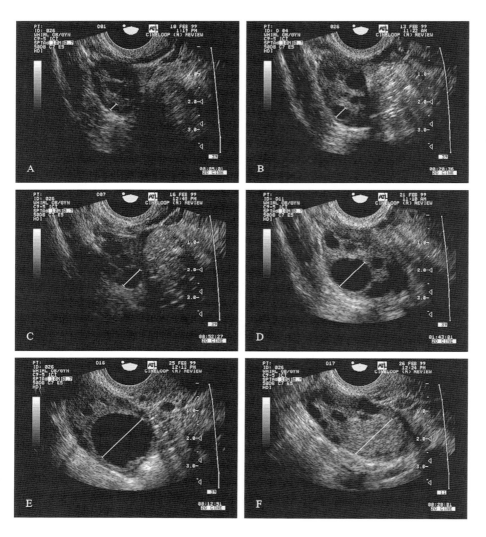

Fig. 29.3 Serial transvaginal ultrasonographic images of the right ovary of a research participant on days 1 (A), 4 (B), 7 (C), 11 (D), 16 (E), and 17 (F) of a spontaneous menstrual cycle. The same ovarian follicle is identified throughout the growth phase in A–E. The corresponding corpus luteum on the day of ovulation is shown in F. Reprinted from *Fertility and Sterility*, Vol. 91, Baerwald A, Walker R, Pierson R. Growth rate of ovarian follicles during natural menstrual cycles, oral contraceptives cycles and ovarian stimulation cycles, 440–449, Copyright 2009, with permission from Elsevier.

therapy. As there were low pregnancy rates and oocyte retrieval in the group of women with uniformly low-grade vascularity, the identification of these cycles would be valuable in terms of counseling with regard to the potential outcome in that cycle. Ideally, the identification of these women (who may also be "low recruiters") earlier in the cycle (before hCG) would be helpful. This could allow the cancellation of treatment after careful counseling, on the basis of perifollicular vascular perfusion, and could be cost-effective, both financially and emotionally. However, further longitudinal data would be needed before this form of prospective management of treatment cycles could be applied clinically. The risk of multiple pregnancies and their implications on the health service is also well recognized. Since there were higher multiple pregnancy rates in stimulated intra-uterine insemination (IUI) cycles with uniformly high-grade follicular vascularity, perhaps these cycles in particular should be considered for follicle reduction or even cancellation. This may potentially reduce the number of developmentally competent oocytes that have a higher capability of producing more viable embryos for implantation [7].

Induction of ovulation

In patients whose infertility can be attributed to an ovulation abnormality, ovulation induction is indicated. Ovulation induction is also used in IVF embryo transfer (IVF-ET) to increase the number of oocytes aspirated, which in turn increases the number of fertilized conceptuses that may be transferred, thereby increasing the chance of pregnancy. Commonly used ovulation induction medications include clomiphene citrate, human menopausal gonadotropin, and purified FSH and recombinant gonadotropins. Although all of these medications result in the development of multiple follicles, they act via different mechanisms.

TVS has a vital role in monitoring the follicular growth rate in women receiving ovulation induction medications. In an elegant prospective study, Baerwald et al. [8] compared the growth rate of ovarian follicles during the natural cycle and ovarian stimulation cycles using standardized techniques. While the growth rate in natural cycles was 1.42 mm per day the growth in stimulated cycles was significantly greater, i.e.

1.7 mm per day. Continued research on the effect of greater follicular growth rates and shorter intervals to ovulation is being conducted (Fig. 29.3).

An initial baseline scan of the pelvis is mandatory to rule out ovarian or uterine pathology and assess the ovarian reserve: moreover, one needs to rule out the presence of ovarian cysts.

Objectives of a baseline scan

A. To rule out ovarian or uterine pathology requiring attention prior to beginning infertility treatment (Table 29.1)

A common adnexal finding, endometriosis [9], can be seen in over 30% of women with clinically defined infertility. Endometriosis is defined as the extrauterine presence of endometrial tissue, and is likely due to retrograde menstruation and/or immunologic variations or deficiencies within the peritoneal cavity.

In mild cases, small lesions are often located on the ovarian and peritubular surfaces. Cases of minimal endometriosis are not amenable to ultrasonographic diagnosis. However, in more moderate cases one can visualize an endometrioma, i.e. a cystic structure lined with endometrial epithelium which can involve one or both ovaries, uterosacral ligaments, etc.

Endometrioma may appear as an ovarian cyst with an echo-dense appearance of blood within a cyst; the appearance may range from anechoic to solid, depending on the amount and organization of the blood within the cystic structure. Commonly one can visualize low-level echoes evenly distributed throughout the cyst (Fig. 29.4).

It is important for physicians to familiarize themselves with the ultrasonographic picture of endometrioma in order to avoid aspirating the cyst because of an increased risk of infection, compared with aspiration of a simple cyst.

Since ovarian teratomas are the most common ovarian neoplasm especially in reproductive-age women [10], one may encounter them during a baseline scan; the ultrasonographic findings will depend on which elements are present ectoderm; mesoderm, etc. Very often one can appreciate an echogenic mass with acoustic shadowing. The presence of ectodermal elements gives irregular and variable internal echogenicity (Fig. 29.5).

B. Check ovarian reserve to help identify the ideal treatment protocol

In our clinic a baseline scan involves antral follicle count and evaluation of ovarian volume. The number of antral follicles of at least 2 mm in diameter can be detected using ultrasound imaging; generally follicles that are greater than 2 mm in diameter are highly responsive to gonadotropins; however, some follicles in this size range may be in the early states of atresia. Antral follicle count is performed on days 2–4 of a natural cycle or following pituitary down-regulation. Prospective studies assessing antral follicle count demonstrate that lower counts (fewer than four follicles) are associated with significantly

Table 29.1 Common adnexal masses

Cystic masses	Follicular cyst; corpus/uterus cyst; hydrosalpinx dermoid cyst; endometrioma/hemorrhagic cyst
Solid masses	Fibroma; dysgerminoma; teratoma Carcinoid subserosal fibroid
Complex masses	Dermoid cyst; cyst adenoma; granulosa

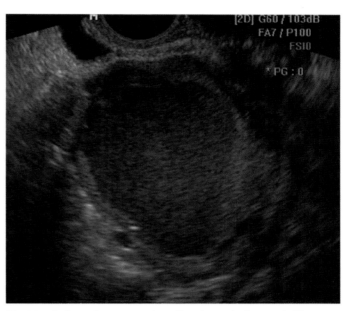

Fig. 29.4 Endometrioma – note the uniform internal echoes typical for endometrioma. Reproduced with permission from *Seminars in Reproductive Medicine*, ©2008, Thieme Medical Publishers.

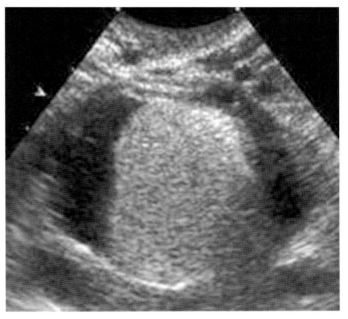

Fig. 29.5 Dermoid cyst (teratoma) with a "hyperechoic ball." © 2008, Elsevier Inc.

Table 29.2 Anovulation-treatment options (based on WHO classification)

	Option I	Option II
Group I: low FSH	GnRH (pulsatile)	Gonadotropins
	Gonadotropins	Bromocriptine
	Bromocriptine	Clomiphene citrate
Group II: normal FSH	Clomiphene citrate	Gonadotropins
		Surgical approach
Group III: high FSH	Ovum donation	

decreased pregnancy rates and increased cycle cancellation rates [11].

Ovarian volume is measured using the formula volume (cm³) = length × width × anterior posterior diameter × 0.53.

It has been shown that ovarian volume is inversely correlated with age. Significant decrease in ovarian volume is observed in women older than 35 years. The prognostic practicality of measuring early follicular ovarian volume is limited because clinically meaningful changes are only manifest at the physiologic extremes [12]. However, ovarian volumes less than 3 cm³ are associated with a significant decrease in clinical pregnancy rates.

C. To identify ovarian cysts

It is important to identify cysts and or hydrosalpinx prior to stimulation since these situations could later be misinterpreted as a developing follicle. Moreover, basal ovarian cyst significantly reduces ovulating events in patients treated with clomiphene citrate [13].

Upon detection of an ovarian cyst, a conservative approach is generally effective. One can wait for a spontaneous menstrual bleed, which indicates that endogenous ovarian hormone levels have returned to base level; if the cyst is not resolving and hormone levels of E_2 are high then cyst aspiration prior to stimulation remains a viable option.

Selection of patients

The ovulatory treatment options are based on the WHO classification with patients separated into three main groups (Table 29.2).

Group I. Hypothalamic-pituitary failure; includes women with primary or secondary amenorrhea, low levels of endogenous gonadotropins, and lack of endogenous estrogen activity. The treatment of choice for this group of patients is gonadotropic therapy.

Group II. Hypothalamic-pituitary dysfunction; includes patients with anovulation associated with a variety of menstrual disorders whose serum gonadotropin levels are within the normal range and who have evidence of endogenous estrogen activity. The treatment of choice for patients belonging to group II is a chlorotrianisene analogue, such as clomiphene citrate.

Group III. Includes patients with high FSH levels; the only viable option for them is ovum donation.

The above classification is based on hormone levels of FSH and estrogens; however, some conclusions can be drawn following a baseline ultrasound evaluation of the endometrium. If the endometrium is thick (7–14 mm) one can conclude that the patient has sufficient ovarian estrogen secretion and normal FSH level (i.e. Group II).

If, on the other hand, the endometrium is thin the patient has low estrogen levels and in this case a single FSH level will differentiate between Group I (low FSH) and Group III (high FSH).

Ovarian location and follicle measurement

Ovaries

The ovaries are located posterior to the broad ligament and anteromedial to the internal iliac vessels, which are easily located and can be used as a landmark for ovarian localization; moving laterally from the endometrial canal will produce an image of the ovary adjacent to the iliac vessels.

The pelvic organs may be scanned either transabdominally or transvaginally. In most infertility units transvaginal ultrasound has become the routine method since it improves spatial resolution; however, it has a smaller field of view. During the transvaginal approach only a few centimeters separate the probe from the ovaries.

The best way to locate the ovaries is to scan along the lateral margin of the uterus in the transverse plane from the fundus to the cervix. In cases where you cannot locate the ovaries, look for them adjacent to the iliac vessels, which are usually easily identified or try to follow the fallopian tube laterally.

In cases when the ovary is high in the pelvis, a transabdominal scan is also necessary; in these situations begin with the abdominal transducer perpendicular at the midline just superior to the symphysis pubis. Once you locate the long axis of the uterus, move the transducer lateral until the ovary is located. Again remember that the internal iliac vessels are located immediately posterior to the ovary.

Follicle

The spatial resolution of transvaginal scans is 2–3 mm, so small follicles can be visualized easily as echo-free structures which usually lie towards the periphery of the more echogenic ovarian tissue. Since the follicles may be flattened in one plane or have their shape altered due to pressure, the internal diameter of the follicle should be measured in three planes and the mean value calculated. The intra-observer standard deviation of transabdominal follicular measurement was reported in one study to be 0.6 mm, and the inter-observer standard deviation 1.2 mm, irrespective of the follicular diameter [14]. Thus, the 95% confidence limits for any particular measurement should be 2.4 mm³ [14], and one would expect transvaginal measurements to confer even greater accuracy [15].

Follicles can be confused with blood vessels, and they can be differentiated by rotating the transducers. If the structure is a vessel, it will appear tubular following rotation.

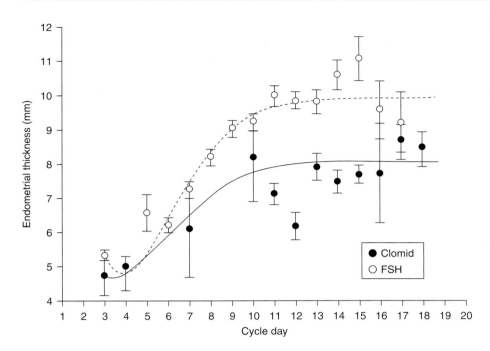

Fig. 29.6 Pattern of follicular phase endometrial development. Comparison of all cycles using CC (Clomid) to those using FSH. Reprinted from *Fertility and Sterility*, Vol. 91, Bromer JG, Aldad DS, Taylor HS. Defining the proliferative phase endometrial defect, 698–704, Copyright 2009, with permission from Elsevier.

A baseline scan should always be done to identify cystic structures which could later be misinterpreted as follicles.

Clomiphene citrate

Clomiphene citrate (CC) is a nonsteroidal triphenylethylene compound currently used as the first choice of treatment for induction of ovulation in anovulatory or oligo-ovulatory women.

Mode of action

The stereoscopic configuration of CC is sufficiently similar to that of β-estradiol to compete with it for available estrogen receptor sites in all estrogen-dependent target cells such as the hypothalamus, pituitary, ovary, uterus, and cervical glands.

The mode of action of CC in the induction of ovulation may be tentatively described as follows. "Blinded" by CC molecules occupying the estrogen receptor sites, the hypothalamus and pituitary are unable to correctly perceive true serum estrogen levels. A false message of insufficient estrogen concentration is registered and acted upon, resulting in exaggerated FSH and LH secretion. The occupation of hypothalamic estrogen receptors by CC is a short-duration, time-limited process. A fair chance exists that, by the time ovarian follicles that are stimulated by the CC-induced gonadotropin elevation reach the pre-ovulatory stage, the hypothalamus is already free of CC influence and ready to perceive the correct steroid signal. From this moment forward, the events are regulated and controlled by the endogenous feedback mechanisms within the hypothalamic–pituitary–ovarian (HPO) axis.

Considering its mode of action, an antiestrogen such as CC should be effective in patients having a hypothalamus capable of releasing pulsatile GnRH, a pituitary gland capable of responding to GnRH, and an ovary containing normal primordial follicles. Clomiphene citrate is most effective when used in patients with hypothalamic-pituitary dysfunction. These patients lack the proper regulation within the HPO axis, but they have some endogenous GnRH secretion and estradiol production. These anovulatory women probably have irregularities in the pulsatile secretion of GnRH, even though they do have fluctuating, detectable levels of gonadotropins and estrogens.

Antiestrogenic effects on the cervix and endometrium (Fig. 29.6)

The antiestrogenic action of CC may exert an adverse effect on the uterus and the cervix. This detrimental effect, caused by the drug's competition for estrogen receptors, is claimed to be one factor responsible for the discrepancy between the ovulation rate (85%) and the pregnancy rate (43%) of women receiving CC treatment. Padma et al. [16] demonstrated, in a prospective crossover study, that the number of follicles at the assumed time of ovulation was significantly higher in patients treated with clomiphene citrate; moreover, the endometrial thickness on the same day was significantly smaller (7.6 mm vs. 8.5 mm). Most investigators report decreased secretion of mucus from the cervical glands caused by antiestrogenic agents such as CC. The antiestrogenic effect on the cervical mucus, when present, is expressed by a decreased amount of mucus, which occurs despite the relatively high levels of estrogens in the circulation. Wolman et al. [17] demonstrated that the cervical mucus can be visualized in many patients around the time of ovulation, using pelvic ultrasound (see Fig. 29.5). In many patients given CC, the cervical mucus does not exhibit any depressed effects. To understand this phenomenon, we must remember that the antiestrogen effect on the hypothalamus will result in elevated

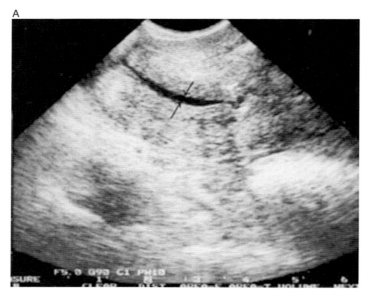
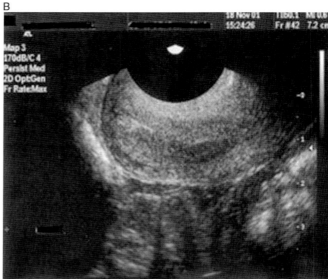

Fig. 29.7 Cervical canal measurement (A) near ovulation and (B) after ovulation. Reprinted from *Fertility and Sterility*, Vol. 92, Wolman I, Birenbaum-Gal T, Jaffa AJ. Cervical mucus status can be accurately estimated by transvaginal ultrasound during fertility evaluation, 1165–1167, Copyright 2009, with permission from Elsevier.

circulating FSH and LH levels. The elevated gonadotropin levels may cause multifollicular development, which in turn, enhances estrogen production. The elevated estrogen levels, 5–10 times higher than in normal cycles, sometimes mask the antiestrogen effect of CC and tamoxifen citrate in the cervix and uterus (Fig. 29.7).

Treatment schema and monitoring of clomiphene citrate therapy

Clomiphene citrate is administered orally in 50 mg tablets. Therapy should be initiated with 50 mg of CC over a period of 5 days, usually starting on the fifth day after the first appearance of spontaneous or progestin-induced menstrual bleeding. Clomiphene citrate dosage is typically increased in subsequent months until ovulatory cycles become evident. Clomiphene citrate-induced ovarian cysts often resolve spontaneously and typically do not require intervention.

In addition to the baseline scan, we advocate cycle monitoring via ultrasonographic evaluation of follicular size, endometrial thickness, and cervical mucus observation. Ultrasound monitoring of patients undergoing ovulation induction cycles will ensure adequate follicular recruitment and identify those patients not responding or with delayed endometrial thickening. In cases where there is concern that cervical mucus is insufficient, often due to the antiestrogenic effect of clomiphene, intrauterine insemination (bypassing the cervix) is probably the best solution. Whenever the endogenous feedback mechanism responsible for the pre-ovulatory LH surge is not properly activated, the midcycle LH peak may consequently be inadequate, ill-timed, or entirely absent. In such instances hCG should be administered to induce ovulation. The optimal timing for hCG ovulation trigger injections is when ultrasonographic measurement of mean follicular diameter is in the range 19–20 mm. Ovulation will occur 34–36 hours following hCG injection, so the IUI is often performed 34 hours later.

Universal agreement is lacking as to when to introduce ultrasonographic cycle monitoring versus less complicated or costly alternatives. However, we agree with the predominant opinion that the additional ultrasound expense is justified by the prevention of protracted periods of ineffective therapy [18].

Gonadotropins

Principles of gonadotropic therapy

In order to optimally stimulate follicular maturation both FSH and LH are required. While FSH content of the pharmacologic preparation is essential for follicular development, final maturation of the follicles and subsequent ovulation are brought about by a pituitary release and circulatory surge of LH. Thus two gonadotropins are required for induction of ovulation: one providing the required amount of FSH and another providing LH or LH-like material (hCG) of sufficient quantity to provoke ovulation and corpus luteum formation. Well-accepted ovulation induction protocols include alterations in the precise ratio of FSH to LH.

Selection of patients

Ideal candidates for ovulation induction with gonadotropins are patients who have low endogenous gonadotropin secretion and are amenorrheic or anovulatory (Group I-WHO). This treatment can also be given to patients with hypothalamic-pituitary dysfunction (Group II), including anovulatory patients associated with a variety of menstrual disorders. The treatment of choice for patients belonging to Group II is clomiphene citrate alone or in conjunction with estrogen and/or hCG. Patients who fail to ovulate or conceive within a reasonable time are considered "clomiphene failures" and can be considered for hMG therapy.

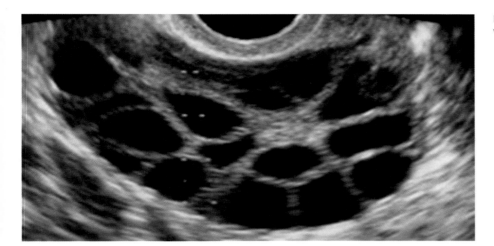

Fig. 29.8 Ovary following 5 days of stimulation with gonadotropins; follicle size 8–12 mm.

Monitoring of therapy

Gonadotropins are given daily by injection in order to stimulate follicular development; ovulation is actually induced by hCG. The daily dose of gonadotropins given in a particular cycle depends upon the ovarian response of the patient in that particular cycle. The response is reflected in a growth of follicles accompanied by biochemical changes mainly with respect to increased synthesis and secretion of steroidal hormones. The follicular enlargement can be visualized by ultrasonographic measurement, while estrogen secretion values can be estimated directly by blood measurement.

Ultrasonographic monitoring of treatment cycles serves to assess the effective dose required to evoke an ovarian response, the length of time required for follicular maturation, and the appropriate time for induction of ovulation. Furthermore, such monitoring should aim to prevent ovarian hyperstimulation syndrome (OHSS), or at least lead to early detection. For these purposes, a combination of ultrasonography and estrogen determination was advocated. Given that exogenous gonadotropic stimulation usually induces the development and growth of several follicles, ultrasonographic monitoring is particularly advisable for these treatment cycles. The levels of estrogens reflect the total estrogen secretion of all growing follicles.

Sonographic visualization may thus discriminate between single and multiple follicular growths, and their measurement may aid in the interpretation of the meaning of the estrogen levels. Evidence is accumulating that follicles with diameters greater than 18–19 mm should be "ovulated." Thus, sonography can be a more precise indicator for the determination of the optimal ovulatory timing. Gonadotropin treatment is often started on the fifth day of spontaneous or induced bleeding. It is safe to start with low doses of gonadotropins with close ultrasonic monitoring to insure appropriate follicular growth and development. Monitoring may be suspended if multiple follicles are developing. If the patient received gonadotropic therapy within the previous 3 months, treatment is usually started at the highest effective dose of the previous course.

Follicular development should be monitored with frequent ultrasound studies (Fig. 29.8). Ultrasound plays a critical role in assessing response to gonadotropins and timing of hCG administration. A baseline ultrasound scan is suggested in the early follicular phase to determine the presence or absence of persistent follicles. Scanning should become more frequent when the follicle reaches 14 mm or greater. When a follicle 18 mm or greater is identified, hMG is discontinued and hCG is administered 24 hours later to cause ovum release. Usually 10 000 units of hCG, injection are given to trigger ovulation.

While in the past it was emphasized that ultrasound scanning should be complementary to estradiol data, Shoham et al. [19,20] have raised the question of whether it is possible to run a successful ovulation induction program based solely on ultrasound monitoring. In their prospective study, monitoring of ovulation induction was performed using serial ultrasound measurements, and correlated with the patient's E_2 concentrations that became available at the end of each cycle. Twenty hypogonadotropic and 29 ultrasonically diagnosed polycystic ovary patients received treatment with gonadotropins. The results of this study demonstrated that transvaginal ultrasound findings including (a) follicular growth, (b) uterine measurements, and (c) endometrial thickness all strongly correlated with serum E_2 concentrations ($P < 0.0001$). Shoham et al. concluded that serial ultrasound examinations used alone (eliminating determination of serum E_2 levels) are an effective monitoring approach for ovulation induction cycles.

The role of ultrasound in assessing complications

The major adverse effects of induction of ovulation are multiple pregnancies and OHSS.

Around 5–8% of clomiphene-induced pregnancies and 15–25% of all pregnancies following gonadotropin-induced ovulation are multiple gestations. While almost all of the multiple gestations conceived on clomiphene will be twins, 30%

Table 29.3 Complications associated with twin pregnancy

Maternal complications	Fetal complications
• Anemia	• Premature delivery
• Pre-eclampsia/eclampsia	• Difficult delivery
• Pre-/postpartum hemorrhage	• Prolapse of an umbilical cord
	• Hypoxia of second twin

of multiple gestations following gonadotropin therapy will be triplets.

Poorly monitored ovulation induction is probably the major cause of the multiple pregnancy epidemics. Table 29.3 summarizes the clinical complications associated with twin pregnancies. It is important to diagnose multiple pregnancies early, in the first trimester, so women who conceive with high-order multiple pregnancies can consider multiple pregnancy reduction.

In cases of twin pregnancy it is recommended by the American Institute of Ultrasound in Medicine (AIUM) to document anmionicity and chorionicity in the early first trimester, so one can prepare for high-risk situations such as a monochorionic twin gestation.

In many countries, triggering of ovulation with hCG is only done if there are no more than two mature follicles around the assumed time of ovulation. Adhering to strict guidelines involving ultrasound monitoring will definitely reduce the incidence of multiples.

Ovarian hyperstimulation is the most serious complication, which in extreme situations is potentially life threatening (see Chapter 37).

It is important to understand the risk factors that can be identified before ovulation is induced. The presence of polycystic ovaries puts the patient at increased risk; we have shown that a decrease in the fraction of mature follicles and an increase in the fraction of very small follicles around the assumed time of ovulation correlates with an augmented risk for the development of severe stimulation of the ovaries. Our data suggest [21] that ultrasonography is of good predictive value in the occurrence of clinically moderate to severe ovarian hyperstimulation in women treated by hMG and hCG. Even with estrogen levels within accepted normal limits, it is suggested that hMG/hCG administration should be interrupted in the presence of 11 or more pre-ovulatory follicles, especially if most of them are immature (<9 mm).

Final remarks

Ultrasound is the most powerful tool to monitor normal and stimulated cycles; predictions of the assumed time of ovulation allow optimal timing of various procedures such as insemination, ovum aspiration, etc.

In stimulated cycles, sonographic detection of too many follicles allows withholding of hCG induction thus preventing hyperstimulation.

In the past, ovulation function was monitored by estradiol estimation. Since the development of sophisticated ultrasonographic techniques, monitoring of ovarian follicular growth by ultrasound has become a routine addition to estradiol measurement in most clinics.

Accumulating data from the Cochran Database [22] indicate that there is no evidence from randomized trials to support cycle monitoring by ultrasound plus serum estradiol as being more efficacious, in terms of live-birth outcomes and pregnancy rates, than cycle monitoring by ultrasound alone.

As far as OHSS is concerned, a randomized trial with a sufficiently large sample is needed. Until such a trial is considered, ultrasound plus serum estradiol may need to be retained as a precautionary good practice point.

References

1. Broekmans FJM, Ziegler DD, Howles CM, Gougeon A, Trew G, Olivennes F. The antral follicle count: practical recommendations for better standardization. *Fertil Steril* 2010; **94**(3): 1044–1051.

2. Pallares P, Letelier C, Gonzalez-Bulnes A. Progress toward "in vitro virtual histology" of ovarian follicles and corpora lutea by ultrasound biomicroscopy. *Fertil Steril* 2009; **91**(2): 624–626.

3. Shrestha SM, Costello MF, Sjoblom P, et al. Doppler ultrasound assessment of follicular vascularity in the early follicular phase and its relationship with outcome of in-vitro fertilization. *J Assist Reprod Genet* 2006; **23**(4): 161–169.

4. Coulam CB, Goodman C, Rinehart JS. Colour Doppler indices of follicular blood flow as predictors of pregnancy after in vitro fertilization and embryo transfer. *Hum Reprod* 1999; **14**(8): 1979–1982.

5. Nargund G, Bourne T, Doyle P, et al. Associations between ultrasound indices of follicular blood flow, oocyte recovery and preimplantation embryo quality. *Hum Reprod* 1996; **11**(1): 109–113.

6. Jayaprakasan K, Al-Hasie H, Jayaprakasan, R, et al. The three-dimensional ultrasonographic ovarian vascularity of women developing poor ovarian response during assisted reproduction treatment and its predictive value. *Fertil Steril* 2009; **92**(6): 1862–1869.

7. Bhal PS, Pugh ND, Gregory L, O'Brien S, Shaw RW. Peri-follicular vascularity as a potential variable affecting outcome in stimulated intrauterine insemination treatment cycles: a study using transvaginal power Doppler. *Hum Reprod* 2001; **16**(8): 1682–1689.

8. Baerwald A, Walker R, Pierson R. Growth rate of ovarian follicles during natural menstrual cycles, oral contraceptives cycles and ovarian stimulation cycles. *Fertil Steril* 2009; **91**(2): 440–449.

9. Kinkel K, Frei KA, Balleyguier C, et al. Diagnosis of endometriosis with imaging: a review. *Eur Radiol* 2006; **16**: 285.

10. de Silva KS, Kanumakala S, Grover SR, et al. Ovarian lesions in children and adolescents-an 11 year review. *J Pediatr Endocrinol Metab* 2004; **17**: 951.

11. Frattearelli JL, Levi AJ, Miller BT, Segars JH. A prospective assessment of predictive value of basal antral follicles in in-vitro fertilization cycles. *Fertil Steril* 2003; **80**: 350–355.

12. Hendriks DJ, Ben-Willem JM, Laszlo FJ, Egbert R, Broekmans FJM. Antral follicle count in the prediction of poor ovarian response and pregnancy after in vitro fertilization: a meta-

analysis and comparison with basal follicle-stimulating hormone level. *Fertil Steril* 2005; **83**(2): 291–301.

13. Csokmay JM, Frattarelli JL. Basal ovarian cysts and clomiphene citrate ovulation induction cycles. *Obstet Gynecol* 2006; **107**(6): 1292–1296.

14. Eissa MK, Hudson K, Docker MF, Sawers RS, Newton JR. Ultrasound follicular diameter measurement: and assessment of inter-observer and intra-observer variation. *Fertil Steril* 1985; **44**: 751–754.

15. Gonzalez CJ, Curson R, Parsons J. Transabdominal versus transvaginal ultrasound screening of ovarian follicles: are they comparable. *Fertil Steril* 1988; **50**:657.

16. Jirge PR, Patil RS. Comparison of endocrine and ultrasound profiles during ovulation induction with clomiphene citrate and letrozole in ovulatory volunteer women. *Fertil Steril* 2010; **93**(1): 174–183.

17. Wolman I, Birenbaum-Gal T, Jaffa AJ. Cervical mucus status can be accurately estimated by transvaginal ultrasound during fertility evaluation. *Fertil Steril* 2009; **92**: 1165–1167.

18. Homburg R, Clomiphene citrate – End of an era? *Hum Reprod* 2005; **20**: 2043–2051.

19. Shoham Z, DiCarlos C, Patel A, Conway GS, Jacobs HS. Is it possible to run a successful ovulation induction program based solely on ultrasound monitoring? The importance of endometrial measurements. *Fertil Steril* 1992; **56**: 836–841.

20. Shoham Z. Ultrasound is the only monitoring modality necessary for ovulation induction. OBGyn.net; July 21, 2011.

21. Blankstein J, Shalev J, Saadone, Kokia J, et al. Ovarian hyperstimulation syndrome; Prediction by number and size of preovulatory follicles. *Fertil Steril* 1987; **47**: 597–602.

22. Kwan I, Bhattacharya S, et al. (Systemic Review) Cochrane Menstrual Disorders and Sub-fertility Group (MDSG). *Database of Systematic Reviews*, 2008; 4.

Ultrasound-guided fallopian tube catheterization

Shawy Z. A. Badawy and Beverly A. Spirt

Introduction

The fallopian tubes were first accurately described in 1561 by the Italian anatomist and surgeon Gabriel Fallopio, for whom they are named [1,2]. However, it was not until the next century that their function was understood. Reinier de Graaf, the seventeenth-century Dutch anatomist and physician who is considered the founder of modern reproductive biology, and who is best remembered for his description of ovarian follicles, was probably the first to comprehend the role of the fallopian tubes [3,4]. He was familiar with pathological conditions such as ectopic pregnancy, and concluded in his tractate on the female reproductive system, published in 1672, that the egg is transferred from the ovary to the uterus via the fallopian tube. The function of the fallopian tube is now known to be far more complex. It not only serves as a conduit for the ovum, the sperm, and the early embryo, but also provides the necessary environment for both conception and development of the early embryo.

The fallopian tubes lie within the free edge of the broad ligament, extending from the cornua of the uterus to the ovaries. They are approximately 10 cm in length, and are composed of three layers: the external serosal layer, an intermediate muscle layer, and the internal mucosal layer. The tubes are considered to have four segments: the trumpet-shaped infundibulum with its fringed (fimbriated) ends that sweep over the ovary at ovulation; the relatively dilated ampulla, which is 3–5 mm in diameter and 5–8 cm in length, constituting the longest portion of the fallopian tube; the isthmus, which has the narrowest lumen (<1 mm in diameter) and the thickest muscle layer; and the interstitial (intramural) portion, which is approximately 1 mm in diameter and extends through the wall of the uterus to the endometrial cavity.

The endosalpinx contains two types of cell, ciliated cells and non-ciliated secretory cells. Both of these cell types are affected by hormonal status: estrogen, progesterone, and prostaglandin. The ciliary cells, which comprise the majority of the cells and are most numerous in the distal portion of the tube, are tallest at midcycle. Prior to ovulation, the ciliary motion creates a negative pressure that effectively aspirates the oocyte from the surface of the ovary into the fallopian tube. The continuous motion of the cilia creates a current from the distal to the proximal portion of the fallopian tube, facilitating the movement of the oocyte toward the uterus. The second type of cell secretes tubal fluid that is rich in glycol protein, in order to support the needs of the oocyte and the sperm [5–7]. The secretory cells are longest at midcycle, when maximal secretion occurs.

Pathology of the fallopian tube

Tubal disease is the most common cause of female infertility. The most significant pathology affecting the fallopian tube results from infection. There has been an increased incidence of salpingitis as a result of an increase in sexually transmitted diseases, mainly due to gonorrhea and chlamydia. While in some cases the infection is silent, in the majority of cases the patient presents with symptoms of fever, abdominal pain, and leukocytosis [8].

Infection of the fallopian tube leads to destruction of the endosalpinx with formation of intraluminal adhesions. The infection may extend across the tubal wall with formation of peritubal adhesions that will lead to narrowing of the tubal lumen. In severe cases the fimbriated end of the tube becomes agglutinated and closed, resulting in hydrosalpinx or pyosalpinx [9,10].

Salpingitis isthmica nodosa is a diffuse lesion that primarily involves the isthmus of the fallopian tube, and is often bilateral. The etiology is unclear; it is felt to be an acquired condition, likely on a mechanical basis [11]. It is characterized by hyperplasia of the myosalpinx, with diverticula of the endosalpinx projecting into the muscle; this results in marked narrowing and obstruction of the tubal lumen [12].

Endometriosis may affect any portion of the fallopian tube. If it affects the proximal portion of the tube, the condition may mimic salpingitis isthmica nodosa and may lead to complete obstruction of the tube at that site. In addition, tubal dysfunction may be due to biological changes in peritoneal fluid that contains high levels of prostaglandins in these patients [13].

Proximal tubal obstruction is present in about 20–30% of patients with tubal disease. The most common cause of

Ultrasonography in Gynecology, ed. Botros R. M. B. Rizk and Elizabeth E. Puscheck. Published by Cambridge University Press. © Cambridge University Press 2015.

obstruction of the interstitial portion of the fallopian tube is spasm of the tube that could be due to stress, excess prostaglandins, or the use of cold radiopaque contrast during hysterosalpingography. In addition, debris has been reported to be a factor in obstruction of the interstitial portion of the tube [14,15].

Assessment of tubal patency

Hysterosalpingography is the standard screening examination to evaluate tubal patency. This is an outpatient procedure and is performed during the proliferative phase of the menstrual cycle following the completion of the menstrual period. Patients are instructed to take 600–800 mg of ibuprofen about 1–2 hours before the procedure. The patient is brought to the radiology suite and is placed in the dorsal lithotomy position. The vagina is evaluated with a speculum. The cervix and vagina are washed with an antiseptic lotion. A hysterosalpingogram catheter is inserted through the cervix into the uterine cavity, and the balloon is inflated in the lower uterine segment. The speculum is removed and the patient is placed in the supine position. Water-soluble radiopaque contrast is slowly injected into the uterus under fluoroscopic visualization. The contrast may be at room temperature, or it may be warmed in order to prevent uterine or tubal spasm. If either or both of the tubes are not opacified, turning the patient prone may be useful. The contrast injection is discontinued when spillage into the peritoneal cavity is visualized, or when intravasation occurs.

Intravasation may be caused by increased intrauterine pressure due to tubal occlusion or by excessive injection pressure. Recent pregnancy, uterine or tubal surgery, or curettage may predispose to venous intravasation via defects in the endometrium or endosalpinx. Therefore, hysterosalpingography should not be performed until 6 weeks post-procedure.

Hysterosalpingography is contraindicated if there is active pelvic infection. If the patient has a history of allergic reaction to contrast, nonionic contrast should be used [16]. Premedication with steroids or antihistamines should be considered. However, such patients are not usually considered to be at increased risk when contrast is administered via a nonvascular route. Venous intravasation, which may occur during hysterosalpingography in up to 7% of patients [17], may theoretically result in a reaction to contrast.

Tubal catheterization

Interstitial tubal obstruction is diagnosed when contrast is not visualized in the fallopian tube beyond the tubocornual junction during hysterosalpingography. These patients are candidates for tubal catheterization to confirm the presence of interstitial obstruction and to assess the remainder of the tube. Tubal catheterization can be performed in several ways. Hysteroscopic cannulation may be performed under general anesthesia in conjunction with laparoscopy. Fluoroscopic or ultrasound-guided tubal catheterization with selective salpingography can be performed with or without sedation.

In 1985, Platia and Krudy reported using a 3-French catheter under fluoroscopic visualization to clear fallopian tubes that were proximally occluded [18]. A method for tubal catheterization using angiographic techniques to evaluate and recanalize the fallopian tube was described in 1987 by Thurmond et al. [19]. The success of this method was such that in 1993 the American Society for Reproductive Medicine recommended in its guidelines that fluoroscopically guided tubal catheterization with selective salpingography and recanalization be performed in patients with proximal obstruction of the fallopian tube demonstrated at hysterosalpingography before other invasive methods to treat infertility are used [20].

As with hysterosalpingography, the procedure is scheduled during the follicular phase of the menstrual cycle. The patient may be pretreated with antibiotics and sedated. The procedure is performed by the interventional radiologist, often in conjunction with the gynecologist, with the gynecologist placing the hysterosalpingography catheter using sterile technique. After inflating the intrauterine balloon, the radiologist injects contrast into the uterine cavity. With sedation and analgesia, contrast can be injected with increased pressure that can overcome tubal spasm, thus resolving some cases of apparent obstruction. If there is persistent proximal obstruction, coaxial catheters and guide wires are used to clear the obstruction and recanalize the tube. Following recanalization, contrast is injected into the tube to better delineate the tubal anatomy and pathology.

The patient usually experiences mild uterine cramping and vaginal bleeding with this procedure. Perforation of the tube occurs in about 4% of cases; this is usually related to the severity of the underlying tubal pathology. No additional treatment or monitoring is needed if perforation occurs [21,22].

Thurmond reported a successful fallopian tube recanalization rate of 95% in a series of 20 women with documented bilateral proximal tubal occlusion and no additional tubal pathology; 47% of these patients conceived in an average of 4 months following tubal recanalization; all were intrauterine pregnancies. There is a reocclusion rate of approximately 50% in patients who do not become pregnant within 6 months of the procedure [22]. In that situation, repeat recanalization can be performed.

Confino et al., in a multicenter study, described a successful recanalization rate of 92% using a transcervical balloon tuboplasty catheter designed according to the same principle as arterial balloon catheters, with fluoroscopic guidance. The pregnancy rate was 34%, including one ectopic pregnancy [23]. This procedure was not as widely accepted as the catheter/guide wire method.

The average absorbed radiation dose to the ovaries in fluoroscopically guided tubal catheterization is estimated to be 8.5 mGy ± 5.6 (0.85 rad ± 0.56), based on an average fluoroscopy time of 8.5 minutes, with an average of 14 spot films obtained [24]. This dose is in the same range as an intravenous pyelogram or barium enema.

Use of ultrasound for assessment and treatment of tubal factor infertility

Ultrasound is usually the modality of choice for examinations and procedures involving the reproductive organs because of the lack of ionizing radiation. During the past three decades, infertility specialists have used ultrasonography for evaluation of the uterus and for assessment of follicular development and maturation in assisted reproductive technology. The fallopian tubes, however, are not well visualized at sonography unless they are abnormal, or unless they are outlined by fluid.

Saline infusion sonohysterography (SIS) is a valuable means of defining intrauterine lesions, and has become an established procedure for the study of patients with abnormal uterine bleeding. Patency of at least one fallopian tube can be indirectly established during a sonohysterogram if free fluid is visualized following the injection of saline that had not been visualized prior to the injection. Microbubble contrast agents such as Albunex allow direct visualization of flow through the fallopian tubes and have been used to evaluate tubal patency and to catheterize the fallopian tubes with more specific results [25–28].

In the late 1980s and early 1990s, methods of ultrasound-guided fallopian tube catheterization were developed for gamete intrafallopian transfer (GIFT), for embryo transfer, and for fallopian tube recanalization with varying degrees of success. One such method, using outer and inner catheters, was developed by Jansen et al. [29,30,31]. Using transvaginal ultrasound guidance, Jansen placed an outer 5.5F Teflon catheter at the tubocornual junction. Following this, an inner 3F Teflon catheter with a tapered distal end was placed 3–4 cm beyond the tubocornual junction, at the junction of the ampulla and the isthmus. The second catheter was not placed unless tubal patency was confirmed by ultrasound visualization of small bubbles of 5% carbon dioxide in air that had been injected into the catheter, moving freely from the catheter through the adnexa. In a series of five patients who underwent embryo transfer with this method, one became pregnant [30]. Of a series of 35 patients in whom GIFT was performed, 6 became pregnant.

Lisse and Sydow reported a series of 41 patients, wherein 21 out of 38 fallopian tubes (55%) were successfully recanalized using ultrasound guidance along with "tactile sensation" when placing the catheter [32]. Of the patients who were successfully recanalized, 5 became pregnant (32%). Reocclusion rate was 43%. The tactile method requires significant experience and is not easily reproducible. This method has been more recently applied [33] in a group of 50 patients; 84% of fallopian tubes were successfully catheterized with ultrasound guidance, and 63% using tactile sensation. The total pregnancy rate was 16%, with no significant difference between the two groups.

Thurmond et al. [34] and Breckenridge and Schinfeld [35] began with a catheter system designed by Jansen and Anderson, consisting of an outer catheter with an obturator, and an inner catheter with a guide wire to cannulate the fallopian tube. Both groups subsequently modified the procedure, and both switched from transvaginal to transabdominal ultrasound guidance. The transvaginal probe tended to dislodge the catheter in some cases and, in combination with the speculum, tenaculum, and catheters, was cumbersome and uncomfortable for the patient. The full bladder that is required for the transabdominal approach served to straighten the uterus, making it easier to insert the catheter.

Ultrasound-guided catheterization of the fallopian tubes has not proven to be as popular and as widely used as the fluoroscopically guided procedure. Limitations to the technique include poor visualization of smaller catheters with sonography, poor visualization of the fallopian tubes, and poor differentiation between guide wires, gas, and larger catheters, which are all echogenic. While the procedure is easier to perform with transabdominal ultrasound, the resolution is significantly better with transvaginal ultrasound.

In conclusion, fallopian tube catheterization and recanalization is the procedure of choice in the initial management of proximal or interstitial tubal obstruction, and is recommended prior to invasive procedures such as IVF or tuboplasty. Several technologies are available. Fluoroscopically guided selective salpingography and fallopian tube recanalization has proven to be successful in more than 90% of cases, and is the most widely used technique. While ultrasound-guided fallopian tube catheterization has been used with some success in GIFT procedures, laparoscopy is the standard technique for that procedure at this time.

References

1. Siegler AM. A review of early contributions to the development of tuboplasty. In: Siegler AM, Ansari AH, Chesley C. (Eds.) *The Fallopian Tube. Basic Studies and Clinical Contributions*. Futura Publishing Co.; 1986: 359–368.

2. Speert H. Obstetric-gynecologic eponyms: Gabriele Falloppio and the fallopian tubes. *Obstet Gynecol* 1955; **6**(4): 467–470.

3. Ankum WM, Houtzager HL, Bleker OP. Reinier de Graaf (1641–1673) and the Fallopian tube. *Hum Reprod Update* 1996; **2**(4): 365–369.

4. Houtzager HL. Reinier de Graaf and his contribution to reproductive biology. *Eur J Obstet Gynecol* 2000; **90**: 125–127.

5. Eddy CA, Pauerstein CJ. Anatomy and physiology of the fallopian tube. *Clin Obstet Gynecol* 1980; **23**(4): 1177–1193.

6. Hershlag A, Diamond MP, DeChreney AH. Tubal physiology: an appraisal. *J Gynecol Surg* 1989; **5**: 2–25.

7. Verhage HG, Bareither ML, Jaffe RC, et al. Cyclic changes in ciliation, secretion, and cell height of the oviductal epithelium in women. *Am J Anat* 1979; **156**: 505.

8. Patton DL, Moore DE, Spadoni LR, Soules MR, Halbert SA, Wang SP. A comparison of the fallopian tubes' response to overt and silent salpingitis. *Obstet Gynecol* 1989; **73**(4): 622.

9. Mardh PA. An overview of infectious agents of salpingitis, their biology and recent advances in methods of detection. *Am J Obstet Gynecol* 1980; **138**: 933.

10. Westrem L. Incidence, prevalence and trends of acute pelvic inflammatory disease and its consequences in industrialized countries. *Am J Obstet Gynecol* 1980; **138**: 880.

11. Honore LH. Pathology of the Fallopian tube. In: Fox H (Ed.) *Haines and Taylor Obstetrical and Gynaecological Pathology*, 3rd edn. Edinburgh: Churchill Livingstone; 1987: 479–518.

12. Creasy JL, Clark RL, Cuttino JT, Greff TR: Salpingitis isthmica nodosa: radiologic and clinical correlates. *Radiology* 1985; **154**: 597–600.

13. Badawy SZA. Endometriosis of the fallopian tube and factors leading to infertility. In: Siegler AM, Ansari AH, Chesley C. (Eds.) *The Fallopian Tube. Basic Studies and Clinical Contributions* Futura Publishing Co.; 1986: 219–223.

14. Fortier KJ, Haney AF. The pathologic spectrum of uterotubal junction obstruction. *Obstet Gynecol* 1985; **65**: 93–98.

15. Sulak PJ, Letterie GS, Coddington CC, Hayslip CC, Woodward JE, Klein TA. Histology of proximal tubal occlusion. *Fertil Steril* 1987; **48**: 437–440.

16. Badawy SZA, Singer SJ, Etman A. Hysterosalpingography. In: Rizk BRMB (Ed.) *Ultrasonography in Reproductive Medicine and Infertility*. Cambridge University Press; 2010; 22–33.

17. Thurmond AS, Winfield A. Hysterosalpingography Part I: procedure and normal findings. In: Taveras JM, Ferrucci JT (Eds.) *Radiology: Diagnosis Imaging Intervention*. Philadelphia: J. B. Lippincott; 1992: 1–7.

18. Platia MP, Krudy AG. Transvaginal fluoroscopic recanalization of a proximally occluded oviduct. *Fertil Steril* 1985; **44**: 604–706.

19. Thurmond AS, Novy M, Uchida BT, Bosch J. Fallopian tube obstruction: selective salpingography and recanalization: Work in Progress. *Radiology* 1987; **163**: 511–514.

20. Guidelines for Practice. Birmingham, AL. American Fertility Society. September 1993.

21. Thurmond AS, Rosch J. Nonsurgical fallopian tube recanalization for treatment of infertility. *Radiology* 1990; **174**: 371–374.

22. Thurmond AS, Fallopian tube catheterization. *Semin Radiol* 2008; **25**(4): 425–431.

23. Confino E, Turkaspa I, DeCherney A, et al. Transcervical balloon tuboplasty – a multicenter study. *JAMA* 1990; **264**: 2079–2082.

24. Hedgpeth PL, Thurmond AS, Fry R, et al. Radiographic fallopian tube recanalization: absorbed ovarian radiation dose. *Radiology* 1991; **180**: 121–122.

25. Korell M, Seehaus D, Strowitzki T, Hepp H. Radiologic versus ultrasound fallopian tube imaging. Painfulness of examination and diagnostic reliability of hysterosalpingography and hysterosalpingo-contrast-ultrasonography with Echovist 200. *Ultraschall Med* 1997; **18**(1): 3–7.

26. Balen FG, Allen CM, Siddle NC, Lees WR. Ultrasound contrast hysterosalpingography. Evaluation as an outpatient procedure. *Br J Radiol* 1993; **66**: 592–599.

27. Session DR, Lerner JP, Tehen CK, Kelly AC. Ultrasound-guided fallopian tube cannulation using Akbybex. *Fertil Steril* 1997; **67**: 972–974.

28. Exacoustos C, Zupi E et al. Contrast-tuned imaging and second-generation contrast agent Sonovue: a new ultrasound approach to evaluation of tubal patency. *J Minim Invasive Gynecol* 2009; **16**(4): 437–444.

29. Jansen RPS, Anderson JC. Catheterisation of the fallopian tubes from the vagina. *Lancet* 1987; **2**: 209–310.

30. Jansen RPS, Anderson JC, Sutherland PD. Nonoperative embryo transfer to the fallopian tube. *N Engl J Med* 1987; **319**(5): 288–291.

31. Jansen RPS, Anderson JC, Radomic I, et al. Pregnancies after ultrasound-guided fallopian insemination with cryostored donor semen. *Fertil Steril* 1988; **49**(5):900–902.

32. Lisse K, Sydow P. Fallopian tube catheterization and recanalization under ultrasonic observation. A simplified technique to evaluate tubal patency and open proximally obstructed tubes. *Fertil Steril* 1991; **56**: 198–201.

33. Rahimunnioa S, Tanwar R, Prasad S. Ultrasound versus tactile cannulation in the treatment of proximal tubal obstruction. *Int J Gynaecol Obstet* 2009; **196**: 216–217.

34. Thurmond AS, Patton PE, Hector DM, Jones MK. US-guided fallopian tube catheterization. *Radiology* 1991; **180**(2): 571–572.

35. Breckenridge JW, Schinfeld, JS. Technique for US-guided fallopian tube catheterization. *Radiology* 1991; **180**(2): 569–570.

Chapter

31

Ultrasound imaging of fibroids and infertility

Terri L. Woodard, Samuel Johnson and Elizabeth E. Puscheck

Introduction

Uterine fibroids are benign monoclonal tumors [1] that occur in up to 60% of reproductive age women and 80% of women during their lifetime [2]. While many women with fibroids are asymptomatic, the clinical presentation and symptoms can vary and include menorrhagia, pelvic pressure, bowel and urinary complaints, pain, and infertility. Fibroids are the leading cause of hysterectomy and are a significant public health care burden, estimated to exceed 34 billion dollars annually in the United States [3] (Figs 31.1 and 31.2).

Diagnosis of fibroids

Ultrasound is the method of choice to initially evaluate the uterus for fibroids. Typically, transvaginal ultrasound is the best method to identify the presence of fibroids in the uterus, since the transvaginal probe can get closer to the uterus than the abdominal sector probe. However, if the uterus is greatly enlarged (i.e. 14 weeks size or greater), then transabdominal ultrasound would be better to evaluate the uterus in its

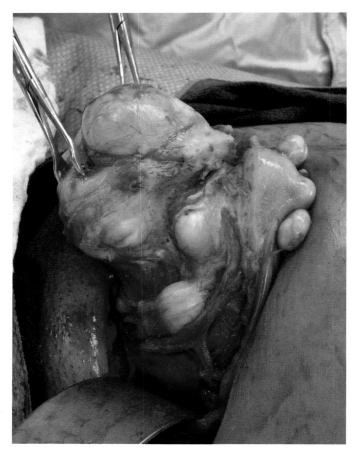

Fig. 31.2 Multiple fibroids during myomectomy showing submucous, intramural and subserous fibroids. Courtesy of Botros Rizk.

entirety. Early fibroids may just distort the serosal border and make the uterus look bulky. The classic appearance of fibroids on ultrasound is a smooth circular pattern with shadowing, since the fibroid is denser than the surrounding myometrium and it is difficult for the sound waves to penetrate the fibroid (Fig. 31.3). Surgical specimens when bifurcated demonstrate the density of fibroids very well (Fig. 31.4). Some fibroids may not be hyperechoic and may mostly blend in with

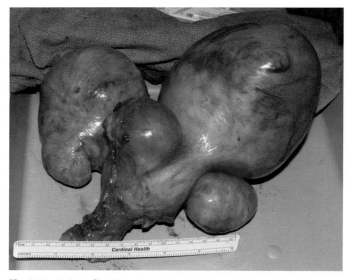

Fig. 31.1 Multiple fibroids on hysterectomy specimen.

Ultrasonography in Gynecology, ed. Botros R. M. B. Rizk and Elizabeth E. Puscheck. Published by Cambridge University Press. © Cambridge University Press 2015.

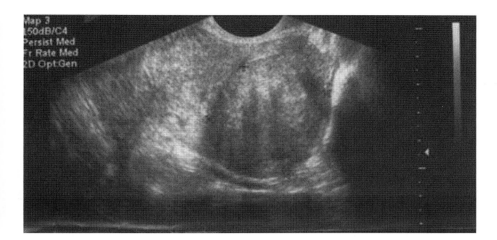

Fig. 31.3 Well-circumscribed fibroid with sound wave drop-outs through the fibroid attributed to its density.

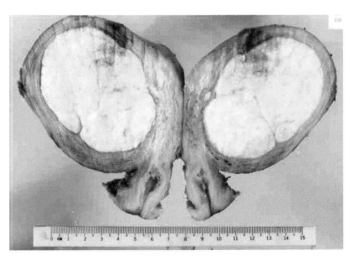

Fig. 31.4 Fibroid on bifurcation at time from hysterectomy specimen. Note the white appearance consistent with its density and the lack of vascularity within the fibroid.

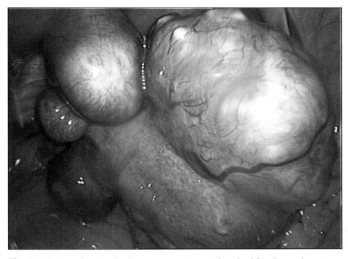

Fig. 31.6 Note that on this laparoscopy picture that the blood vessels are found on the surface of the fibroids.

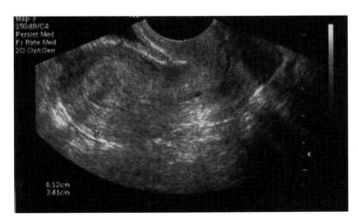

Fig. 31.5 Ultrasound of the uterus with an abnormality noted centrally. The borders are not clear. There is little to no shadowing.

the myometrium, plus they have indistinct borders making them difficult to identify (Fig. 31.5). Doppler can help since the blood vessels are usually pushed to the side (Figs 31.6 and 31.7). Calcifications may surround the outer surface of

the fibroid over time and these calcifications appear white on ultrasound. These calcifications are much more difficult for sound waves to penetrate and resultant significant shadowing limits the ultrasound evaluation.

Multiple fibroids and/or calcifications can make visualization of these fibroids difficult. Tips on improving visualization that most ultrasound machines have include:

1. Use the "Optimize" button if your machine has one. This does multiple adjustments concurrently.
2. Turn off the "Harmonics." This will allow for deeper penetration.
3. Change the probe to a lower frequency so greater depth (e.g. from 6–12 MHz to 5–9 MHz for a vaginal probe). Remember that the higher the frequency, the shorter the focal length and vice versa, the lower the frequency, the longer the focal length (more penetration into the fibroid).
4. Many machines allow you to change focal length.
5. Add more foci.

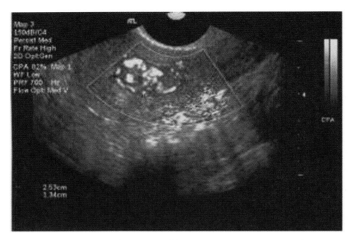

Fig. 31.7 This ultrasound image is of the same uterus as in Fig. 31.6 but power Doppler was applied. Note the increased vasculature on the surface of the fibroid, which is very different to the surrounding myometrium.

6. Change probes (from transvaginal to transabdominal).

If visualization is still difficult, then changing to a different modality (e.g. MRI) can be very helpful for fibroid mapping.

On the ultrasound report, the number, size, and location of each fibroid should be noted for patients with infertility. Those that impinge the uterine cavity will need further evaluation since this impacts fertility significantly. A number of methods are available to assess the uterine cavity, including hysterosalpingogram, saline infusion sonohysterogram, and hysteroscopy.

The association between fibroids and infertility

Depending on the method used for diagnosis, fibroids are estimated to occur in 5–77% of women [4]. More importantly, it has been estimated that 5–10% of infertile women have a fibroid and the presence of a fibroid(s) is the sole abnormal finding in 1–2.4% of them [5]. This may become increasingly important, as women are delaying childbearing and presenting at an older age, when fibroids have been exposed to a longer duration of estrogen which causes the fibroid to grow and discovery to be more likely.

It is recognized and accepted that fibroids can potentially impact fertility; therefore, the presence of fibroids should be sought during the workup for infertility. The extent to which fibroids impair fertility is debatable because of the heterogeneity of the condition in terms of size, number, and location. Additionally, many studies of the impact of fibroids on fertility have been confounded by age and other factors [6,7].

It is generally accepted that submucosal fibroids and intramural fibroids that distort the uterine cavity decrease implantation and pregnancy and that patients with these fibroids may benefit from myomectomy [7]. However, it is less clear whether intramural fibroids that do not distort the cavity have

negative effects on implantation and pregnancy rates. While it has been shown that the degree to which fibroids impact fertility is dependent upon the type of fibroid (i.e. subserosal vs. transmural vs. submucosal), it is less clear how the size and number of fibroids influence fertility outcomes. Thus, the management of fibroids in the setting of infertility remains controversial.

Theoretical mechanisms of how fibroids cause infertility

Fibroids have been hypothesized to impair fertility in a number of ways. Several mechanisms have been proposed: (1) large or multiple fibroids may cause anatomical distortion that prevents proper ovum pick-up and embryo transport by the tubes; (2) they may interfere with normal implantation of the embryo; (3) the normal pattern of uterine contractility may be altered, inhibiting gamete transport [8]; (4) alterations in endometrial blood supply may mechanically or biochemically interfere with implantation [9]; and (5) they may cause localized endometrial inflammation or secrete vasoactive substances that interfere with gamete/embryo survival [10].

Fibroid type and impact on fertility
Subserosal fibroids

Subserosal fibroids (Fig. 31.8) are those where more than 50% of the fibroid extends beyond the serosal surface of the uterus; they do not distort the endometrial cavity. Subserosal fibroids can be either sessile (attached to its base without a stalk) or pedunculated (attached by a stalk). It has been suggested that these types of fibroid could potentially impact fertility by disrupting uterine peristalsis [11]. However, in large-scale studies, they do not appear to significantly impact fertility outcomes. A systematic review of 11 trials evaluating the effect of fibroids that included subserosal tumors demonstrated no effect on clinical pregnancy (odds ratio [OR] 1.0; 95% CI 0.8–1.2) or delivery (OR 0.9; 95%CI 0.7–1.1) [7]. Furthermore, they have not been found to effect implantation and clinical pregnancy in women undergoing assisted reproductive technology (ART) treatment [12,13].

Intramural fibroids

Intramural fibroids are those that have less than 50% of their largest diameter protruding into the serosal surface of the uterus; they may or may not distort the endometrial cavity. Typically, intramural fibroids do not enter the uterine cavity but may distort it. Studies of intramural fibroids that do not distort the endometrial cavity and infertility have been conflicting; Somigliana et al. [14] evaluated 80 cases of intramural fibroids (10–50 mm), 39 cases of subserosal fibroids, and 119 controls. Uterine cavities were evaluated with hysteroscopy to exclude any uterine cavity distortion by fibroids. The results suggested that intramural fibroids did not negatively effect pregnancy,

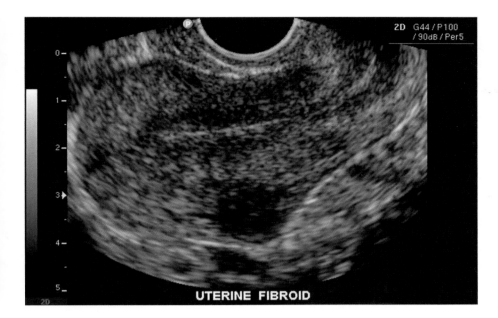

Fig. 31.8 This uterine image demonstrates a hypoechoic fibroid located subserosally. It is an early subserosal fibroid.

implantation, and delivery in ART cycles (OR 1.41 [95% CI 0.67–2.98]; 1.75 [95% CI 0.90–3.39]; 1.36 [95% CI 0.58–3.15], respectively) [14]. Similar findings have been reported in other trials with autologous in vitro fertilization (IVF) [15] and oocyte recipient populations [16]. However, there are studies that suggest a negative impact on ART outcomes, including a prospective trial that demonstrated a reduction in implantation and ongoing pregnancy compared with controls (implantation: 11.9% vs. 20.2%; $P = 0.018$; ongoing pregnancy: 15.1% vs. 28.3%; $P = 0.003$) [17,18].

Intramural fibroids that distort the endometrial cavity are more likely to be associated with reduced fertility and an increased miscarriage rate (MR). There are multiple mechanisms by which this may occur. Intramural fibroids may promote an inflammatory reaction within the endometrium and/or higher monocyte chemotactic protein-1 (MCP-1), and macrophage accumulation may interfere with implantation or increase risk of miscarriage [18]. Finally, they may cause abnormal uterine peristalsis during the mid-luteal phase, which may prohibit implantation [19].

The largest review on the topic demonstrated the negative impact of intramural fibroids. In this review, heterogeneity of the available studies was minimized by performing multiple sensitivity analyses based on age, order of treatment cycle, and study design. These sub-analyses all demonstrated a negative impact of non cavity-distorting, intramural fibroids on ART outcomes [20]. This detrimental impact appears to be related to size, as fibroids larger than 3 cm have been shown to have detrimental affects on ART outcomes [13,21]. While it appears that intramural fibroids (distorting and nondistorting) may have a negative effect on fertility and miscarriage rates, there is insufficient evidence to determine whether myomectomy

absolutely improves these outcomes. Removal of intramural fibroids >5 cm may be of benefit, with up to a 50% improvement in live birth rate [22].

Submucosal fibroids

Submucosal fibroids are fibroids that project into the endometrial cavity; they can be further subdivided into three subtypes (Figs 31.9, 31.10, and 31.11): type 0, which are pedunculated fibroids that do not exhibit any intramural extension; type I, which are sessile and have less than 50% intramural extension into the myometrium (more than 50% in the uterine cavity); and type II, which are sessile and have more than 50% intramural extension (less than 50% in the uterine cavity) [23]. Submucosal fibroids and particularly the type 0 fibroid are most strongly associated with reduced fertility and an increased miscarriage rate. Systematic reviews have indicated that the presence of submucosal fibroids correlates with a decrease in implantation by 60–70% compared with patients without fibroids and a 70% decrease in clinical pregnancy [16,24,25]. A potential mechanism by which this occurs is through a global decrease in endometrial HOX gene expression [26]. Unlike intramural fibroids, myomectomy for submucosal fibroids definitely improves fertility outcomes.

Impact of size of fibroid

There are limited data on how the size of fibroids impacts fertility and pregnancy outcomes. While fibroids larger than 3 cm have been shown to have detrimental affects on ART outcomes [13,21], a prospective case-control study of women with asymptomatic intramural or subserosal fibroids measuring 50 mm or less compared with controls revealed no significant difference

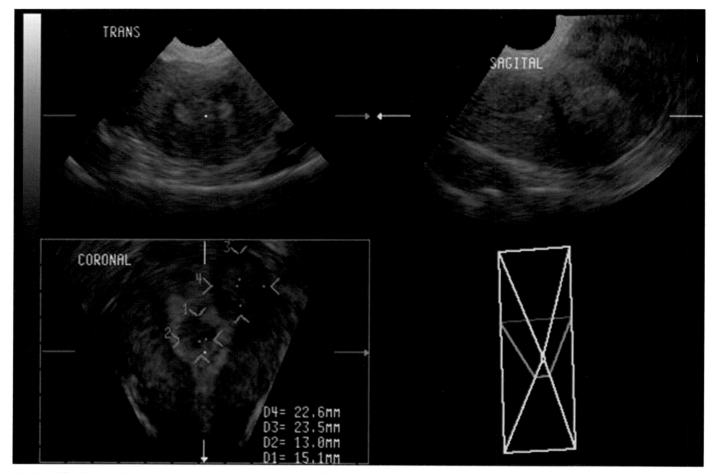

Fig. 31.9 This ultrasound image is notable for submucosal fibroids. It a 3D ultrasound of the uterus performed in the luteal phase which shows the endometrium as a hyperechoic or whiter appearance and demonstrates the location of the fibroids in relationship to the uterine cavity without using an invasive contrast material. The lower left panel shows number calipers measuring fibroids: Numbers 1 and 2 identify the submucosal fibroid, which is completely in the uterine cavity with the hyperechoic (white) endometrium surrounding it, consistent with a type 0 submucosal fibroid. Numbers 3 and 4 identify a fibroid that is mostly in the myometrium with less than 50% in the uterine cavity, so it is consistent with a submucosal fibroid, type II. Courtesy of Leeber Cohen.

in IVF success rates [14]. Interestingly, hyperstimulation during IVF does not appear to influence the size of small fibroids (2 cm or less) [27].

Impact of number of fibroids

There are limited data on how the number of fibroids impacts fertility and pregnancy outcomes. A recent study by Bozdag and colleagues examined the reproductive performance of women having a single intramural fibroid and an intact endometrium (confirmed by hysteroscopy) versus controls, with all patients undergoing IVF with intracytoplasmic sperm injection (ICSI) [28]. All had severe male-factor infertility. Implantation rates and clinical pregnancy rates were virtually identical for the two groups. In addition, size of the fibroid (ranging from 5 to 43 mm) had no effect on outcome. In a case-control study of women with subserosal or intramural fibroids going through IVF, there was not a significant relationship between clinical outcomes and the number or size of the fibroids [14].

Fibroids and pregnancy

Evaluation of women with first trimester ultrasounds demonstrated that the prevalence of uterine fibroids in pregnancy is approximately 10% [29]. Patients with uterine fibroids identified on first trimester sonogram were twice as likely to have a pregnancy loss compared with controls (14% vs. 7.6%) [30]. Studies of patients undergoing ART have also demonstrated an increased miscarriage rate in patients with uterine fibroids. A meta-analysis of retrospective and prospective cohort trials evaluating the impact of fibroids on miscarriage in patients undergoing IVF showed that patients with fibroids have approximately twice the loss rate of controls (15.3% vs. 7.7%) [25].

Fibroids may have other impacts on pregnancy and outcomes. Women with large uterine fibroids in pregnancy are at significantly increased risk for delivery at an earlier gestational age compared with women with small or no fibroids, as well as obstetric complications including excess blood loss and increased frequency of postpartum blood transfusion [31]. In addition, women with

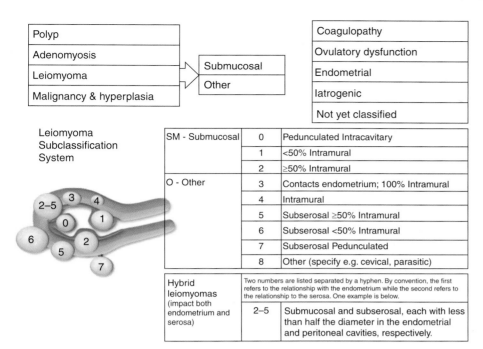

Fig. 31.10 Fibroid mapping.

fibroids have a higher incidence of cesarean delivery [32–35] and abnormal placentation [36] associated with abruption, placenta previa, and intrauterine growth retardation (IUGR). When large fibroids are found on ultrasound, the patient should be appropriately counseled regarding these risks.

Evaluation of fibroids in the setting of infertility

The standard infertility workup includes an evaluation of the uterus and the uterine cavity. A transvaginal ultrasound (TVUS) is often performed as a baseline in the early follicular phase. In addition to evaluating the ovaries and determining the antral follicle count (AFC), this ultrasound should also evaluate the uterus for anomalies and fibroids. The endometrial lining is hyperechoic in relation to the myometrium and can be used to identify the location of the fibroid. If the endometrial lining appears to be abnormal, further investigation is warranted either by performing the ultrasound in the luteal phase of the woman's menstrual cycle when the endometrium is thickened and homogeneously hyperechoic or by another imaging technique. Potential alternative methods of evaluation include hysterosalpingogram (HSG), saline infusion sonohysterography (SIS), MRI, and hysteroscopy. Hysteroscopy remains the gold standard for the evaluation of the uterine cavity; however, it is invasive and carries the risk of perforation, infection, and bleeding. HSG, while providing the added benefit of being able to visualize tubal morphology, contour and patency, yields a lower sensitivity and specificity compared with other modalities. In addition, an HSG requires exposure to dye and radiation. Ultrasound assessment of the uterine cavity, including SIS, is a much more sensitive method to identify the fibroid and its impact on the uterine cavity, as has been discussed in another chapter.

A prospective study comparing TVUS, SIS, and diagnostic hysteroscopy revealed that SIS was better than TVUS for detection of both polyps and fibroids [37]. Similarly, in a study comparing the accuracy of TVUS, SIS, and hysteroscopy for uterine pathologies among infertile women, SIS appeared to be superior to TVUS alone for the detection of submucosal fibroids [38].

There has been interest in adding the technology of three-dimensional ultrasound to saline infusion sonohysterography (3D-SIS) to improve detection and diagnosis. 3D-SIS has been shown to have good agreement with diagnostic hysteroscopy for the classification of submucosal fibroids [39]. While 3D ultrasound renderings improve visualization of the uterine fundus and aid in identification or exclusion of a fundal contour abnormality, they do not increase the detection of endometrial abnormalities [40]. In contrast, in a study of 180 women who had a normal TVUS and HSG during their infertility workup, it was found that 3D-SIS was comparable to diagnostic hysteroscopy for the diagnosis of intrauterine lesions and was superior to 2D-SIS [41].

Treatment of fibroids in the setting of infertility

The impact of fibroids on fertility and miscarriage rate is a topic of great debate. Given all the controversy, which women should be treated and how?

The management of women who present with infertility and fibroids depends largely on the clinical presentation. While there are many treatment options that exist for women with fibroids, some are not indicated in women who wish to conceive. For instance, medications such as GnRH agonists, while effective, are not of practical use because they require long-term use and delay time to conception. Hysterectomy – the definitive

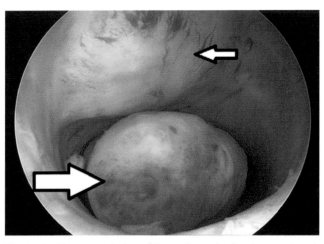

Fig. 31.11 Hysteroscopic view of the uterine cavity showing a pedunculated submucous fibroid (large arrow) and type 1 submucous fibroid (small arrow). Courtesy of Botros Rizk.

treatment for fibroids – also precludes conception and would require use of a surrogate or gestational carrier. Newer and less invasive technologies such as uterine artery embolization are efficacious; however, the potential effects on fertility are not predictable, so this therapy should be avoided in women who desire to conceive. There are several investigational treatments that hold promise for the treatment of uterine fibroids; currently these are utilized in clinical trials and patients should be counseled appropriately, since the long-term reproductive consequences are unknown at present.

Traditional surgical methods

Hysteroscopic myomectomy

Hysteroscopic myomectomy is the first line of therapy for the treatment of submucosal fibroids. Removal of submucosal fibroids has been shown to improve clinical pregnancy rates and decrease miscarriage rates [42]. Although it is a minimally invasive outpatient procedure, risks include perforation, fluid overload, bleeding, infection, and rarely, development of Asherman's syndrome. Several types of surgical instruments including the resectoscope, morcellator, and vaporizing electrode can facilitate removal. A randomized trial was conducted among 204 women with unexplained infertility and at least one submucous myoma [43]. The patients received either hysteroscopic myomectomy or diagnostic hysteroscopy alone, and no other fertility treatments were administered. Subsequent pregnancy rates were 63.4% for the myomectomy group and 28.2% for controls; the relative risk of pregnancy with myomectomy was 2.1 (95% CI 1.5–2.9) [43].

Abdominal myomectomy

Abdominal myomectomy is indicated for women with multiple fibroids and/or a significantly enlarged uterus. It is a major surgical procedure and is associated with the risk of bleeding, infection, and damage to other anatomical structures. In addition, it may result in intrauterine scarring that interferes with implantation and/or intraperitoneal scarring that negatively impacts tubo-ovarian function.

Laparoscopic myomectomy

Laparoscopic myomectomy provides a minimally invasive option for removal of fibroids; however, it requires the same thoughtful approach as abdominal myomectomy [6]. While laparoscopic myomectomy results in less pain, shorter hospitalization, and shorter recovery [44], operative time may be longer and there may be more blood loss [44,45].

The only randomized comparison of abdominal versus laparoscopic myomectomy for fertility [46] found no significant difference in reproductive outcomes between groups. Furthermore, recurrence rates appear to be similar to that seen with abdominal myomectomy [47]. The benefits of laparoscopic myomectomy include better cosmesis and fewer adhesions [48, 49]. While there has been the concern for uterine rupture, this appears to be a rare event for either approach [49].

Robotic-assisted laparoscopic myomectomy

Robotic-assisted laparoscopic myomectomy (RALM) may improve the surgical procedure by allowing the surgeon to remain seated comfortably while visualizing the abdominal and the pelvic cavities in a 3D view. It also allows for increased dexterity and precision during the procedure [6]. When compared with traditional laparoscopic myomectomy, there was no difference in blood loss, hospitalization time, and postoperative complications; however, mean surgical time was significantly longer (234 compared with 203 minutes for laparoscopic myomectomies) [50]. A more recent study also demonstrated an increased operative time, but there was a significant decrease in blood loss, change in hematocrit concentration on postoperative day 1, length of stay, number of days to regular diet, and febrile morbidity in robotic-assisted myomectomies compared with traditional laparoscopic myomectomy [51].

Other treatment methods: Uterine artery embolization

Uterine artery embolization (UAE) involves the intra-arterial infusion of embolization particles through a femoral artery catheter, which produces ischemia resulting in decreased size of fibroids. Its efficacy reaches 80–90% for improvement in menorrhagia, pain, and bulk-related symptoms [52]. However, the impact of UAE on fertility or miscarriage rates remains to be determined. Some note a 5% rate of ovarian failure [53]. In one study, 23 patients out of 102 who underwent UAE were actively attempting conception and 14 (61%) succeeded spontaneously, with one additional patient undergoing ART. Two patients (13%) had spontaneous abortions and the rest of the pregnancies were uncomplicated term deliveries [54]. Additionally, other studies have demonstrated an increased risk of obstetric complications such as first trimester pregnancy loss, fetal malpresentation, abnormal placentation, IUGR, and preterm delivery [55–59]. Despite these risks some providers have been offering UAE to patients desiring fertility, particularly if hysterectomy or repeat myomectomy are the only options. In general, it is not recommended that patients attempt conception after UAE, and UAE should not be offered as an alternative therapy to patients interested in future fertility until more extensive safety data are collected.

Treatment methods utilizing ultrasound

Hysteroscopic myomectomy under ultrasound guidance

Hysteroscopic myomectomy can be performed under ultrasound guidance. The use of intraoperative ultrasound in this setting has not been robustly evaluated, but it has been shown to decrease operative time and complication rates in dilation and curettage procedures. Intraoperative ultrasound also reduces recurrence and reoperation rates after hysteroscopy by facilitating more complete resection of uterine myomas [60].

MRI-guided focused ultrasound

MRI-guided focused ultrasound (MRgFUS) is another minimally invasive method of treating fibroids that was approved by the Food and Drug Administration (FDA) in 2004. With this method, high-intensity ultrasound waves pass through the abdominal wall and are focused to a particular target point within the fibroid, causing a temperature rise. This results in coagulative necrosis within seconds. By using MRI, accurate tissue targeting and controlled localized thermal ablation is achieved [61]. Treatment consists of consecutive exposures to focused ultrasound energy (sonications). MRgFUS is feasible, safe, and appears to have an efficacy that is comparable to other treatment modalities [62]. Pregnancies have been reported [63–65] and the FDA changed the labeling of the device in 2009 to take into account desire for future pregnancy but not to have this as an absolute contraindication. At least 51 pregnancies have occurred in women who have had this treatment; the mean time to conception was 8 months. Pregnancy outcomes included a 41% live birth rate and a 28% spontaneous abortion rate. The mean birth weight was 3.3 kg, and the vaginal delivery rate was 64% [66].

Percutaneous ultrasound-guided radiofrequency ablation

Percutaneous ultrasound-guided radiofrequency ablation (US-gRFA) has been found to reduce fibroid symptoms and size, even in women with larger fibroids up to 8 cm. One study showed that it is a safe and effective treatment that yields significant improvement in symptoms as well as decreased size of fibroids [67]. Another recent study also revealed a significant improvement in symptoms and size over a 9-month period [68]. While approved in other countries, this electrosurgical radiofrequency ablation system is currently being investigated in the United States (Halt Medical). With this procedure, a laparoscopic surgery is performed during which intra-abdominal ultrasound will guide RF ablation of uterine fibroids. Given its investigational status, it is contraindicated in patients desiring fertility.

Conclusion

Fibroids are a common gynecologic condition that have variable effects of fertility. There are multiple mechanisms by which fibroids may affect fertility status; however, the degree to which this occurs is dependent on many factors, including fibroid location and possibly size and number. Fibroids are easily diagnosed using ultrasound technology and this should be the first evaluation method. It is accepted that submucosal fibroids negatively impact fertility and pregnancy outcomes and that these negative consequences can be reversed by removal. It appears that all intramural fibroids may negatively impact fertility, especially if they are larger than 3 cm; however, their removal may not improve fertility. Removing fibroids larger than 5 cm may improve live birth rate and may reduce some of the obstetric complications; however, the true effect of myomectomy in the remainder of these cases is less clear. In addition to traditional surgical techniques for removal, newer techniques that employ ultrasound have been developed and show great promise for the treatment of fibroids. Further studies are needed to clarify the optimal treatment for women wishing to conceive.

References

1. Bowden W, Skorupski J, Kovanci E, Rajkovic A. Detection of novel copy number variants in uterine leiomyomas using high-resolution SNP arrays. *Mol Hum Reprod* 2009; **15**(9): 563–568.

2. Laughlin SK, Schroeder JC, Baird DD. New directions in the epidemiology of uterine fibroids. *Semin Reprod Med* 2010; **28**(3): 204–217.

3. Cardozo ER, Clark AD, Banks NK, Henne MB, Stegmann BJ, Segars JH. The estimated annual cost of uterine leiomyomata in the United States. *Am J Obstet Gynecol.* 2012; **206**(3): 211 e211–219.

4. Lethaby A, Hickey M, Garry R, Penninx J. Endometrial resection/ablation techniques for heavy menstrual bleeding. *Cochrane Database Syst Rev* 2009(4): CD001501.

5. Donnez J, Jadoul P. What are the implications of myomas on fertility? A need for a debate? *Hum Reprod* 2002; **17**(6): 1424–1430.

6. Olive DL. The surgical treatment of fibroids for infertility. *Semin Reprod Med* 2011; **29**(2): 113–123.

7. Somigliana E, Vercellini P, Daguati R, Pasin R, De Giorgi O, Crosignani PG. Fibroids and female reproduction: a critical analysis of the evidence. *Hum Reprod Update* 2007; **13**(5): 465–476.

8. Orisaka M, Kurokawa T, Shukunami K, et al. A comparison of uterine peristalsis in women with normal uteri and uterine leiomyoma by cine magnetic resonance imaging. *Eur J Obstet Gynecol Reprod Biol* 2007; **135**(1): 111–115.

9. Ng EH, Ho PC. Doppler ultrasound examination of uterine arteries on the day of oocyte retrieval in patients with uterine fibroids undergoing IVF. *Hum Reprod* 2002; **17**(3): 765–770.

10. Richards PA, Richards PD, Tiltman AJ. The ultrastructure of fibromyomatous myometrium and its relationship to infertility. *Hum Reprod Update* 1998; **4**(5): 520–525.

11. Nishino M, Togashi K, Nakai A, et al. Uterine contractions evaluated on cine MR imaging in patients with uterine leiomyomas. *Eur J Radiol* 2005; **53**(1): 142–146.

12. Eldar-Geva T, Meagher S, Healy DL, MacLachlan V, Breheny S, Wood C. Effect of intramural, subserosal, and submucosal uterine fibroids on the outcome of assisted reproductive technology treatment. *Fertil Steril* 1998; **70**(4): 687–691.

13. Healy DL. Impact of uterine fibroids on ART outcome. *Environ Health Perspect* 2000; **108**(Suppl 5): 845–847.

14. Somigliana E, De Benedictis S, Vercellini P, et al. Fibroids not encroaching the endometrial cavity and IVF success rate: a prospective study. *Hum Reprod* 2011; **26**(4): 834–839.

15. Farhi J, Ashkenazi J, Feldberg D, Dicker D, Orvieto R, Ben Rafael Z. Effect of uterine leiomyomata on the results of in-vitro fertilization treatment. *Hum Reprod* 1995; **10**(10): 2576–2578.

16. Klatsky PC, Lane DE, Ryan IP, Fujimoto VY. The effect of fibroids without cavity involvement on ART outcomes independent of ovarian age. *Hum Reprod* 2007; **22**(2): 521–526.

17. Hart R, Khalaf Y, Yeong CT, Seed P, Taylor A, Braude P. A prospective controlled study of the effect of intramural uterine fibroids on the outcome of assisted conception. *Hum Reprod* 2001; **16**(11): 2411–2417.

18. Miura S, Khan KN, Kitajima M, et al. Differential infiltration of macrophages and prostaglandin production by different uterine leiomyomas. *Hum Reprod* 2006; **21**(10): 2545–2554.

19. Yoshino O, Hayashi T, Osuga Y, et al. Decreased pregnancy rate is linked to abnormal uterine peristalsis caused by intramural fibroids. *Hum Reprod* 2010; **25**(10): 2475–2479.

20. Sunkara SK, Khairy M, El-Toukhy T, Khalaf Y, Coomarasamy A. The effect of intramural fibroids without uterine cavity involvement on the outcome of IVF treatment: a systematic review and meta-analysis. *Hum Reprod* 2010; **25**(2): 418–429.

21. Stovall DW, Parrish SB, Van Voorhis BJ, Hahn SJ, Sparks AE, Syrop CH. Uterine leiomyomas reduce the efficacy of assisted reproduction cycles: results of a matched follow-up study. *Hum Reprod* 1998; **13**(1): 192–197.

22. Bulletti C, DE Ziegler D, Levi Setti P, Cicinelli E, Polli V, Stefanetti M. Myomas, pregnancy outcome, and in vitro fertilization. *Ann N Y Acad Sci* 2004; **1034**: 84–92.

23. Wamsteker K, Emanuel MH, de Kruif JH. Transcervical hysteroscopic resection of submucous fibroids for abnormal uterine bleeding: results regarding the degree of intramural extension. *Obstet Gynecol* 1993; **82**(5): 736–740.

24. Pritts EA. Fibroids and infertility: a systematic review of the evidence. *Obstet Gynecol Surv* 2001; **56**(8): 483–491.

25. Klatsky PC, Tran ND, Caughey AB, Fujimoto VY. Fibroids and reproductive outcomes: a systematic literature review from conception to delivery. *Am J Obstet Gynecol* 2008; **198**(4): 357–366.

26. Rackow BW, Taylor HS. Submucosal uterine leiomyomas have a global effect on molecular determinants of endometrial receptivity. *Fertil Steril* 2010; **93**(6): 2027–2034.

27. Benaglia L, Somigliana E, de Benedictis S, et al. Hyperstimulation during IVF cycles does not modify dimensions of small subserosal and intramural leiomyomas. *Fertil Steril* 2011; **95**(8): 2489–2491.

28. Bozdag G, Esinler I, Boynukalin K, Aksu T, Gunalp S, Gurgan T. Single intramural leiomyoma with normal hysteroscopic findings does not affect ICSI-embryo transfer outcome. *Reprod Biomed Online* 2009; **19**(2): 276–280.

29. Laughlin SK, Baird DD, Savitz DA, Herring AH, Hartmann KE. Prevalence of uterine leiomyomas in the first trimester of pregnancy: an ultrasound-screening study. *Obstet Gynecol* 2009; **113**(3): 630–635.

30. Benson CB, Chow JS, Chang-Lee W, Hill JA, 3rd, Doubilet PM. Outcome of pregnancies in women with uterine leiomyomas identified by sonography in the first trimester. *J Clin Ultrasound* 2001; **29**(5): 261–264.

31. Shavell VI, Thakur M, Sawant A, et al. Adverse obstetric outcomes associated with sonographically identified large uterine fibroids. *Fertil Steril* 2012; **97**(1): 107–110.

32. Vergani P, Locatelli A, Ghidini A, Andreani M, Sala F, Pezzullo JC. Large uterine leiomyomata and risk of cesarean delivery. *Obstet Gynecol* 2007; **109**(2 Pt 1): 410–414.

33. Coronado GD, Marshall LM, Schwartz SM. Complications in pregnancy, labor, and delivery with uterine leiomyomas: a population-based study. *Obstet Gynecol* 2000; **95**(5): 764–769.

34. Roberts WE, Fulp KS, Morrison JC, Martin JN, Jr. The impact of leiomyomas on pregnancy. *Aust N Z J Obstet Gynaecol* 1999; **39**(1): 43–47.

35. Vergani P, Ghidini A, Strobelt N, et al. Do uterine leiomyomas influence pregnancy outcome? *Am J Perinatol* 1994; **11**(5): 356–358.

36. Stout MJ, Odibo AO, Graseck AS, Macones GA, Crane JP, Cahill AG. Leiomyomas at routine second-trimester ultrasound examination and adverse obstetric outcomes. *Obstet Gynecol* 2010; **116**(5): 1056–1063.

37. Grimbizis GF, Tsolakidis D, Mikos T, et al. A prospective comparison of transvaginal ultrasound, saline infusion sonohysterography, and diagnostic hysteroscopy in the evaluation of endometrial pathology. *Fertil Steril* 2010; **94**(7): 2720–2725.

38. Bingol B, Gunenc MZ, Gedikbasi A, Guner H, Tasdemir S, Tiras B. Comparison of diagnostic accuracy of saline infusion sonohysterography, transvaginal sonography and hysteroscopy in postmenopausal bleeding. *Arch Gynecol Obstet* 2011; **284**(1): 111–117.

39. Salim R, Lee C, Davies A, Jolaoso B, Ofuasia E, Jurkovic D. A comparative study of three-dimensional saline infusion sonohysterography and diagnostic hysteroscopy for the classification of submucous fibroids. *Hum Reprod* 2005; **20**(1): 253–257.

40. Ghate SV, Crockett MM, Boyd BK, Paulson EK. Sonohysterography: do 3D reconstructed images provide additional value? *AJR Am J Roentgenol* 2008; **190**(4): W227–233.

41. El-Sherbiny W, Nasr AS. Value of 3-dimensional sonohysterography in infertility work-up. *J Minim Invasive Gynecol* 2011; **18**(1): 54–58.

42. Roy KK, Singla S, Baruah J, Sharma JB, Kumar S, Singh N. Reproductive outcome following hysteroscopic myomectomy in patients with infertility and recurrent abortions. *Arch Gynecol Obstet* 2010; **282**(5): 553–560.

43. Shokeir T, El-Shafei M, Yousef H, Allam AF, Sadek E. Submucous myomas and their implications in the pregnancy rates of patients with otherwise unexplained primary infertility undergoing hysteroscopic myomectomy: a randomized matched control study. *Fertil Steril* 2010; **94**(2): 724–729.

44. Mais V, Ajossa S, Guerriero S, Mascia M, Solla E, Melis GB. Laparoscopic versus abdominal myomectomy: a prospective, randomized trial to evaluate benefits in early outcome. *Am J Obstet Gynecol* 1996; **174**(2): 654–658.

45. Stringer NH, Walker JC, Meyer PM. Comparison of 49 laparoscopic myomectomies with 49 open myomectomies. *J Am Assoc Gynecol Laparosc* 1997; **4**(4): 457–464.

46. Seracchioli R, Rossi S, Govoni F, et al. Fertility and obstetric outcome after laparoscopic myomectomy of large myomata: a randomized comparison with abdominal myomectomy. *Hum Reprod* 2000; **15**(12): 2663–2668.

47. Rossetti A, Sizzi O, Soranna L, Cucinelli F, Mancuso S, Lanzone A. Long-term results of laparoscopic myomectomy: recurrence rate in comparison with abdominal myomectomy. *Hum Reprod* 2001; **16**(4): 770–774.

48. Dubuisso JB, Fauconnier A, Babaki-Fard K, Chapron C. Laparoscopic myomectomy: a current view. *Hum Reprod Update* 2000; **6**(6): 588–594.

49. Seracchioli R, Manuzzi L, Vianello F, et al. Obstetric and delivery outcome of pregnancies achieved after laparoscopic myomectomy. *Fertil Steril* 2006; **86**(1): 159–165.

50. Nezhat CH, Rogers JD. Robot-assisted laparoscopic trachelectomy after supracervical hysterectomy. *Fertil Steril* 2008; **90**(3): 850 e851–853.

51. Ascher-Walsh CJ, Capes TL. Robot-assisted laparoscopic myomectomy is an improvement over laparotomy in women with a limited number of myomas. *J Minim Invasive Gynecol* 2010; **17**(3): 306–310.

52. Hirst A, Dutton S, Wu O, et al. A multi-centre retrospective cohort study comparing the efficacy, safety and cost-effectiveness of hysterectomy and uterine artery embolisation for the treatment of symptomatic uterine fibroids. The HOPEFUL study. *Health Technol Assess* 2008; **12**(5): 1–248, iii.

53. Spies JB, Spector A, Roth AR, Baker CM, Mauro L, Murphy-Skrynarz K. Complications after uterine artery embolization for leiomyomas. *Obstet Gynecol* 2002; **100**(5 Pt 1): 873–880.

54. Firouznia K, Ghanaati H, Sanaati M, Jalali AH, Shakiba M. Pregnancy after uterine artery embolization for symptomatic fibroids: a series of 15 pregnancies. *AJR Am J Roentgenol* 2009; **192**(6): 1588–1592.

55. Homer H, Saridogan E. Uterine artery embolization for fibroids is associated with an increased risk of miscarriage. *Fertil Steril* 2010; **94**(1): 324–330.

56. Holub Z, Mara M, Kuzel D, Jabor A, Maskova J, Eim J. Pregnancy outcomes after uterine artery occlusion: prospective multicentric study. *Fertil Steril* 2008; **90**(5): 1886–1891.

57. Goldberg J, Pereira L, Berghella V, et al. Pregnancy outcomes after treatment for fibromyomata: uterine artery embolization versus laparoscopic myomectomy. *Am J Obstet Gynecol* 2004; **191**(1): 18–21.

58. Lichtinger M, Burbank F, Hallson L, Herbert S, Uyeno J, Jones M. The time course of myometrial ischemia and reperfusion after laparoscopic uterine artery occlusion – theoretical implications. *J Am Assoc Gynecol Laparosc* 2003; **10**(4): 554–563; quiz 564–556.

59. Vilos GA, Vilos EC, Abu-Rafea B, Hollett-Caines J, Romano W. Transvaginal Doppler-guided uterine artery occlusion for the treatment of symptomatic fibroids: summary results from two pilot studies. *J Obstet Gynaecol Can* 2010; **32**(2): 149–154.

60. Criniti A, Lin PC. Applications of intraoperative ultrasound in gynecological surgery. *Curr Opin Obstet Gynecol* 2005; **17**(4): 339–342.

61. Hindley J, Gedroyc WM, Regan L, et al. MRI guidance of focused ultrasound therapy of uterine fibroids: early results. *AJR Am J Roentgenol* 2004; **183**(6): 1713–1719.

62. Chapman A, ter Haar G. Thermal ablation of uterine fibroids using MR-guided focused ultrasound-a truly non-invasive treatment modality. *Eur Radiol* 2007; **17**(10): 2505–2511.

63. Morita Y, Ito N, Ohashi H. Pregnancy following MR-guided focused ultrasound surgery for a uterine fibroid. *Int J Gynaecol Obstet* 2007; **99**(1): 56–57.

64. Hanstede MM, Tempany CM, Stewart EA. Focused ultrasound surgery of intramural leiomyomas may facilitate fertility: a case report. *Fertil Steril* 2007; **88**(2): 497 e495–497.

65. Gavrilova-Jordan LP, Rose CH, Traynor KD, Brost BC, Gostout BS. Successful term pregnancy following MR-guided focused ultrasound treatment of uterine leiomyoma. *J Perinatol* 2007; **27**(1): 59–61.

66. Rabinovici J, David M, Fukunishi H, Morita Y, Gostout BS, Stewart EA. Pregnancy outcome after magnetic resonance-guided focused ultrasound surgery (MRgFUS) for conservative treatment of uterine fibroids. *Fertil Steril* 2010; **93**(1): 199–209.

67. Carrafiello G, Recaldini C, Fontana F, et al. Ultrasound-guided radiofrequency thermal ablation of uterine fibroids: medium-term follow-up. *Cardiovasc Intervent Radiol* 2010; **33**(1): 113–119.

68. Iversen H, Lenz S, Dueholm M. Ultrasound-guided radiofrequency ablation of symptomatic uterine fibroids: short-term evaluation of treatment on quality of life and symptom severity. *Ultrasound Obstet Gynecol* 2012; **40**(4): 445–451.

32

Ultrasound imaging and IVF embryo transfer

Misty M. Blanchette Porter

Introduction

Improvement in the pregnancy rate with in vitro fertilization (IVF) and embryo transfer (ET) has resulted from the careful evaluation of each step of the process. The use of ultrasound (US) to evaluate the patient for potential ovarian response, monitor follicular development in response to gonadotropin stimulation, perform oocyte retrieval (OR), and guide ET has contributed significantly to the progress made in improving the outcomes in ART treatment. US-guided outpatient OR has become the standard of care. Transvaginal ultrasound (TVUS) guided oocyte retrievals are overall safe, but may result in severe and life-threatening complications for the patient. This chapter will focus on the utilization of TVUS in the performance of the assessment of the antral follicle count (AFC) as a marker for potential ovarian response to stimulation protocols, the use and limitations of automated follicular monitoring computerized programs, complications of USOR, and the use of transabdominal (TA) and transvaginal (TV) ultrasound to assist in transcervical ET in assisted reproductive technology (ART) cycles.

Ovarian AFC to assess ovarian response

Early in the follicular phase of the menstrual cycle, a cohort of fluid-filled, 2–10 mm, selectable follicles are believed to reflect ovarian reserve [1] (Fig. 32.1). A proportion of these antral follicles have been shown to be highly responsive to gonadotropins, and thus, reflective of the oocyte yield during ART treatment cycles [2]. A low, or high, AFC has been associated with an increased risk for poor, or hyper-ovarian, response to gonadotropin therapy [3,4]. Given the ease and reliability of measurement by TVUS, the AFC is often used as one marker of potential ovarian responsiveness [2], may be helpful in counseling patients about the risk of cycle cancellation, and useful in the determination of the stimulation protocol [5] (Figs 32.2 and 32.3).

While the predictive value of the AFC remains unchanged across the menstrual cycle [6], by convention the AFC has been measured between days 2 and 4 of a spontaneous menstrual bleed (with or without short-term GnRH agonist therapy) or an oral contraceptive withdrawal bleed. Obtaining an AFC

consists of counting all small follicles in the range of 2–10 mm as visualized by TVUS within both ovaries. In the interest of improving inter-observer reproducibility, basic clinical and technical requirements for assessment of the AFC have been suggested [1] (Table 32.1).

Although chronologic age is the most important predictor of qualitative and quantitative ovarian function, the correlation between AFC and reproductive age is well established. Autopsy and surgical specimen studies have shown that the number of antral follicles is related to the number of primordial follicles within the ovaries [7]. Specifically, the number of small antral follicles decreases with age similarly to the number of remaining ovarian primordial follicles [7]. The AFC has been shown to decline in a linear fashion with age [8] (Fig. 32.4), with an annual loss reported of 0.35–0.95 antral follicles/year [8–11]. Indeed, a strong positive correlation exists between the AFC and the extent of the follicular pool, and has been shown to be a simple method for predicting the occurrence of menopause and the duration of the reproductive life span [12].

Limitations of use of the AFC to predict ovarian responsiveness include inclusion of follicles that may be in the process of atresia, inter-cycle variability of the AFC, and use of the AFC in patients who may have artificially reduced ovarian follicle counts such as those with endometriosis, previous ovarian surgery, or unilateral oophorectomy [1].

Ovarian volume

A large-scale study has shown that ovarian volume (OV) is inversely correlated with age with a statistically significant decrease in OV with increasing age (Table 32.2) [13]. A statistically significant decrease in OV is noted in women older than 30 years of age [13]. However, use of the OV to predict ovarian responsiveness is limited in a clinically meaningful way as the change in OV appears to be limited to the extremes of reproductive life [14]. Ovarian volume is calculated by utilizing a simplified formula for a prolate ellipse. It is recognized that any calculation of the volume of a sphere or prolate ellipse ($0.5 \times$ length $\times$ width $\times$ thickness) based on two-dimensional (2D)

Ultrasonography in Gynecology, ed. Botros R. M. B. Rizk and Elizabeth E. Puscheck. Published by Cambridge University Press. © Cambridge University Press 2015.

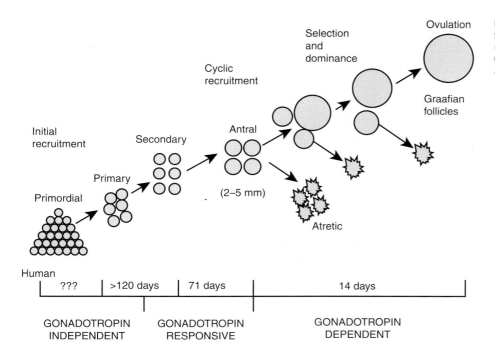

Fig. 32.1 A representation of follicle development from primordial to the post-ovulatory status. (Adapted with permission from Broekmans. Copyright 2000, The Endocrine Society. © 2010 American Society for Reproductive Medicine.)

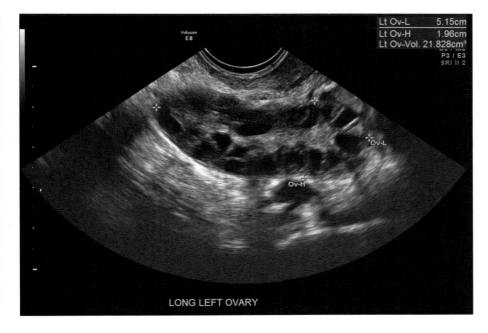

Fig. 32.2 Cross-section of an ovary with a high antral follicle count and ovarian volume.

measurements assumes a degree of regularity of the ovary, and can be misleading in the presence of an ovarian cyst. The predictive value of the OV to assess poor response may be a useful, easily obtained additional piece of information, but has been shown to be inferior to AFC [14].

Automated volume count for follicular assessment

Follicular development during gonadotropin stimulation has traditionally been performed with serial TV (2D US scans.

The follicular measurement has been taken as the mean of two (or three) orthogonal follicular diameters and calculated as the mean follicular diameter (MFD; Fig. 32.5). In the highly stimulated ovary with multiple follicles, the process of manual measurement is time-consuming, and may be imprecise because the follicular shape can be irregular. Intra- and inter-observer variability can contribute to the potential for errors in the assessment of the follicular pool [15], alter the timing of human chorionic gonadotropin (hCG) administration, and possibly lead to a decrease in mature oocytes obtained.

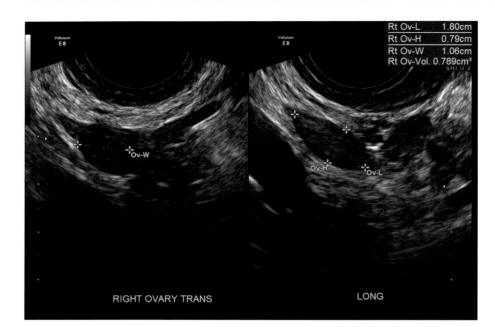

Rt Ov-L	1.80cm
Rt Ov-H	0.79cm
Rt Ov-W	1.06cm
Rt Ov-Vol.	0.789cm³

RIGHT OVARY TRANS

LONG

Fig. 32.3 Cross-section of an ovary with a low antral follicle count and ovarian volume.

Table 32.1 The basic clinical and technical requirements for assessment of the antral follicle count in clinical practice

Clinical considerations

Select patients with regular menstrual cycles with no coexisting pathologic condition that could technically affect the counting of follicles, such as ovarian endometriosis or previous ovarian surgery

Count follicles between days 2 and 4 of a spontaneous menstrual or oral contraceptive cycle to avoid the effect of intra-cycle variation

Include all antral follicles of 2–10 mm in diameter

Technical considerations

A limited number of personnel, appropriately trained in transvaginal sonography, should perform AFCs in each unit

Real-time two-dimensional imaging is adequate

Use a transvaginal transducer

Use a probe with a minimum frequency of 7 MHz, which is maintained in an adequate condition and able to resolve a structure of 2 mm in diameter

Use a systematic process for counting antral follicles:

1. Identify the ovary

2. Explore the dimensions in two planes (perform a scout sweep)

3. Decide on the direction of the sweep to measure and count follicles

4. Measure the largest follicle in two dimensions

A. If the largest follicle is ≤10 mm in diameter:

  i. Start to count from outer ovarian margin of the sweep to the opposite margin

  ii. Consider every round or oval transonic structure within the ovarian margins to be a follicle

  iii. Repeat the procedure with the contralateral ovary

  iv. Combine the number of follicles in each ovary to obtain the AFC

Clinical considerations

B. If the largest follicle is >10 mm in diameter:

  i. Further ascertain the size range of the follicles by measuring each sequentially smaller follicle, in turn, until a follicle with a diameter of ≤10 mm is found

  ii. Perform a total count (as described) regardless of follicle diameter

  iii. Subtract the number of follicles of >10 mm from the total follicle count

From Broekmans, *Fertil Steril*, 94(3), Table 1.

Sonography-based Automated Volume Count (SonoAVC: General Electric Medical Systems, Kretz Ultrasound, Waukesha, WI) is a software program that automatically identifies and quantifies the size of any hypoechoic region captured within a three-dimensional (3D) ovarian volume. The use of SonoAVC provides estimates of follicular dimensions in the stimulated ovary. These measurements include the largest diameters in three orthogonal plans (dx, dy, dz), the MFD, the volume of the follicle, and the volume-based diameter (*dv*) of the follicle. The MFD is the arithmetic mean of the three longest orthogonal diameters, and *dv* is defined as the diameter of a perfect sphere with the same volume as the follicle that is measured. After calculation of the actual volume of a follicle, SonoAVC calculates the diameter of a perfect sphere which has the same volume as the follicle by using the relaxed sphere diameter formula, and reports the value as *dv* (Figs 32.6 and 32.7).

To apply SonoAVC a 3D volume is acquired during a TVUS examination. The volume captures the entire ovary in one complete volume sweep. The user then adjusts the region of interest (ROI) box over the entire ovary, excluding extraneous extra-ovarian structures.

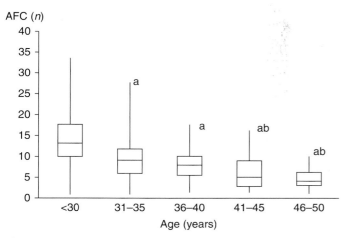

AFC (n)

x-axis: Age (years): <30, 31–35, 36–40, 41–45, 46–50

Fig. 32.4 Women were categorized in the following groups based on age: ≤30 years (n = 68), 31–35 years (n = 76), 36–40 years (n = 96), 41–45 years (n = 92), and 46–50 years (n = 30). The horizontal line represents the median, the box represents the 25th and 75th centiles, and the vertical line represents the lowest and highest values. ANOVA indicated a statistically significant difference in AFC values between the groups (F ratio 41 907; P < 0.001). a = P < 0.05 vs. age group ≤30 years; b = P < 0.05 vs. age groups ≤30, 31–35, and 36–40 years. (© 2011 American Society for Reproductive Medicine. La Marca, *Fertil Steril* 2011; 95: 684–685.)

Table 32.2 Ovarian volumes in relationship to age

Age (years)	Number	Volume (cm³)
<30	444	6.6 ± 0.19
30–39	3 259	6.1 ± 0.06
40–49	9 963	4.8 ± 0.03
50–59	24 321	2.6 ± 0.01
60–69	15 678	2.1 ± 0.01
>70	2 226	1.8 ± 0.01

From Pavlik et al., Ovarian volume related to age. *Gynecol Oncol* 2000; 77: 410–412.

Upon completing automated analysis, and prior to generating a report of follicular measurements, post-processing evaluation of the ovarian volume set is imperative to avoid erroneous data. The ovarian images must be manually rotated 360° to identify errors. The program can erroneously include extra-ovarian structures such as free fluid, blood vessels, paraovarian or paratubal cysts, and hydrosalpinges that then can be incorrectly included in the follicular count. Post-image acquisition image assessment can identify the erroneous fluid collections and the measurements can be removed from the final dataset. Follicles that were overlooked can be added to the count, and follicles with thin follicular walls that were identified as a single follicle can be separated in the post-processing volume assessment. Follicles and their corresponding measurements are color coded for interpretation in the work sheet.

The use of SonoAVC has been demonstrated to provide reliable and valid measurements of follicular size greater than 6 mm, and most accurate for follicles ≥12 mm. Use of SonoAVC does not appear to improve, or detract from, the outcome of ART when used to determine the timing of oocyte maturation and OR [16]. The observed measurements may, however, vary slightly from those obtained from the traditional 2D orthogonal measurements.

In a study on 100 women undergoing controlled ovarian stimulation for IVF the MFD determined by three 2D orthogonal measurements was compared to SonoAVC-generated MFD and *dv* [17]. When the two methods of measurement were compared, the SonoAVC MFD and *dv* were almost the same for total number of follicles >14 mm, while for the 10–13 mm follicular pool SonoAVC-based measurement was 1.1 higher for MFD, and 1.3 higher for *dv* [17]. As the total number of follicles counted increased, the limits of agreement for the two methods were wider [17]. In summary, Ata et al. suggested that SonoAVC MFD values tend to be greater than manual measurements (~1 mm), and the *dv* measurements yield a slightly

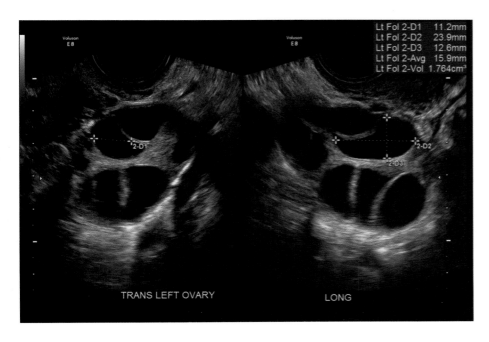

Lt Fol 2-D1   11.2mm
Lt Fol 2-D2   23.9mm
Lt Fol 2-D3   12.6mm
Lt Fol 2-Avg 15.9mm
Lt Fol 2-Vol 1.764cm³

Fig. 32.5 Measurement of a follicle by three orthogonal measurements in a stimulated ovary.

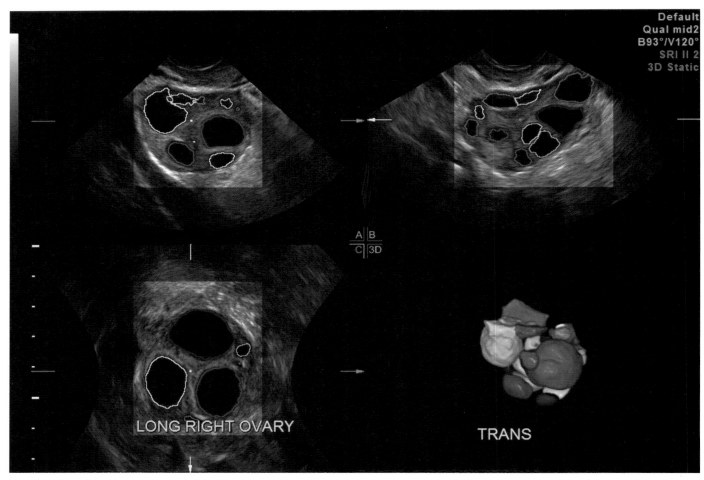

Fig. 32.6 Three-dimensional volume acquisitions for the use of a software program to obtain automated follicular measurements. Each follicle is color-coded.

Fig. 32.7 Table generated by the automated follicular monitoring program to correlate color-coded follicle with measurements.

Ovary:	Left						Ovary:	Right				
Total#:	24						Total#:	0				
Nr.	d(V) mm	dx mm	dy mm	dz mm	mn. d mm	V cm³	Nr.	d(V) mm	dx mm	dy mm	dz mm	mn. d mm	V cm³
1	13.8	20.1	16.3	9.4	15.3	1.38						
2	11.5	14.4	12.2	10.0	12.2	0.81						
3	11.0	14.1	10.5	9.2	11.3	0.69						
4	10.3	16.8	13.7	6.4	12.3	0.58						
5	10.1	14.4	11.0	7.4	10.9	0.54						
6	9.4	13.6	9.3	7.7	10.2	0.44						
7	9.1	11.7	11.3	6.8	10.0	0.39						
8	8.7	13.2	9.7	5.8	9.5	0.35						
9	8.7	11.1	9.5	6.9	9.2	0.34						
10	7.8	10.7	8.2	6.1	8.3	0.25						
11	7.1	8.8	7.3	6.0	7.4	0.19						
12	7.0	8.0	7.5	6.0	7.2	0.18						
13	6.5	11.3	8.6	3.2	7.7	0.14						
14	6.4	11.0	6.1	5.0	7.4	0.13						
15	6.2	8.1	6.3	5.3	6.6	0.13						
16	5.8	9.1	6.6	3.7	6.5	0.10						
17	5.1	6.6	5.7	3.7	5.3	0.07						

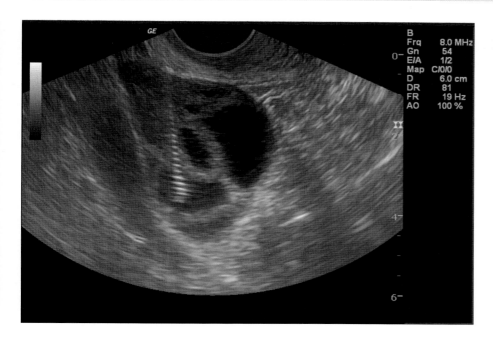

Fig. 32.8 Transvaginal ultrasound of stimulated ovary with scored IVF needle present within a follicle.

higher number of smaller sizes [17]. These differences could lead to shifting of the timing of hCG administration and oocyte retrieval, with hCG criteria potentially reached earlier with SonoAVC MFD and later with SonoAVC *dv* [17].

Observed potential advantages of the use of SonoAVC include a decreased length of time for the scan [18] (average 7.6 minutes per patient), the potential for decreasing inter- and intra-operator error, being ergonomically more efficient for the sonographer, potentially less discomfort for the patient, a reporting page that automatically tracks follicular growth, and a means of standardizing measurements across institutions for research purposes. Besides the time and skill necessary to process the volume datasets, the application of this program requires the use of a US machine equipped with the appropriate software, and a 5- to 9-MHz TV probe.

Oocyte retrieval

The use of TVUS guidance for the aspiration of follicles was first reported in 1982 [19]. Because of its simplicity, effectiveness, and relative safety, TVOR has become the standard for the acquisition of oocytes in ART cycles (Fig. 32.8). Indeed the majority of oocyte retrievals, whether transvaginal, -abdominal, -myometrial, or -vesicular, are now performed in an outpatient setting, under paracervical block, conscious sedation, or general anesthesia. Use of the beveled, single-lumen IVF (16–17 gauge) needle allows for a highly efficient and effective process, typically in less than half the time needed for a double-lumen needle.

Complications from a TVOR are unusual. Observational studies evaluating the rates of complications associated with this procedure have shown low rates of serious complications [20–22]. Vaginal bleeding and pelvic abscess remain the most frequent complications, although intra-abdominal

hemorrhage necessitating admission and/or surgery may occur. Complications from anesthesia are rare and reports are isolated to patients with underlying cardiovascular conditions [23]. Injury to the bowel, such as puncture resulting in a perforated appendix, appears to be very rare [24], or may cause minor problems and therefore remain undetected [20]. Damage to the ureter, ureteral obstruction, ureterovaginal fistula, and pseudoaneurysm of the bladder, have been described [25–29]. Patients with urogenital tract injury typically present with abdominal pain, irritative urinary symptoms, and leukocytosis in the setting of a negative urine culture [27]. Injury to the genital urinary tract should be suspected when patients present with severe abdominal pain in the absence of a hemoperitoneum, and/or the presence of hematuria.

The average estimated blood loss from a TVOR is reported as 230 mL [30]. Minor vaginal bleeding responsive to pressure (2.8%) less frequently requires a suture, and appears to be the most common complication associated with TVOR [20]. While hemorrhage requiring laparoscopy (0.6–0.2%) [22,31], laparotomy (0.07%) [32], and transfusion (0.08%) [33] have been reported, they are infrequent complications (Fig. 32.9). The diagnosis of a bleeding disorder, such as essential thrombocytopenia [34], or a deficiency of a coagulation factor [35], should be entertained in the event of a severe intra-abdominal hemorrhage following TVOR.

The incidence of pelvic infection following TVOR has been reported at a rate of 0.1–0.6% [20,36], 0.003% for ovarian abscess [22], half of which were classified as severe with pelvic abscess formation. Three different mechanisms have been suggested to be etiologic in the development of these infections: (1) direct inoculation of vaginal microorganisms; (2) reactivation of a latent pelvic infection; and (3) direct colonic injury [34]. Patients with a history of endometriosis, pelvic inflammatory disease, pelvic adhesions, and prior pelvic surgery appear to be

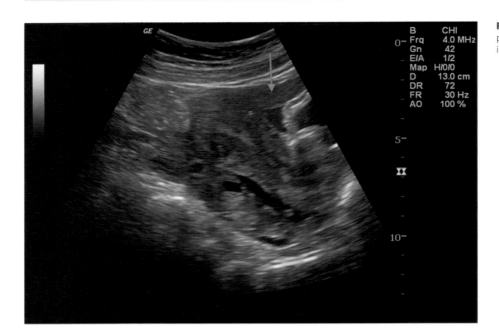

Fig. 32.9 Transabdominal ultrasound of the pelvis with evidence of echogenic and hypoechoic intraperitoneal free fluid surrounding the uterus.

at highest risk [31]. The routine use of prophylactic antibiotics remains controversial. However, their use in high-risk groups should be entertained.

Common symptoms and signs of post-TVOR infection include fever, vaginal discharge, abdominal or pelvic pain, leukocytosis, and presence of a pelvic mass on exam and/or ultrasound [20,37,38]. The interval between TVOR and symptom onset is highly variable (mean 38.5 days; median 22.5 days, range 1–320 days) [37]. Pelvic abscess formation may be life-threatening and require drainage, laparoscopy, or laparotomy [20,37,38]. Leakage, or rupture, of a tubo-ovarian abscess can result in fulminant disseminated intravascular coagulation, and multi-system failure. A pre-existing endometrioma or hydro-salpinx may increase the risk of abscess formation. Pregnancy in the setting of a pelvic abscess following TVOR is an unusual clinical scenario, but consideration should be given to aggressive management, as preterm delivery and infant death has been reported as a result of a partial treatment [39].

Cases of pseudoaneurysm of the iliac artery [40], mesenteric vein thrombosis [41], and venous thromboembolism [42] (VTE) have been described. The incidence of first-trimester VTE in relation to IVF has been reported at 0.2%, rising to 1.7% in the case of women with ovarian hyperstimulation syndrome (OHSS) who received hospitalization [43].

Death related to IVF is reportedly rare. In a large cohort study conducted in the Netherlands, all deaths within one year of IVF between 1984 and 2008 were evaluated [44]. Six deaths were directly attributed to IVF (6/100 000), and 17 (42.5/100 000) deaths were directly attributed to the IVF pregnancy [44]. In this study, three women died as a result of complications from OHSS (Fig. 32.10), two of whom had polycystic ovarian syndrome (PCOS). Two of these three deaths were attributed to adult respiratory distress syndrome and multi-organ failure, the third as a result of a cerebrovascular thrombosis. All of the patients with OHSS had all their embryos cryopreserved. Two

women died of sepsis, and one death was attributed to a dose error of local anesthetic medication given just prior to oocyte retrieval [44].

The overall mortality of patients undergoing IVF (6/100 000) was lower than the general population (31/100 000) [44]. The most likely explanation given for the lower overall mortality of IVF patients as compared with the general population of women in the Netherlands was the "healthy women effect," i.e. women eligible for IVF treatment are healthier and have higher socio-economic status than the general population. The maternal mortality rate (MMR) (42.5/100 000) was higher in IVF pregnancies than the MMR in the general population in the Netherlands (12.1/100 000 1993–2005) [44]. The higher MMR in IVF pregnancies can be attributed to an "unhealthy women effect": IVF patients are older, and have higher rates of multiple pregnancy and cesarean section [44].

Embryo transfer

Transcervical ET was initially performed blindly. In the traditional "clinical touch" technique, the catheter is advanced through the endocervical canal until the tip of the catheter is perceived to make contact with the top of the endometrial cavity. The catheter is then withdrawn 5–10 mm, and the embryo(s) injected. This technique relies upon the dexterity and tactile ability of the operator.

Limitations of the "clinical touch" technique have been recognized. Even when placed by an experienced clinician, tactile placement of the catheter has been demonstrated to be unreliable, with marked discrepancies between feel and the actual position of the catheter noted [45]. Utilizing TVUS to assess placement of the tip of the catheter after it was threaded by "clinical touch," Woolcott and Stanger demonstrated that the tip of the catheter was inadvertently placed near the opening of the fallopian tube (7.4%), abutting the fundal endometrium (17.4%), or below the

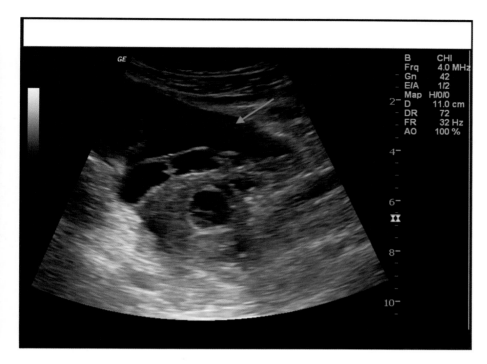

Fig. 32.10 Transabdominal ultrasound of the pelvis revealing free fluid within the pelvis in a patient with ovarian hyperstimulation syndrome.

surface of the endometrium (24.8%), even when perceived to be accurately placed by experienced clinicians [45].

With the recognition that contact with the uterine fundus can provoke bleeding and induce uterine contractions [46], and that blood on the tip of the ET catheter was associated with a significant reduction in the clinical pregnancy rate per transfer (14.3% with blood vs. 52.4% without blood) [47], interest evolved in refining the technique of ET. The advent of high-resolution US allowed for enhancement in the definition and detail of pelvic structures. With an interest in improving catheter placement, two-dimensional transabdominal ultrasound (2D TAUS) to assist ET was first utilized in 1985 [48]. Yet many clinics continued to rely on a modified "blind" transfer technique modified by avoiding contact with the fundus and placing embryos in the mid-lower cavity as established by tactile perception of just passing the internal os, or by prior measurement, by mock or trial embryo transfer, or pre-cycle uterine sounding.

Mock transfer

ET procedures are often classified as either "easy" or "difficult." Easy transfers are often defined as those in which no difficulty in negotiating the cervix is encountered, and fundal contact is avoided. An abundance of literature suggests that the overall "ease" of the ET is strongly correlated with pregnancy outcome [49–51]. Although somewhat subjective, "difficult" transfers are often defined as those that are time-consuming, when cervical stenosis is encountered, when blood or mucus is detected upon the catheter, when use of a firmer catheter is required, or successful completion of the ET involves additional instrumentation such as a tenaculum [52].

The use of the mock, or trial, transfer has gained wide acceptance and can be performed at any time before the actual ET. The two most common times of performing the mock

transfer are before starting ovarian stimulation, and immediately before the actual transfer. In pre-cycle trial transfers, the catheter is often advanced through the cervix to the uterine fundus, and the depth and configuration of the cervix and uterine cavity documented. Notation can be made with regard to the type of speculum, type of catheter, use of a stylet, ease of catheterizing the cervix, direction and curve of the catheter, and angle of the uterocervical junction and fundus. The sounding of the uterus can be done blindly.

Interest increased in performing US-guided ET when it was demonstrated that when done without confirmatory imaging, the length measurement obtained on pre-cycle uterine sounding can be highly inaccurate. In a prospective study, Shamonki et al. demonstrated that even in highly experienced hands, 19.1% of patients had a discrepancy of ≥1.5 cm, and 29.9% of patients had a discrepancy of ≥1 cm, when uterine cavity measurements obtained at the time of actual ultrasound-guided (UG)-ET were compared to those previously obtained during an office mock transfer. These authors suggested a major benefit to UG-ET over traditional "blind" transfer in that US allows for a more accurate placement of embryos within the cavity. Another clear benefit in performing mock transfer is the ability to identify those individuals with a stenotic cervix who might benefit from pre-ET treatment with a laminaria, pre-cycle cervical dilation, or surgical correction [53].

Mock performed at time of transfer

A trial transfer may also be performed just prior to the actual ET. Often under ultrasound guidance, the catheter should only be advanced to just past the internal os. Passing the catheter further into the fundus risks disrupting the endometrial lining and introducing mucus and bacteria into the endometrial cavity. The catheter can then be removed and the embryos loaded and transferred. Alternatively, steadying a stylet or the outer sheath of a catheter at trial transfer, and then loading a soft inner ET catheter can prevent endometrial trauma. Known as the "afterloading" technique, the inner catheter is then advanced to the desired transfer depth.

Technique of optimizing visualization for transabdominal ultrasound-guided embryo transfer

While no evidenced-based international protocol exists for ET, certain elements are considered fundamental in performing the procedure (Table 32.3) [54]. The patient is placed in a modified

Table 32.3 Protocol for embryo transfer

Trial transfer prior to controlled ovarian hyperstimulation
Ultrasound guidance, full bladder for transabdominal, bladder empty for transvaginal
Cervical lavage and/or gentle removal of excess mucus
Soft catheter, 30 μL volume, with "air lock" microbubbles either side of embryo column, and a continuous fluid column to the syringe
Gentle insertion of the catheter with minimal manipulation to negotiate the cervix
Use of ultrasonography to avoid catheter tip disrupting the endometrium or touching the fundus
Injection of embryos slowly and >1.5–2.0 cm from the fundal endometrial surface
Withdraw catheter slowly
Inspection of the catheter by the embryologist for blood, mucus, or retained embryos

Adapted from Schoolcraft et al., Embryo transfer: techniques and variables affecting success. *Fertil Steril* 2001;76: 863–870.

dorso-lithotomy position with a comfortably full bladder. For TAUS-guided ET, the bladder should be filled so that the dome reaches just above the level of the top of the uterine fundus. This provides the appropriate acoustic window for viewing the endometrial cavity without displacing the uterus out of the pelvis from an overly distended bladder. A full bladder may also act to passively straighten the fundus [55], and may reduce the uterocervical angle.

A 2D TA scan is performed utilizing a 3.5–5 MHz transducer to locate the midsagittal plane of the uterus aligning the fundus and the cervix (Figs 32.11 and 32.12). The angle of the uterus within the pelvis relative to midline, and the angle of the uterus within the axial plane (antero-, retro-, or mid position) are noted. The image is then magnified to include the inferior half of the bladder, the entire uterine fundus, and upper portion of the cervix. The uterocervical angle is noted and the transfer catheter and/or outer sheath can be pre-molded to approximate that angle. The angle to which the catheter should be molded can be calculated by measurement of uterocervical angle as determined by US or visual estimation. In cases where the uterocervical angle is noted to be especially sharp, the bill of the speculum, or an instrument such as a ring forceps, can be used to gently elevate or displace the cervix to decrease the severity of the angle.

Scatter of the ultrasound waves can obscure visualization of the cervix and lower uterine segment by the speculum. This may be corrected by gently withdrawing the speculum several millimeters, or excluding the lower portion of the cervix in the view created by magnification of the uterine image. The endometrium may be difficult to image on TAUS in the setting of obesity, and in the patient with a sharply retroverted uterus. Increasing the depth of the focal zone of the transducer while decreasing the overall image depth, narrowing the size of the probe sector width, and altering the contrast of

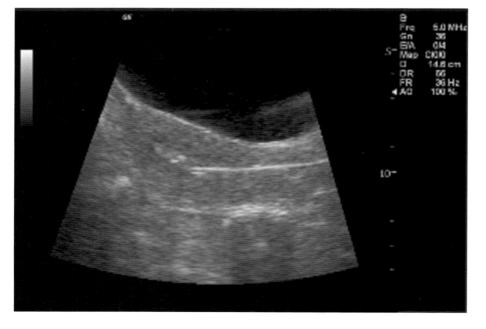

Fig. 32.11 Transabdominal ultrasound guidance of an embryo transfer with a soft catheter present and echogenic air seen within the endometrial cavity.

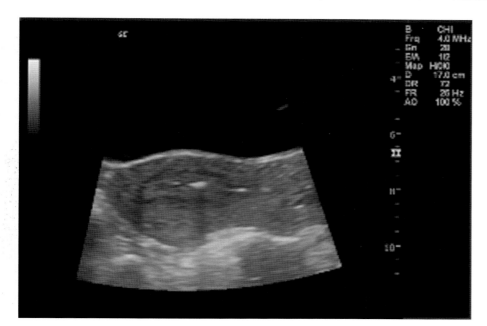

Fig. 32.12 Echogenic micro air bubble in the mid uterine cavity demonstrating the appropriate site within the endometrial cavity for delivery of the column of fluid within the catheter for embryo delivery.

the image can aid visualization of the endometrium in these situations. Obtaining a transverse view of the cervix, and noting the course and deviation of the endocervical echo may improve negotiation of a tortuous cervix. Additionally, noting the position of the transducer relative to midline on the anterior abdominal wall can facilitate placement of the catheter by aiming the tip in the same direction. US guidance can be especially helpful in uteri distorted by fibroids or those with cesarean section scar defects in which the catheter can get hung up or misdirected [52].

Prior to transcervical ET, the cervix and vagina are cleansed with a sterile medium, and excess mucus in the endocervical canal carefully extracted. Gentle cleansing with a buffered medium is thought to decrease the likelihood of the introduction of cervical blood, mucus, and bacterial contamination within the endometrial cavity. Blood or mucus on the catheter tip has been associated with a higher incidence of embryo retention within the catheter [50], and may increase the likelihood of misplacement of the embryos within the uterus [49].

Pelvic infection is an uncommon complication of IVF/ET. However, subclinical infection of the endometrium from the transfer procedure has been implicated as a possible cause of failure of embryo implantation. Cervical mucus can be a source of bacterial contamination, and patients with culture-positive catheter tips have been shown to have lower clinical pregnancy rates (29.6% vs. 57%) [56]. Antibiotics (ceftriaxone and metronidazole) at the time of retrieval are associated with a reduction of positive cultures of catheter tips at transfer [57]. Following preparation of the cervix and vagina, the embryos are loaded, the tip of the catheter is advanced under US guidance into the mid-uterine cavity, and the embryos are deposited by gently pushing the plunger on the syringe.

Transvaginal ultrasound-guided embryo transfer

Transvaginal (TV) ultrasound-guided ET was first described in the 1990s [45]. A large retrospective Japanese study revealed higher pregnancy and implantation rates with TVUS guidance in 846 ART cycles [58]. Transvaginal US-guided ET is performed utilizing a protocol adapted from the Kato Ladies Clinic [58]. In brief, the position and angle of the uterus and cervical canal are noted by TVUS. A vaginal speculum is placed, and the cervix cleansed. The transfer procedure is performed using a two-stage technique ("afterloading") in collaboration with the embryologist. A Kitazato ET Long catheter (no. 233340; Kitazato Medical Co., Ltd., Tokyo, Japan) is composed of a semi-rigid, 20-cm long, 3F, precurved (30°) outer sheath with a soft obturator and very thin, hyperflexible, 40-cm long, soft silicone inner catheter. The outer sheath with a small ball-shaped tip is inserted into the cervix to the internal os under US guidance. The speculum can be removed, or left in place. A TVUS probe is maintained, or reinserted, in the vagina while the catheter position is maintained. The position of the tip of the introducer at the internal os is confirmed by TVUS. The soft obturator is removed and the embryos are loaded into the soft inner catheter. The loaded transfer catheter is then inserted into the introducer (outer sheath), and the tip of the catheter placed at the desired level within the endometrial cavity and embryo(s) are injected. The instrumentation is removed and the catheter inspected.

To date two randomized clinical trials have been published to compare abdominal versus transvaginal ultrasound-guided ET [59,60]. In both studies there was no difference in implantation or clinical pregnancy rates in either group [59,60].

Reported advantages of TVUS guidance are better visualization of the cervico-uterine angle, improved visualization of the catheter tip (especially in the retroverted uterus or the obese patient), no need for an additional skilled staff member to assist with US guidance, and less patient discomfort as TVUS guidance does not require a full bladder [60]. Total duration of transfer was noted to be longer in the TVUS-guided ET group as compared with the TAUS-guided transfer group (154 ± 119 vs. 85 ± 76 seconds) [60].

Ultrasound and the detection of air bubble position

Transfer catheters are commonly loaded utilizing a "three drop technique," in which the drop of medium containing the embryo(s) is encompassed on either side by a micro-air bubble. These microbubbles are responsible for the "transfer flash" that is observed at the time of deposition of the embryo(s), and is an often-stated advantage of US-guided ET. The position and direction of flow of the microbubble collection can be observed. Retrograde flow of the air–fluid column may indicate coiling of the catheter and result in the embryo(s) being expelled from the uterus.

It has been suggested that the relative position of the air bubbles within the cavity may represent the area of eventual embryo implantation. In a prospective study utilizing 3D US to document catheter tip placement, Baba et al. demonstrated that 80% of gestational sacs seen on US were located at the area of the original air bubble location [61]. Furthermore, Woolcott and Stanger examined the effect of standing immediately after transfer on the location of the air–embryo fluid column interface [62]. These authors demonstrated that no movement of the embryo-associated air was seen in 94% of transfers, with movement <1.0 cm seen in 4.0%, and 1.0–5.0 cm seen in 2.0% of all transfers [62]. However, splitting of the air column within the uterus has been noted [63] and may be influenced by uterine contractions and uterine cavity contour. It is reasonable to assume that, as the embryo is heavier than air and has a different surface tension, the air bubble location may not represent the location of the embryo(s). In this case, the site of eventual implantation may be dependent upon random movement of the embryo within the cavity.

Uterine contractility

Real-time TVUS in connection with advanced audiovisual and computer technology has made the systematic investigation of endometrial contractile activity possible. Images are recorded over a period of several minutes and are then digitalized online. The uterine contraction frequency is then assessed utilizing a time-mode graph generated electronically and 3D reconstruction. In the time-mode graphs, uterine contraction frequency can be identified as the number of vertical displacements of the myometrial–endometrial interface and the uterine cavity line over time [64] (Fig. 32.13).

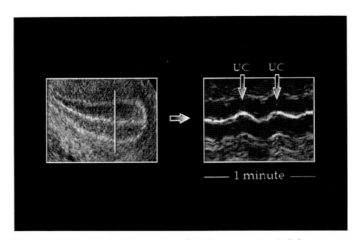

Fig. 32.13 Computerized assessment of uterine contraction (UC) frequency. After determining the uterine section to be analyzed (left panel), time-dependent changes in endomyometrial interfaces corresponding to UC were assessed (right panel). (Adapted from Fanchin R et al. Uterine contractions at the time of embryo transfer alter pregnancy rates after in-vitro fertilization. *Hum Reprod* 1998; 13(7): 1968–1974.)

In a study comparing uterine contractility with an "easy" (atraumatic) versus "difficult" mock transfer, Lesny et al. demonstrated that touching the fundus with the catheter induced a marked increase in strong, random waves generated in the fundus, and was associated with a higher frequency of junctional zone and fundo-cervical contractions [46]. With an atraumatic mock transfer, uterine contractions did not change and an echogenic contrast placed in the fundus remained in the upper uterus [46]. In the difficult transfer, contrast was seen to relocate from the fundus to the cervix in four patients, and toward the fallopian tubes in two patients [46]. In a separate study, these same investigators reported that a tenaculum applied to the cervix during mock transfer increased uterine contractions [65]. It is therefore reasonable to conclude that touching the fundus may lead to uterine contractions, which may conceivably lead to extrusion of the embryos from the uterine cavity and a decrease in pregnancy rates.

Indeed a marked and stepwise decrease in clinical and ongoing pregnancy rates, as well as in implantation rates, has been demonstrated with an increase in uterine contraction frequency (Fig. 32.14) [64]. Further, a significant negative correlation between plasma progesterone concentrations measured just before ET and uterine contraction frequency was identified [64]. In a separate study these investigators demonstrated that uterine contraction decreased progressively, and was nearly quiescent at the time of blastocyst transfer, suggesting that uterine relaxation could play a role in blastocyst implantation [66].

Optimal depth of embryo transfer

The best location to place the embryos within the endometrial cavity continues to be a topic of debate. In surgical specimens, implantation has been shown to take place predominantly in the upper half of the uterine cavity [67]. The optimal point to place the tip of the catheter under US guidance is not clear, but

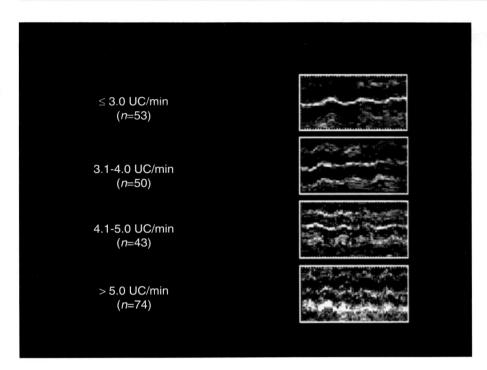

≤ 3.0 UC/min
(*n*=53)

3.1–4.0 UC/min
(*n*=50)

4.1–5.0 UC/min
(*n*=43)

> 5.0 UC/min
(*n*=74)

Fig. 32.14 Stepwise decrease in clinical pregnancy rates from the lowest to the highest uterine contraction (UC) frequency groups ($P <$ 0.001; ANOVA). (Adapted from Fanchin R et al. Uterine contractions at the time of embryo transfer alter pregnancy rates after in-vitro fertilization. *Hum Reprod* 1998; 13(7): 1968–1974.)

it appears that a mid-uterine transfer location may provide the best pregnancy rates [68].

The definition of a mid-uterine cavity transfer point continues to be a topic of discussion. Some authors define the optimal location for transfer as a point defined as the distance from the fundal endometrial surface into the cavity [68], while others utilize a calculated point of transfer based upon length of the entire endometrial cavity [69]. In a prospective randomized trial, Coroleu et al. defined the optimal point of transfer as 15–20 mm from the apex of the endometrial echo [68]. In contrast, Frankfurter et al. noted that transfers directed toward the lower-to-middle uterine segment experienced a better clinic pregnancy rate (39.6% lower-mid vs. 31.2% fundal) [69].

US guidance in training programs

One benefit of UG-ET may also be in enhancing the training of fellows in reproductive endocrinology and infertility (REI). Pregnancy rates, and therefore, the outcome of the ART cycle may hinge on the technique and proficiency with which the procedure is performed. While it is clear that many factors such as instrumentation and placement of the catheter influence outcome, provider technique is often cited as a critical variable [70]. In a survey of current fellows and recent graduates of REI fellowships, 44% of respondents reported that they did not perform any ETs during their fellowship training [71]. The reason cited for lack of training in ET was that only attendings performed transfers at these programs (83%), and that patients were unwilling to let fellows perform the transfer (33%) [71].

While no set guidelines exist for the number of ETs to be performed to ensure proficiency, training programs can adopt models of parallel skill to serve as simulation for ET. Techniques

such as intrauterine insemination (IUI) and mock transfer may impart the essential skill needed to establish pregnancy rates similar to experienced providers. Demonstration of successful catheter placement on several mock ETs may improve hand–eye coordination, allow for learning to negotiate a "difficult transfer" at a less critical time, and confer experience without detracting from patient care. Certainly the ability to demonstrate under US guidance appropriate catheter tip placement within the uterine cavity at the time of ET would reassure both patient and attending staff.

Meta-analysis of prospective randomized trials of ET

In a 2007 meta-analysis of 20 studies, Abou-Setta et al. reported on both primary (clinical pregnancy, ongoing pregnancy, and live-birth rates) and secondary (implantation, multiple pregnancies, and miscarriage rates) outcome measures encompassing 5968 ET cycles [72]. With regard to primary outcome measures, there was a significantly increased chance of a clinical pregnancy (odds ratio [OR] 1.50, 95% confidence interval [CI] 1.34–1.68), live birth (OR 1.78, 95% CI 1.19–2.67), and ongoing pregnancy (OR 1.51, 95% CI 1.31–1.74) with US guidance as compared with the standard clinical touch method [72].

With regard to secondary outcome measures, these authors demonstrated a significantly increased likelihood of embryo implantation after US guidance compared with the clinical touch method (OR 1.35, 95% CI 1.22–1.50) [72]. The rates of multiple and ectopic pregnancy, and spontaneous miscarriage in the two groups were similar [72]. After further analysis of the data, these authors confirmed that the use of instrumentation (e.g. stylet, tenaculum, dilation) was higher with the "clinical touch" method, as compared with those ETs performed under US guidance [72]. The presence of blood, mucus, and/or retained embryos was not significantly different between the two groups.

In a recent updated meta-analysis, Brown et al. reported on the data analysis of 17 available studies comparing US guidance to "clinical touch" for ET [73]. These authors confirmed a significantly higher ongoing pregnancy rate for women undergoing UG-ET than for those undergoing ET by "clinical touch" (OR 1.38, 95% CI 1.16–1.64; $P < 0.0003$) [73].

Three- and four-dimensional ultrasound-guided embryo transfer

The use of 3D and 4D ("real-time" 3D) ultrasonography for ET has been described [74,75]. Although use of this new technology has not been shown to improve placement of the catheter or pregnancy rates [75], the benefit of its application may be in the ability to observe deflection of the catheter in a third dimension. Indeed, in situations where the uterine cavity shape may be altered such as in the case of müllerian anomalies, increased clarity of the fundal endometrial contour may be of benefit in obtaining a measurement of the mid-cavity.

Conclusion

The use of US in the process of ART has improved the efficiency and effectiveness of the OR and ET procedures. The use of US to assess AFC and ovarian volume may inform pre-ART patient counseling and selection of medication protocols. The use of automated follicular monitoring may decrease the time needed for the follicular monitoring scan, improve sonographer ergonomics, and decrease intra-and inter-observer variability.

TVUS OR has become the mainstay of treatment and is a relatively safe and effective process. The pregnancy rate after ET is dependent upon multiple factors such as embryo quality [76,77], endometrial receptivity [78], and the technique of the transfer itself. While an estimated 85% of all couples undergoing IVF/ICSI will reach this stage of treatment, only one-third of them will achieve ongoing pregnancy. Uterine contractions, the presence of blood on the catheter, retained embryos, and the difficulty of transfer all influence the success rate of the IVF/ICSI treatment. While it is clear that with an experienced operator the "clinical touch" method of ET affords adequate pregnancy rates [79], current evidence from meta-analyses indicates a benefit from utilizing 2D TAUS in guiding catheter placement. The mechanism whereby US-guided ET improves clinical pregnancy, ongoing pregnancy, and live birth rate is unclear. Possible explanations include increasing the ease of ET by noting and measuring the uterocervical angle [80], positioning the tip within the mid-uterine cavity, avoiding the fundus [54], and decreasing the need for instrumentation [72].

The greatest benefits of UG-ET may be in increasing the ease of transfer, facilitating the placement of soft catheters, and being able to identify the tip of the transfer catheter. The optimal depth of transfer remains open to debate. Associated benefits include direct visual reassurance for the patient and the physician, and identification of pelvic ascites in the setting of enlarged ovaries signaling early-onset ovarian hyperstimulation syndrome that may preclude transfer.

References

1. Broekmans FJ, de Ziegler D, Howles CM, Gougeon A, Trew G, Olivennes F. The antral follicle count: practical recommendations for better standardization. *Fertil Steril* 2010; **94**: 1044–1051.

2. Frattarelli JL, Lauria-Costab DF, Miller BT, Bergh PA, Scott RT. Basal antral follicle number and mean ovarian diameter predict cycle cancellation and ovarian responsiveness in assisted reproductive technology cycles. *Fertil Steril* 2000; **74**: 512–517.

3. Kwee J, Elting ME, Schats R, McDonnell J, Lambalk CB. Ovarian volume and antral follicle count for the prediction of low and hyper responders with in vitro fertilization. *Reprod Biol Endocrinol* 2007; **5**: 9.

4. Papanikolaou EG, Humaidan P, Polyzos NP, Tarlatzis B. Identification of the high-risk patient for ovarian hyperstimulation syndrome. *Semin Reprod Med* 2010; **28**: 458–462.

5. Hsu A, Arny M, Knee AB, et al. Antral follicle count in clinical practice: analyzing clinical relevance. *Fertil Steril* 2011; **95**: 474–479.

6. Rombauts L, Onwude JL, Chew HW, Vollenhoven BJ. The predictive value of antral follicle count remains unchanged across the menstrual cycle. *Fertil Steril* 2011; **96**: 1514–1518.

7. Faddy MJ, Gosden RG, Gougeon A, Richardson SJ, Nelson JF. Accelerated disappearance of ovarian follicles in mid-life: implications for forecasting menopause. *Hum Reprod* 1992; **7**: 1342–1346.

8. La Marca A, Spada E, Sighinolfi G, et al. Age-specific nomogram for the decline in antral follicle count throughout the reproductive period. *Fertil Steril* 2011; **95**: 684–688.

9. Ng EH, Yeung WS, Fong DY, Ho PC. Effects of age on hormonal and ultrasound markers of ovarian reserve in Chinese women with proven fertility. *Hum Reprod* 2003; **18**: 2169–2174.

10. Ruess ML, Kline J, Santos R, Levin B, Timor-Tritsch I. Age and the ovarian follicle pool assessed with transvaginal ultrasonography. *Am J Obstet Gynecol* 1996; **174**: 624–627.

11. Scheffer GJ, Broekmans FJ, Dorland M, et al. Antral follicle counts by transvaginal ultrasonography are related to age in women with proven natural fertility. *Fertil Steril* 1999; **72**: 845–851.

12. Broekmans FJ, Faddy MJ, Scheffer G, te Velde ER. Antral follicle counts are related to age at natural fertility loss and age at menopause. *Menopause* 2004; **11**: 607–614.

13. Pavlik EJ, DePriest PD, Gallion HH, et al. Ovarian volume related to age. *Gynecol Oncol* 2000; **77**: 410–412.

14. Hendriks DJ, Kwee J, Mol BW, te Velde ER, Broekmans FJ. Ultrasonography as a tool for the prediction of outcome in IVF patients: a comparative meta-analysis of ovarian volume and antral follicle count. *Fertil Steril* 2007; **87**: 764–775.

15. Forman RG, Robinson J, Yudkin P, Egan D, Reynolds K, Barlow DH. What is the true follicular diameter: an assessment of

the reproducibility of transvaginal ultrasound monitoring in stimulated cycles. *Fertil Steril* 1991; **56**: 989–992.

16. Raine-Fenning N, Deb S, Jayaprakasan K, Clewes J, Hopkisson J, Campbell B. Timing of oocyte maturation and egg collection during controlled ovarian stimulation: a randomized controlled trial evaluating manual and automated measurements of follicle diameter. *Fertil Steril* 2010; **94**: 184–188.

17. Ata B, Seyhan A, Reinblatt SL, Shalom-Paz E, Krishnamurthy S, Tan SL. Comparison of automated and manual follicle monitoring in an unrestricted population of 100 women undergoing controlled ovarian stimulation for IVF. *Hum Reprod* 2011; **26**: 127–133.

18. Deutch TD, Joergner I, Matson DO, et al. Automated assessment of ovarian follicles using a novel three-dimensional ultrasound software. *Fertil Steril* 2009; **92**: 1562–1568.

19. Lenz S, Lauritsen JG. Ultrasonically guided percutaneous aspiration of human follicles under local anesthesia: a new method of collecting oocytes for in vitro fertilization. *Fertil Steril* 1982; **38**: 673–677.

20. Ludwig AK, Glawatz M, Griesinger G, Diedrich K, Ludwig M. Perioperative and post-operative complications of transvaginal ultrasound-guided oocyte retrieval: prospective study of >1000 oocyte retrievals. *Hum Reprod* 2006; **21**: 3235–3240.

21. Bodri D, Guillen JJ, Polo A, Trullenque M, Esteve C, Coll O. Complications related to ovarian stimulation and oocyte retrieval in 4052 oocyte donor cycles. *Reprod Biomed Online* 2008; **17**: 237–243.

22. Aragona C, Mohamed MA, Espinola MS, et al. Clinical complications after transvaginal oocyte retrieval in 7,098 IVF cycles. *Fertil Steril* 2011; **95**: 293–294.

23. Ayestaran C, Matorras R, Gomez S, Arce D, Rodriguez-Escudero F. Severe bradycardia and bradypnea following vaginal oocyte retrieval: a possible toxic effect of paracervical mepivacaine. *Eur J Obstet Gynecol Reprod Biol* 2000; **91**: 71–73.

24. Roest J, Mous HV, Zeilmaker GH, Verhoeff A. The incidence of major clinical complications in a Dutch transport IVF programme. *Hum Reprod Update* 1996; **2**: 345–353.

25. von Eye Corleta H, Moretto M, D'Avila AM, Berger M. Immediate ureterovaginal fistula secondary to oocyte retrieval – a case report. *Fertil Steril* 2008; **90**: 2006.e1–3.

26. Jayakrishnan K, Raman VK, Vijayalakshmi VK, Baheti S, Nambiar D. Massive hematuria with hemodynamic instability – complication of oocyte retrieval. *Fertil Steril* 2011; **96**: e22–24.

27. Fiori O, Cornet D, Darai E, Antoine JM, Bazot M. Uro-retroperitoneum after ultrasound-guided transvaginal follicle puncture in an oocyte donor: a case report. *Hum Reprod* 2006; **21**: 2969–2971.

28. Miller PB, Price T, Nichols JE, Jr., Hill L. Acute ureteral obstruction following transvaginal oocyte retrieval for IVF. *Hum Reprod* 2002; **17**: 137–138.

29. Fugita OE, Kavoussi L. Laparoscopic ureteral reimplantation for ureteral lesion secondary to transvaginal ultrasonography for oocyte retrieval. *Urology* 2001; **58**: 281.

30. Dessole S, Rubattu G, Ambrosini G, Miele M, Nardelli GB, Cherchi PL. Blood loss following noncomplicated transvaginal oocyte retrieval for in vitro fertilization. *Fertil Steril* 2001; **76**: 205–206.

31. Govaerts I, Devreker F, Delbaere A, Revelard P, Englert Y. Short-term medical complications of 1500 oocyte retrievals for in vitro fertilization and embryo transfer. *Eur J Obstet Gynecol Reprod Biol* 1998; **77**: 239–243.

32. Bennett SJ, Waterstone JJ, Cheng WC, Parsons J. Complications of transvaginal ultrasound-directed follicle aspiration: a review of 2670 consecutive procedures. *J Assist Reprod Genet* 1993; **10**: 72–77.

33. Dicker D, Ashkenazi J, Feldberg D, Levy T, Dekel A, Ben-Rafael Z. Severe abdominal complications after transvaginal ultrasonographically guided retrieval of oocytes for in vitro fertilization and embryo transfer. *Fertil Steril* 1993; **59**: 1313–1315.

34. El-Shawarby SA, Margara RA, Trew GH, Laffan MA, Lavery SA. Thrombocythemia and hemoperitoneum after transvaginal oocyte retrieval for in vitro fertilization. *Fertil Steril* 2004; **82**: 735–737.

35. Battaglia C, Regnani G, Giulini S, Madgar L, Genazzani AD, Volpe A. Severe intraabdominal bleeding after transvaginal oocyte retrieval for IVF-ET and coagulation factor XI deficiency: a case report. *J Assist Reprod Genet* 2001; **18**: 178–181.

36. Ashkenazi J, Farhi J, Dicker D, Feldberg D, Shalev J, Ben-Rafael Z. Acute pelvic inflammatory disease after oocyte retrieval: adverse effects on the results of implantation. *Fertil Steril* 1994; **61**: 526–528.

37. Sharpe K, Karovitch AJ, Claman P, Suh KN. Transvaginal oocyte retrieval for in vitro fertilization complicated by ovarian abscess during pregnancy. *Fertil Steril* 2006; **86**: 219.e11–13.

38. Kelada E, Ghani R. Bilateral ovarian abscesses following transvaginal oocyte retrieval for IVF: a case report and review of literature. *J Assist Reprod Genet* 2007; **24**: 143–145.

39. Matsunaga Y, Fukushima K, Nozaki M, et al. A case of pregnancy complicated by the development of a tubo-ovarian abscess following in vitro fertilization and embryo transfer. *Am J Perinatol* 2003; **20**: 277–282.

40. Bozdag G, Basaran A, Cil B, Esinler I, Yarali H. An oocyte pick-up procedure complicated with pseudoaneurysm of the internal iliac artery. *Fertil Steril* 2008; **90**: 2004.e11–13.

41. Dorais J, Jones K, Hammoud A, Gibson M, Johnstone E, Peterson CM. A superior mesenteric vein thrombosis associated with in vitro fertilization. *Fertil Steril* 2011; **95**: 804.e11–13.

42. Chan WS, Ginsberg JS. A review of upper extremity deep vein thrombosis in pregnancy: unmasking the 'ART' behind the clot. *J Thromb Haemost* 2006; **4**: 1673–1677.

43. Rova K, Passmark H, Lindqvist PG. Venous thromboembolism in relation to in vitro fertilization: an approach to determining the incidence and increase in risk in successful cycles. *Fertil Steril* 2012; **97**: 95–100.

44. Braat DD, Schutte JM, Bernardus RE, Mooij TM, van Leeuwen FE. Maternal death related to IVF in the Netherlands 1984–2008. *Hum Reprod* 2010; **25**: 1782–1786.

45. Woolcott R, Stanger J. Potentially important variables identified by transvaginal ultrasound-guided embryo transfer. *Hum Reprod* 1997; **12**: 963–966.

46. Lesny P, Killick SR, Tetlow RL, Robinson J, Maguiness SD. Embryo transfer – can we learn anything new from the observation of junctional zone contractions? *Hum Reprod* 1998; **13**: 1540–1546.

47. Goudas VT, Hammitt DG, Damario MA, Session DR, Singh AP, Dumesic DA. Blood on the embryo transfer catheter is associated

with decreased rates of embryo implantation and clinical pregnancy with the use of in vitro fertilization-embryo transfer. *Fertil Steril* 1998; **70**: 878–882.

48. Strickler RC, Christianson C, Crane JP, Curato A, Knight AB, Yang V. Ultrasound guidance for human embryo transfer. *Fertil Steril* 1985; **43**: 54–61.

49. Mansour R, Aboulghar M, Serour G. Dummy embryo transfer: a technique that minimizes the problems of embryo transfer and improves the pregnancy rate in human in vitro fertilization. *Fertil Steril* 1990; **54**: 678–681.

50. Visser DS, Fourie FL, Kruger HF. Multiple attempts at embryo transfer: effect on pregnancy outcome in an in vitro fertilization and embryo transfer program. *J Assist Reprod Genet* 1993; **10**: 37–43.

51. Tomas C, Tikkinen K, Tuomivaara L, Tapanainen JS, Martikainen H. The degree of difficulty of embryo transfer is an independent factor for predicting pregnancy. *Hum Reprod* 2002; **17**: 2632–2635.

52. Mains L, Van Voorhis BJ. Optimizing the technique of embryo transfer. *Fertil Steril* 2010; **94**: 785–790.

53. Noyes N. Hysteroscopic cervical canal shaving: a new therapy for cervical stenosis before embryo transfer in patients undergoing in vitro fertilization. *Fertil Steril* 1999; **71**: 965–966.

54. Schoolcraft WB, Surrey ES, Gardner DK. Embryo transfer: techniques and variables affecting success. *Fertil Steril* 2001; **76**: 863–870.

55. Abou-Setta AM. Effect of passive uterine straightening during embryo transfer: a systematic review and meta-analysis. *Acta Obstet Gynecol Scand* 2007; **86**: 516–522.

56. Egbase PE, al-Sharhan M, al-Othman S, al-Mutawa M, Udo EE, Grudzinskas JG. Incidence of microbial growth from the tip of the embryo transfer catheter after embryo transfer in relation to clinical pregnancy rate following in-vitro fertilization and embryo transfer. *Hum Reprod* 1996; **11**: 1687–1689.

57. Moore DE, Soules MR, Klein NA, Fujimoto VY, Agnew KJ, Eschenbach DA. Bacteria in the transfer catheter tip influence the live-birth rate after in vitro fertilization. *Fertil Steril* 2000; **74**: 1118–1124.

58. Kojima K, Nomiyama M, Kumamoto T, Matsumoto Y, Iwasaka T. Transvaginal ultrasound-guided embryo transfer improves pregnancy and implantation rates after IVF. *Hum Reprod* 2001; **16**: 2578–2582.

59. Porat N, Boehnlein LM, Schouweiler CM, Kang J, Lindheim SR. Interim analysis of a randomized clinical trial comparing abdominal versus transvaginal ultrasound-guided embryo transfer. *J Obstet Gynaecol Res* 2010; **36**: 384–392.

60. Bodri D, Colodron M, Garcia D, Obradors A, Vernaeve V, Coll O. Transvaginal versus transabdominal ultrasound guidance for embryo transfer in donor oocyte recipients: a randomized clinical trial. *Fertil Steril* 2011; **95**: 2263–2268, 8.e1.

61. Baba K, Ishihara O, Hayashi N, Saitoh M, Taya J, Kinoshita K. Where does the embryo implant after embryo transfer in humans? *Fertil Steril* 2000; **73**: 123–125.

62. Woolcott R, Stanger J. Ultrasound tracking of the movement of embryo-associated air bubbles on standing after transfer. *Hum Reprod* 1998; **13**: 2107–2109.

63. Confino E, Zhang J, Risquez F. Air bubble migration is a random event post embryo transfer. *J Assist Reprod Genet* 2007; **24**: 223–226.

64. Fanchin R, Righini C, Olivennes F, Taylor S, de Ziegler D, Frydman R. Uterine contractions at the time of embryo transfer alter pregnancy rates after in-vitro fertilization. *Hum Reprod* 1998; **13**: 1968–1974.

65. Lesny P, Killick SR, Robinson J, Raven G, Maguiness SD. Junctional zone contractions and embryo transfer: is it safe to use a tenaculum? *Hum Reprod* 1999; **14**: 2367–2370.

66. Fanchin R, Ayoubi JM, Righini C, Olivennes F, Schonauer LM, Frydman R. Uterine contractility decreases at the time of blastocyst transfers. *Hum Reprod* 2001; **16**: 1115–1119.

67. Adams EC, Hertig AT, Rock J. A description of 34 human ova within the first 17 days of development. *Am J Anat* 1956; **98**: 435–493.

68. Coroleu B, Barri PN, Carreras O, et al. The influence of the depth of embryo replacement into the uterine cavity on implantation rates after IVF: a controlled, ultrasound-guided study. *Hum Reprod* 2002; **17**: 341–346.

69. Frankfurter D, Trimarchi JB, Silva CP, Keefe DL. Middle to lower uterine segment embryo transfer improves implantation and pregnancy rates compared with fundal embryo transfer. *Fertil Steril* 2004; **81**: 1273–1277.

70. Karande VC, Morris R, Chapman C, Rinehart J, Gleicher N. Impact of the "physician factor" on pregnancy rates in a large assisted reproductive technology program: do too many cooks spoil the broth? *Fertil Steril* 1999; **71**: 1001–1009.

71. Wittenberger MD, Catherino WH, Armstrong AY. Role of embryo transfer in fellowship training. *Fertil Steril* 2007; **88**: 1014–1015.

72. Abou-Setta AM, Mansour RT, Al-Inany HG, Aboulghar MM, Aboulghar MA, Serour GI. Among women undergoing embryo transfer, is the probability of pregnancy and live birth improved with ultrasound guidance over clinical touch alone? A systemic review and meta-analysis of prospective randomized trials. *Fertil Steril* 2007; **88**: 333–341.

73. Brown J, Buckingham K, Abou-Setta AM, Buckett W. Ultrasound versus 'clinical touch' for catheter guidance during embryo transfer in women. *Cochrane Database Syst Rev* 2010: CD006107.

74. Letterie GS. Three-dimensional ultrasound-guided embryo transfer: a preliminary study. *Am J Obstet Gynecol* 2005; **192**: 1983–7; discussion 7–8.

75. Gergely RZ, DeUgarte CM, Danzer H, Surrey M, Hill D, DeCherney AH. Three dimensional/four dimensional ultrasound-guided embryo transfer using the maximal implantation potential point. *Fertil Steril* 2005; **84**: 500–503.

76. De Neubourg D, Gerris J, Mangelschots K, Van Royen E, Vercruyssen M, Elseviers M. Single top quality embryo transfer as a model for prediction of early pregnancy outcome. *Hum Reprod* 2004; **19**: 1476–1479.

77. Roseboom TJ, Vermeiden JP, Schoute E, Lens JW, Schats R. The probability of pregnancy after embryo transfer is affected by the age of the patient, cause of infertility, number of embryos transferred and the average morphology score, as revealed by multiple logistic regression analysis. *Hum Reprod* 1995; **10**: 3035–3041.

78. Hoozemans DA, Schats R, Lambalk CB, Homburg R, Hompes PG. Human embryo implantation: current knowledge and clinical implications in assisted reproductive technology. *Reprod Biomed Online* 2004; **9**: 692–715.

79. Flisser E, Grifo JA. Is what we clearly see really so obvious? Ultrasonography and transcervical embryo transfer – a review. *Fertil Steril* 2007; **87**: 1–5.

80. Sallam HN, Agameya AF, Rahman AF, Ezzeldin F, Sallam AN. Ultrasound measurement of the uterocervical angle before embryo transfer: a prospective controlled study. *Hum Reprod* 2002; **17**: 1767–1772.

Chapter

33

Ultrasound to monitor difficult embryo transfers

Gautam N. Allahbadia and Rubina Merchant

Introduction

Embryo transfer is a significant step in the assisted reproductive technology (ART) protocol that ultimately determines the success of the entire treatment. Although much of the published data that evaluates these factors is conflicting or confounded and there is no consensus on the optimal technique of embryo transfer (ET), there is good and consistent evidence to support the fact that several technical factors significantly impact the results. Optimizing the "ease" of the transfer with a mock transfer prior to the actual ET, ultrasound guidance, and the use of soft catheters [1–6] facilitates a gentle, atraumatic ET by avoiding trauma to the endometrium and the stimulation of uterine junctional zone (JZ) contractions. Junctional zone contractions are associated with a negative outcome and factors that increase JZ contractions should be avoided [7]. Evidence also supports the removal of cervical mucus to avoid inadvertent removal of the embryo during catheter withdrawal, avoidance of blood and bacterial contamination, deposition of embryos in the mid-portion of the uterus, avoiding negative pressure from the catheter, and completion of the procedure in a timely manner in optimizing pregnancy and implantation rates [1–3,6]. Prior knowledge of the uterocervical angulation and uterine cavity length by ultrasound can optimize the embryo transfer technique and may reduce the rate of ectopic pregnancies [3,5]. However, the value of a mock transfer a few days before the actual procedure has been challenged as the position of the uterus may change [6]. A trial catheterization on the day of ET could prevent most of the unanticipated procedural difficulties during the transfer [4]. It is important to ensure that the embryo transfer catheter has passed the internal cervical os and that the embryos are delivered gently inside the uterine cavity [5]. Progesterone administration, starting on the day of oocyte retrieval induces a decrease in uterine contraction frequency on the day of ET (embryo transfer) [4]. Air in the catheter, immediate removal of the catheter, performing two transfers in the same cycle, prolonged bed rest, sexual intercourse after embryo transfers or the use of sildenafil do not significantly impact the results [2].

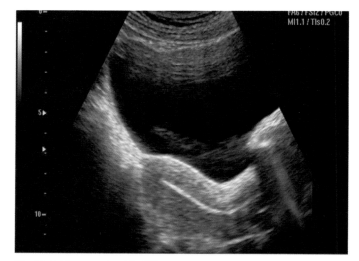

Fig. 33.1 Ultrasound -guided ET.

Clinical discussion

Ultrasound-guided ET (Fig. 33.1)

Failure to achieve a live birth following ART has often been attributed to the embryo transfer stage due to lack of good-quality embryo(s), lack of uterine receptivity, or the transfer technique itself. The success of ET is dependent upon multiple factors including embryo quality, proper endometrial receptivity, and the technique by which the embryos are transferred [8]. Optimizing the technique of ET, with the use of ultrasound guidance for proper catheter placement in the endometrial cavity, has been suggested as a more effective technique of embryo transfer than "clinical touch" [9]. Several studies have attempted to compare the ART outcome following ultrasound-guided ET (USG-ET) and the clinical touch method. The results of these studies are presented in Table 33.1. Though no standard evidence-based protocol exists, and wide variation exists in the studies that evaluated the role of ultrasound, USG-ET has been shown to significantly increase the chance of embryo implantation, ongoing pregnancy, and live birth and to improve the

Table 33.1 Summary of pregnancy outcomes following a comparison between ultrasound-guided ET and the clinical touch method

Study	Study design	Total patients/ cycles	Ultrasound-guided ET				Clinical touch ET				Significance
			(n)	PR (%)	IR	OPR (%)	(n)	PR	IR	OPR	P
Coroleu et al., 2000 [10]	Prospective	362	182	50.0*	25.3†		180	33.7	18.1		*P < 0.002 †P < 0.05
Wood et al., 2000 [11]		518 cycles		38.0 CPR/T				25			P < 0.002
Matorras et al., 2002 [12]	Prospective randomized (computer-generated random table) trial	515	255	26.3	11.1		260	18.1	7.5		P < 0.05 (PR and IR)
Prapas et al., 2001 [13]	Prospective	433	433	47.0			636	36.0			P < 0.001
Kojima et al., 2001 [15]	Retrospective	846 cycles		28.9	15.2			13.1	7.0		P < 0.01
Lindheim et al., 1999 [16]	Retrospective	137		63.1	28.8			36.1	18.4		P < 0.05
Kan et al., 1999 [36]	Prospective control study	187	93	37.8	20.4		94	28.9	16.2		NS
Kosmas et al., 2007 [22]	Randomized, double-blind controlled trial	300		53.3				51.3			NS
Tang et al., 2001 [26]	Prospective randomized, controlled trial (fresh + frozen ET)	400	400	26.0	15.3*	23.5	400	22.5	12.0*	19.0	NS P = 0.048*
Eskandar et al., 2008 [14]	Prospective, single-operator randomized, controlled trial	183	183	40.98	40.98	40.98	190	28.42		28.42	Significant
Mirkin et al., 2003 [34]	Retrospective analysis	823 ET	367	48.0	22.0		456	44.0	20.0		NS
Lambers et al., 2006 [23]	Prospective study	730 ET	367 ET	35.1	24.3	31.1	363 ET based on previous ultrasonographic length measurement	33.9	24.2	29.5	NS
de Camargo Martins et al., 2004 [25]		100	50	42.0	19.6		50	16.3			P = 0.51 IR P = 0.29 PR
García-Velasco et al., 2002 [27]	Prospective randomized, controlled trial	374		59.9	30.6			55.1	26.3		NS

PR, pregnancy rate; IR, implantation rate; ET, embryo transfer; CPR/T, clinical pregnancy rate/transfer; NS, non-significant.

ease of transfer in a majority of these randomized controlled trials [8, 10–16].

Several systematic reviews and randomized controlled trials comparing USG-ET with embryo transfer by clinical touch alone have demonstrated a significantly increased chance of clinical pregnancy, embryo implantation, ongoing pregnancy and live birth following USG-ET compared with the clinical touch method [9,17–20] with no effect on the incidence of ectopic pregnancy, multiple pregnancy, or miscarriage rate [20]. The 25% chance of pregnancy using clinical touch increased to 32% following USG-ET [17]. With regard to the technique, studies have also proved that transvaginal USG-ET results in an overall increase in embryo implantation and pregnancy rates compared with the use of the clinical touch method in patients with previous in vitro fertilization (IVF) failure following clinical touch ET [21], with no significant difference in ectopic pregnancy rates [15]. Although technically difficult, its use may maximize the chances of achieving a successful pregnancy outcome [15]. However, the Cochrane Database Systematic Reviews, conducted in 2007 [17] and recently in 2010 that included 17 randomized controlled trials [2], concluded that the studies were limited by their quality, with only one or two studies reporting details of both computerized randomization techniques and adequate allocation concealment [9,17].

In contrast, a few studies, that compared USG-ET with the clinical touch method, failed to show any superior benefit of the use of transabdominal ultrasound to perform embryo transfer in terms of the pregnancy outcome [22–28]. There was no significant difference in the incidence of easy transfers, clinical pregnancy rates, ongoing pregnancy rates, or incidences of ectopic pregnancy, miscarriage, and multiple pregnancy rates following USG-ET and the clinical touch method [26, 27]. Flisser et al. [28] concluded that the clinical touch method of embryo transfer yields equivalent results to transabdominal ultrasound-guided embryo placement in the hands of the experienced operator; however, in patients with a prior history of difficult uterine sounding or embryo transfer, transabdominal ultrasound guidance may still play a role [28]. Comparing ET with a K-J-SPPE echo tip soft catheter (ultrasound-guided ET) and the traditional K-Soft catheter (clinical touch) in a randomized, double-blind controlled trial on 300 women, Kosmas et al. [22] also found no additional benefit of USG-ET in terms of overall clinical pregnancy and embryo implantation rates when ET was performed by an experienced operator. In contrast, Harris et al. [24] reported similar outcomes in terms of pregnancy and live birth rates following ET performed by experienced and inexperienced sonologists, suggesting that the clinical experience of the person performing ultrasound guidance during IVF-ET does not have an effect on clinical outcome and the use of an assistant without formal ultrasound training during IVF-ET is a reasonable option [24].

Dealing only with patients identified as likely to have an easy transfer after mock transfer, de Camargo Martins et al. [25] concluded that as long as previous mock transfers are routinely performed during a cycle preceding assisted reproduction and

the clinician considers transfer to be easy, ultrasound does not benefit the process of embryo transfer [25]. Ultrasonographic guidance does not show any benefit in terms of pregnancy and implantation rates compared with previous ultrasonographic length measurement, another precise and atraumatic transfer technique [23]. Though Tang et al. [26] reported a slightly significant difference in the implantation rate in favor of the USG-guided technique, suggesting a significant improvement in implantation rate following the use of ultrasound guidance during embryo transfer, the study included both fresh and frozen ETs, which could confound and impact the results. While demonstrating a significantly higher overall pregnancy rate following USG-ET than the tactile assessment ("clinical feel") method (47% vs. 36%; $P < 0.001$), Prapas et al. [13] additionally observed that ultrasound assistance in embryo transfer on days 3 and 4 significantly improved pregnancy rates in IVF but had no impact on day 5 [13].

Difficult transfers

Embryo transfer is considered difficult if it was time-consuming, the catheter met great resistance, there was a need to change the catheter, if sounding or cervical dilatation was needed, or if blood was found in any part of the catheter [29]. Tomás et al. [29] evaluated the degree of difficulty of embryo transfer as an independent factor for predicting pregnancy after taking into account the other confounding variables. Embryo transfer was classified as easy (2821), intermediate (1644), or difficult (342). The authors observed that easy or intermediate transfers resulted in a 1.7-fold higher pregnancy rate than difficult transfers ($P < 0.0001$; 95% confidence interval [CI] 1.3–2.2), suggesting that the degree of difficulty of embryo transfer is an independent factor as regards achieving pregnancy after IVF/ICSI [29]. Judging an "easy" transfer to be an atraumatic insertion of the catheter without touching the uterine fundus, Lesny et al. [30] mimicked a "difficult" embryo transfer by deliberately touching the uterine fundus twice with the soft end of the cannula. Junctional zone contractility was evaluated by recorded transvaginal scan images, digitized and converted into five times the normal speed. Echovist bolus (30 μL) was used to represent embryos and transfer medium. While easy mock embryo transfers did not change the endometrial mechanical activity and the Echovist bolus remained in the upper part of the uterine cavity and was not dispersed after 45 minutes, a difficult procedure generated strong random waves in the fundal area and waves from fundus to cervix which relocated the Echovist in six out of seven cases; from the upper part of the uterus towards the cervix (four cases) and into fallopian tubes (two patients), confirming that the mechanical activity of the uterus is capable of relocating intrauterine embryos and that this activity depends on physical stimulation. Lesny et al. concluded that junctional zone contractions can be implicated in cases of IVF-ET failure or ectopic gestation [30].

Hence, all efforts should be made to avoid difficult embryo transfers provoking bleeding, uterine contractions, and the retention of the embryo in the cervix, or even its expulsion [3,29,31]. Physicians should be alert to the factors associated with ET and should use a stepwise approach in difficult transfers [29]. Identifying appropriate ultrasound-guided simulation training techniques in ET would ensure adequate fellowship training without affecting the outcome of ART cycles [8].

Ultrasound-guided ET for difficult transfers

Ultrasound guidance is reported to significantly increase the frequency of easy transfers [12,19] and decrease the incidence of difficult transfers and endometrial injury [32], possibly due to a decrease in cervical and uterine trauma [12].

Evaluation of the guiding cannula and transfer catheter placement in relation to the endometrial surface and uterine fundus during embryo transfer and the impact of subendometrial myometrial contraction have demonstrated that tactile assessment of embryo transfer catheter placement is unreliable. It was observed that following clinical touch ET, the outer guiding catheter inadvertently abutted the fundal endometrium in 17.4% of transfers, indented the endometrium in 24.8%, and the transfer catheter embedded in the endometrium in 33.1%. Unavoidable subendometrial transfers occurred in 22.3% of transfers. Ultrasound-guided transfer avoided accidental tubal transfer in 7.4% of transfers [33].

According to Mirkin et al. [34], though USG-ET yielded higher, but not statistically significant, clinical pregnancy (48% vs. 44%) and implantation rates (22% vs. 20%) with similar incidences of multiple and ectopic pregnancies, the frequency of negative factors typically associated with difficult transfers, such as the requirement of a tenaculum, and presence of blood or mucus on the catheter tip, was significantly lower in the ultrasound-guided group in comparison with the clinical touch group. Ultrasound-guided embryo transfer was associated with a significantly increased ease of transfer performance; 95% of the transfers were rated as very easy in the ultrasound guidance group compared with 87% in the clinical touch group. Mirkin et al. concluded that ultrasound guidance facilitates embryo transfer and in combination with the use of a soft catheter should be implemented to optimize embryo transfer results [34]. Using an ovum donation model to eliminate confounding variables, Lindheim et al. [16] reported significantly improved implantation and pregnancy rates following USG-ET in cycles with easy transfers (28.8% vs. 18.4% and 63.1% vs. 36.1%, respectively; $P < 0.05$) without impacting multiple pregnancy rates. Difficult ET was defined as requiring at least two attempts and/or the presence of blood on the catheter and/or taking >5 min. The authors concluded that USG-ET is simple and reassuring and appears to significantly improve pregnancy outcomes in ovum donation cycles by optimizing the placement of embryos [16].

Transfers requiring cervical dilatation that were classified as difficult or impossible ($n = 281$) yielded a 17.4% pregnancy rate/transfer following ET and an 18% pregnancy rate/transfer following transmyometrial-transvaginal ET for difficult transfers ($n = 50$). Following the adoption of USG-ET ($n = 74$), the pregnancy rate/transfer increased to 28.4%, suggesting that the use of ultrasonography for embryo transfer is beneficial in an IVF program [35]. Though Kan et al. [36] observed no significant difference in the pregnancy and implantation rates when USG-ET was used, they observed that in the subgroup where the clinician rated the transfer procedure as difficult, there appeared to be a substantial improvement in the pregnancy rate in the group that used ultrasound (54.5% vs. 10.0%; not significant). They concluded that though their results were not statistically significant, USG-ET should be used in clinically difficult embryo transfers and in older women, as it appears to improve the pregnancy rate over clinical touch transfers [36].

Significance of USG for ET

Abdominal ultrasound facilitates the measurement of the uterocervical angle. Molding the embryo transfer catheter according to the uterocervical angle is reported to result in significantly increased clinical pregnancy (OR 1.57, 95% CI 1.08–2.27) and implantation rates (OR 1.47, 95% CI 1.10–1.96) and significantly decreased incidence of difficult (OR 0.25, 95% CI 0.16–0.40) and bloody transfers (OR 0.71, 95% CI 0.50–0.99) compared with the "clinical feel" method ($n = 320$) [37]. Fig. 33.2A and B illustrate molding of the embryo transfer catheter according to the uterocervical angle.

Abdominal ultrasound facilitates the accurate evaluation of the uterine position and cavity length before the actual embryo transfer. Ultrasound measurement of cavity depth from the vaginal stripe to the fundus before embryo transfer (Fig. 33.3) is clinically useful to determine the depth beyond which catheter insertion should not occur. Pope et al. [38] observed that cavity depth by ultrasound differed from cavity depth by mock transfer by at least 10 mm in >30% of cases. The transfer distance from the fundus (TDF) by US was highly predictive of the pregnancy rate; TDF by mock was not predictive of pregnancy rate. Pope et al. concluded that for every additional millimeter embryos are deposited away from the fundus, the odds of clinical pregnancy increase by 11% [38].

An interesting study by Henne and Milki [39] on the comparison between uterine position at real embryo transfer and mock embryo transfer in 585 patients revealed that in 2% of the patients, an anteverted (AV) uterus at mock embryo transfer became retroverted (RV), while an RV uterus in 55% of the patients on mock embryo transfer converted to AV at real embryo transfer ($P < 0.0001$), suggesting that an RV uterus at mock embryo transfer will often change position at real embryo transfer. Hence, an accurate knowledge of the uterine position at the time of embryo transfer by routine ultrasound guidance is essential to prevent misdirecting the embryo transfer catheter. Additionally, patients with an RV uterus at mock embryo transfer should still present with a full bladder for embryo transfer, since a significant number will convert to an AV position [39]. Though the mock transfer may predict a difficult embryo transfer, it is an inaccurate predictor of the final

A

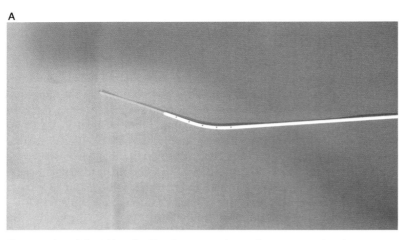

B

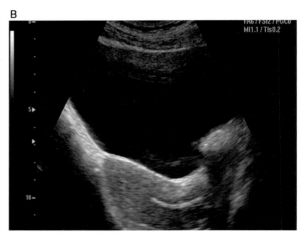

Fig. 33.2 (A and B) Molding the ET catheter according to the uterocervical angle.

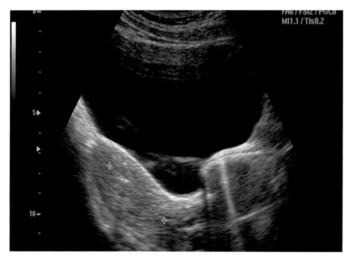

Fig. 33.3 Ultrasound-guided measurement of cavity from internal os to fundus.

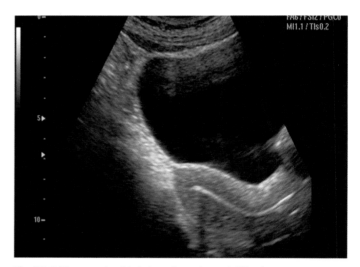

Fig. 33.4 Ultrasound-guided view of an echogenic ET catheter.

embryo transfer depth as the uterine depth has been shown to significantly differ (≥1 cm) between the blind pre-cycle mock transfer measurement and the ultrasound-guided embryo transfer measurement [40].

Ultrasound guidance facilitates visualization of the catheter tip during embryo transfer and the position of embryo deposition. Wood et al. [11] considered ultrasound visualization to be excellent/good when the catheter could be followed from the cervix to the fundus by transabdominal ultrasound with the retention of the embryo-containing fluid droplet, but fair/poor if visualization could not document the sequence of events. They reported significantly higher clinical pregnancy (CP) rates following ET with soft (Frydman or Wallace) catheters compared with hard (Tefcat, Tom Cat, or Norfolk) catheters (36% vs.17%, respectively; $P < 0.0001$) and significantly higher CP rates following USG-ET compared with ET without ultrasound guidance (38% vs. 25%; $P < 0.002$), respectively. A statistically significant difference was also noted when visualization ranks were compared. CP rates per transfer were

significantly higher in all excellent/good ultrasound-guided transfers compared with fair/poor transfers (41.5% vs. 16.7%; $P < 0.038$). The authors concluded that performance of embryo transfer with a soft catheter under ultrasound guidance with good visualization resulted in a significant increase in clinical pregnancy rates [11].

Several prospective randomized controlled trials have reported that USG-ET with an echogenic catheter simplifies ET by facilitating catheter identification under ultrasound, thus decreasing the duration of the embryo transfer without definite benefit in terms of the pregnancy outcome when compared with the standard soft catheter [41,42] (Fig. 33.4). In a prospective, randomized study on 175 patients, Allahbadia et al. [41] compared the performance of the SureView ultrasonic embryo transfer catheter (Fig. 33.5) with the classic Wallace catheter during USG-ET. They concluded that the SureView catheter with its ultrasonic contrast properties significantly enhances catheter visualization by enabling consistent visualization of the echo-dense tip and the entire length of the SureView catheter under ultrasound guidance, thus simplifying

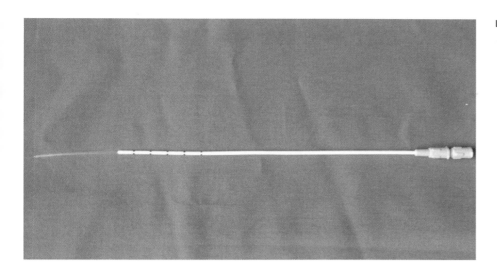

Fig. 33.5 SureView embryo transfer catheter.

USG-ET without significant influence on pregnancy rates [41]. Arriving at a similar conclusion, Coroleu et al. [42] additionally observed that USG-ET with an echogenic Wallace catheter by a single health care provider resulted in a significant increase ($P < 0.01$) in the number of twin pregnancies, reflecting a significant increase in the implantation rate in this group (37.1% vs. 23.2%) as compared with the standard soft Wallace catheter group (23.2%). Following USG-ET by a single physician with a standardized technique, Karande et al. [43] concluded that the Cook Echo-Tip catheter with its echogenic tip simplifies USG-ET, minimizing the need for catheter movement to identify the tip, but pregnancy success rates are similar to those obtained when a Wallace catheter is used.

Easy visualization of the outer sheath of the catheter through the cervix and into the lower uterine segment due to the outer sheath's thickness, immediate identification of the echodense catheter tip under transabdominal ultrasonographic guidance with minimal movement of the catheter or ultrasonographic transducer, and easy tracking during passage through the entire uterine cavity into the fundal region all reduce the need to move the catheter for identification, providing a method for precise, atraumatic ET [44]. Fig. 33.6 illustrates ultrasound visualization of the catheter tip and position of embryo deposition.

With regard to the modality used, though two-dimensional ultrasound-guided embryo transfer continues to be the standard for image-guided transfers, studies have reported the superiority of three-dimensional ultrasound for seeking an optimal transfer area in the uterine cavity, precision in catheter tip placement, and thus, the embryo transfer technique with a positive impact on overall pregnancy rates and fewer complications [45,46].

The potential to visualize the embryo transfer associated air bubbles is, according to Lambers et al. [47], one of the main benefits of USG-ET. In an analysis of 367 consecutive USG-ETs, they demonstrated that when the relative position of the air bubbles was in the fundal half of the endometrial plate, pregnancy rates were significantly higher compared with the

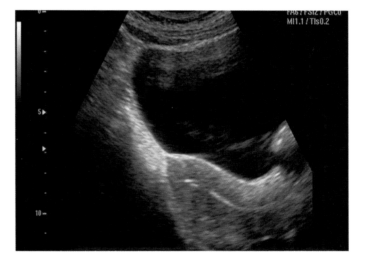

Fig. 33.6 Visualization of the catheter tip and position of embryo deposition.

lower half of the endometrial plate (43.0% vs. 24.4%, respectively; $P = 0.002$) [47]. However, Confino et al. [48] challenged the significance of embryo transfer-associated air bubbles and suggested that the air bubble location following ET is the presumable placement spot of embryos, and air bubble migration, assessed by bubble migration analysis 30 minutes following ET, is a random event post-embryo transfer without visible gravity effect, suggestive of active uterine contractions and a possibly large "window" of embryo placement [48].

Conclusion

Though numerous studies evaluating the pregnancy outcomes following USG-ET and the traditional clinical touch method thus far have differed in technique, catheters used, patient indications, study design, and outcome measures, and have divided opinions, the numerous undoubted advantages provided by ultrasound guidance in facilitating an easy, atraumatic, vision-guided transfer, with adequate knowledge of uterine size and position and depth of catheter placement, makes USG-ET a reliable technique with a positive impact on pregnancy outcomes. Regarding the variables associated with embryo transfer success, using an atraumatic transfer technique, avoiding a difficult transfer, and a stepwise approach in dealing with such a transfer would maximize embryo implantation and avoid failure at ET. The benefits offered by USG-ET clearly decrease the incidence of difficult transfers, its associated complications, and inadvertent failure following ET. Larger, well-designed, prospective randomized controlled trials with careful attention to details, such as standardized protocols, technique, outcome measures, and reporting, are warranted to establish the indispensable role of ultrasound guidance in embryo transfer, and especially, in difficult transfers.

References

1. Mains L, Van Voorhis BJ. Optimizing the technique of embryo transfer. *Fertil Steril* 2010; **94**(3): 785–790.

2. Levi Setti PE, Albani E, Cavagna M, Bulletti C, Colombo GV, Negri L. The impact of embryo transfer on implantation – a review. *Placenta* 2003; **24**(Suppl B): S20–26.

3. Schoolcraft WB, Surrey ES, Gardner DK. Embryo transfer: techniques and variables affecting success. *Fertil Steril* 2001; **76**(5): 863–870.

4. Frydman R. [Impact of embryo transfer techniques on implantation rates]. [Article in French] *J Gynecol Obstet Biol Reprod* (Paris) 2004; **33**(1 Pt 2): S36–39.

5. Mansour RT, Aboulghar MA. Optimizing the embryo transfer technique. *Hum Reprod* 2002; **17**(5): 1149–1153.

6. Sallam HN. Embryo transfer: factors involved in optimizing the success. *Curr Opin Obstet Gynecol* 2005; **17**(3): 289–298.

7. Biervliet FP, Lesny P, Maguiness SD, Robinson J, Killick SR. Transmyometrial embryo transfer and junctional zone contractions. *Hum Reprod* 2002; **17**(2): 347–350.

8. Porter MB. Ultrasound in assisted reproductive technology. *Semin Reprod Med* 2008; **26**(3): 266–276.

9. Brown J, Buckingham K, Abou-Setta AM, Buckett W. Ultrasound versus 'clinical touch' for catheter guidance during embryo transfer in women. *Cochrane Database Syst Rev* 2010; **20**(1): CD006107.

10. Coroleu B, Carreras O, Veiga A, et al. Embryo transfer under ultrasound guidance improves pregnancy rates after in-vitro fertilization. *Hum Reprod* 2000; **15**(3): 616–620.

11. Wood EG, Batzer FR, Go KJ, Gutmann JN, Corson SL. Ultrasound-guided soft catheter embryo transfers will improve pregnancy rates in in-vitro fertilization. *Hum Reprod* 2000; **15**(1): 107–112.

12. Matorras R, Urquijo E, Mendoza R, Corcóstegui B, Expósito A, Rodríguez-Escudero FJ. Ultrasound-guided embryo transfer improves pregnancy rates and increases the frequency of easy transfers. *Hum Reprod* 2002; **17**(7): 1762–1766.

13. Prapas Y, Prapas N, Hatziparasidou A, Vanderzwalmen P, Nijs M, Prapa S, Vlassis G. Ultrasound-guided embryo transfer maximizes the IVF results on day 3 and day 4 embryo transfer but has no impact on day 5. *Hum Reprod* 2001; **16**(9): 1904–1908.

14. Eskandar M, Abou-Setta AM, Almushait MA, El-Amin M, Mohmad SE. Ultrasound guidance during embryo transfer: a prospective, single-operator, randomized, controlled trial. *Fertil Steril* 2008; **90**(4): 1187–1190.

15. Kojima K, Nomiyama M, Kumamoto T, Matsumoto Y, Iwasaka T. Transvaginal ultrasound-guided embryo transfer improves pregnancy and implantation rates after IVF. *Hum Reprod* 2001; **16**(12): 2578–2582.

16. Lindheim SR, Cohen MA, Sauer MV. Ultrasound guided embryo transfer significantly improves pregnancy rates in women undergoing oocyte donation. *Int J Gynaecol Obstet* 1999; **66**(3): 281–284.

17. Brown JA, Buckingham K, Abou-Setta A, Buckett W. Ultrasound versus 'clinical touch' for catheter guidance during embryo transfer in women. *Cochrane Database Syst Rev* 2007; **24**(1): CD006107.

18. Buckett WM. A meta-analysis of ultrasound-guided versus clinical touch embryo transfer. *Fertil Steril* 2003; **80**(4): 1037–1041.

19. Abou-Setta AM, Mansour RT, Al-Inany HG, Aboulghar MM, Aboulghar MA, Serour GI. Among women undergoing embryo transfer, is the probability of pregnancy and live birth improved with ultrasound guidance over clinical touch alone? A systemic review and meta-analysis of prospective randomized trials. *Fertil Steril* 2007; **88**(2): 333–341.

20. Sallam HN, Sadek SS. Ultrasound-guided embryo transfer: a meta-analysis of randomized controlled trials. *Fertil Steril* 2003; **80**(4): 1042–1046.

21. Anderson RE, Nugent NL, Gregg AT, Nunn SL, Behr BR. Transvaginal ultrasound-guided embryo transfer improves outcome in patients with previous failed in vitro fertilization cycles. *Fertil Steril* 2002; **77**(4): 769–775.

22. Kosmas IP, Janssens R, De Munck L, et al. Ultrasound-guided embryo transfer does not offer any benefit in clinical outcome: a randomized controlled trial. *Hum Reprod* 2007; **22**(5): 1327–1334.

23. Lambers MJ, Dogan E, Kostelijk H, Lens JW, Schats R, Hompes PG. Ultrasonographic-guided embryo transfer does not enhance pregnancy rates compared with embryo transfer based on previous uterine length measurement. *Fertil Steril* 2006; **86**(4): 867–872.

24. Harris ID, Styer AK, Petrozza JC. Ultrasonographer experience does not impact outcomes following ultrasound-guided embryo transfer. *Fertil Steril* 2009; **92**(3): 918–922.

25. de Camargo Martins AM, Baruffi RL, Mauri AL, et al. Ultrasound guidance is not necessary during easy embryo transfers. *J Assist Reprod Genet* 2004; **21**(12): 421–425.

26. Tang OS, Ng EH, So WW, Ho PC. Ultrasound-guided embryo transfer: a prospective randomized controlled trial. *Hum Reprod* 2001; **16**(11): 2310–2315.

27. García-Velasco JA, Isaza V, Martinez-Salazar J, et al. Transabdominal ultrasound-guided embryo transfer does not increase pregnancy rates in oocyte recipients. *Fertil Steril* 2002; **78**(3): 534–539.

28. Flisser E, Grifo JA, Krey LC, Noyes N. Transabdominal ultrasound-assisted embryo transfer and pregnancy outcome. *Fertil Steril* 2006; **85**(2): 353–357.

29. Tomás C, Tikkinen K, Tuomivaara L, Tapanainen JS, Martikainen H. The degree of difficulty of embryo transfer is an independent factor for predicting pregnancy. *Hum Reprod* 2002; **17**(10): 2632–2635.

30. Lesny P, Killick SR, Tetlow RL, Robinson J, Maguiness SD. Embryo transfer – can we learn anything new from the observation of junctional zone contractions? *Hum Reprod* 1998; **13**(6): 1540–1546.

31. Aubriot FX. [Difficult embryo transfer: what can be done in practice?].[Article in French] *Gynecol Obstet Fertil* 2003; **31**(2): 157–161.

32. Aboulfotouh I, Abou-Setta AM, Khattab S, Mohsen IA, Askalani A, el-Din RE. Firm versus soft embryo transfer catheters under ultrasound guidance: does catheter choice really influence the pregnancy rates? *Fertil Steril* 2008; **89**(5): 1261–1262.

33. Woolcott R, Stanger J. Potentially important variables identified by transvaginal ultrasound-guided embryo transfer. *Hum Reprod* 1997; **12**(5): 963–966.

34. Mirkin S, Jones EL, Mayer JF, Stadtmauer L, Gibbons WE, Oehninger S. Impact of transabdominal ultrasound guidance on performance and outcome of transcervical uterine embryo transfer. *J Assist Reprod Genet* 2003; **20**(8): 318–322.

35. Broussin B, Jayot S, Subtil D, et al. [Difficult embryo transfers: contribution of echography]. [Article in French] *Contracept Fertil Sex* 1998; **26**(7–8): 492–497.

36. Kan AK, Abdalla HI, Gafar AH, Nappi L, Ogunyemi BO, Thomas A, Ola-ojo OO. Embryo transfer: ultrasound-guided versus clinical touch. *Hum Reprod* 1999; **14**(5): 1259–1261.

37. Sallam HN, Agameya AF, Rahman AF, Ezzeldin F, Sallam AN. Ultrasound measurement of the uterocervical angle before embryo transfer: a prospective controlled study. *Hum Reprod* 2002; **17**(7): 1767–1772.

38. Pope CS, Cook EK, Arny M, Novak A, Grow DR. Influence of embryo transfer depth on in vitro fertilization and embryo transfer outcomes. *Fertil Steril* 2004; **81**(1): 51–58.

39. Henne MB, Milki AA. Uterine position at real embryo transfer compared with mock embryo transfer. *Hum Reprod* 2004; **19**(3): 570–572.

40. Miller KL, Frattarelli JL. The pre-cycle blind mock embryo transfer is an inaccurate predictor of anticipated embryo transfer depth. *J Assist Reprod Genet* 2007; **24**(2–3): 77–82.

41. Allahbadia GN, Kadam K, Gandhi G, et al. Embryo transfer using the SureView catheter-beacon in the womb. *Fertil Steril* 2010; **93**(2): 344–350.

42. Coroleu B, Barri PN, Carreras O, et al. Effect of using an echogenic catheter for ultrasound-guided embryo transfer in an IVF programme: a prospective, randomized, controlled study. *Hum Reprod* 2006; **21**(7): 1809–1815.

43. Karande V, Hazlett D, Vietzke M, Gleicher N. A prospective randomized comparison of the Wallace catheter and the Cook Echo-Tip catheter for ultrasound-guided embryo transfer. *Fertil Steril* 2002; **77**(4): 826–830.

44. Letterie GS, Marshall L, Angle M. A new coaxial catheter system with an echodense tip for ultrasonographically guided embryo transfer. *Fertil Steril* 1999; **72**(2): 266–268.

45. Baba K, Ishihara O, Hayashi N, Saitoh M, Taya J, Kinoshita K. Three-dimensional ultrasound in embryo transfer. *Ultrasound Obstet Gynecol* 2000; **16**(4): 372–373.

46. Letterie GS. Three-dimensional ultrasound-guided embryo transfer: a preliminary study. *Am J Obstet Gynecol* 2005; **192**(6): 1983–1987.

47. Lambers MJ, Dogan E, Lens JW, Schats R, Hompes PG. The position of transferred air bubbles after embryo transfer is related to pregnancy rate. *Fertil Steril* 2007; **88**(1): 68–73.

48. Confino E, Zhang J, Risquez F. Air bubble migration is a random event post embryo transfer. *J Assist Reprod Genet* 2007; **24**(6): 223–226.

Ultrasound to detect congenital anomalies after ART

Carrie Warshak and David F. Lewis

Since their inception in the late 1970s, assisted reproductive technologies (ARTs) have become a widely available means of enabling infertile couples an opportunity at childbearing. A recent study from the United States National Birth Defects Prevention Study (NBDPS) reported that between the years 1997 and 2004, 4.2% of women delivering live-born infants had conceived with the assistance of maternal fertility treatment, with 1% conceiving via ART [1]. In fact, over 3 500 000 children worldwide were born after use of ART. ART is a term referring to multiple invasive techniques of egg retrieval and subsequent return of gametes or embryos to the female reproductive tract to facilitate conception and subsequent pregnancy. Common procedures include in vitro fertilization (IVF), the technique of egg and sperm retrieval with fertilization outside the body; intracytoplasmic sperm injection (ICSI), in which a single sperm is directly injected into a processed ovum used to enhance conception in cases of male infertility factor; zygote intrafallopian transfer (ZIFT), which entails egg removal and fertilization in vitro with return to the fallopian tube; and gamete intrafallopian transfer (GIFT), in which unfertilized male and female gametes are manually placed within the fallopian tubes to facilitate conception. As technologies have expanded, so too have concerns regarding associations of ART and congenital anomalies.

Several large epidemiological studies conducted in the United States [2–5], Canada [6], Sweden [7], France [8], Belgium [9,10], Israel [11], Saudi Arabia [12], Australia [13], China [14], and Japan [15] have evaluated the association between ART and congenital anomalies. The results of these studies are conflicting. Several reported no increased risk of anomalies with ART over pregnancies following natural conception (NC) [3,8,11,13,14]. Others demonstrated increased risk of a major anomaly in general, or specific birth defects. Olson et al. in 2005 found IVF was associated with a 30% increase in risk of a major birth defect (odds ratio [OR] 1.3, 95% CI 1.00–1.67) [4]. In this study cardiovascular, musculoskeletal, and syndromic anomalies appeared to be at increased risk in pregnancies conceived by ART. Similarly, Reefhuis et al. also found an increased risk of anomalies with ART [5]. This case control study compared mothers of fetuses with a major birth defect to control mothers of fetuses who did not have a major birth defect. After controlling for multiple potential confounders, including maternal age, investigators found an increased risk of cardiac septal defects, cleft lip/palate, and gastrointestinal atresias.

Other retrospective cohort studies have found similar results. A Canadian trial reported by El-Chaar et al. also found a significant association between infertility treatment and the risk of birth defects [6]. This retrospective cohort study had a prevalence of birth defects of 2.91% with any fertility treatment compared with 1.86% in the non-ART population (OR 1.55, 95% CI 1.11–4.77). Again it appeared infertility treatment increased anomaly rates for cardiovascular, gastrointestinal, and musculoskeletal anomalies disproportionately. The authors found that 3.45% of women undergoing IVF had an infant with a birth defect compared with 1.86% of women who conceived naturally.

Similarly, a Swedish study also demonstrated an increased risk of cardiovascular malformations, limb reduction defects, neural tube defects, and gastrointestinal atresias [7]. Interestingly, this study evaluated two study periods (1982 to March 31, 2001 and April 2001 to end of 2006) and found that some defects, such as cardiovascular malformations and limb reduction defects were consistently higher in both study periods, while others such as neural tube defects, cardiac septal defects, and esophageal atresias, although still at increased risk over controls, seemed to have improvements in risk in the second time period, suggesting the ability to reduce this risk with improved techniques or experience. In fact, for anomalies such as anal or small bowel atresias and hypospadias, this risk became nonsignificant in the second study time period.

Meta-analyses have examined whether forms of ART increase the risk of congenital anomalies [16–18]. The first, reported by Hansen et al. in 2005, compared the rate of anomalies between IVF pregnancies and those following natural conception (NC) [16]. They identified seven studies reporting outcomes on 14 900 children that met inclusion criteria. They found women who had undergone ART were at a 30–40% increased risk of a birth defect, with two-thirds of the studies reporting at least a 25% increase in risk. Depending upon the underlying prevalence of birth defects (considered to be 1–4% of all births) the "number needed to harm" by the use of ART is between 62 and 250.

A meta-analysis by Lie et al., also published in 2005, examined whether ICSI increased the risk of birth defects compared to the use of IVF alone [17]. Four studies reporting outcomes on 5395 children met inclusion criteria for the systematic review. This review did not demonstrate an increased risk for either general birth defects or categories of birth defects in women undergoing ICSI over IVF alone. A similar meta-analysis by Rimm et al., published in 2004, compared the rate of anomalies between patients undergoing ICSI or IVF and NC [18]. This review included 19 studies and over 3.5 million infants. When the IVF and ICSI patients were pooled, an increased risk for anomalies was seen (OR 1.29, 95% CI 1.01–1.67).

Studies in this field are plagued by several methodological limitations: small numbers of anomalous fetuses, lack of suitable control groups, heterogeneity of ART therapies and techniques, and ascertainment, recall, and reporting bias. It has yet to be demonstrated whether or not the factors causing parental infertility are responsible for any observed increased risk in anomalies, and not necessarily the ART techniques themselves. In addition, most studies to date have analyzed data regarding anomalies at birth, without consideration of rates of prenatal detection and termination of pregnancy that may be different between patients undergoing ART and NC. It is likely there are key differences in this area given patients undergoing ART by definition have extensive care prior to conception, a fact that may increase factors such as folic acid supplementation, which should actually lower their risk of certain anomalies such as neural tube defects. In addition, this group is generally screened for other factors that also have an impact on the rate of anomalies such as karyotypical abnormalities and diabetes. On the other hand, this group is more likely to undergo earlier ultrasound evaluation of the pregnancy, enabling the earlier detection of anomalies and thereby potentially increasing the rate of interrupted pregnancies that may not reach a gestational age at which data would be reported in many of the above studies. There are few data to facilitate a better understanding of these important considerations.

One of the major criticisms of the epidemiological research in this area is the diversity of the ART treatments being studied. Often any ART procedure is compared to NC, without consideration for the specific nature of the intervention. Only recently have investigators began to evaluate specific techniques more individually to reduce the heterogeneity inherent to studies in this field. Several small series have reported that there is no clear association between ICSI and the rate of anomalies when compared with traditional IVF or NC [12,19–22] However, large prospective trials comparing a cohort of children born following ICSI versus a cohort of either IVF or NC controls have demonstrated conflicting results. Bonduelle et al. found no association between ICSI and anomalies, except in cases of aneuploidy (see below), when compared to those conceived via IVF [23].

A second prospective report from 59 centers in Germany found ICSI to have comparable risk to IVF, but with increased risks of anomalies over NC (relative risk [RR] 1.25,95% CI 1.11–1.40) [24]. Similarly, Hansen et al. also published a large prospective cohort study in 2002 that demonstrated that 8.6% of infants born to women after ICSI had anomalies, a rate that was similar to that of infants whose mothers had undergone IVF (9.0%) but nearly twice as high as for infants conceived naturally (4.2%: $P < 0.001$) [13]. In particular, this study found increased risks of cardiovascular, urogenital, musculoskeletal, and chromosomal anomalies in infants whose mothers had undergone IVF with or without ICSI. Long-term studies of the development of children born after IVF with or without ICSI have demonstrated similar neurodevelopment outcomes at 5 years of life [25,26]

Similarly, cryopreservation of embryos, slow freezing, and vitrification of early cleavage stage embryos have been analyzed to determine whether these processes increase the rate of anomalies as compared to that of fresh embryo transfers. Concerns have arisen, in large part, because of preservative solutions that are often used in these processes. An initial small case control study in 1995 conducted in the UK provided early reassurance that cryopreservation did not appear to increase the risk of anomalies when compared to normally conceived controls [27]. More recently, several small series have also reported similar rates of minor and major birth defects between infants born after cryopreservation and vitrification and those arising from fresh embryo IVF cycles [28–30]. One large trial comparing cryopreservation to fresh embryo transfer and IVF to ICSI found a significantly increased risk which was most prominent in the setting of cryopreservation and ICSI [31]. In this study, cryopreservation versus fresh embryo IVF had similar rates of anomalies; however, cryopreservation with ICSI had twice the rate of malformations as cryopreservation with IVF or fresh ICSI. In some studies the risk of anomalies and/or growth abnormalities seemed to be lower in frozen embryos compared with fresh embryo transfers [29,30].

A recent Australian study warrants consideration as to the direction in which future research should go so that investigators may elucidate which anomalies have an increased risk, and why, and to consider whether changes in techniques, media, procedures, etc. may ameliorate this risk [32]. This study considered over 27 000 births in Australia, comparing those resulting from IVF or IVF/ICSI to those conceived without ART, matched for maternal age and year of birth. This study was unique in that it compared the study groups not by system or specific anomaly, but rather by classifying birth defects according to pathological mechanism. A primary goal of the study was to evaluate the category of anomalies known as "defects of blastogenesis." This was based upon the observation that several of the anomalies which have more consistently been identified as ones for which ART incurs a higher risk, such as neural tube defects, abdominal wall defects, and gastrointestinal atresias, are defects of blastogenesis. Although the authors state that the etiologies for these disorders are largely unknown, it is known that "as a group these defects tend to affect the midline and mesoderm, involve two or more developmental fields, be severe, and be without sex differences in occurrence," consistent with the pattern of increased anomalies seen with ART. The study investigators grouped birth defects according to known categories such as genetic (monogenetic, chromosomal, or disorder of imprinting), teratogenic, and syndromic. Any anomaly not explained by the above mechanisms was then considered as to whether it was a blastogenesis defect, multiple malformation, or isolated malformation by an investigator blinded to the method of conception. Similar to prior studies, the authors found an increased risk of anomalies when comparing ART to non-ART controls (adjusted OR 1.36, 95% CI 1.19–1.55). Also similar to prior reports as outlined above, there was a small increase in risk associated with fresh embryo transfer as compared with thawed embryos, though not significant (adjusted OR 1.15, 95% CI 0.93–1.48). ICSI did not appear to increase this baseline risk further when compared to traditional IVF (adjusted OR 1.19, 95% CI 0.96–1.48). As hypothesized by the authors, the rate of anomalies classified as defects in blastogenesis was substantially higher in ART pregnancies over non-ART pregnancies (adjusted OR 2.80, 95% CI 1.63–4.81). The fresh embryo transfers appeared to be the subgroup of ART at highest rate of vulnerability (adjusted OR 3.65, 95% CI 2.02–6.59) and in fact those embryos that had undergone cryopreservation had similar rates of blastogenesis defects as non-ART controls. Studies such as this will be instrumental as we move forward to better understand the mechanisms contributing to higher rates of anomalies in ART pregnancies in an effort to improve prevention of these birth defects.

Aneuploidy

Since its inception and as advances in ART have occurred, a focus of concern has been on whether ART increases the risk of chromosomal aneuploidy. Owing to the multitude of inherent confounding variables that plague research in this area, this has been a challenging question for investigators to address. It is well established that women who undergo ART are older, on average, than those undergoing NC. In addition, male factors contributing to infertility are also believed to increase risk of aneuploidy in the offspring. Whether other factors leading to infertility also contribute to the risk of aneuploidy is an area of current investigation.

Two large population-based cohort studies, both published in 2002, raised concern for an increased risk of chromosomal aneuploidy in fetuses after ART [13,23]. Hansen et al. found rates of chromosomal anomalies in fetuses reaching 20 weeks gestation to be 0.2, 0.7, and 1.0% in fetuses conceived via NC, IVF, and ICSI, respectively ($P < 0.05$) [13]. Subsequent to this publication, Bonduelle similarly reported an increased risk of aneuploidy, but found this was an increase in rate of aneuploidy with ICSI specifically over IVF (1.6 vs. 0.5%, respectively; $P < 0.007$) [23]. These investigators found that the observed increase in chromosomal aneuploidies seemed to stem mainly from an increase in sex chromosome anomalies. Multiple subsequent

studies looking at both rate of aneuploidy in spontaneous abortuses and fetuses have confirmed this increased risk of sex chromosome aneuploidy with ICSI [33–35]. Other studies have found this risk is particularly high after testicular sperm extraction, with aneuploidy rates of 80% in this category of ART [36]. An elevated follicle-stimulating hormone level has been shown to be predictive of aneuploidy in the fetus [37]. In addition, the timing of oocyte maturation also appears to play a role in the elevation of risk of aneuploidy, with embryos derived from in vivo maturation of oocytes or maturation within 24 hours having a lower risk of aneuploidy than those matured 48 hours after collection [38]. Finally, simply being a "poor responder," defined as producing fewer than four oocytes, does not appear to be an independent risk factor for aneuploidy [39].

It is generally recommended that patients who have undergone ART be offered aneuploidy screening. The American College of Obstetrics and Gynecology recommends all women be offered aneuploidy screening [40]. First trimester screening, using both nuchal translucency and serum analytes (free beta-hCG and PAPP-A), is ideal in this population for several reasons. Patients having undergone ART by definition present early in the pregnancy for prenatal care, averting a considerable hurdle to offering early screening. First trimester screening has a superior detection rate, as high as 87% as an isolated screening modality and over 90% when combined with a midtrimester genetic sonogram, for a false-positive rate of 5%, ideal for a population in which advanced maternal age is more common [41]. Nuchal translucency measurement is not only an effective screening tool for autosomal aneuploidies, such as trisomy 21, but it offers an early screen for sex chromosome disorders, such as monosomy X, or Turner's syndrome, in that many fetuses with monosomy X will present with evidence of a cystic hygroma when they are imaged in the first trimester (Fig. 34.1). In addition, a thickened nuchal translucency screening has been shown to be associated with congenital heart defects, a specific group of anomalies for which fetuses conceived via ART are at risk (see below) [42,43]. In addition, given a possible increased risk of neural tube defects, early ultrasound screening offers an early opportunity to detect such anomalies as neural tube defects and even spina bifida in some cases (Fig. 34.2). Pregnancies conceived via ART have also been shown to have increased hCG and lower alpha-fetoprotein (AFP) levels, which increases the false-positive rate with second trimester serum screening, such as the triple screen or quad screen [44–47]. For all of these reasons, patients who have undergone ART should be offered first trimester screening.

Neural tube defects

Since Lancaster's original report in 1987, the association between ART and neural tube defects (NTDs) has been extensively studied, with contradictory results [48]. Prior to this study, an association between ovulation induction with clomiphene citrate and NTD had been reported in several small series and it was noted that in fact clomiphene had been used for ovulation induction

A

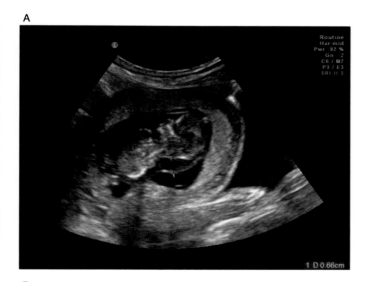

B

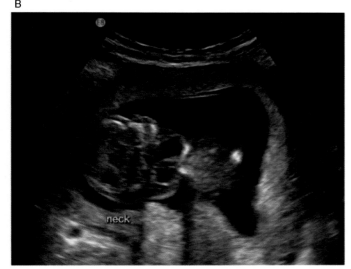

Fig. 34.1 Cystic hygroma. (A) Sagittal view of cystic hygroma demonstrating the marked thickening (6.6 mm) of the nuchal translucency at 11 weeks. (B) Oblique view demonstrating the multiple septations that characterize a cystic hygroma.

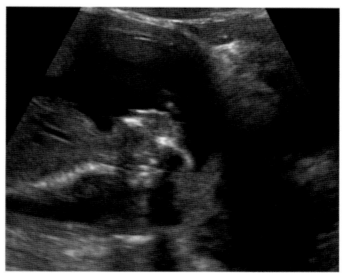

Fig. 34.2 Fetal anencephaly through a sagittal view of the fetal profile.

in 98% of Lancaster's Australian IVF pregnancies. While subsequent research has largely refuted an association between clomiphene citrate per se and NTDs, whether IVF increases this risk remains highly debated. The largest study to date was reported by Kallen in 2005 and included data on over 20 000 ART pregnancies in comparison to all births during the same period in Sweden [49]. This study found an increased risk of anencephaly (RR 7.6, 95% CI 2.5–7.7) and an increased risk of spina bifida (RR 5.1, 3.4–7.8). There were no cases of encephalocele among ART pregnancies. Therefore the total calculated risk for any NTD was found to be a nearly five-fold increase in risk (RR 4.8, 95% CI 3.3–6.9). Similarly, other studies have also reported an increased risk of NTD after ART [50].

However, other studies have not confirmed these findings [6,51]. In addition, ICSI has not been found to have a consistently increased risk of NTD over IVF [17,52,53]. A study comparing cryopreservation of embryos to use of fresh embryos also did not find an increased risk of NTD following cryopreservation [54].

Given the possible association between NTDs and either infertility, ovarian stimulation, and/or ART, careful examination of the fetal spine is indicated in pregnancies conceived following ART. There are three subtypes of neural tube defects: anencephaly (absence of cranial vault and telencephalon), spina bifida (protrusion of the meninges and possibly segments of the spinal cord through the spinal column), and encephalocele (partial defect in the fetal skull). Sonographic diagnosis is based upon an absence of the fetal cranium, and is usually possible after 10 weeks' gestation.

The diagnosis of spina bifida relies on abnormal imaging in the spine and cranium. Imaging of the spine in sagittal sections can often demonstrate protrusion of a cystic structure or soft tissue mass beyond the normally visualized parallel lines of the vertebral bodies. Often abnormal curvatures of the spine (kyphosis or lordosis) may also be seen in relation to the lesion. Transverse, axial views of the spine may also demonstrate a splaying of the vertebral bodies at the level of the spinal lesion. Examination of fetal cranium often raises suspicion of the presence of spina bifida. Nearly all cases of spina bifida have associated Arnold–Chiari malformations, which consist of displacement to varying degrees of the cerebellar vermis, fourth ventricle, and upper brainstem posteriorly. This displacement causes a "banana sign," which describes the typical appearance of the cisterna magna as its central component is tugged posteriorly and caudally. These forces also cause a characteristic appearance of the cranium known as a "lemon sign" as the temporal regions of the cranium are pulled posteriorly, creating a concavity of the anterior skull bilaterally. The sensitivity of these cranial signs for the detection of neural tube defects exceeds 99% [55]. The ability to discover the actual spinal lesion can prove to be much more challenging depending upon the size of the abnormality, the contents of the meningeal sac, the position of the fetus, and other limitations such as maternal body habitus.

Finally, fetal encephaloceles are uncommon anomalies. Their appearance is highly variable depending upon the location and severity of the pathology. Often other associated fetal anomalies, such as ventriculomegaly, are detected, leading to a more extensive search for defects at which time the encephalocele is detected with either ultrasound or fetal MRI.

Cardiovascular anomalies

Lancaster's original report also raised concerns of a possible association between IVF and congenital heart defects, in particular transposition of the great vessels (TGV) [48]. He noted that out of nearly 1700 IVF pregnancies, 4 had TGV ($P < 0.0034$). Unlike the case with NTDs, the increased risk of congenital heart defect has been consistently demonstrated in multiple trials of varying study designs, spanning an extended time period and many populations [5,6,13,17,49,56–60]. The strength of this association has been found to range between an almost two-fold to a five-fold increased risk [56,61]. As with other associated anomalies, it is unclear whether the ART procedure itself is the causal force, or other entities inherent to infertile couples. Some of this risk appears to be related to a higher incidence of multiple gestation [57,69]. Neither ICSI nor cryopreservation appears to increase the risk over IVF alone [17,23].

As outlined above, increased nuchal translucency thickness has been correlated with the presence of congenital heart defects and therefore should be considered as an early screening approach in pregnancies achieved through ART [42,43,62,63]. Improving technology in ultrasound equipment and use of transvaginal cardiac imaging has enabled an earlier evaluation of the structure of the heart with improving sensitivity for the diagnosis of heart defects, even into the first trimester.

However, at this time it is the midtrimester anatomical evaluation that is key for the detection of heart anomalies. In fact, in light of the consistently demonstrated increased cardiac malformation risk, ART exposure is included in the American Institute of Ultrasound in Medicine (AIUM) recommendations for referral for fetal echocardiogram [64]. Several studies have subcategorized heart defects to specify which defects occur at increased rates after ART [5,49,56,57, 60]. These studies indicate that septal defects and malformations of the outflow tracts and ventriculoarterial connections, such as TGV and tetralogy of Fallot (TOF), are the congenital heart diseases at highest risk after ART and therefore imaging the heart should be directed toward the detection of these entities.

An essential component of any evaluation of the heart is a basic four-chamber view. All of the following should be considered while examining this view [65]:

1. The fetal situs is normal. The fetal heart should point toward the left side of the chest with an axis at approximately 45 degrees and should be located in a mid position in the chest.

2. The heart should occupy 35–50% of the thoracic cavity. The heart circumference to thoracic circumference, which is obtainable in a routine four-chamber view, should be less than 0.5.

3. The size of the two atria should be similar. The leaflet of the foramen ovale should be seen in the left atrium. An intra-atrial septum should be visualized, often as an essential component of the normal crux between the atrioventricular valves, the atrial septum, and the ventricular septum.

4. The two ventricles should be equal in size and contractility. A detailed examination of the septum with grayscale and a color Doppler examination should be performed to insure absence of a jet of flow across this septum.

5. The atrioventricular valves should be seen, with the tricuspid valve inserting more apically on the ventricular septum.

The four-chamber heart view is likely to detect many congenital cardiac abnormalities including heterotaxy syndromes, septal defects, ventricular hypoplasias, and valve abnormalities. Given the consistent associations of septal defects with ART, attention to this view of the heart, and in particular to the septum, should be paid in pregnancies conceived via ART.

However, many relatively common and significant anomalies of the heart may masquerade behind a normal four-chamber view of the heart, such as TOF or TGV. It is for this reason that a more extensive evaluation of the heart is recommended, particularly in higher-risk patients such as those who have undergone ART. Right and left outflow views have a higher detection rate for abnormalities of the great vessels, such as TOF and TGV, known to occur at higher rates after ART (Fig. 34.3). In addition, extended views through the upper mediastinum, such as the three-vessel view and three-vessel tracheal view, further improve the detection rate of anomalies of the great vessels.

One of the more consistently demonstrated anomalies of the heart after ART is TGV [48, 60]. A hallmark feature of TGV is the inability to obtain a normal right outflow view of the heart resulting from the great vessels running in parallel in the upper mediastinum. For this reason, in this view, both arteries will be seen in cross-section and in close proximity to one other. The visualization of the parallel coursing of the great vessels through the upper mediastinum is a key feature of TGV and is best seen by tracing the origin of these vessels from their associated ventricles. Abnormalities in the three-vessel tracheal view will be pronounced as only the aorta is likely to be visualized. Finally, more subtle findings, such as the characteristic branching of the pulmonary trunk after exit from the left ventricle, in the left outflow view will usually be evident though easily missed without a high index of suspicion [65].

Another more commonly associated abnormality of the heart that appears to be related to ART is TOF, which consists

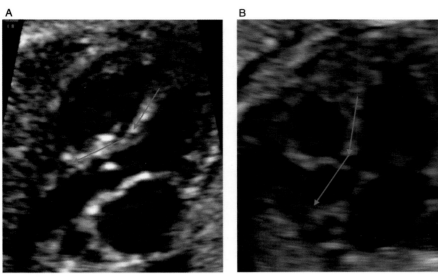

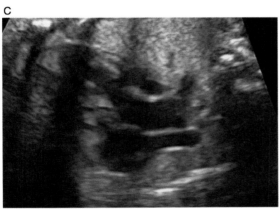

Fig. 34.3 Congenital heart defects which have been demonstrated to be at increased risk after ART. (A) Normal five-chamber view of the heart. (B) Five-chamber view demonstrating alterations seen with tetralogy of Fallot. (Courtesy of Alfred Abuhamad, A Practical Guide to Fetal Echocardiography, 2009.) (C) Transposition of the great vessels: note the parallel path of the pulmonary trunk and ascending aorta.

of the concurrent presence of an overriding aorta, infundibular pulmonary stenosis, ventricular septal defect (VSD), and compensatory right ventricular hypertrophy seen after chronic exposure to the resulting circulatory changes from the aberrant cardiac anatomy. Like TGV, this anomaly can often go undetected after a basic examination of the heart. Sometimes the four-chamber view of the heart will reveal a VSD, if this VSD is large. The preferred cardiac view for the detection of TOF is the five-chamber, or left outflow, view [65]. In this view the aorta is shifted slightly to the right and may be mildly dilated. Ventricular septal defects may also be visualized. Also in the five-chamber view, one of the hallmark signs of the presence of TOF may be seen: a blunting of the normally wide angle between the ventricular septum and the anterior wall of the ascending aorta, which runs nearly in parallel with the ventricular septum.

Given the consistent association of congenital heart defects with ART and the importance of its prenatal detection, we recommend a detailed examination of the heart by a center with expertise in fetal cardiac imaging in these patients. If fetal cardiac abnormalities are suspected, or if imaging is suboptimal, further assessment by a pediatric cardiologist may be indicated.

Gastrointestinal anomalies

Gastrointestinal (GI) anomalies are a broad category of anomalies typically including clefts of the lip and/or palate, ventral wall defects, and bowel atresias or stenoses, with diverse inheritance patterns and physiological etiologies. Nonetheless, given the rarity of these anomalies, for the purposes of evaluation they are often analyzed collectively. Not surprisingly, findings from such studies are also diverse. Some studies have found increased rates of GI anomalies, in particular with GI atresias [5,6,49,50,56,66]. In these reports, the rate of GI atresias is increased two- to nine-fold. Clefts appear to have a less substantial increase in risk, with many of the above studies not demonstrating an increase in risk to at most a two-fold increased risk [5,49]. Omphaloceles have been demonstrated to have a three-fold increased risk [50] with a nearly two-fold increased risk for ventral wall defects in general [49]. Other studies did not see such an association between GI anomalies and ART; however, these were studies inadequately powered to detect an increase in risk of these less common pathologies [57,58].

It should be noted that unlike neural tube defects that tend to follow a polygenic inheritance pattern and are in some ways related to folic acid metabolism or congenital heart defects which are also polygenic, the anomalies commonly grouped as "gastrointestinal" are far more diverse. Clefts appear to be multi-factorial with both a genetic and environmental influence to risk and result when there is a failure of the normal fusion of the maxillary processes. The development of the GI tract entails a proliferatory phase of the lining epithelium, followed by a period of canalization. It is believed a failure of this canalization process is the causative mechanism for bowel stenoses and atresias. Abdominal wall defects themselves are a pathologically diverse entity. Omphaloceles are either caused by a failure of the normal retraction of the developing bowel back into the abdominal cavity or a failure of the abdominal wall to develop over the bowel structure or some combination of the two. These anomalies are more likely to be syndromic. Alternatively, fetal gastroschisis is believed to result from a vascular accident leading to abdominal wall ischemia and subsequent herniation of the bowel contents into the amniotic cavity. Given the multitude of pathological mechanisms, it is unlikely that any teratogenic exposure, including ART, would increase the risk of all entities. In light of this, although they are commonly grouped under the umbrella of "gastrointestinal anomalies" this grouping likely dilutes the underlying effect, increasing the probability of a type II error.

There are multiple ways to screen for the presence of such anomalies. Maternal AFP is likely to be elevated in patients carrying a fetus with abdominal wall defects and clefts of the lip and/or palate and therefore the AFP is a useful screening tool. The amniotic fluid volume, as measured by either a deepest vertical pocket or an amniotic fluid index, often demonstrates polyhydramnios in alimentary tract atresias or abdominal wall defects given the mechanical obstruction to passage of GI contents. The sonographically visualized "stomach bubble" may be absent in cases that prevent effective fetal swallowing, such as esophageal atresias, obstructions of gastric filling as may occur when the stomach is herniated in abdominal wall defects, or rarely with severe clefts. All of the above entities may be indirect signs of an underlying pathology which would warrant more detailed evaluation.

Direct examination of the lip and palate is best accomplished through visualization of these structures in two perpendicular planes. Coronal views though the face can be helpful in assessing whether the lip is intact. In a transverse axial plane, the alveolar ridge in the maxilla can be imaged, with clefts being seen as defects in the normally continuous alveolar buds, communicating with the surrounding amniotic cavity. When a cleft is suspected on routine ultrasound, three-dimensional imaging can often provide greater detail and a more comprehensive examination of the deformity. This may be medically helpful for counseling patients regarding the prognosis for the fetus and for predicting the extent of surgical repair that would be anticipated. In addition, in light of the nature of facial clefts, three-dimensional imaging may also be instrumental for helping parents and family develop a comfort with the anticipated appearance of their child.

Alimentary atresias are uncommon birth defects. One of the more common sites of atresia is in the distal esophagus. Most

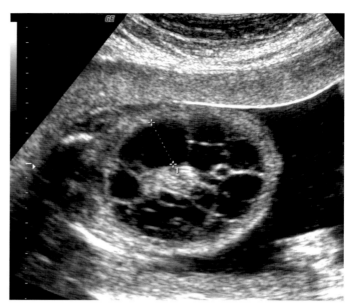

Fig. 34.4 Alimentary atresia. Note the dilated loops of bowel, the largest of which measures 1.56 cm in diameter.

often, the presence of a distal esophageal atresia is inferred secondary to an absent stomach bubble and marked polyhydramnios. On occasion the esophagus can be seen to be dilated, but given expulsion of GI contents retrograde through the oral cavity, this is commonly not seen. In one study, ART increased the risk of esophageal atresias over six-fold (OR 6.8, 95% CI 2.8–15.5) [5,50,66].

More distal GI atresias have also been seen to be associated with ART, in particular small bowel atresias [49,50] and anorectal atresias [5,49,50], with most studies reporting a three- to four-fold increased risk. Detection of these anomalies is challenging. Many fetuses with distal GI atresias will appear within normal limits at the midtrimester examination, although later in pregnancy most will be detected with routine imaging. While they may be associated with polyhydramnios, as a general rule the more distal the lesion, the less likely it is there will be polyhydramnios given fetal bowel absorption of the GI contents. Most often bowel atresias or strictures present as a tubular cystic structure in the fetal abdomen (Fig. 34.4). On occasion, there will be associated abdominal ascites, which is indicative of bowel rupture. These can be similar in appearance to urogenital abnormalities, such as a dilated ureter, which must be distinguished with real-time imaging.

The data reporting an association of abdominal wall defects are less convincing, with most studies that specifically evaluate this category of anomalies showing a mild increase in risk [49,50]. Screening for these anomalies is straightforward and an integral part of the fetal ultrasound assessment. An axial view through the fetal abdomen at the level of the umbilical cord insertion is sufficient for the detection of most abdominal wall defects. An omphalocele is seen as a mass of variable size at the base of the abdominal cord insertion. It is typically contained within a thick protective membrane and is more solid in appearance than a gastroschisis. In addition, the umbilical arteries are usually able to be seen diverging around the mass as they course into the fetal abdomen. Conversely, a fetal gastroschisis typically herniates to the right of the umbilical cord and freely extrudes into the amniotic cavity without a covering membrane.

Genitourinary anomalies

Similar to gastrointestinal anomalies, those often categorized within the subgroup "genitourinary anomalies" are a heterogeneous group with respect to pathogenesis and therefore vulnerability to any teratogenic effects of ART. There are few data to suggest an increase in renal anomalies or urological tract abnormalities following ART. However, an increased incidence of hypospadias in fetuses conceived via ART has been a fairly consistent finding, with a two- to three-fold increase in risk specifically following ICSI [5,29,49,67]. Ultrasound is poorly sensitive for the detection of this anomaly. Mild hypospadias involving only an abnormal location of the urethral orifice onto the ventral shaft of the penis is unlikely to be detected prenatally. However, more severe hypospadias may present as a micropenis or an abnormally curved appearance.

Other genetic disorders

While most of the above associations are based only upon a superficial categorization of organ systems, other associations have been demonstrated based more upon physiologic mechanisms of pathological disease. For instance, an epigenetic process called imprinting occurs during embryogenesis and entails, for reasons not well understood, one parental gene, maternal or paternal, becoming inactivated by DNA methylation. Maternal imprinting of a gene silences the maternal allele, whereas paternal imprinting silences the paternal allele. The two commonly described examples of this category of genetic disease are Beckwith–Wiedemann syndrome (BWS) and the deletions of a common region on chromosome 15 that lead to either Angelman syndrome or Prader–Willi syndrome. It has been delineated that an allele in a region on chromosome 15 normally undergoes maternal imprinting early in development, thereby silencing the maternal allele. If the corresponding paternal allele is abnormally deleted, the syndrome known as Prader–Willi syndrome develops which is characterized by severe developmental delay, short stature, hypotonia, and obesity. Conversely, a second allele in the same region of chromosome 15 is paternally imprinted, leading to exclusive maternal transcription. When there is a genetic deletion of this maternal allele, Angelman syndrome results characterized by severe developmental delay, ataxic gait, seizure disorder, and inappropriate laughter.

Beckwith–Wiedemann syndrome is another disorder that appears to be related to abnormalities in DNA methylation at imprinting sites of the genome. This syndrome is characterized by organomegaly, macrosomia, macroglossia, omphalocele, and a predisposition to tumors, such as adrenocorticoid

and Wilms tumors, as well as other tumors. The genetic locus implicated in this genetic disease resides on chromosome 11, in close approximation to the WT1 allele. It is theorized that the gene encoding insulin-like growth factor, which resides in this region and normally undergoes maternal imprinting, is abnormally methylated, disturbing the process of imprinting, and the subsequent over expression of maternally derived insulin-like growth factor leads to BWS.

Several studies have described a possible relationship between imprinting disorders and ART [68–74]. These studies are limited to several small series which compared the rate of ART in patients that have diagnosed BWS to the expected rate, as well as questionnaire studies. The strength of this association is, however, fairly constant – around a three- to four-fold increased risk. These studies have not controlled for potentially important confounding variables such as increased maternal or paternal age, increased rates of multiple gestation, and the presence of an underlying diagnosis of infertility. One study which attempted to ascertain the relationship between BWS and infertility specifically concluded the increased risk of BWS following ART could be explained by the concurrent diagnosis of infertility and not necessarily the ART procedures themselves [75]. The largest cohort study, derived from the Danish birth registry, did not support the presence of this association [76]. Clearly, further study is warranted in this highly debated area. Similarly, there are few data regarding the possible association between Angelman syndrome and ART. The data in this area are limited again to small series [77,78].

There are no characteristic findings of Angelman syndrome on ultrasound, and therefore the ability to prenatally diagnose this disease is very limited. BWS, however, may have sonographically evident findings making this syndrome more amenable to prenatal diagnosis. In the midtrimester, the diagnosis is most likely to be suspected because of the discovery of an omphalocele. As the pregnancy progresses, the findings of macroglossia and macrosomia are more likely to be appreciated. Organomegaly, usually involving the kidneys, spleen, liver, pancreas, and/or adrenal glands, can be more challenging to detect during routine ultrasound screening (Fig. 34.5). Given the association of omphalocele with other chromosomal and genetic syndromes, analysis of the fetal karyotype is recommended. The presence of a normal karyotype, particularly in conjunction with other suspicious findings as above, should prompt an evaluation for BWS, which may be confirmed with further genetic testing of the cultured amniocytes.

Other ultrasound considerations

Several other obstetrical outcomes have been associated with ART, which should be considered during prenatal imaging. While an association between ART and multiple gestation is expected to lead to increased growth abnormalities in fetuses of such pregnancies, the association of low birth weight (LBW) with ART even in singletons has been consistently demonstrated [79–85]. Again a limitation of these studies is the relative inability to truly determine a causative relationship with the ART procedures specifically because of the multiple confounding variables. However, many of these cohort studies have controlled for variables such as maternal age, parity, and concurrent conditions and this association has fairly consistently been demonstrated. Whether unknown factors related to both infertility leading to ART and impaired fetal growth exist remains to be determined.

Other obstetrical outcomes, such as a higher rate of preeclampsia, placenta previa, abruption, and preterm delivery,

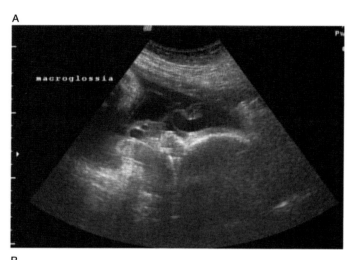

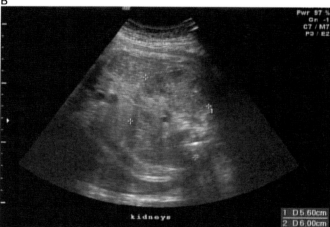

Fig. 34.5 Beckwith–Wiedemann syndrome. (A) Macroglossia. (B) Organomegaly as demonstrated by massively enlarged fetal kidneys that are otherwise normal in appearance.

have also been observed [85,86]. Given these concerns, patients that have undone ART should be considered for serial growth scans to monitor fetal growth and screen for these potential complications of pregnancy.

In conclusion, one of the most important endeavors of a physician is in the area of preventative care. This effort is particularly important when providing care for a woman who desires to conceive. The infertile couple expends a significant amount of time, energy, emotion, and finance to achieve their goal. Therefore, we in the health care industry have an obligation to provide the infertile couple with the appropriate care to assist them in delivering a healthy baby. Preconception care sets the stage for providing this opportunity. An exhaustive discussion of preventative care is beyond the scope of this chapter, though some of the more pertinent aspects should be considered. The prevention of birth defects can include a detailed history to assess for risk factors for genetic disease with genetic counseling as indicated and consideration for preimplantation genetic diagnosis as indicated. Preconceptional workup for underlying conditions known to have a direct impact on embryogenesis such as karyotypical abnormalities or diabetes, for example, should be undertaken. Proactive measures known to reduce birth defects such as administration of vaccines, folic acid supplementation, or aggressive diabetes control should be taken prior to proceeding with ART procedures. Changes in lifestyle can also be vitally important. Embracing weight loss and control of chronic illnesses such as diabetes can make significant differences to patient outcomes. Patients should be encouraged to stop smoking and consuming alcohol during this period. Stress has also been related to poor pregnancy outcome and this risk factor should be discussed with the couple so efforts can be made to alleviate stressful situations [87].

There are significant data available that indicate an increased risk of anomalies in children born after ART (Table 34.1). Whether these anomalies are related to the components of the ART process itself or risk factors inherent to patients undergoing ART remains intensely debated. Fortunately, although the relative risk for many anomalies appears increased as outlined above, given the rarity of the associated anomalies the absolute risk for patients undergoing ART remains small. Therefore, screening for these anomalies is indicated as described above, but this should not be considered a deterrent to those considering ART. Continued research to delineate the nature of the increased risk to guide potential advances in therapeutic techniques is needed.

Table 34.1 Studies of congenital abnormalities after ART

Anomaly	Study	Year	n (total/ART)	Increased risk	Relative risk	Confidence interval/P value
Any fetal malformation						
	Halliday JL	2010	27 784/6 946	Yes	1.36	1.19–1.55
	Shevell T	2005	36 052/1 222	No	0.9	0.4–2.0
	Olson CK	2005	10 227/1 462	Yes	1.3	1.0–1.67
	El-Chaar D	2009	60 170/1 399	Yes	1.55	1.03–2.38
	Dhont M	1999	331 068/5 539	Yes	1.8	1.54–2.10
	Merlob P	1986–94	31 007/278	Yes	2.3	P < 0.0001
	Merlob P	1995–2002	53 208/1 632	Yes	1.75	P < 0.0001
	Hansen M	2002	5 138/1 138[a]			
			IVF vs. NC	Yes	2.14	P < 0.001
			ICSI vs. NC	Yes	2.12	P < 0.001
	Fujii M	2010	55 347/1 408	No	1.15	NS
	Bergh T	1999	1.5 million/5 856	Yes	1.39	1.25–1.54
	Kurinczuk JJ	1997	110 874/420[b]	Yes	2.03	1.4–2.93
Aneuploidy	Halliday JL	2010	27 784/6 946	No	1.09	0.71–1.68
	Hansen M	2002	5 138/1 138[a]			
			IVF vs. NC	Yes	3.5	P = 0.03
			ICSI vs. NC	Yes	5	P = 0.05
	Kim JW[c]	2010	382/254	No		P = 0.503
	Bettio D[d]	2008	277/133	No	0.88	NS
Sex chromosome anomalies	Kim JW	2010	382/254	Yes (with ICSI only)	1.53	1.09–2.14
Imprinting disorders	Doornbos ME	2007	4.0 million/[e]	Yes	6.1	P < 0.001
	Sutcliffe AG	2006	[f]	Yes	2.9	1.4–6.3
	DeBaun MR	2003	[g]/65	Yes	5.75	
	Maher ER	2003	[h]	Yes	3.33	P = 0.009
	Gicquel C	2003	[i]	Yes	3.08	1.5–7.3
	Lidegaard O	2005		No		
Anomaly by organ system						
Neural tube defects						
	Kallen B	2010	689 157/15 570	Yes	4.8	3.3–6.9
	Ericson A	2001	1.7 million/9111	Yes	2.9	1.5–5.1
Anencephaly	Kallen B	2010	689 157/15 570	Yes	7.6	2.5–7.7
	Bergh T	1999	1.5 million/5 856	Yes	12.9	3.5–33.0
Spina bifida	Kallen B	2010	689 157/ 15 570	Yes	5.1	3.4–7.8
	Bergh T	1999	1.5 million/5856	No	2.4	0.9–5.01
Cardiovascular defects						
Any heart defect	Ericson A	2001	1.7 million/9 111	No	1.1	0.9–1.4
	Halliday JL	2010	27 784/6 946	No	1.25	0.88–1.79
	Wen SW	2010	2 954/1 044	Yes	2.75	P < 0.01
	Kallen B	2010	689 157/15 570	Yes	2.1	1.6–2.8
	Bahtiyar MO	2010	749/[g]	Yes	2.52	
	El-Chaar D	2009	61 569	Yes	2.3	1.11–4.77
	Hansen M	2002	5 138/1 138[a]			
			IVF vs. NC	Yes	3	P < 0.001
			ICSI vs. NC	Yes	2.17	

Table 34.1 (cont.)

Anomaly	Study	Year	n (total/ART)	Increased risk	Relative risk	Confidence interval/P value
	Koivurova S	2002	873/304	Yes	4	1.4–11.7
	Kurinczuk JJ	1997	110 874/420[b]	Yes	5.12	2.99–8.77
Septal defects	Tararbit K	2010	9 380/3 847	Yes	1.3	1.0–1.6
	Reefhuis J	2009	4 792/51[j]	Yes	2.7	1.6–4.8
	Kallen B	2010	689 157/ 15 570	Yes	2.6	2.2–3.1
Transposition of the great vessels	Tararbit K	2010	9 380/3 847	No	1.3	0.8–2.3
Tetralogy of Fallot	Reefhuis J	2009	4 792/51[j]	No	2.3	0.7–6.2
Gastrointestinal anomalies						
Any gastrointestinal anomaly	El-Chaar D	2009	61 569	Yes	9.85	3.44–28.44
	Hansen M	2002	5 138/1 138[a]			
	IVF vs. NC			No	1	NS
	ICSI vs. NC			No	1.67	NS
Cleft	Ericson A	2001	1.7 million/9 111	No	1.3	0.8–1.9
	Reefhuis J	2009	4 792/51[j]	Yes	2	1.0–4.0
	Kallen B	2010	689 157/15 570	Yes	2.4	1.9–3.1
	Bergh T	1999	1.5 million/5 856	No	1.3	0.7–2.1
	Kurinczuk JJ	1997	110 874/420[b]	Yes	5.11	1.26–20.80
Ventral wall defects	Ericson A	2001	1.7 million/9 111	Yes	3.3	1.3–6.9
	Kallen B	2010	689 157/15 570	No	1.8	0.9–3.6
	Bergh T	1999	1.5 million/5 856	No	2.3	0.5–6.8
Atresias – esophageal	Ericson A	2001	1.7 million/9 111	Yes	3.5	1.5–6.9
	Reefhuis J	2009	4792/51[j]	Yes	6.8	2.8–15.5
	Kallen B	2010	689 157/15 570	Yes	4	2.6–6.3
	Bergh T	1999	1.5 million/5 856	Yes	3.9	1.4–8.4
Atresia – small gut	Kallen B	2010	689 157/15 570	Yes	6.4	4.2–9.6
Atresias – anorectal	Ericson A	2001	1.7 million/9 111	Yes	3.1	1.3–6.1
	Reefhuis J	2009	4 792/51[j]	Yes	3.4	1.2–8.3
	Kallen B	2010	689 157/ 15 570	Yes	4.7	3.2–6.9
	Bergh T	1999	1.5 million/5 856	No	2.4	0.7–6.2
Genitourinary anomalies						
Any genitourinary anomaly	Hansen M	2002	5 138/1 138[a]			
	IVF vs. NC			Yes	1.86	P = 0.01
	ICSI vs. NC			Yes	1.64	
	Kurinczuk JJ	1997	110 874/420[b]	No	1.33	0.59–2.98
Hypospadias	Kallen B	2010	689 157/15 570	Yes	1.7	1.4–2.1
	Halliday	2010	27 784/6 946	No	1.56	0.93–2.62
	Funke S	2010	15 206/890[b]	Yes	3.97	1.19–13.2
	Reefhuis J	2009	4792/51[j]	Yes	4.6	2.0–10.8
	Ericson A	2001	1.7 million/9 111	Yes	1.5	1.0–2.1
	Bergh T	1999	1.5 million/5 856	No	1.5	0.9–2.3
Musculoskeletal anomalies						
Limb reduction defects	Kallen B	2010	689 157/15 570	No	1.5	0.9–2.5
	Hansen M	2002	5 138/1 138[a]			
	IVF vs. NC			Yes	3	P < 0.001
	ICSI vs. NC			Yes	3	

Table 34.1 *(cont.)*

ART, assisted reproductive technology; IVF, in vitro fertilization; NC, natural conception; ICSI, intracytoplasmic sperm injection; NS, not significant.

[a] Hansen divided into three groups: NC ($n = 4000$)/IVF ($n = 837$)/ICSI ($n = 301$).

[b] ICSI only.

[c] Study by Kim compared three groups after spontaneous abortions: NC ($n = 128$)/IVF ($n = 114$)/ICSI ($n = 140$). The rate of aneuploidy was 48.4, 55.5, and 54.3%, respectively, $P = 0.503$.

[d] Cytogenetic analysis on spontaneous abortions.

[e] The Doornbos study evaluated 71 cases of Beckwith–Wiedemann syndrome versus the Dutch population as a whole.

[f] Sutcliffe studied 79 patients with Beckwith–Wiedemann syndrome, 75 children with Angelman syndrome, and 163 with Prader–Willi syndrome. There was no association of ART with Angelman syndrome or Prader–Willi syndrome.

[g] Study used historical data for control group.

[h] Maher study with 149 children with Beckwith–Wiedemann syndrome, 6 after ART compared to baseline rate of ART in population of 1.2%.

[i] Gicquel studied 149 patients with varying forms of Beckwith–Wiedemann syndrome; 6 had followed ART, for a rate of 4%, which compared to a baseline risk in France of 1.3%.

[j] Reefhuis analyzed data considering singleton or multiple. All results presented correspond only to the singleton pregnancies. There was no increased risk of any of the anomalies studied in multiple pregnancies resulting from ART over natural conception.

References

1. Duwe KN, Reefhuis J, Honein MA, Schieve LA, Rasmussen SA. Epidemiology of fertility treatment use among U.S. women with liveborn infants, 1997–2004. *J Womens Health* 2010; **19**(3): 407–416.

2. Society for Assisted Reproductive Technology and American Society for Reproductive Medicine (ASRM/SART Registry). Assisted reproductive technology in the United States: 1997 results generated from the American Society for Reproductive Medicine/Society for Assisted Reproductive Technology Registry. *Fertil Steril* 2000; **74**(4): 641–653.

3. Shevell T, Malone FD, Vidaver J, et al. Assisted reproductive technology and pregnancy outcome. *Obstet Gynecol* 2005; **106**: 1039–1045.

4. Olson CK, Keppler-Noreuil KM, Romitti PA, et al. *Fertil Steril* 2005; **84**(5): 1308–1315.

5. Reefhuis J, Honein MA, Schieve LA, Correa A, Hobbs CA, Rasmussen SA. Assisted reproductive technology and major structural birth defects in the United States. *Hum Reprod* 2009; **24**(2): 360–366.

6. El-Chaar D, Yang Q, Gao J, et al. Risk of birth defects increased in pregnancies conceived by assisted human reproduction. *Fertil Steril* 2009; **92**(5): 1557–1561.

7. Kallen B, Finnstrom O, Lindam A, Nilsson E, Nygren KG, Otterblad PO. Congenital malformations in infants born after in vitro fertilization in Sweden. *Birth Defects Res A Clin Mol Teratol* 2010; **88**(3): 137–1343.

8. Mayor S. Risk of congenital malformations in children born after assisted reproduction is higher than previously thought. *BMJ* 2010; **340**: c3191.

9. Dhont M, De Sutter P, Ruyssinck G, Martens G, Bekeart A. Perinatal outcome of pregnancies after assisted reproduction: a case-control study. *Am J Obstet Gynecol* 1999; **181**(3): 688–695.

10. Goossens V, Harton G, Moutou C, et al. ESHRE PGD Consortium data collection VIII: cycles from January to December 2005 with pregnancy follow-up to October 2006. *Hum Reprod* 2008; **23**(12): 2629–2645.

11. Merlob P, Sapir O, Sulkes J, Fisch B. The prevalence of major congenital malformations during two periods of time, 1986–1994 and 1995–2002 in newborns conceived by assisted reproduction technology. *Eur J Med Genet* 2005; **48**(1): 5–11.

12. Al-Fifi S, Al-Binali A, Al-Shahrani M, et al. Congenital anomalies and other perinatal outcomes in ICSI vs. naturally conceived pregnancies: a comparative study. *J Assist Reprod Genet* 2009; **26**: 377–381.

13. Hansen M, Kurinczuk J, Bower C, Webb S. The risk of major birth defects after intracytoplasmic sperm injection and in vitro fertilization. *NEJM* 2002; **346**(10): 725–730.

14. Yan J, Huang G, Sun Y, et al. Birth defects after assisted reproductive technologies in China: analysis of 15,405 offspring in seven centers (2004 to 2008). *Fertil Steril* 2011; **95**(1): 458–460.

15. Fujii M, Matsuoka R, Bergel E, van der Poel S, Okai T. Perinatal risk in singleton pregnancies after in vitro fertilization. *Fertil Steril* 2010; **94**(6): 2113–2117.

16. Hansen M, Bower C, Milne E, de Klerk N, Kurinczuk J. Assisted reproductive technologies and the risk of birth defects – a systematic review. *Hum Reprod* 2005; **20**(2): 328–338.

17. Lie R, Lyngstadaas A, Orstavik K, Bakketeig L, Jacobsen G, Tanbo T. Birth defects in children conceived by ICSI compared with children conceived by other IVF-methods; a meta-analysis. *Int J Epidemiol* 2005; **34**: 696–701.

18. Rimm A, Katayama A, Diaz M, Katayama KP. A meta-analysis of controlled studies comparing major malformation rates in IVF and ICSI infants with naturally conceived children. *J Assist Reprod Genet* 2004; **21**(12): 437–443.

19. Hindryckx A, Peeraer K, Debrock S, et al. Has the prevalence of congenital abnormalities after intracytoplasmic sperm injection increased? The Leuven data 1994–2000 and a review of the literature. *Gynecol Obstet Invest* 2010; **70**(1): 11–22.

20. Buckett WM, Chian RC, Holzer H, Dean N, Usher R, Tan SL. Obstetric outcomes and congenital abnormalities after in vitro

maturation, in vitro fertilization and intracytoplasmic sperm injections. *Obstet Gynecol* 2007; **110**(4): 885–891.

21. Knoester M, Helmerhorst FM, Vandenbroucke JP, van der Westerlaken LA, Walther FJ, Veen S. Perinatal outcome, health, growth and medical care utilization of 5- to 8-year old intracytoplasmic sperm injection singletons. *Fertil Steril* 2008; **89**(5): 1133–1146.

22. Palermo GD, Neri Qv, Hariprashad JJ, Davis OK, Veeck LL, Rosenwaks Z. ICSI and its outcome. *Semin Reprod Med* 2000; **18**(2): 161–169.

23. Bonduelle M, Van Assche E, Joris H, et al. Prenatal testing in ICSI pregnancies: incidence of chromosomal anomalies in 1586 karyotypes and relation to sperm parameters. *Hum Reprod* 2002; **17**(10): 2600–2614.

24. Ludwig M, Katalinic A. Malformation rate in fetuses and children conceived after ICSI: results of a prospective cohort study. *Reprod Biomed Online* 2002; **5**(2): 171–178.

25. Ponjaert-Kristoffersen I, Bonduelle M, Barnes J, et al. International collaborative study of intracytoplasmic sperm injection – conceived, in vitro fertilization-conceived and naturally conceived 5-year-old child outcomes: cognitive and motor assessments. *Pediatrics* 2005; **115**: e283–289.

26. Van Steirteghem A, Bonduelle M, Devroey P, Liebaers I. Follow-up of children born after ICSI. *Hum Reprod Update* 2002; **8**(2): 111–116.

27. Sutcliffe AG, Souza SWD, Cadman J, Richards B, McKinlay IA, Lieberman B. Minor congenital anomalies, major congenital malformations and development in children conceived from cryopreserved embryos. *Hum Reprod* 1995; **10**(12): 3332–3337.

28. Chian RC, Huang JY, Tan SL, et al. Obstetric and perinatal outcome in 200 infants conceived from vitrified oocytes. *Reprod Biomed Online* 2008; **16**(5): 608–610.

29. Wennerholm UB, Soderstrom-Anttila V, Bergh C, et al. Children born after cryopreservation of embryos or oocytes: a systematic review of outcome data. *Hum Reprod* 2009; **24**(9): 2158–2172.

30. Wikland M, Hardarson T, Hillensjo T, et al. Obstetrical outcomes after transfer of vitrified blastocysts. *Hum Reprod* 2010; **25**(7): 1699–1707.

31. Belva F, Henriet S, Van den Abbeel E, et al. Neonatal outcome of 937 children born after transfer of cryopreserved embryos obtained by ICSI and IVF and comparison with outcome data of fresh ICSI and IVF cycles. *Hum Reprod* 2008; **23**(10): 2227–2238.

32. Halliday JL, Ukoumunne OC, Baker HW, et al. Increased risk of blastogenesis birth defects, arising in the first 4 weeks of pregnancy, after assisted reproductive technologies. *Hum Reprod* 2010; **25**(1): 59–65.

33. Kushnir VA, Frattarelli JL. Aneuploidy in abortuses following IVF and ICSI. *J Assist Reprod Genet* 2009; **25**(2): 93–97.

34. Kim JW, Lee W, Yoon T, Seok H, Cho J, Kim Y, Lyo S, Shim S. Chromosomal abnormalities in spontaneous abortion after assisted reproductive treatment. *BMC Med Genet* 2010; **11**: 153.

35. Martinez MC, Mendez C, Ferro J, Nicolas M, Serra V, Landeras J. Cytogenetic analysis of early nonviable pregnancies after assisted reproduction treatment. *Fertil Steril* 2010; **93**(1): 289–292.

36. Bettio D, Venci A, Levi Setti PE. Chromosomal abnormalities in miscarriages after different assisted reproduction procedures. *Placenta* 2008; **29**: s126–128.

37. Wu YW, Peng YT, Want B, Zeng YH, Zhuang GL, Zhou CQ. High follicle-stimulating hormone increases aneuploidy in human oocytes matured in vitro. *Fertil Steril* 2011; **95**(1): 99–104.

38. Zhang XY, Ata B, Son WY, Buckett WM, Tan SL, Ao A. Chromosomal abnormality rates in human embryos obtained from in-vitro maturation and IVF treatment cycles. *Reprod Biomed Online* 2010; **21**(4): 552–559.

39. Setti AS, Braga DP, Figueira RD, Azevedo MD, Iaconelli A, Borges E. Are poor responders patients at higher risk for producing aneuploid embryos in vitro? *J Assist Reprod Genet* 2011; **28**(5): 399–404.

40. American Congress of Obstetricians and Gynecologists. Screening for fetal chromosomal abnormalities. *ACPG Practice Bulletin*, Number 77. January 2007.

41. Malone FD, Canick JA, Ball RH, et al. First-trimester or second-trimester screening, or both, for Down's syndrome. *NEJM* 2005; **353**: 2001–2011.

42. Bahado-Singh RO, Wapner R, Thom E, et al. Elevated first-trimester nuchal translucency increases the risk of congenital heart defects. *Am J Obstet Gynecol* 2005; **192**(5): 1357–1361.

43. Makrydimas G, Sotiriadis A, Huggon IC, et al. Nuchal translucency and fetal cardiac defects: a pooled analysis of major fetal echocardiography centers. *Am J Obstet Gynecol* 2005; **192**: 89–95.

44. Barkai G, Goldman B, Reis L, Chaki R, Dor J, Cuckle H. Down's syndrome screening marker levels following assisted reproduction. *Prenat Diagn* 1996; **16**: 1111–1114.

45. Frishman GN, Canick JA, Hogan JW, Hackett RJ, Kellner LH, Saller Jr DN. Serum triple-marker screening in in vitro fertilization and naturally conceived pregnancies. *Obstet Gynecol* 1997; **90**: 98–101.

46. Lam YH, Yeung WS, Tang MH, Ng EH, So WW, Ho PC. Maternal serum alpha-fetoprotein and human chorionic gonadotrophin in pregnancies conceived after intracytoplasmic sperm injection and conventional in vitro fertilization. *Hum Reprod* 1998; **14**: 2120–2123.

47. Maymon R, Dreazen E, Rozinsky S, Bukovsky I, Weinraub Z, Herman A. Comparison of nuchal translucency measurement and mid-gestation serum screening in assisted reproduction versus naturally conceived singleton pregnancies. *Prenatal Diagn* 1999; **19**: 1007–1011.

48. Lancaster PL. Congenital malformations after in-vitro fertilisation. *Lancet* 1987; **330**: 1392–1393.

49. Kallen B, Finnstrom O, Nygren KG, Olausson PO. In vitro fertilization (IVF) in Sweden; risk for congenital malformations after different IVF methods. *Birth Defects Res A Clin Mol Teratol* 2005; **73**(3): 162–169.

50. Ericson A, Kallen B. Congenital malformations in infants born after IVF: a population-based study. *Hum Reprod* 2001; **16**(3): 504–509.

51. Whiteman D, Murphy M, Hey K, O'Donnell M, Goldacre M. Reproductive factors, subfertility, and risk of neural tube defects: a case-control study based on the Oxford Record Linkage Study Register. *Am J Epidemiol* 2000; **152**(9): 823–828.

52. Bonduelle M, Liebaers I, Deketelaere V, et al. Neonatal data on a cohort of 2889 infants born after ICSI (1991–1999) and of 2995 infants born after IVF (1983–1999). *Hum Reprod* 2002; **17**(3): 671–694.

53. Wennerholm UB, Bergh C, Hamberger L, et al. Incidence of congenital malformations in children born after ICSI. *Hum Reprod* 2000; **15**(4): 944–948.

54. Hong-zhen L, Jie Q, Hong-bin C, Xin-na C, Ping L, Cai-hong MA. Comparison of the major malformation rate in children conceived from cyropreserved embryos and fresh embryos. *Chin Med J* 2010; **123**(14): 1893–97.

55. Watson W, Chesier N, Katz V. The role of ultrasound in the evaluation of patients with elevated MSAFP: a review. *Obstet Gynecol* 1991; **78**: 123.

56. Kurinczuk JJ, Bower C. Birth defects in infants conceived by intracytoplasmic sperm injection: an alternative interpretation. *BMJ* 1997; **315**: 1260–1265.

57. Koivurova S, Hartikainen AL, Gissler M, Hemminki E, Sovio U, Jarvelin MR. Neonatal outcome and congenital malformations in children born after in-vitro fertilization. *Hum Reprod* 2002; **17**(5): 1391–1398.

58. Wen SW, Leader A, White RR, et al. A comprehensive assessment of outcomes in pregnancies conceived by in vitro fertilization/ intracytoplasmic sperm injection. *Eur J Obstet Gynecol Reprod Biol* 2010; **150**(2): 160–165.

59. Bahtiyar MO, Campbell K, Dulay AT, et al. Is the rate of congenital heart defects detected by fetal echocardiography among pregnancies conceived by in vitro fertilization really increased? A case-historical control study. *J Ultrasound Med* 2010; **29**(6): 917–922.

60. Tararbit K, Houyel L, Bonnet D, et al. Risk of congenital heart defects associated with assisted reproductive technologies: a population-based evaluation. *Eur Heart J* 2010; **32**(4): 500–508.

61. Williams C, Sutcliffe A, Sebire NJ. Congenital malformations after assisted reproduction: risks and implications for prenatal diagnosis and fetal medicine. *Ultrasound Obstet Gynecol* 2010; **35**: 255–259.

62. Hyett J, Perdu M, Sharland G, et al. Using fetal nuchal translucency to screen for major congenital cardiac defects at 10–14 weeks gestation: population based cohort study. *BMJ* 1999; **318**: 81–85.

63. Hafner E, Schuller T, Metzenvauer M, et al. Increased nuchal translucency and congenital heart defects in a low-risk population. *Prenat Diagn* 2003; **23**: 985–989.

64. AIUM Practice Guideline for the Performance of Fetal Echocardiography. The American Institute of Ultrasound in Medicine. 2010.

65. Abuhamad AZ, Chaoui R. *A Practical Guide to Fetal Echocardiography: Normal And Abnormal Hearts*, 2nd edn. Philadelphia: Lippincott Williams & Wilkins; 2009.

66. Bergh T, Ericson A, Hillensjo T, Nygren KG, Wennerholm UB. Deliveries and children born after in-vitro fertilisation in Sweden 1982–95: a retrospective cohort study. *Lancet* 1999; **354**: 1579–1585.

67. Funke S, Flach E, Kiss I, et al. Male reproductive tract abnormalities: more common after assisted reproduction? *Early Hum Dev* 2010; **86**(9): 547–550.

68. Olivennes F, Mannaerts B, Struijs M, Bonduelle M, Devroey P. Perinatal outcome of pregnancy after GnRH antagonist (ganirelix) treatment during ovarian stimulation for conventional IVF or ICSI: a preliminary report. *Hum Reprod* 2001; **16**(8): 1588–1591.

69. DeBaun MR, Niemitz EL, Feinberg AP. Association of in vitro fertilization with Beckwith-Wiedemann Syndrome and epigenic alterations of *LIT1* and *H19*. *Am J Hum Genet* 2003; **72**: 156–160.

70. Maher ER, Brueton LA, Bowdin SC, et al. Beckwith-Wiedemann syndrome and assisted reproductive technology (ART). *J Med Genet* 2003; **40**: 62–64.

71. Gicquel C, Gaston V, Mandelbaum J, Siffroi JP, Flahault A, Le Bouc Y. In vitro fertilization may increase the risk of Beckwith-Wiedemann Syndrome related to the abnormal imprinting of the *KCNQ1OT* gene. *Am J Hum Genet* 2003; **72**: 1338–1341.

72. Chang AS, Moley KH, Wangler M, Feinberg AP, Dehaun MR. Association between Beckwith-Wiedemann syndrome and assisted reproductive technology: a case series of 19 patients. *Fertil Steril* 2005; **83**(2): 349–354.

73. Sutcliffe AG, Peters CJ, Bowdin S, et al. Assisted reproductive therapies and imprinting disorders – a preliminary British survey. *Hum Reprod* 2006; **21**(4): 1009–1011.

74. Wilkins-Haug L, Porter A, Hawley P, Benson CB. Isolated fetal omphalocele, Beckwith-Wiedemann syndrome, and assisted reproductive technologies. *Birth Defects Res A Clin Mol Teratol* 2009; **85**(1): 58–62.

75. Doornbos ME, Maas SM, McDonnell J, Vermeiden JPW, Henneham CM. Infertility, assisted reproduction technologies and imprinting disturbances: a Dutch study. *Hum Reprod* 2007; **22**(9): 2476–2480.

76. Lidegaard, O, Pinborg A, Andersen AN. Imprinting diseases and IVF: Danish national IVF cohort study. *Hum Reprod* 2005; **20**(4): 950–954.

77. Cox GF, Burger J, Lip V, et al. Intracytoplasmic sperm injection may increase the risk of imprinting defects. *Am J Hum Genet* 2002; **71**: 162–164.

78. Orstavik KH, Eiklid K, van der Hagen CB, et al. Another case of imprinting defect in a girl with Angelman syndrome who was conceived by intracytoplasmic sperm injection. *Am J Hum Genet* 2003; **72**: 218–219.

79. Westergaard HB, Johansen AM, Erb K, Andersen AN. Danish national In-Vitro Fertilization Registry 1994 and 1995: a controlled study of births, malformations and cytogenetic findings. *Hum Reprod* 1999; **14**: 1896–1902.

80. Schieve LA, Meikle SF, Ferre C, Peterson HB, Jeng G, Wilcox LS. Low and very low birth weight in infants conceived with use of assisted reproductive technology. *NEJM* 2002; **346**(10): 731–737.

81. Klemetti R, Gissler M, Hemminki E. Comparison of perinatal health of children born after IVF in Finland in the early and late 1990s. *Hum Reprod* 2002; **17**(8): 2192–2198.

82. Schieve LA, Rasmussen SA, Buck GM, Schendel DE, Reynolds MA, Wright VC. Are children born after assisted reproductive technology at increased risk for adverse health outcomes? *Am J Obstet Gynecol* 2004; **103**(6): 1154–1163.

83. Jackson RA, Gibson KA, Wu YW. Perinatal outcomes in singletons following in vitro fertilization: A meta-analysis. *Am J Obstet Gynecol* 2004; **103**(3): 551–563.

84. Zhu JL, Obel C, Hammer Bech B, Olsen J, Basso O. Infertility, infertility treatment and fetal growth restriction. *Obstet Gynecol* 2007; **110**(6): 1326–1334.

85. Helmerhorst FM, Perquin DAM, Donker D, Keirse M. Perinatal outcome of singletons and twins after assisted conception: a systematic review of controlled studies. *BMJ* 2004; **328**(7434): 261.

86. Pandian Z, Bhattacharya S, Templeton A. Review of unexplained infertility and obstetric outcome: a 10 year review. *Hum Reprod* 2001; **16**(12): 2593–2597.

87. Curtis M, Abelman S, Schulkin J, Williams JL, Fassett EM. Do we practice what we preach? A review of actual clinical practice with regards to preconception care guidelines. *Matern Child Health J* 2006; **10**: S53–58.

Chapter

35

Ultrasound to detect multiple pregnancies after ART

Julie M. Sroga, Carrie Warshak and David F. Lewis

Assisted reproductive technology (ART) is defined as a group of therapies using manipulation of gametes within a laboratory setting in order to achieve pregnancy [1]. The first successful delivery resulting from in vitro fertilization (IVF) in the United States occurred in 1981 with the birth of Elizabeth Carr [2]. Since 1981 the use of ART has steadily increased to 148 055 ART cycles in 2007 resulting in approximately 1% of all births in the United States [3]. ART technologies have vastly improved over the past three decades allowing for higher implantation and delivery rates. More recently, though, investigation has been focusing on the negative outcomes resulting from ART including complications of multiple gestations and ovarian hyperstimulation syndrome [4].

The rate of multiple gestations rose 70% from 1980 to 2004 and the rate of triplet or greater pregnancies increased 400% between 1980 and 1998 [5]. The marked increase, especially of triplet and higher order births, was universally thought to be the result of ART. However, some of the increase is associated with advanced age at childbearing, the greater use of gonadotropins for ovulation induction (OI), as well as the use of controlled ovarian hyperstimulation (COH) to develop two or more follicles using clomiphene citrate [1,5,6]. As of 2004, 35.8% of births resulting from ART were multiples and 3.8% were higher-order multiple births (HOMB) [7]. In response to the increasing complications of multiple gestation and HOMB, the American Society for Reproductive Medicine (ASRM) issued embryo transfer guidelines beginning in 1998. Those guidelines were made more stringent in 1999, recommending that no more than two embryos should be transferred in patients less than 35 years of age with a good prognosis [8]. As of 2001, more than two-thirds of patients had embryo transfers with three or more embryos [1]. By 2008 that number had decreased to only 13% in patients less than 35 years old [3]. The downward trend is reflected in the decrease in HOMB by approximately 20% since 1998, with the twinning rate remaining constant since 2004 [5,9]. Recently the use of elective single embryo transfer (eSET) has been recommended as an option for patients with good prognosis in order to reduce the number of multiple gestations including twins. The process for eSET involves culturing embryos to the blastocyst stage and transferring a single blastocyst into the receptive uterus. Thurin et al. reported pregnancy rates of 42% in double embryo transfer patients versus 38% in eSET patients, with multiple rates of 33.1% versus 0.8%, respectively [10]. Other reports have indicated that eSET may slightly decrease overall pregnancy rates but significantly reduces the rate of twins and HOMB [11].

Twin pregnancies as well as HOMB present unique challenges for both the obstetrician and patient during prenatal care and delivery. Maternal risks include higher incidence of hypertension, anemia, placental abruption, placenta previa, preterm labor, cesarean section delivery, and death [7]. Multiples represent only 3% of live births, but are responsible for 17% of preterm deliveries less than 37 weeks gestation, 23% of preterm deliveries less than 32 weeks gestation, and 26% of very low birth weight deliveries [4]. Neonates are at higher risk for prematurity and subsequently for neurologic impairments, anomalies, and death.

Ultrasound technology has improved immensely over the past several decades and has transformed the obstetric management of multiple gestation pregnancies. First trimester ultrasound following ART procedures allows for early detection of the number and location of gestational sacs as well as viability of each fetus and for determination of the chorionicity and amnionicity of the multiples. An early and complete obstetric ultrasound allows for appropriate testing and management of the pregnancy throughout prenatal care.

Etiology of multiples resulting from ART

Multiple gestations are distinct from singleton pregnancies because two or more fetuses with a single placenta or multiple placentas are present within the pregnant uterus. Zygosity further characterizes these pregnancies. Monozygotic gestations result from a single fertilized embryo splitting to form two or more separate embryos derived from one zygote. In dizygotic or trizygotic (quadzygotic, pentazygotic, etc.) gestations, each embryo is the result of a single sperm fertilizing a single egg. The majority of multiple gestations resulting from ART are multizygotic rather than monozygotic secondary to transferring of multiple fertilized embryos at the time of embryo transfer [12].

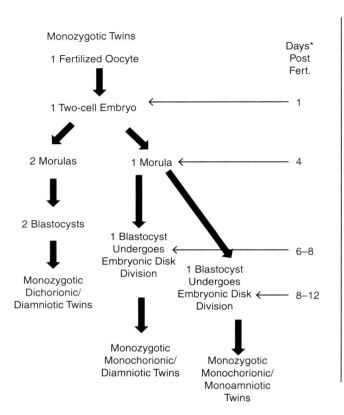

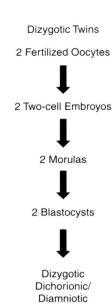

Fig. 35.1 Mechanism of twinning.

The incidence of monozygotic twinning has been reported to be two to twelve times higher than the natural occurrence of 0.4% in spontaneous conceptions [12,13]. In addition, several cases of monozygotic triplets have been reported following ART procedures. At least two cases of monozygotic triplets have been reported following single blastocyst transfer [14]. This increase is thought to be the result of zona pellucida manipulation (assisted hatching) during ART as well as extended culture to the blastocyst stage prior to embryo transfer [12,14].

The type of placentation is most predictive of complications occurring in multiple gestation pregnancies [15,16]. The stage of cleavage of the monozygotic embryo determines the type of placentation (Fig. 35.1). Three types of placentation exist: dichorionic-diamnionic (cleavage occurring days 0–3, about 1/3), monochorionic-diamnionic (cleavage days 4–8, about 2/3), and monochorionic-monoamnionic (occurring days 9–12, less than 1%) [17]. Almost all dizygotic twins have dichorionic-diamnionic placentation. The occurrence of monochorionic dizygotic twins is extremely rare in spontaneous conception [17]. Following ART procedures, a number of reports have noted increased incidence of monochorionic dizygotic twin gestation likely resulting from fusion of the two blastocysts' outer cell mass prior to implantation [17]. The monochorionic placenta, despite zygosity, has an increased rate of pregnancy complications including twin–twin transfusion syndrome (TTTS), congenital anomalies, intrauterine growth retardation (IUGR), and mortality associated with fetal loss [18]. Because the rate of complications in multiple gestations is directly correlated to placentation, an accurate assessment of chorionicity and amnionicity should be performed for all multiple gestations, specifically in the first trimester when diagnosis is most easily made.

Ultrasonography to diagnose and characterize multiple gestations following ART

Components of the first trimester obstetric ultrasound

Technological advances in ultrasonography have allowed obstetricians to detect and characterize multiple gestations within the first trimester and to provide better counseling, surveillance, and testing throughout pregnancy. Prior to routine ultrasound, the majority of multiples were discovered at the time of delivery [19]. Indications for performance of a first trimester ultrasound following ART include: determining the number and location of gestational sacs, confirmation of gestational age following embryo transfer, detection of markers predictive of pregnancy failure, evaluation of maternal vaginal bleeding or pain, visualization of the adnexa, and providing information prior to invasive procedures (e.g. selective reduction or chorionic villus sampling) [20]. In 1967, Kratochwil and Eisenhut reported the first transvaginal ultrasound (TVUS) demonstrating an early intrauterine pregnancy [21]. Since that time, high-resolution ultrasound imaging has enabled sonographers to evaluate in vivo the progression of early human embryologic development. TVUS is superior to transabdominal ultrasound (TAUS) during the early first trimester. Typically with TVUS, structures can be visualized earlier in the pregnancy and with greater accuracy than with TAUS performed at the same time [22].

Every obstetrical scan should start with a complete evaluation of the uterus. This evaluation should be performed by viewing the uterus in multiple planes including sagittal or longitudinal and transverse. Within the sagittal plane, the ultrasound probe should sweep completely from the patient's right to left (or vice versa). Following this evaluation, the probe should be turned to the transverse view and moved from the cervix to the uterine fundus. At the uterine fundus, in the transverse view, again a sweep from right to left should be performed to evaluate both of the cornua. Utilizing this technique allows the sonographer to accurately determine the number and location of intrauterine gestational sacs (Fig. 35.2) but also evaluates for complications including cervical and cornual ectopic pregnancy. Following uterine evaluation, the adnexa should be visualized. In the transverse fundal plane, the ultrasound probe should be moved laterally to both right and left sides to visualize each adnexa. Following a fresh autologous ART cycle, multiple corpus luteal cysts resulting from COH may be present within each ovary, which may also still be enlarged at the time of the first trimester ultrasound. Following embryo transfer with a donor embryo or frozen embryo, typically the corpus luteal cyst is absent from the ovaries, with exogenous progesterone and estrogen administered to provide pregnancy support until the placenta provides these hormones at the 9–10th weeks of gestation [23]. The area adjacent to the ovary and the uterus should be carefully visualized to evaluate for ectopic pregnancies. Complete documentation including measurements of the ovaries and adnexal masses should be performed for monitoring purposes during the pregnancy.

Identifying and evaluating the gestational sac(s)

Structures visualized during the first obstetric ultrasound following ART procedures are determined by the timing of the first ultrasound (Table 35.1). Typically a serum human chorionic gonadotropin (hCG) level is drawn 15–17 days post-oocyte retrieval or 10–15 days post-embryo transfer depending on the stage of embryo transfer. Subsequent ultrasound is performed 1–2 weeks later. Visualization of the gestational sac is the first definitive sign of pregnancy, which should be noted with transvaginal ultrasound (TVUS) between 4.1 and 4.4 weeks of gestational age (GA). The number, location, and character (i.e. regularly shaped or irregularly shaped) of each gestational sac should be documented during the uterine evaluation. Traditionally, the sac closest to the cervix has been identified as A, with each subsequent letter applied to the remaining sacs moving from the cervix to the fundus. Once the number of gestational sacs has been determined, each sac should be evaluated separately for documentation of the early stages of fetal development as well as signs of pregnancy failure.

With TVUS, the secondary yolk sac (SYS) can be seen as early as the beginning of the fifth gestational week and is almost always seen by 5.5 weeks GA [24]. The SYS is the first anatomic structure visualized within the gestational sac. Its presence confirms intrauterine pregnancy as opposed to a pseudosac noted in ectopic pregnancies [25]. Within each sac, the number of SYSs should be documented in each early sonogram up to 10–12 weeks of gestation. After that time the SYS becomes difficult to visualize. The number of SYSs contributes to chorionicity determination during the first trimester. When the mean sac diameter reaches 5–12 mm, typically the embryonic disk of 1–2 mm in length can be observed with TVUS [26]. The number of embryonic disks should be quantified as well as any fetal cardiac activity. Between the fifth and sixth weeks GA, the fetal heart rate can be visualized and is typically slow ranging between 100 and 115 beats per minute (BPM). Then the heart rate increases to 140–170 BPM by 8 weeks of GA [27].

From early ultrasound occurring between 5 and 6 weeks of GA, the final number of embryos and early embryonic structures may not accurately depict the final number of viable fetuses. When ultrasound was performed between 5.0 and 5.9 weeks of GA, Doubliet and Benson found in 325 multiple gestations that 11% of dichorionic twin gestations and 86% of monochorionic twin gestations were initially identified as singletons. Evaluation of higher-order multiples also revealed that 16% of pregnancies were initially undercounted. Therefore if the initial ultrasound following ART therapy is performed between 5.0 and 5.9 weeks, then the number and location of gestational sacs and early embryonic structures should be confirmed with a repeat ultrasound 1–2 weeks later in order to accurately determine the number of viable fetuses as well as the amnionicity and chorionicity [28].

Determining chorionicity and amnionicity

Determining the chorionicity in multifetal pregnancies is extremely important. This procedure is much easier to complete in the first and second trimesters than later in pregnancy. In monozygotic gestations, the type of placentation is determined by the timing of the division of the zygote. Early division (first three days) results in a dichorionic-diamniotic set of monozygotic twins. If the division occurs between 4 and 7 days post-fertilization, then monochorionic-diamniotic twins develop. This is the most common type of monozygotic twins comprising 75% of all monozygotic twins. In monochorionic-monoamniotic twins, the division occurs between 8 and 12 days.

With the advent of high-resolution ultrasound, determining the chorionicity of twins has become much easier (Table 35.2). The lambda sign was first described by Bessis and Papernik in 1981 [29]. This is an echo-dense area between the two layers of the chorion. Later this was called the "twin peak" sign [30]. These two signs are very sensitive in early pregnancy, but this sensitivity decreases dramatically as the pregnancy progresses (Fig. 35.3).

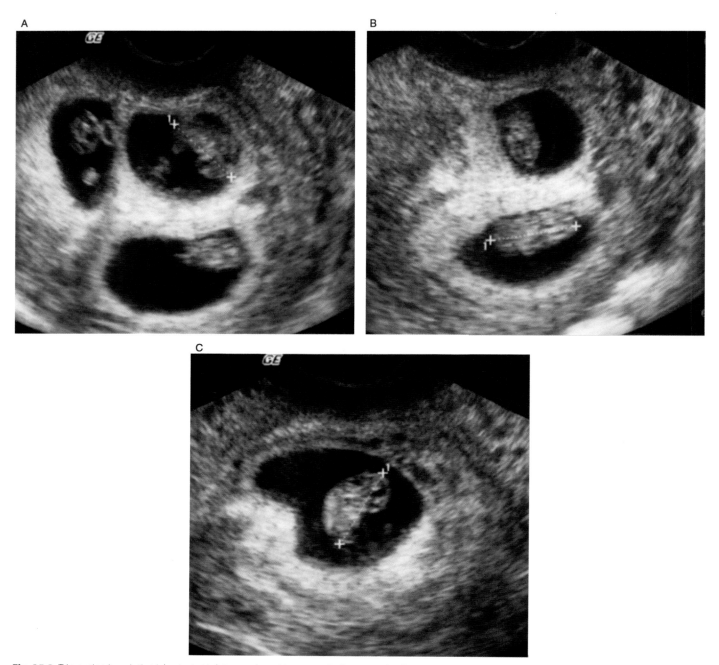

Fig. 35.2 Trizygotic triamniotic trichorionic triplet gestation with transvaginal sonography demonstrating the importance of thorough inspection of all planes for complete visualization. (A) View of all fetuses in a single plane. (B) View of only two fetuses in this plane. (C) Single fetus visualized in this plane.

The dividing membrane in monochorionic gestations has been described with the "T" sign in early pregnancy. This is a thin membrane extending from a single placenta (Fig. 35.4). Both the T sign and the twin peaks sign have been found to be very sensitive in several studies. Wood et al. [31] reported a sensitivity of 94%, a specificity of 88%, a PPV of 97%, and a NPV of 78% in one series for the twin peak sign. Others have had similar results [32]. Similar sonographic evaluation of membrane thickness, and use of lambda and T signs can be applied to higher-order multiple gestations to determine chorionicity and amnionicity (Fig. 35.5).

Other techniques have been described to determine chorionicity, including thickness of the intertwine membrane [33]. Others have suggested counting the layers in the intertwine membrane [34]. Recently vaginal probe ultrasound using 3D imaging has been used, and the results appear promising [35]. This technique can be utilized very early. Large series prospectively collected are lacking utilizing these techniques.

In conclusion, determining the chorionicity in multifetal pregnancies is very important. It is easy to do in early gestation. The "lambda or twin peak" sign can be used to determine a dichorionic pregnancy. In a monochorionic gestation one will

Table 35.1 Components of standard first trimester ultrasound

Structures during first trimester[a]	Gestational age for visualization (weeks)[b]
Gestation sac and location	5.0
Secondary yolk sac (SYS)	5.5
Crown–rump length measurement	6.0
Fetal cardiac activity	6.0–6.5
Fetal number	6.0–6.5
Determining amnionicity and chorionicity of multiples	8.0[c]
Uterus, adnexal, and cul-de-sac evaluation	Each TVUS

[a] Based on American Institute of Ultrasound in Medicine.
[b] Based on Benson, CB, Doubliet PM: Fetal measurements-normal and abnormal growth. In: Rumack CM, Wilson S, Charboneau JW et al. (Eds.) *Diagnostic Ultrasound*, 3rd edn. St. Louis: Elsevier Mosby, 2005, pp. 1493–1512.
[c] Dividing membrane is not typically visualized until 8.0 weeks GA. Based on Bromley B, Benacerraf B. Using yolk sacs to determine amnionicity in early first trimester monochorionic twins. *J Ultrasound Med* 1998; **17**: 199.

see the "T" sign. These two ultrasonographic signs have stood the test of time and appear to have the sensitivity and specificity to help the clinician make this important determination. Diagnosing monochorionic gestations earlier allows obstetricians to change their management plans in extremely high-risk pregnancies.

Complications of ART associated with multiples

Pregnancy loss and multiple gestations following ART

Approximately 10–40% of twin pregnancies result in a singleton live birth [36–38]. This outcome is due to an occurrence known as the "vanishing" twin. The loss or "vanishing" of a fetus can affect twin pregnancies resulting in a singleton as well as higher-order multiple gestations, resulting in the loss of one or more fetuses. Vaginal bleeding does not always accompany the loss of a "vanishing" fetus, and therefore ultrasound surveillance may be the only sign that fetal loss has occurred. The "vanishing" twin phenomenon is more likely to occur in diamnionic monochorionic twins when the initial ultrasound is performed prior to 8 weeks of gestation [39]. Diamnionic dichorionic twins are more likely to result in live birth of two neonates as compared with diamnionic monochorionic twins [39]. Around 10–15% of singletons from IVF were initially noted to be multiple gestations [37,38].

Spontaneous reduction in multiple pregnancies resulting from ART is more evident in iatrogenic pregnancies that typically undergo an earlier TVUS between 5.5 and 6 weeks in order to confirm intrauterine pregnancy. Patients with triplets or more often consider iatrogenic selective reduction procedures which are typically performed between 11 and 13 weeks. The

physician and patient typically make the decision for selective reduction several weeks prior to the timing of the procedure [40]. Repeat ultrasound is important prior to the procedure to determine whether spontaneous reduction has occurred and to decide whether the planned reduction procedure is necessary. The incidence of spontaneous reduction of one or more fetuses prior to the 12th week of gestation occurred in 36% of twin, 53% of triplet, and 65% of quadruplet pregnancies [37]. The spontaneous reduction rate is inversely proportional to gestational age, but directly proportional to maternal age. The frequency of spontaneous loss of one or more gestational sacs was decreased following ovulation induction with clomiphene citrate or gonadotropins without ART and with IVF/gamete intrafallopian tube transfers when compared with spontaneously conceived multiples. However, the incidence of spontaneous loss of singleton gestations was slightly higher following ovulation induction or ART than in spontaneous conceptions [40].

Although complications such as preterm delivery, low birth weight, and very low birth rate in multiple gestation pregnancies are typically inversely related to the number of fetuses, many authors believe that the initial number of implanting sacs may affect outcomes at the time of delivery. Dickey et al. reported that regardless of the final birth number, pregnancy length and birth weight inversely correlated with the initial number of gestational sacs [37]. Luke et al. also reported that pregnancies with three or more initial heartbeats resulting in delivery of twins were more likely to deliver preterm and have lower birth weights than those twin deliveries with only two initial heartbeats [41]. Others have reported that increased incidence of preterm delivery and low birth weight in the surviving twin were only noted when the fetal demise occurred at more than 8 weeks of GA [38]. Authors classified the timing of spontaneous reduction as early (<8 weeks), intermediate (8–21 weeks), or late (>22 weeks) and found that an increased incidence of complications, including delivery prior to 32 weeks, neonatal intensive care stay more than 28 days, and neurological sequelae, were only noted in either intermediate or late loss. In general, if the spontaneous loss of twin occurs prior to 8 weeks of gestation the resulting clinical outcomes are similar for the surviving twin when compared to singletons [19]. In addition, a study investigated the effect of the "vanishing" twin on a first trimester screening test for Down's syndrome and found that testing is equally predictive in spontaneously conceived singletons versus singletons resulting from a spontaneous loss [42]. The "vanishing" gestation phenomenon emphasizes the importance of accurate, thorough, and sequential ultrasound throughout pregnancy in multiple gestations.

Early, high-resolution TVUS has provided fundamental clues about the pathophysiology and epidemiology of early pregnancy loss and given insight into normal and abnormal fetal development. Early ultrasound can evaluate the progression and characterization of embryonic structures once the initial gestational sac is visualized in order to predict the possibility of fetal loss. Once an initial sac is seen, the risk of miscarriage is approximately 11% [43]. The gestational sac grows

Table 35.2 First trimester ultrasonography to determine chorionicity and amnionicity in twins[a]

Placentation	Gestational sacs	Yolk sacs	Embryos/Sacs	Amnionic cavities	T sign	Lambda sign
Dichorionic/Diamnniotic	2	2	1	2	No	Yes
Monochorionic/ Diamnionic	1	2	2	2	Yes	No
Monochorionic/ Diamnionic	1	1/partially divided	2	1	No	No

[a] Based on Egan JFX, Borgida AF: Ultrasound evaluation of multiple pregnancies [19].

A

B

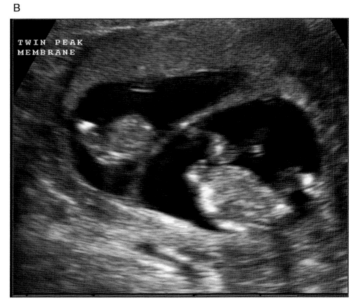

Fig. 35.3 First trimester transvaginal ultrasound image of dichorionic diamniotic twin gestation. (A) Two visible distinct chorionic sacs should be seen by 7 weeks of GA. (B) The lambda or twin peak sign should be visible by 10–14 weeks' gestation. The lambda sign is a triangular projection of tissue with the same echogenicity as the placenta. The thick membrane containing four total layers consists of two chorions sandwiched between two amnions.

at a rate of approximately 1 mm/day in mean diameter. Serial ultrasounds demonstrated slower growth in those pregnancies that ultimately resulted in miscarriage [22]. A smaller than expected gestational sac can also be a predictor of impending pregnancy failure. Studies have also demonstrated that a variety of early gestational sac sizes have been noted in normal early pregnancy. Oh et al. reported in very early pregnancy that gestational sac diameter is not a predictor of outcomes until after 5 weeks of GA [44]. A small gestational sac as a single marker has high variability for prediction of pregnancy failure and is dependent on other factors such as accuracy of pregnancy dating and clinical symptoms of miscarriage [22]. Measurements of the SYS have also been utilized as signs for predicting miscarriage, but their utility is limited. This is supported by the fact that the SYS can persist following embryonic demise. The variation that also occurs in the sonographic measurement and appearance of the SYS in abnormal pregnancies likely results from the embryonic demise itself [22]. Once the fetal pole has developed up to 5 mm in crown–rump length (CRL), the risk of miscarriage decreases to 7.2% and continues to decrease as

the fetal pole grows appropriately [43]. Retarded growth of the embryo once visualized may be associated with increased risk of fetal loss, but evidence is conflicting as is the evidence for gestational sac (GS):CRL ratio for predicting fetal loss [45]. Asynchrony between multiple GS or fetal pole size may also indicate pregnancy failure in one or more of the gestations (Fig. 35.6). Bradycardia and/or abnormal patterns in the fetal heart rate have been associated with fetal demise, specifically if this occurs at 6–8 weeks of GA [46]. Other sonographic findings such as an abnormally shaped GS, abnormal echogenicity of the placenta, or the presence of a subchorionic hematoma (SCH) have all been examined for prediction of miscarriage with variable results. SCH results from blood accumulation between the chorionic membrane and myometrium visualized as a crescent-shaped, echo-free area on ultrasound. Once an SCH is visualized, the risk of miscarriage is 4–33% [47]. Data to understand the natural progression and obstetric outcomes in pregnancies with an SCH are limited. Many of the sonographic findings associated with fetal loss are "soft" markers for prediction of miscarriage when considered in isolation. The physician

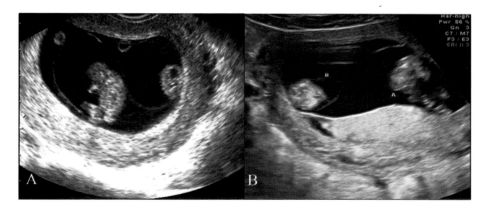

Fig. 35.4 First trimester transvaginal ultrasound image of a monochorionic diamniotic twin gestation. (A) In monochorionic pregnancies, a single chorionic sac can be seen with two visible yolk sacs. Sufficient amniotic fluid should be present by the eighth week for distinct amnions to been seen. (B) The T sign should also be present by 10–14 weeks and is a thin membrane with two layers containing only amnion. Look for the insertion into the chorionic plate at a 90° angle.

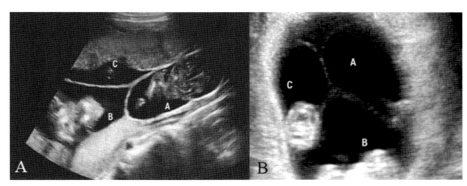

Fig. 35.5 First trimester transvaginal ultrasound image of triplet gestations. (A) Triamniotic trichorionic triplet gestation. Notice the thick membrane containing a chorion and amnion for each fetus. (B) Triamniotic monochorionic triplets with a thin membrane containing only amnion for each fetus.

must evaluate all the ultrasound findings in conjunction with clinical symptoms (e.g. bleeding, pain) to counsel the patient for the risk of loss of one or more embryos as well as to help define the plan of care (e.g. need for selective reduction procedures in HOM pregnancy or dilation and curettage).

Heterotopic pregnancy

Heterotopic pregnancy is defined as the presence of an ectopic pregnancy in conjunction with an intrauterine pregnancy (IUP). The incidence in natural conception is very rare, occurring in only 3.3–6.4 per 100 000 naturally conceived pregnancies [48]. Along with the overall risk of multiple conceptions following ART, the risk of heterotopic pregnancies has also increased to 152 per 100 000 ART pregnancies [49]. This increased incidence is not surprising since many patients undergoing ART have tubal pathology which increases the risk of ectopic pregnancies [50]. The transfer of multiple embryos during ART also contributes to this increased rate. Heterotopic pregnancy can result in serious morbidity for the patient. Due to the presence of an IUP, the diagnosis of heterotopic pregnancy is often delayed. Maternal complications such as tubal rupture, hypovolemia, and blood product transfusions can result. In addition, delay of diagnosis and the resulting maternal sequelae can impact the IUP resulting in fetal loss. Clayton et al. reported that heterotopic pregnancy most likely will result in spontaneous or induced abortion of the intrauterine pregnancy. This conclusion was determined by an analysis of 207 heterotopic pregnancies versus 132 660 intrauterine-only pregnancies [50].

But they also reported that in those heterotopic pregnancies where the IUP continued, the obstetric complications such as preterm birth and low birth weight were not increased.

When a patient presents with pain and a viable IUP, ultrasonic inspection of the adnexa is crucial to the diagnosis and management of heterotopic pregnancy. Visualization of an extrauterine live embryo and an IUP are the most specific findings for the diagnosis. If an extrauterine live embryo is not seen in a pregnant patient with pain then an evaluation of the pelvis for other markers of an ectopic embryo should be performed, including detection of cul-de-sac fluid and/or an adnexal mass. However, it is important to differentiate an ovarian cyst from a tubal mass. A simple apparent anechogenic cyst is unlikely to be an ectopic pregnancy. A corpus luteum can be distinguished from the ectopic ring because the wall is less echogenic than endometrium. Sequential ultrasound and close clinical monitoring will be crucial in making the diagnosis if the ultrasonic findings are not initially diagnostic.

Cervical ectopic is a rare form of ectopic pregnancy, with the overall incidence ranging from 1:2500 to 1:12 000 in spontaneous conceptions [51], but it accounts for 0.1% of ART pregnancies and 3.7% of ART ectopic pregnancies [52]. The presence of a cervical ectopic pregnancy with a viable IUP is extremely rare, but has been demonstrated following ART procedures (Fig. 35.7) [52,53]. This form of ectopic pregnancy is extremely dangerous and can result in delayed diagnosis secondary to the viable IUP. If the diagnosis is delayed, the patient can present with severe maternal hemorrhage requiring emergency hysterectomy, transfusion of blood products, and other morbidities [53]. Termination of the cervical pregnancy is the recommended therapy in order to avoid these morbidities. Earlier sonographic detection of cervical pregnancies has shifted therapy to more conservative approaches including medical therapy alone (methotrexate, potassium chloride [KCl], RU-486) or combined with minimally invasive surgery in order to preserve the uterus for future fertility. Treatment of the cervical ectopic in the presence of a viable IUP in ART patients presents a unique challenge where the physician must weigh the patient's desire for maintaining the viable IUP against the risk of significant morbidity from the cervical ectopic pregnancy. Selective KCl injection of the cervical pregnancy presents the best option for maintaining the IUP, but this therapy can result in the increasing size and vascularity of the placenta or may cause the placenta to behave in a similar way to a placenta accreta resulting in maternal morbidity [54]. Monteagudo et al. reported a case of selected KCl injection of cervical pregnancy while the IUP was delivered at 34 weeks' gestation via cesarean section. The patient received methotrexate post partum until complete resolution of the cervical pregnancy [54]. However, other cases with management of nonviable cervical ectopics resulted in loss of both cervical pregnancy and IUP during monitoring [52,53]. Management of cervical ectopic pregnancy alone or in conjunction with an IUP is best accomplished by early diagnosis with a thorough initial ultrasound, close monitoring of the patient with serial ultrasounds to evaluate progression or resolution of the cervical pregnancy, and appropriate counseling of the patient in order to determine treatment strategy to minimize risks.

Ovarian hyperstimulation syndrome and multiple gestations

Ovarian hyperstimulation syndrome (OHSS) is a rare complication that typically occurs following superovulation with either intrauterine insemination procedures or ART. OHSS can present with moderate or severe symptoms as well as early or late onset after completion of ovarian stimulation. The pathophysiological hallmark of OHSS is increased vascular permeability allowing for redistribution of intravascular fluid into third-space compartments [55]. Moderate symptoms include nausea, vomiting, tissue fluid accumulation, and weight gain. Decreased urine output, shortness of breath, and venous thromboembolism are associated with severe OHSS and typically require hospitalization for close monitoring and supportive care of the patient [55,56]. Risk factors for OHSS include a large number of follicular cysts, elevated estradiol, young age, polycystic ovarian syndrome, and previous history of OHSS [55]. After the evaluation of 214 219 ART cycles, Luke et al. [56] reported that patients with OHSS are 1.98 times more likely to achieve live birth and those with severe OHSS are 2.68 more likely to have a live birth. Furthermore, those with OHSS were 58% more

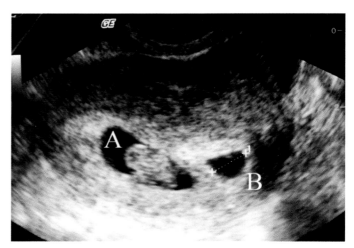

Fig. 35.6 Transvaginal ultrasound 6 weeks following embryo transfer of two cleavage-stage embryos. Image shows viable 8 weeks' gestation (A) and second empty gestational sac (B).

likely to have a multiple gestation. If the patients experienced severe OHSS, 86% were more likely to have a multiple gestation [56]. OHSS is also associated with higher rates of complications including fetal loss, low birth weight, and preterm birth [56]. Cycles resulting in pregnancy often prolong symptoms of OHSS [55]. Patients diagnosed with OHSS must be closely followed for signs of worsening disease state as well as monitoring of the viability of any fetuses. Typical ultrasound findings include pelvic and abdominal ascites in addition to enlarged ovaries with multiple corpus luteum cysts. Interventions including hospitalization, paracentesis, or thoracocentesis are determined by the clinical state of the patient and her symptoms rather than by ultrasound findings. Since patients with multiple gestations are at higher risk of developing OHSS and complications affecting the pregnancy, the reproductive endocrinologist should attempt to minimize OHSS by decreasing the number of embryos transferred or transferring no embryos during the fresh cycle in patients with risk factors for OHSS.

Conclusion

ART procedures have allowed couples who previously were unable to conceive the opportunity for conception by overcoming obstacles such as tubal occlusion or severe male-factor infertility. As technologies have improved for optimizing pregnancy rates with ART, so have the risks of twins, higher-order multiple gestations, and complications including heterotopic pregnancy and OHSS. In the future, the increased use of eSET with improved embryo culture may help to continue to reduce the incidence of multiples following ART. Until that time, early and sequential transvaginal ultrasound is the reproductive endocrinologist's and obstetrician's best tool for appropriate diagnosis and management of multiple gestations and complications resulting from ART.

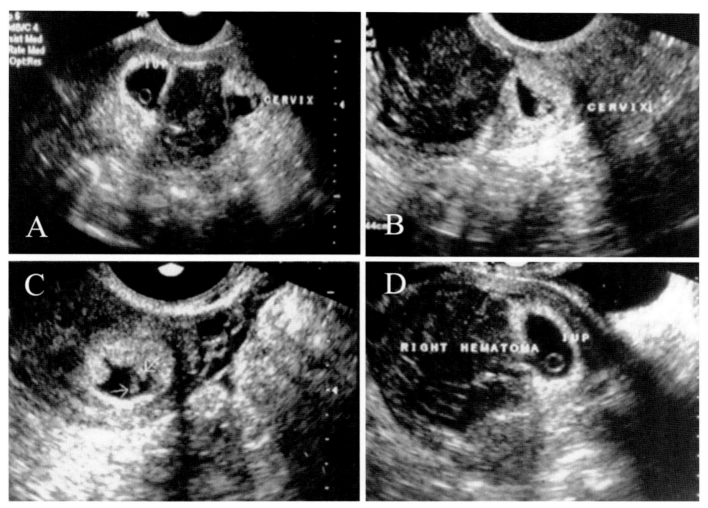

Fig. 35.7 Transvaginal sonography. (A) Sagittal view of intrauterine pregnancy with subchorionic hematoma and heterotopic cervical pregnancy. (B) Sagittal view of cervical pregnancy with fetal pole. (C) Oblique view of cervical gestational sac with two fetal poles (arrows). (D) Transverse view of subchorionic hematoma in conjunction with IUP. (With kind permission from Springer Science+Business Media: *Journal of Assisted Reproduction and Genetics*, Combined intrauterine, tubal, and cervical pregnancies following in vitro fertilization and embryo transfer, Vol. **18**; 2001, p. 350, Mor E, Lindheim SR, Lerner J, Sauer MV, Figure 1.)

References

1. Wilson EE. Assisted reproductive technologies and multiple gestations. *Clin Perinatol* 2005; **32**: 315–328.

2. Jones Jr HW, Jones GS, Andrews MC, et al. The program for in vitro fertilization at Norfolk. *Fertil Steril* 1982; **34**: 14–21.

3. CDC, American Society for Reproductive Medicine, Society for Assisted Reproductive Technology. *2007 Assisted Reproductive Technology Success Rates: National Summary and Fertility Clinic Reports.* Atlanta: US Department of Health and Human Services, Centers for Disease Control and Prevention; 2009.

4. Van Voorhis BJ. Outcomes from assisted reproductive technology. *Obstet Gynecol* 2006; **107**: 183–200.

5. Martin JA, Hamilton BE, Sutton PD. Births: Final Data for 2007. *National Vital Statistics Reports* 2010; **58**: 1–86.

6. Dickey R. The relative contribution of assisted reproductive technologies and ovulation induction to multiple births in the United States 5 years after the Society for Assisted Reproductive Technology/American Society for Reproductive Medicine recommendation to limit the number of embryos transferred. *Fertil Steril* 2007; **88**: 1554–1561.

7. Rebar RW, DeCherney AH. Assisted reproductive technology in the United States. *N Engl J Med* 2004; **350**: 1603–1604.

8. American Society for Reproductive Medicine. *Guidelines on Number of Embryos Transferred.* Birmingham (AL): American Society for Reproductive Medicine; 1999.

9. Jain T, Missmer S, Hornstein M. Trends in embryo-transfer practice and outcomes of the use of assisted reproductive technology in the United States. *N Engl J Med* 2004; **350**: 1639–1645.

10. Thurin A, Hausken J, Hillensjo T, et al. Elective single-embryo transfer versus double-embryo transfer in in vitro fertilization. *N Engl J Med* 2004; **351**: 2392–2402.

11. Pandian Z, Bhattacharya S, Ozturk O, et al. Number of embryos for transfer following in-vitro fertilization or intra-cytoplasmic sperm injection. *Cochrane Database Syst Rev* 2009; **15**: CD003416.

12. Aston KI, Peterson CM, Carrell DT. Monozygotic twinning associated with assisted reproductive technologies: a review. *Reproduction* 2008; **136**: 377–386.

13. Chang HJ, Lee JR, Jee BC, et al. Impact of blastocyst transfer on offspring sex ratio and the monozygotic twinning rate: a systematic review and meta-analysis. *Fertil Steril* 2008; **91**: 2381–2390.

14. Dessolle L, Allaoua D, Freour T. Monozygotic triplet pregnancies after single blastocyst transfer: two cases and literature review. *Reprod BioMed Online* 2010; **2**: 283–289.

15. Carroll SGM, Soothill PW Abdel-Fattah SA, et al. Prediction of chorionicity in twin pregnancies at 10–14 weeks of gestation. *Br J Obstet Gynecol* 2002; **109**: 182–186.

16. Dube J, Dodds L, Armson BA. Does chorionicity or zygosity predict adverse perinatal outcomes in twins? *Am J Obstet Gynecol* 2002; **186**: 579–583.

17. Miura K, Niikawa N. Do monochorionic dizygotic twins increase after pregnancy by assisted reproductive technology? *J Hum Genet* 2005; **50**: 1–6.

18. Hall JG. Twinning. *Lancet* 2003; **362**: 735–743.

19. Egan JFX, Borgida AF. Ultrasound evaluation of multiple pregnancies. In: Callen PW (edr.) *Ultrasonography in Obstetrics and Gynecology*, 5th edn. Philadelphia: Saunders Elsevier; 2008: 266–296.

20. American Institute of Ultrasound in Medicine: AIUM Practice Guideline for the performance of an antepartum obstetric ultrasound examination. *J Ultrasound Med* 2010; **29**: 157–166.

21. Kratochwil A, Eisenhut L. The earliest detection of fetal heart activity by ultrasound. *Geburtshilfe Frauenheikd* 1967; **27**: 176–180.

22. Jauniaux E, Johns J, Burton GJ. The role of ultrasound imaging in diagnosing and investigating early pregnancy failure. *Ultrasound Obstet Gynecol* 2005; **25**: 613–624.

23. Mesiano S. The endocrinology of human pregnancy and fetoplacental neuroendocrine development In: Strauss J, Berbieri R, eds. *Yen and Jaffe's Reproductive Endocrinology*, 6th edn. Philadelphia: Saunders Elsevier; 2009: 248–281.

24. Levi CS, Lyons EA, Lindsay DJ. Early diagnosis of nonviable pregnancy with transvaginal US. *Radiology* 1988; **167**: 383–385.

25. Rowling SE, Langer JE, Coleman BG, et al. Sonography during early pregnancy: Dependence of threshold and discriminatory values on transvaginal transducer frequency. *AJR Am J Roentgenol* 1999; **172**: 983–988.

26. Hadlock FP, Shah YP, Kanon DJ, et al. Fetal crown-rump length: reevaluation of relation to menstrual age (5–18 weeks) with high-resolution real-time US. *Radiology* 1992; **182**: 501–505.

27. Doubliet PM, Benson CB. Outcome of first-trimester pregnancies with slow embryonic heart rate at 6–7 weeks gestation and normal heart rate by 8 weeks at US. *Radiology* 2005; **236**: 643–646.

28. Doubliet PM, Benson CB. "Appearing twin": undercounting of multiple gestation on early first trimester sonograms. *J Ultrasound Med* 1998; **17**: 199–203.

29. Bessis R, Papernik E. Echographic imagery of amniotic membranes in twin pregnancies. *Twin Research 3: Twin Biology and Multiple Pregnancy*. New York: Alan R. Liss;183–187: 1981.

30. Finberg HJ. The twin peak sign: reliable evidence of dichorionic twinning. *J Ultrasound Med* 1992; **11**: 571–577.

31. Wood SL, St Onge R, Connors G, Elliot PD. Evaluation of the twin peak or lambda sign in determining chorionicity in multiple pregnancy. *Obstet Gynecol* 1996; **88**: 6–9.

32. Kurtz AB, Wapner RJ, Mata J, Johnson A, Morgan P. Twin pregnancies: accuracy of first trimester abdominal US in predicting chorionicity and amnionicity. *Radiology* 1992; **185**: 759–762.

33. Winn HN, Gabrielli S, Reece EA, Roberts JA, Salafia C, Hobbins JC. Ultrasonographic criteria for the prenatal diagnosis of placental chorionicity in twin gestations. *Am J Obstet Gynecol* 1989; **161**: 1540–1542.

34. Monteagudo A, Timor-Tritsch IE. Second and third trimester ultrasound evaluation of chorionicity and amnionicity in twin pregnancy – a simple algorithm. *J. Reprod Med* 2000; **45**: 476–479.

35. Babinszki A, Mukherjee T, Kerenyi T, Berkowitz RL, Copperman AB. Diagnosing amnionicity at 6 weeks of pregnancy with transvaginal three-dimensional ultrasonography: case report. *Fertil Steril* 1999; **71**: 1161–1164.

36. Landy HJ, Weiner S, Corsno SL, et al. The "vanishing twin": ultrasonographic assessment of fetal disappearance in the first trimester. *Am J Obstet Gynecol* 1986; **155**: 14–19.

37. Dickey RP, Taylor SN, Lu PY, et al. Spontaneous reduction of multiple pregnancy: incidence and effect on outcome. *Am J Obstet Gynecol* 2002; **78**: 77–83.

38. Pinborg A, Lidegaard O, la Cour Freiesleben N, et al. Consequences of vanishing twins in IVF/ICSI pregnancies. *Hum Reprod* 2005; **20**: 2821–2829.

39. Benson CB, Doubliet PM, Laks MP. Outcome of twin gestations following sonographic demonstration of two heart beats in the first trimester. *Ultrasound Obstet Gynecol* 1993; **1**: 343–345.

40. Dickey RP. Embryonic loss in iatrogenic multiples. *Obstet Gynecol Clin N Am* 2005; **32**: 17–27.

41. Luke B, Brown M, Grainger D. The effect of early fetal losses on twin assisted-conception pregnancy outcomes. *Fertil Steril* 2009; **91**: 2586–2592.

42. Gjerris AC, Loft A, Pinborg A. The effect of a 'vanishing twin' on biochemical and ultrasound first trimester screening makrers for Down's syndrome in pregnancies conceived by assisted reproductive technology. *Hum Reprod* 2009; **24**: 55–62.

43. Goldstein SR, Wolfson R. Transvaginal ultrasonographic measurement of early embryonic size as a means of assessing gestational age. *J Ultrasound Med* 1994; **12**: 27–31.

44. Oh JS, Wright G, Coulam CB. Gestational sac diameter in very early pregnancy as a predictor of fetal outcome. *Ultrasound Obstet Gynecol* 2002; **20**: 267–269.

45. Choong S, Rombaust L, Ugoni A, et al. Ultrasound prediction of risk of spontaneous miscarriage in live embryos from assisted conceptions. *Ultrasound Obstet Gynecol* 2003; **22**: 571–577.

46. Benson CB, Doubliet PM. Slow embryonic heart rate in early first trimester: indicator of poor pregnancy outcome. *Radiology* 1994; **192**: 343–344.

47. Pearlston M, Baxi L Subchorionic hematoma: a review. *Obstet Gynecol Surv* 1993; **48**: 65–68.

48. Richards SR, Stempel LE, Carlton BD. Heterotopic pregnancy: reappraisal of incidence. *Am J Obstet Gynecol* 1982; **112**: 928–930.

49. Clayton HB, Schieve LA, Peterson HB, et al. Risk of ectopic pregnancy among women who underwent ART, United State, 1999–2001. *Obstet Gynecol* 2006; **107**: 595–604.

50. Clayton HB, Schieve LA, Peterson HB, et at. Risk of heterotopic and intrauterine-only pregnancy outcomes after assisted reproductive technologies in the United State, 1999–2002. *Fertil Steril* 2007; **87**: 303–309.

51. Ushakov FB, Elchalal U, Aceman PJ, et al. Cervical pregnancy: past and future. *Obstet Gynecol Surv* 1997; **52**: 45–59.

52. Mor E, Lindheim SR, Lerner J, et al. Combined intrauterine, tubal, and cervical pregnancies following in vitro fertilization and embryo transfer. *J Assist Reprod Genet* 2001; **18**: 349–351.

53. Fruscalzo A, Mai M, Lobbeka K, et al. A combined intrauterine and cervical pregnancy diagnosed in the 13th gestational week: which type of management is more feasible and successful? *Fertil Steril* 2008; **89**: 456.e13–16.

54. Monteagudo A, Tarricone NJ, Timor-Tritsch ET, Lerner JP. Successful transvaginal ultrasound-guided puncture and injection of a cervical pregnancy in a patient with simultaneous intrauterine pregnancy and a history of a previous cervical pregnancy. *Ultrasound Obstet Gynecol* 1996; **8**: 381–386.

55. The Practice Committee of the American Society for Reproductive Medicine. Ovarian hyperstimulation syndrome. *Fertil Steril* 2008; **90**(S3): S188–193.

56. Luke B, Brown M, Morbeck D, et al. Factors associated with ovarian hyperstimulation syndrome (OHSS) and its effect on assisted reproductive technology (ART) treatment and outcome. *Fertil Steril* 2010; **94**: 1399–1404.

Ultrasound and pregnancy outcome after ICSI

Ehab Abu Marar

Intracytoplasmic sperm injection (ICSI), being injection of spermatozoa inside the mature oocyte microscopically, is an idea which came to assisted reproduction technology (ART) after it was found that the fertilization rate was low with the conventional in vitro fertilization (IVF) method. The importance of ICSI became apparent during the 1960s when different groups were investigating whether fertilization rates could be improved by directly injecting spermatozoa into the unfertilized oocyte; in animal experiments some groups, but not others, were able to show that they could be improved. Yanagimachi and his team demonstrated at the animal model level that hamster nuclei can develop into pronuclei after microinjection into homologous eggs, and a similar result was obtained when freeze-dried human spermatozoa were injected into a hamster egg [1].

After the noteworthy success of ART, clinicians started thinking out about how to bypass the difficulties confronting their aim of successful oocyte fertilization. This appeared to be a paramount necessity especially after the disappointing results obtained with the procedures of zona drilling, partial zonal dissection (PZD), and subzonal sperm injection (SUZI). A successful human ICSI technique was first developed in the early 1990s at Free University of Brussels, Belgium, by Palermo under the supervision of Van Steirteghem and Devroey [2,3]. Cases which had a limited number of progressively motile spermatozoa with normal morphology were extensively investigated for help, but faced the risk of an increasing incidence of congenital abnormalities. The predominant usage of ICSI in cases of severe male subfertility was confronted by the hypothesis that impaired morphology and motility or immature spermatozoa might lead to a higher risk of congenital abnormalities.

Aside from that, the introduction of ICSI opened the way for other developments such as the use of epididymal and testicular spermatozoa extraction followed by ICSI, leading to a significant improvement in results in many cases that represented a big challenge for fertility specialists. Cases such as azoospermia, whether obstructive or non-obstructive, have the advantage of being in one way or another independent of the three main semen parameters, which are number, morphology, and motility of spermatozoa, as reported by Nagy et al.

[4], who achieved a high fertilization rate in cases of extreme male-factor infertility.

Some authors started to compare the outcomes after ICSI with those after IVF, believing that any new method should be investigated and compared with existing ones before being extensively applied. However, some authors considered this comparison unfair because IVF cases are a heterogeneous group of patients and both partners are usually infertile, whereas ICSI cases are an almost entirely homogeneous group as the female partners are often fertile [5]. Concerning the pregnancy characteristics and perinatal outcome issue, Govaerts et al. [6] concluded that there is no rise in the number of pathologies after ICSI compared with IVF. They found no ectopic pregnancies in the ICSI group in their study, suggesting that the finding of ectopic pregnancy cases by other investigators supports the idea that tubal damage is the underlying cause of infertility itself. Concerning the safety of ICSI, Govaerts et al. also found that the rate of pregnancy complications including prematurity, low birth weight, small for gestational age, and hypertension in singleton pregnancies is comparable in ICSI and in the general population. Furthermore, congenital malformations and karyotype abnormalities were no more frequent in the ICSI group than the IVF group.

Other authors focused on other aspects such as the continuity of ICSI evaluation. Taking the cumulative delivery rates post-ICSI procedure as a parameter for consideration, and for patient counseling purposes, Osmanagaoglu et al. [7] carried out a retrospective study of 498 infertile Belgian women. They performed a 5-year follow-up of the women, who were <37 years old at the time of their first ICSI cycle, and all the ICSI cycles in this study used oocyte retrieval and fresh ejaculated spermatogen. Their outcome measure was any delivery after 25 weeks gestation after categorizing them into groups according to age. The number of analyzed cycles was 963; drop-out rates increased as the number of cycles increased (drop-out rate was 20% per cycle until the fifth cycle, increasing to more than 30% after that). The mean delivery rate per cycle was found to be 31%. For all patients, the average number of cycles required for delivery was 3.15. The increment of cumulative delivery rate was seen in the first three cycles, reaching a plateau by the sixth cycle. The real delivery rate after six cycles was 60%, whereas the expected was 86%. With increasing age of the female partner, the pregnancy rate decreased significantly, whereas sperm quality had no influence on the rate of delivery.

Referring to the cumulative ongoing pregnancy rate in ICSI cycles, Jee et al. [8] performed a study over a period of 6 years on 260 infertile couples considering the ongoing pregnancy as one maintained until 12 weeks of gestation and their results demonstrated an overall ongoing pregnancy rate of 13.5% per cycle and 26.9% per couple. Cumulatively, an increment in the ongoing pregnancy rate could be achieved if the number of cycles increased, rising from 15% after one cycle to 54.9% after six cycles, but no further increase was detected after seven cycles. Again, age was an adverse factor as the cumulative ongoing pregnancy rate decreased with increasing female partner age after five consecutive cycles. The rate was found to be 61.8% in women at 30 years old or less, decreasing to 51.7% in women between 31 and 35 years old, and to 15.3% in women aged 36 years or more. The decline in the success rate with advancing age was attributed to embryonic aneuploidy, decreased ovarian responsiveness to gonadotropins, and low embryo implantation rate in older women. The sperm origin did not affect the outcome of ICSI as regards cumulative ongoing pregnancy rate.

It should also be mentioned that the low success rate found by some researchers after ICSI was correlated to the fact that cases of ICSI were done after failed conventional IVF, a fact that adversely affects ICSI results in general.

Devroey et al. [9] presented a case-controlled study of 71 women ≥40 years old, who were compared to women <40 years old, both groups undergoing ICSI and having similar semen characteristics; the authors concluded that for embryonic implantation prediction, female age is a negative factor. They found that the number of cumulus cells, replaced embryos, implantation rate, and delivery rate were all lower in the older age group.

Aytoz et al. [10], in a retrospective study, investigated the effect of sperm origin and quality on pregnancy outcome after ICSI. The study was conducted on pregnant patients who conceived after ICSI of ejaculated, epididymal, and testicular sperm. Results in the ejaculated sperm group indicated that more intrauterine deaths occurred when sperm had severe defects, whereas fewer intrauterine deaths were found in the moderately defective sperm groups. In addition, the rate of multiple pregnancy, preterm deliveries, low birth weight deliveries, and early perinatal mortality were found to be higher after ICSI than after natural conception. Also perinatal deaths and very low birth weight infants were significantly lower in the ejaculated sperm group than in the epididymal sperm group (5.5–9.1% vs. 20.3%; $P = 0.001$, and 1.1–1.3% vs. 11.9%; $P < 0.001$, respectively).

Before starting treatment for infertility, many factors have to be considered such as the infertility background, the hormonal stimulation protocol and its effects, and the exposure to prematurity and low birth weight. In the Netherlands the

perinatal outcome in singletons was assessed by Knoester et al. [11], who demonstrated their experience in a follow-up study, through focusing on pregnancy and perinatal outcome, congenital malformations and dysmorphic features, general health, growth, and medical care deployment up to the age of 5–8 years between ICSI, IVF, and natural conception groups of children. They selected ICSI-conceived singletons, and collected information about their general health, the pregnancy course, and birth-related issues through a questionnaire. Concerning the children's physical examination, an investigator and geneticist, who were blinded to the mode of conception, counted and categorized the congenital malformations according to whether they were minor or major, and the dysmorphic features as well. However, they found a similarity in distribution of pregnancy complications between the IVF and ICSI groups except for gestational diabetes, which was found to be greater in the IVF group than the ICSI group ($P = 0.04$). Prematurity and the vanishing twin syndrome, which were more frequent in the ICSI group, played a major role in making a difference between the ICSI and the natural conception group, and birth weight was again found to be lower in the ICSI than the natural conception group. The birth parameters were similar in IVF and ICSI groups. The prevalence of minor malformations and dysmorphic features did not differ between the three groups. Estimation of major malformations was not possible due to the small size of the cohorts. The authors found that ICSI children did not differ from other groups in general health up to examination at 5–8 years. They stated that all IVF-born children, whether with or without ICSI, need more medical care, pointing out that multiple birth, prematurity, fertility background, and higher parental concern might be the causes, rather than the IVF procedure itself. They concluded that in a comparison of ICSI and IVF singletons at 5–8 years old, no risk increment was found regarding pregnancy, perinatal period, congenital malformations, general health, growth, and medical care provided. On top of that, ICSI children were found to be prone to less favorable perinatal outcomes than natural-conception children, although both groups had a similar long-term outcome.

Lewis and Klonoff-Cohen [12] reviewed the literature concerning ICSI adverse outcomes and factors affecting its success. They pointed out what other authors [13] had drawn attention to, that in bypassing a critical step in the fertilization process, ICSI throws out the spontaneous selective process done by sperm, speculating that doing so might lead to transmission of defective genetic material. However, Lewis and Klonoff-Cohen postulated that there was no conclusive evidence that congenital malformations were found more frequently after ICSI than after spontaneous conception. They also drew attention to the procedural effects on outcome after ICSI, finding that the quality and quantity of the oocyte plays a major role in that regard rather than the ICSI procedure itself. No difference was found between the uses of fresh or frozen-thawed spermatozoa. In contrast to that, advanced maternal age has been found to have a detrimental effect on ICSI outcome in a direct and indirect way. Alrayyes et al. [14] compared women with an age cut-off of 37 years. In their study, 39% of older women were found to produce fewer than three embryos, the factor that considerably lowers fertilization, pregnancy, and implantation rates in older women. Women less than 37 years old had higher implantation when compared with those aged 37 years or more (11.4% vs. 6.6%; $P = 0.02$), higher pregnancy rate (47% vs. 26%; $P = 0.004$), and higher ongoing pregnancy rates (40% vs. 19%; $P = 0.004$). They also assumed that the two main sperm parameters affecting ICSI outcome are sperm motility and morphology, though data in that regard are controversial. Finally they concluded that to date the long-term prognosis of ICSI-conceived children is promising as most studies on this subject do not report higher congenital abnormalities, developmental delay, or lower intelligence. Some studies have demonstrated a link between de novo chromosomal aberrations and ICSI. However, the only factor that permanently worsens ICSI outcome to date is maternal age.

Fauque et al. [15] studied embryo quality to demonstrate whether pregnancy outcome and live birth after IVF and ICSI could be affected accordingly. Characterization of embryos having the highest implantation chances contributed significantly in the analysis of homogeneous embryo transfers, the definition of homogeneous transfer being the transfer of embryos with similar morphology. After scoring the blastomeres, the authors observed that implantation and birth rates were increased when four-cell embryos were transferred on day 2, in contrast with those embryos having more or less blastomeres transferred on the same day. They elucidated that embryo quality is of utmost importance in determining pregnancy and implantation rate, and that live birth capability and pregnancy outcome is dependent on the embryo cleavage stage as well as the integrity of blastomeres on the second developmental day. Consequently, too rapid or too slow cleavage during the first two days of development might negatively affect the chances of implantation. The morphological aspects of the early embryo affect the implantation rate and pregnancy outcome, with higher birth rates after transfers of four-cell embryos with low fragmentation.

A Swedish group including Hamberger [16] illustrated the indications for ICSI after dividing them into non-existent, relative, and absolute. They also demonstrated the benefit of presenting the IVF method as first choice in cases of total sperm count exceeding 0.8 million and morphology of >5% normal forms, or normal semen analysis. The combination of IVF and ICSI was pointed out in cases of total sperm count of <0.8 million or morphology of <5% normal forms, not dropping the idea that such split technique is done as long as oocyte number exceeds 10. ICSI was strongly recommended by them in cases of no or poor fertilization following two IVF cycles, epididymal/testicular spermatozoa, globozoospermia, immotile spermatozoa, poor survival frozen–thawed spermatozoa, and cases necessitating preimplantation genetic diagnosis (PGD), as spermatozoa stuck to the zona pellucida during conventional IVF may contaminate the biopsy taken.

Congenital abnormalities in ICSI children

The assumption that ICSI increases the risk of congenital abnormalities has been disputed by some authors such as Wennerholm et al. [17], who investigated 210 infants in an observational study conducted in Sweden and found that ICSI has a lower risk than other IVF techniques not associated with it, regarding congenital malformations. Because of the paramount importance gained by ICSI in fertility treatment worldwide, and more specifically in cases related to severe male infertility, its safety has been regularly assessed.

After 7 years of using ICSI, Bonduelle et al. [18], presented their team's work associated with follow-up of 1987 children at 2 months, 1 year, and 2 years. They did not find a higher incidence of any malformations in children born by ICSI compared with children born by natural conception. They suggested that chromosomal aberrations might be considered as a consequence post-oligoasthenoteratozoospermia, which per se has a high frequency of chromosomal aberrations, and so is categorized as a risk factor for ICSI. Their figure of a 2.3% malformation rate was within the expected range when compared to registers of children born after assisted reproduction and registers of general population malformations in the late 1990s. However, they referred to the neonatal data stating that prematurity, low birth weight, and very low birth weight are caused mainly by multiple pregnancy itself. Included was a counseling message to reassure patients planning to undergo fertility treatment that there was not higher incidence of congenital malformations in ICSI-born children, which was also demonstrated by Lewis and Klonoff-Cohen [12] in their work.

Again, regarding malformations and specifically the major ones, such as cardiac defects (Fig. 36.1), spina bifida, and cleft lip and palate, a multicenter, prospective cohort control study was conducted by Ludwig and Katalinic in Germany [19]. The authors recruited patients who were less than 16 weeks pregnant from 59 centers across Germany to evaluate the risk of major malformations linked to ICSI, ending up with 2687 pregnancies and 3372 children and fetuses in the ICSI group. Children in both spontaneously conceived and ICSI-conceived groups underwent the same standard criteria examination for assessment in regard to major malformations after the first 8 weeks of life. In the ICSI cohort 8.6% of infants had major malformations, the risk being the same whether the spermatozoa were testicular, epididymal, or post-ejaculation, and in the control cohort 6.9% of infants had major malformations. Based on these figures, the authors stated that children born after ICSI have an increased risk of major malformations compared with those conceived after spontaneous conception. Parental factors such as genetic background leading to infertility and the ICSI technique were assumed to be the causes of this increased risk in the ICSI infants group. Additionally, the weaknesses of their study were pointed out by the authors: no nationwide control group was included, not all ICSI pregnancies in Germany were included, examination time was different for the two groups (median 38 days for ICSI and median day 7 for control group),

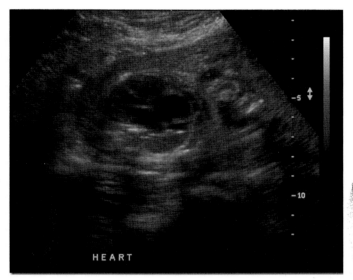

Fig. 36.1 Cardiomegaly.

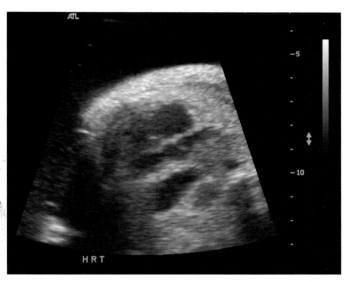

Fig. 36.2 Diaphragmatic hernia.

a blind study would have been more optimal, and the period of birth was different for the two groups (1998–2000 in the ICSI group, 1990–1998 in the control group). We might add to those weaknesses that maternal age was higher in the ICSI group as were multiple births, both of which could have influenced results in favor of the control group.

The same group led another prospective, multicenter, controlled, German nationwide cohort study to determine the pregnancy course as well as the major malformation (Fig. 36.2) rate for babies born following ICSI technique, comparing them to babies born after spontaneous conception [20]. They recruited 3198 pregnancies in the ICSI group, but after some participants dropped out, 2687 pregnancies and 3372 children were included. After recruitment, by contacting the couples to make sure that the pregnancy was ongoing at 16 weeks of gestation, a standardized examination was done on all children in both groups. Cases of live births, premature births, stillbirths, and spontaneous abortions from the 16th week of pregnancy were all included. The major malformation rate difference found in this study differs from the previous one by same group, due to the fact that the definition was modified by excluding some previously included cases such as patent ductus arteriosus and patent foramen ovale from the analysis. The major malformation rate was found to be 8.7% and 6.1% in the ICSI cohort and population-based control cohort, respectively. More precisely, this increased risk was found in the singleton pregnancy subgroup (8.9% vs. 6.0%), whereas in the twins subgroup it was 8.5% vs. 11.2%. In the chromosomal abnormalities group, the risk of rate increment was found to be mainly in the gastrointestinal tract (Fig. 36.3), kidneys, and the urinary tract; however, cardiac malformations (Fig. 36.4) were also found more frequently in the ICSI than in the control group of children. Invasive prenatal diagnostic procedures such as amniocentesis and chorionic villous sampling were done more frequently in the ICSI than in the control group of children (26.2% vs. 7.7%).

Cesarean section delivery rate was higher in the ICSI group, while spontaneous vaginal delivery was higher in the control group. Birth weight was found to be lower in the ICSI group, reflecting the gestational age at which delivery was taking place in favor of the control group of children. It should also be mentioned that the parents of the ICSI group had more sociodemographic risk factors (maternal and paternal age) than the parents of the control group, and this increase in risk factors for major malformations affects the final findings of the study; adjustment of the main risk factors would lead to the figure of 2% (which was set as the sample size calculation for relevant difference) being missed. The male genetic factor is believed to play a role in these findings due to Y chromosome microdeletions, as suggested by some other authors [21]. The authors of the German study [19] concluded by raising the question of whether the risk of major malformations found in their study arose from infertility-linked risks such as uterine, endometrial, placental, or even endocrine factors or whether the IVF, ICSI technique per se was the source. They also recommended counseling for infertile couples regarding the increment risk of parameters like pregnancy course, outcome, and major malformations compared to spontaneously conceived pregnancies. Providers should also keep in mind that such risks might be linked to one or both of the couple's fertility factor status, not excluding procedure-related risks as well.

In Belgium, Hindryckx et al. [22] investigated whether prevalence of congenital abnormalities increased after ICSI in the period between 1994 and 2000 after reviewing the literature. They followed 172 pregnancies after performing 776 cycles of ICSI, and found that major congenital malformations at birth occurred in 9/150 (6.0%), including 5 singleton children 5/99 (5%), 3 children of twin pregnancy 3/61 (3.3%), and 1 of triplet pregnancy 1/6 (1.6%); the total malformations rate was found to be 6.5%. After assuming that the additional risks which could be expected to be found were due to the use of

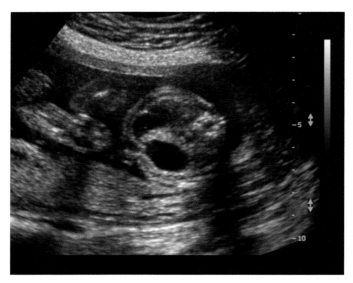

Fig. 36.3 Duodenal atresia.

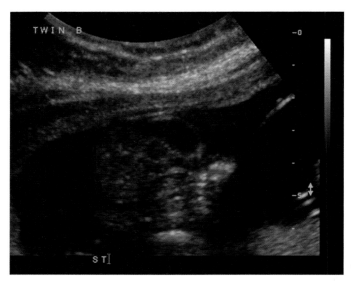

Fig. 36.4 Ectopia cordis.

poor-quality sperm, and the invasive nature of the ICSI procedure, they found their figures were comparable to the literature mentioned and reviewed. They also inquired about the potential risks to future fertility of the ICSI children. The study resulted in 132 deliveries, and termination of pregnancy was done in two cases (2/134, 1.5%) due to anencephaly and multiple congenital anomalies; two (3.6%) de novo chromosomal abnormalities were found. However, their study was conducted on a group that was too small to achieve the 80% power needed for a significance level of 0.05.

We can finally conclude that more studies are still needed especially for sexual development follow-up for ICSI children. The results given to date are reassuring, indicating that the major malformation rate is increased after ICSI compared with natural conception, but not when compared with IVF.

ICSI efficacy

Whatever was mentioned referring to the safety of ICSI, others went further in demonstrating its efficacy even after the failure of the conventional IVF method. Benadiva et al. [23] showed that ICSI overcomes previous fertilization failure with conventional IVF by evaluating its outcome subsequently. They performed ICSI on 25 patients who had unexplained fertilization failure after conventional IVF and on another 87 patients with male-factor infertility and compared both groups. The results were good enough that all patients with previous failed conventional IVF achieved fertilization by the ICSI technique, having figures for fertilization rate, implantation rate per embryo, and delivery rate per cycle that were not significantly different from the male-factor infertility group. The pregnancy rate was found to be 72% after using the same protocol of ovarian stimulation, the same ICSI technique, and embryo transfer policy as well. The authors found it conceivable that differences could exist between their results and others' due to

the improved oocyte quality in their study. They also pointed out the unclear or insufficient information about patients in other studies in whom fertilization trials failed. Their findings in favor of ICSI could be used for counseling and encouraging patients to try a second cycle of ICSI especially after unexplained failed fertilization.

The idea of ICSI treatment extension beyond male-factor infertility couples was in the mind of many clinicians who were enthusiastic about this novel technique. They believed that other groups of patients might benefit from ICSI and it should not be limited to male-factor infertility couples. After conducting a prospective controlled study on 35 patients who had non-male-factor infertility, Khamsi et al. [24] substantiated that it is justifiable that some oocytes would be a subject of ICSI. As they were expecting to improve embryo quality and make their fertilization rates higher after enrolling their patients, 50% of their retrieved oocytes underwent ICSI and the remaining 50% were subjected to conventional IVF. A better fertilization rate per retrieved oocyte was found for ICSI compared with conventional IVF and good-quality embryos at 48 hours after oocyte retrieval were found to be better formed after ICSI. The oocyte scoring was based upon oocyte–cumulus complex size, which did not differ between the two groups. The figures regarding fertilization rate were 57.2% and 71.3% for conventional IVF and ICSI, respectively, and good-quality embryos per fertilized oocyte were 82% in conventional IVF and 90% in the ICSI group. Consequently Khamsi et al. found it reasonable to counsel patients about the benefit of ICSI in their oocytes.

Despite all these promising results, there are others who found that performing ICSI as a standard procedure and dropping conventional IVF is not the best policy. Bhattacharya et al. [25] led a multicenter randomized controlled trial in which they compared ICSI and conventional IVF in non-male-factor infertility couples. Their primary outcome showed the implantation

Table 36.1 Indications for ICSI

Severe male-factor infertility

Male excretory duct obstruction

Oligozoospermia

Teratozoospermia

Asthenozoospermia

Necrozoospermia

Frozen–thawed sperms due to male disease

Ejaculatory disorders

Congenital bilateral absence of vas deferens

Young's syndrome

Bilateral ejaculatory duct obstruction

Artificial insemination with donor spermatozoa

Recurrent conventional IVF failure

Idiopathic infertility

Advanced maternal age

Preimplantation genetic diagnosis (PGD)

rate and the secondary one showed pregnancy as well as fertilization rate related to each treatment group, whereas analysis was done by intention to treat. After illustrating the trials and opinions of others like Fishel and colleagues [26], who found that ICSI should have been considered the treatment of choice in all cases of assisted reproduction, and they followed a standard laboratory protocol for both techniques. Implantation rate after traditional IVF was higher than that after ICSI; fertilization rate per retrieved oocyte was significantly higher in IVF than ICSI: 58% for the IVF group versus 47% for the ICSI group.

They also found that the fertilization rate of inseminated oocytes was lower in the IVF group than in the ICSI group of patients. Accordingly, the authors stated that there is no clinical benefit after ICSI usage if such couples are suitable for conventional IVF as is the case in non-male-factor infertility. But we should keep in mind that failed fertilization could be avoided through the ICSI technique. ICSI indications are listed in Table 36.1.

One of the outstanding advantages of ICSI is in preventing fertilization failure to a certain extent, in comparison with the traditional IVF method in which as many as one-third of treatment cycles result in fertilization failure. That high fertilization failure rate as well as patient stress, treatment expenses, and clinician disappointment after standard IVF in almost all centers providing this service, presented ICSI as an empirical but demanded technology. Hershlag et al. [27] carried out a prospective cohort study to determine whether ICSI could prevent fertilization failure in a group with unexplained infertility and in a group with borderline semen. They built the diagnosis of unexplained infertility upon the criteria of regular menstrual cycle, normal anatomical cavity of the uterus, fallopian tubes found open, endometriosis evidence being ruled out, and normal semen analysis according to World Health Organization

criteria [28]. None of the ICSI couples in the unexplained infertility group experienced fertilization failure, whereas 10 out of 60 (16.7%) IVF couples in this group did not achieve fertilization. After this statistically significant difference, on the other hand, there was no significant difference in the fertilization rate in the borderline sperm group of patients between those who underwent ICSI or IVF treatment method.

Finally, Hershlag et al. [27] concluded that in cases of unexplained infertility, elimination of fertilization failure could be enhanced when the ICSI-IVF insemination split is involved.

Rescue ICSI that consists of performing the technique in cases where conventional IVF fails to accomplish fertilization after 18 hours, did not gain the desired acceptance because of the theoretical risk of genetic abnormalities [29]. All these challenges were found to be evaded by ICSI application which may minimize the dilemma of fertilization failure.

Efforts were carried out by others to make the ICSI technique more efficient or to minimize its failure rate, an example being the application of assisted oocyte activation in cases of fertilization failure. Oocyte activation deficiency was mainly proposed as the cause of that defect in the oocyte which leads to fertilization failure. Such activation in the oocyte depends on both sperm and oocyte-related activating factors. That deficiency was mainly found in oocytes which fail to fertilize after undergoing the ICSI technique [30]. Heindryckx et al. [31] suggested a diagnostic test for oocytes that failed to achieve fertilization after ICSI, especially to find out whether the defect is sperm or oocyte related. They presented the mouse oocyte activation test to detect the exact cause of fertilization failure, mentioning that combined treatment of ICSI and artificially induced activation might be beneficial. Artificial activation could be through agents that prolong calcium (Ca) rise in animal oocytes such as ethanol or Ca ionophores. The results were promising as the fertilization rate was 14% in 50 cycles and no pregnancy rate was established in cases without assisted oocyte activation. After applying their suggested diagnostic test and method on 30 patients they found that with assisted oocyte activation applied, fertilization increased to 75% and pregnancy rate rose to 33%, demonstrating that such a test and technique could be of value for patients who experienced low or no fertilization in previous ICSI treatment cycles. Of note, no major or minor congenital malformations were found in pregnancies which continued to term.

Some authors have shown that such assisted oocyte activation is of no great value, when commencing by ICSI in difficult cases such as globozoospermia. This rare but severe male infertility disorder was first depicted by Schirren et al. [32]. In cases of globozoospermia, ICSI leads to a poor fertilization rate. In a case report described by Bechoua et al. [33], the authors showed that ICSI can still give successful results despite the sperm's disturbed head shape which was assumed to disable the process of fertilization as such sperm lack oocyte activation capacity, which is necessary to fertilize the oocyte. They did not exclude the role of assisted oocyte activation, but conception resulted without it.

ICSI technique

After making sure of semen availability and its analysis, the spermatozoa which are to be injected into the cytoplasm of the collected oocytes are selected. Then the ICSI procedure is carried out on metaphase II oocytes, preferably to be performed after complete assessment of the available retrieved oocyte, namely intact zona pellucida as well as marking the presence or absence of germinal vesicles and polar body. With the assistance of two bent needles with an angle of approximately 30–40 degrees, the two pipettes should be fixed in a straight line with horizontal alignment if possible. Under the 200–400 magnification microscope, heated stage at 37°C, and covering the prepared droplets with light mineral oil for temperature maintenance and droplet stability, then work can be initiated. Priming of the micropipettes with medium before use is of great benefit as it prevents the gametes from coming into contact with oil or air.

With the help of negative pressure created by the micromanipulator device pipette, oocyte fixation is done. At the same time, while the oocyte is attached gently but firmly to the holding pipette, work on keeping the polar body at 6 or 12 o'clock is done. Immobilization of the spermatozoon could be done either by a quick movement of the capillary via the tail or by pressing the tail of the sperm cell downward to the bottom of the dish, after which the single live spermatozoon is ready to be aspirated smoothly, tail first into the injection pipette. Movement of the spermatozoon along the pipette and bringing it to rest at its very tip is the following step. Introduction at the 3 o'clock position of the injection pipette containing the spermatozoon is done gently into the cytoplasm through the zona pellucida by softly pricking the middle of the oocyte, and then releasing the spermatozoon to pass into the cytoplasm with the least possible amount of medium [28]. After the procedure is completed, oocyte washing and storing takes place in approximately 25 μL microdrops of B2 medium on a Petri dish and is stored at 37°C in an incubator containing 5% CO_2.

Assessment of fertilization takes place 16–18 hours after the procedure is completed. Normally fertilized oocytes are those having two fragmented individualized polar bodies, with two visible pronuclei [29].

Acknowledgment

The author would like to thank Dr. Fayez Nasrallah.

References

1. Elder K., Dale B. *In-Vitro Fertilization*, 2nd edn. Cambridge University Press;2000: 228.

2. Palermo G, Joris H, Devroey P, Van Steirteghem AC. Pregnancies after intracytoplasmic injection of single spermatozoon into an oocyte. *Lancet* 1992; **340**(8810): 17–18.

3. Van Steirteghem AC, Liu J, Joris H, et al. Higher success rate by intracytoplasmic sperm injection than by subzonal insemination. Report of a second series of 300 consecutive treatment cycles. *Hum Reprod* 1993; **8**(7): 1055–1060.

4. Nagy ZP, Liu J, Joris H, et al. The result of intracytoplasmic sperm injection is not related to any of the three basic sperm parameters. *Hum Reprod* 1995; **10**(5): 1123–1129.

5. Wisanto, A., Magnus, M., Bonduelle, M., et al. Obstetric outcome of 424 pregnancies after intracytoplasmic sperm injection. *Hum. Reprod* 1995; **10**: 2713–2718.

6. Govaerts I, Devreker F, Koenig I, Place I, Van den Bergh M, Englert Y. Comparison of pregnancy outcome after intracytoplasmic sperm injection and in-vitro fertilization. *Hum Reprod* 1998; **13**(6): 1514–1518.

7. Osmanagaoglu K, Tournaye H, Camus M, Vandervorst M, Van Steirteghem A, Devroey P. Cumulative delivery rates after intracytoplasmic sperm injection: 5 year follow-up of 498 patients. *Hum Reprod* 1999; **14**(10): 2651–2655.

8. Jee BC, Ku SY, Suh CS, et al. Cumulative ongoing pregnancy rate in intracytoplasmic sperm injection cycles. *J Obstet Gynaecol Res* 2004; **30**(5): 372–376.

9. Devroey P, Godoy H, Smitz J, et al. Female age predicts embryonic implantation after ICSI: a case-controlled study. *Hum Reprod* 1996; **11**(6): 1324–1327.

10. Aytoz A, Camus M, Tournaye H, Bonduelle M, Van Steirteghem A, Devroey P. Outcome of pregnancies after intracytoplasmic sperm injection and the effect of sperm origin and quality on this outcome. *Fertil Steril* 1998; **70**(3): 500–505.

11. Knoester M, Helmerhorst FM, Vandenbroucke JP, et al. Leiden Artificial Reproductive Techniques Follow-up Project (L-art-FUP). Perinatal outcome, health, growth, and medical care utilization of 5- to 8-year-old intracytoplasmic sperm injection singletons. *Fertil Steril* 2008; **89**(5): 1133–1146.

12. Lewis S, Klonoff-Cohen H. What factors affect intracytoplasmic sperm injection outcomes? *Obstet Gynecol Surv* 2005; **60**(2): 111–123.

13. Thielemans BF, Spiessens C, D'Hooghe T, Vanderschueren D, Legius E. Genetic abnormalities and male infertility. A comprehensive review. *Eur J Obstet Gynecol Reprod Biol* 1998; **81**(2): 217–225.

14. Alrayyes S, Fakih H, Khan I. Effect of age and cycle responsiveness in patients undergoing intracytoplasmic sperm injection. *Fertil Steril* 1997; **68**(1): 123–127.

15. Fauque P, Léandri R, Merlet F, et al. Pregnancy outcome and live birth after IVF and ICSI according to embryo quality. *J Assist Reprod Genet* 2007; **24**(5): 159–165.

16. Hamberger L, Lundin K, Sjögren A, Söderlund B. Indications for intracytoplasmic sperm injection. *Hum Reprod* 1998; **13**(Suppl 1): 128–133.

17. Wennerholm UB, Bergh C, Hamberger L, et al. Obstetric and perinatal outcome of pregnancies following intracytoplasmic sperm injection. *Hum Reprod* 1996; **11**(5): 1113–1119.

18. Bonduelle M, Camus M, De Vos A, et al. Seven years of intracytoplasmic sperm injection and follow-up of 1987 subsequent children. *Hum Reprod* 1999; **14**(Suppl 1): 243–264.

19. Ludwig M, Katalinic A. Malformation rate in fetuses and children conceived after ICSI: results of a prospective cohort study. *Reprod Biomed Online* 2002; **5**(2): 171–178.

20. Katalinic A, Rösch C, Ludwig M. German ICSI Follow-Up Study Group. Pregnancy course and outcome after intracytoplasmic sperm injection: a controlled, prospective cohort study. *Fertil Steril* 2004; **81**(6): 1604–1616.

21. Patsalis PC, Sismani C, Quintana-Murci L, Taleb-Bekkouche F, Krausz C, McElreavey K. Effects of transmission of Y chromosome AZFc deletions. *Lancet* 2002; **360**(9341): 1222–1224.

22. Hindryckx A, Peeraer K, Debrock S, et al. Has the prevalence of congenital abnormalities after intracytoplasmic sperm injection increased? The Leuven data 1994–2000 and a review of the literature. *Gynecol Obstet Invest* 2010; **70**(1): 11–22.

23. Benadiva CA, Nulsen J, Siano L, Jennings J, Givargis HB, Maier D. Intracytoplasmic sperm injection overcomes previous fertilization failure with conventional in vitro fertilization. *Fertil Steril* 1999; **72**(6): 1041–1044.

24. Khamsi F, Yavas Y, Roberge S, Wong JC, Lacanna IC, Endman M. Intracytoplasmic sperm injection increased fertilization and good-quality embryo formation in patients with non-male factor indications for in vitro fertilization: a prospective randomized study. *Fertil Steril* 2001; **75**(2): 342–347.

25. Bhattacharya S, Hamilton MPR, Shaaban M, et al. Conventional in-vitro fertilisation versus intracytoplasmic sperm injection for the treatment of non-male-factor infertility: a randomised controlled trial. *Lancet* 2001; **357**(9274):2075–2079.

26. Fishel S, Aslam I, Lisi F, et al. Should ICSI be the treatment of choice for all cases of in-vitro conception? *Hum Reprod* 2000; **15**(6): 1278–1283.

27. Hershlag A, Paine T, Kvapil G, Feng H, Napolitano B. In vitro fertilization-intracytoplasmic sperm injection split: an insemination method to prevent fertilization failure. *Fertil Steril* 2002;**77**(2): 229–232.

28. World Health Organization. *Laboratory Manual for the Examination of Human Semen and Semen-Cervical Mucus Interaction*, 3rd edn. New York: Cambridge University Press; 1993: 3p26.

29. Nagy ZP, Staessen C, Liu J, Joris H, Devroey P, Van Steirteghem AC. Prospective, auto-controlled study on reinsemination of failed-fertilized oocytes by intracytoplasmic sperm injection. *Fertil Steril* 1995; **64**(6): 1130–1135.

30. Sousa M, Tesarik J. Ultrastructural analysis of fertilization failure after intracytoplasmic sperm injection. *Hum Reprod* 1994; **9**(12): 2374–2380.

31. Heindryckx B, De Gheselle S, Gerris J, Dhont M, De Sutter P. Efficiency of assisted oocyte activation as a solution for failed intracytoplasmic sperm injection. *Reprod Biomed Online* 2008; **17**(5): 662–668.

32. Schirren C, Laudahn G, Hartmann E, Heinze I, Richter E. Untersuchungen zur Korrelation morphologischer und biochemischer Meßgrößen im menschlichen Ejakulat bei verschiedenen andrologischen Diagnosen. *Andrologia* 1975; **7**(2): 117–125.

33. Bechoua S, Chiron A, Delcleve-Paulhac S, Sagot P, Jimenez C. Fertilisation and pregnancy outcome after ICSI in globozoospermic patients without assisted oocyte activation. *Andrologia* 2009; **41**(1): 55–58.

Chapter

37

The role of ultrasound imaging in the prediction, prevention, and management of ovarian hyperstimulation syndrome

Botros R. M. B. Rizk

Ovarian hyperstimulation syndrome

A grave iatrogenic complication that arises from ovarian stimulation is ovarian hyperstimulation syndrome (OHSS). OHSS typically presents with (a) bilateral multiple follicular and thecal lutein ovarian cysts (Figs 37.1–37.3), (b) an acute shift in distribution of body fluid which results in ascites (Fig. 37.4(A–F), and (c) pleural effusion (Fig. 37.5) [1–8]. In mild forms of OHSS, a patient may complain of distension and discomfort. The severe form of OHSS, however, can be accompanied by the following serious complications: hemoconcentration, thromboembolism, renal failure, and adult respiratory distress syndrome [9,10].

The onset of ovarian hyperstimulation varies from early to late (Fig. 37.6). Specifically, in early onset, OHSS presents 3–7 days after the ovulatory dose of human chorionic gonadotropin (hCG), while in late onset, it presents 12–17 days after hCG administration (Fig. 37.6). Early-onset OHSS occurs with an excessive pre-ovulatory response to stimulation, while late-onset OHSS occurs with pregnancy, particularly multiple pregnancy [11,12]. The etiology of ovarian hyperstimulation is spontaneous or iatrogenic, although most often it is iatrogenic due to gonadotropin ovarian stimulation (Fig. 37.7). More rarely, a spontaneous case of OHSS can result from follicle-stimulating hormone (FSH) receptor mutations [13]. Additionally, the clinical presentation of ovarian hyperstimulation can be moderate or severe.

Pathophysiology of OHSS

To explain the pathophysiology of OHSS requires addressing two phenomena: the presence of multiple hemorrhagic follicular and theca lutein cysts and acute body fluid shifts that result in ascites and pleural effusion. Increased capillary permeability appears to result in the body fluid shifts.

The role of vascular endothelial growth factor (VEGF) and interleukins in the pathogenesis of OHSS was explored by Rizk et al. [14] and Pellicer et al. [15]. Although researchers have examined numerous mediators, the bulk of fluid leakage is due to VEGF production by the granulosa cells and the endothelial cells (Fig. 37.8A and B). There are four

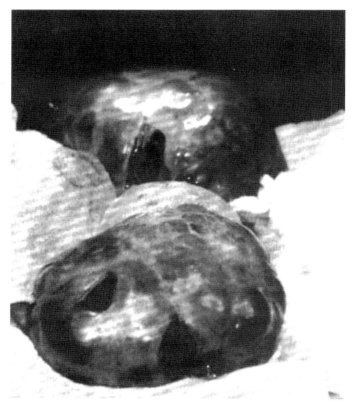

Fig. 37.1 Hyperstimulated ovaries. Reproduced with permission from Schenker JG. Ovarian hyperstimulation syndrome. In: Wallach EE, Zacur HA, *Reproductive Medicine and Surgery*: Mosby, St. Louis, Baltimore, 1995; Chapter 35, p. 654.

dimeric forms (A–D) in the VEGF family. Additionally, the VEGF family includes placental growth factors that all bind in their own way to the three VEGF receptors (VEGF-R 1–3), which are expressed on endothelial cells. The current research indicates that VEGF-A stimulation of VEGF-R-2 results in increased capillary permeability and fluid leakage (Figs 37.9 and 37.10).

Ultrasonography in Gynecology, ed. Botros R. M. B. Rizk and Elizabeth E. Puscheck. Published by Cambridge University Press. © Cambridge University Press 2015.

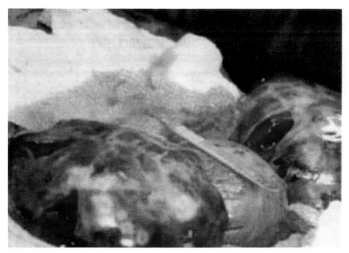

Fig. 37.2 Hyperstimulated ovaries. Reproduced with permission from Serour G. Ovarian hyperstimulation syndrome. In: Gerris J, Delvigne A, Olivenness F, *Ovarian Hyperstimulation Syndrome*: Informa Healthcare, Abingdon, Oxon, UK, 2006; Chapter 1, p. 4.

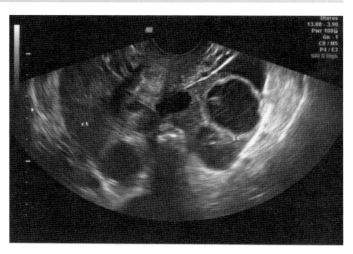

Fig. 37.3 Bilateral enlarged cystic ovaries.

Factors predicting ovarian hyperstimulation syndrome

Accurate prediction is the foundation for successful prevention of OHSS (Table 37.1). Rizk and Smitz [16] found that prediction of OHSS depended on factors identified before ovarian stimulation, which included history of previous OHSS and polycystic ovarian syndrome[17]. Other factors are age, allergies, hyperinsulinism, body mass index, and FSH receptor mutations [17].

The greatest predictors of OHSS during ovarian stimulation include a sharp rise in estradiol or high levels when a large number of follicles are present or oocytes retrieved (Fig. 37.11A–D). Other important factors that help predict OHSS are increased blood flow to the ovaries as well as increased ovarian stromal blood flow (Figs 37.12–37.14A and B). Additionally, pregnancy (Fig. 37.15), and specifically multiple pregnancies, will add to the risk of developing OHSS (Fig. 37.16).

Ultrasonography in prediction of OHSS

Ultrasound criteria for the diagnosis of polycystic ovarian syndrome

Nagamani and Chilvers have carefully considered the use of ultrasonography in diagnosing PCOS [18].

Baseline necklace sign appearance

Appropriately diagnosing polycystic ovaries (PCO) upon ultrasound examination (i.e. the necklace sign) plays a crucial role in predicting OHSS (Table 37.2) [16,17]. In a Belgian multicenter study, such a diagnosis improved the prediction of OHSS to 79% [17].

Laparoscopy, laparotomy, and histologic evaluation were the previous methods used to visualize PCO before ultrasonography

became widely available (Fig. 37.17A and B). Presently, ultrasonography is the most popular method used to evaluate ovarian morphology in patients who have polycystic ovarian syndrome (PCOS). The Rotterdam criteria, which are the gold standard for diagnosing PCO, use antral follicle number and ovarian volume. Other criteria used for diagnosing PCOS, which are still debated by researchers, include stromal echogenicity, stromal volume, ovarian blood flow, and uterine blood flow [18].

Judy Adams proposed the original PCOS definition based on transabdominal ultrasound in 1986. Transabdominal ultrasonography has since been replaced by transvaginal ultrasonography due to its increased resolution: a 3.5 MHz transabdominal transducer did not detect PCO in patients with PCOS whereas a 7.5 MHz transvaginal probe did [19]. For transvaginal examination of the ovaries, the use of a high-frequency probe is advisable. The high-frequency probe has increased resolution, although there is decreased penetration depth. Such a decrease is acceptable, however, due to the ovaries being near to the transducer in the cul-de-sac. Three-dimensional ultrasonography helps with the assessment of antral follicle count (AFC), ovarian volume measurements, and stromal echogenicity.

Antral follicle count

For diagnosing PCOS, the consensus of ESHRE/ASRM embraced the inclusion of PCO on ultrasound as one of the PCOS diagnostic criteria. The Rotterdam criteria to diagnose PCO are 12+ follicles measuring 2–9 mm in diameter in each ovary and/or enlarged ovarian volume of >10 mL. Usually, the follicles are arranged peripherally around the solid ovarian stroma. A single PCO meets the criterion of ovarian morphology for diagnosing PCOS. For multifollicular ovaries, usually 6+ follicles are 4–10 mm in size with normal ovarian stroma. Multifollicular ovaries often arise in the typical early follicular phase, puberty, hypothalamic amenorrhea, hyperthyroidism, and hyperprolactinemia. An AFC that is between 9 and 35 has been observed to be notably more common in women who have PCOS than in normal women, who have 1 to 10 follicles.

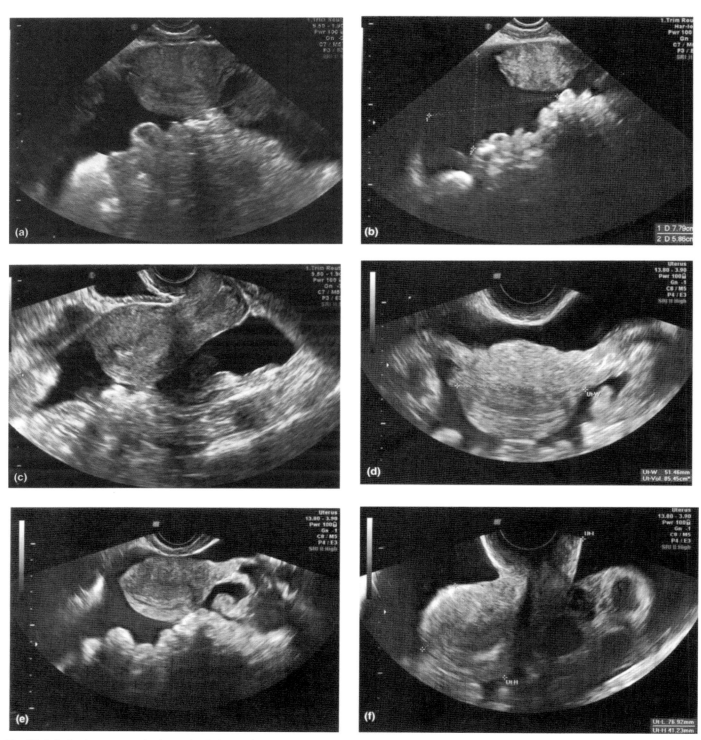

Fig. 37.4 Ascites in severe ovarian hyperstimulation syndrome.

Ovarian volume

Patients with PCO have ovaries that are characteristically enlarged and spherical. As a substitute for stromal hypertrophy, ovarian volume is measured. Given that the Rotterdam criteria for PCO require an ovarian volume of >10 mL, the most frequently used equation to determine ovarian volume is length × width × height × 0.5. Three-D ultrasonography assists clinicians in the computation of ovarian volume.

Stromal area

Stromal hypertrophy is typical of ovarian androgenic dysfunction. In women who have hyperthecosis, the ovarian stroma

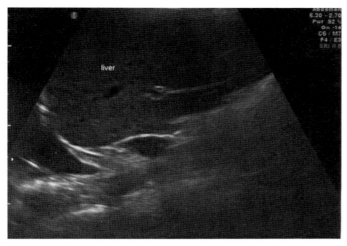

Fig. 37.5 Right pleural effusion in OHSS.

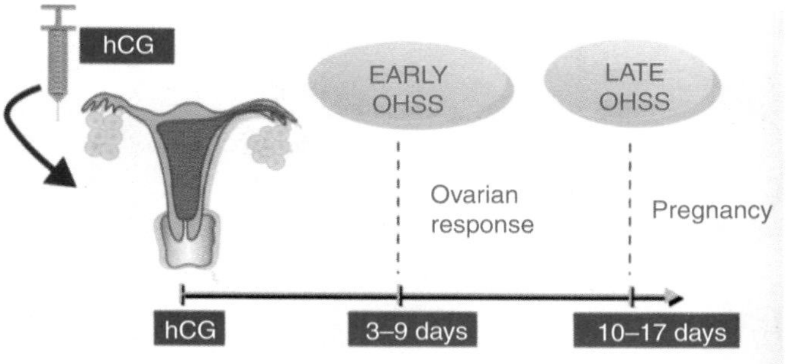

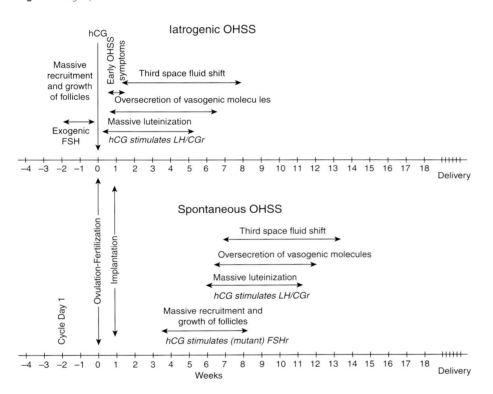

Fig. 37.6 Classification of ovarian hyperstimulation syndrome: early and late.

Fig. 37.7 Chronological development of iatrogenic and spontaneous OHSS. Reproduced with permission from Delbaere et al. (2004). *Hum Reprod* 19: 486–489.

replaces the whole ovary (Fig. 37.18A–C). It was proposed that ovarian hypertrophy associated with an ovarian area of greater than 0.5, unilaterally or bilaterally, indicates PCOS.

Stromal echogenicity

Stromal echogenicity was considered to be an important marker for PCOS. More recent studies challenge this concept. Therefore, ultrasonography of ovarian stromal echogenicity in routine ultrasounds is not warranted.

Vascularity

Doppler analysis of stromal vascularity was not included in the Rotterdam criteria, since results were controversial.

Baseline ovarian volume and the prediction of OHSS

Danninger et al. examined baseline ovarian volume before stimulation in order to study whether it appropriately predicts the risk of OHSS [20]. The researchers used 3D volumetric ultrasound to assess the ovaries before ovarian stimulation as well as on the day of hCG injection. A significant correlation between baseline ovarian volume and the subsequent occurrence of OHSS was observed. On the basis of this correlation, Danninger et al. proposed using ovarian volume to detect patients at risk of OHSS.

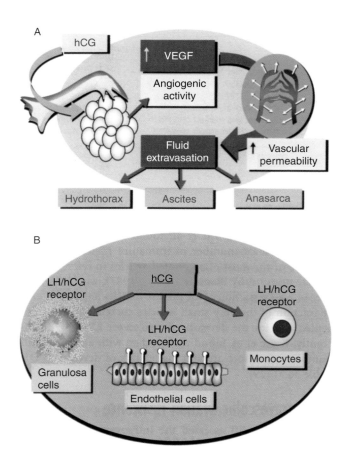

Fig. 37.8 (A and B) Pathophysiology of ovarian hyperstimulation syndrome.

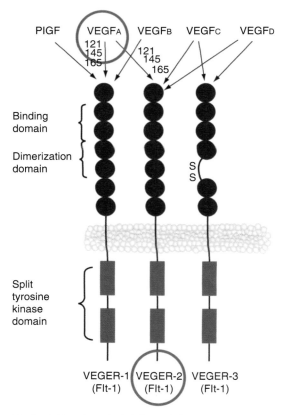

Fig. 37.9 Vascular endothelial growth factor receptors.

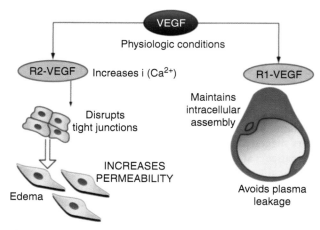

Fig. 37.10 Vascular endothelial growth factor receptors and vascular permeability.

Lass et al. also studied ovarian volume to try and predict ovulation induction response with gonadotropins for WHO group II anovulatory patients in their early follicular phase [21]. The researchers examined retrospective data gathered from two prospective, randomized multicenter studies. The 465 patients were undergoing ovulation induction and Lass et al. observed that the WHO Group II anovulatory women undergoing ovulation induction with low-dose gonadotropin stimulation with medium-sized or large ovaries had a higher risk of OHSS than the women who had small ovaries.

Number and size of follicles during ovarian stimulation

The most crucial role of ultrasonography in prediction of OHSS is to monitor the development of follicles during assisted conception [22,23]. Examining the number, size, and pattern of follicle distribution in helping to predict OHSS, Tal et al. studied OHSS and the mean number of immature follicles and observed a positive correlation [24]. Blankstein et al. also examined this correlation and observed that a decrease in the proportion of mature follicles with an increase in the proportion very small follicles was correlated with an increased risk of severe OHSS development [25]. Kwee et al. found that women who had an AFC of 15+ are at a higher risk of developing OHSS

(Table 37.3) [26]. More recently, Steward et al. concluded that fifteen or more oocytes was associated with a high risk of OHSS [27].

Low intravascular ovarian resistance

Moohan et al. [28] studied the relationship between intraovarian blood flow and severity of OHSS. Thirty women with OHSS and sonographic evidence of ascites after embryo transfer were observed. For the 11 patients who had severe OHSS

Table 37.1 Prediction of ovarian hyperstimulation syndrome (OHSS)

History and physical

1. OHSS in a previous cycle
2. Polycystic ovarian syndrome
3. Young patient
4. Low body mass index
5. Hyperinsulinism
6. Allergies

During ovarian stimulation

1. High serum estradiol, rapid slope of estradiol, and absolute value
2. Ultrasonography
a. Baseline PCO pattern
b. PCO pattern of response to GnRH before gonadotropins
c. Large number of follicles, >20, on each ovary
3. Doppler low intraovarian vascular resistance

Outcome of ART cycles

1. Conception cycles
2. Multiple pregnancy

and 19 patients who had mild OHSS, the researchers calculated the women's resistance to blood flow within their ovaries using transabdominal ultrasound with color flow and pulsed Doppler imaging. The measures of downstream vascular impedance (pulsatility index [PI], resistance index [RI], and the S-D ratio) were notably decreased in the patients with severe OHSS. Over two-thirds of women who had an RI of <0.48 had pleural effusion. Pleural effusion was also reported in over one-half of women who had either a PI of <0.75 or an S-D of <1.92. Even though vascular impedance changes occurred, the blood flow velocity was not significantly different between the two groups. A close relationship was reported between OHSS severity and resistance of intraovarian blood flow. The researchers proposed that assessments of intraovarian vascular resistance in women who are undergoing controlled ovarian hyperstimulation (COH) could assist in the prediction of which specific women were at risk of developing OHSS [28].

The use of both estradiol and ultrasonography provides the best chance of predicting OHSS. Follow-up by ultrasound examination of the leading follicles helps determine

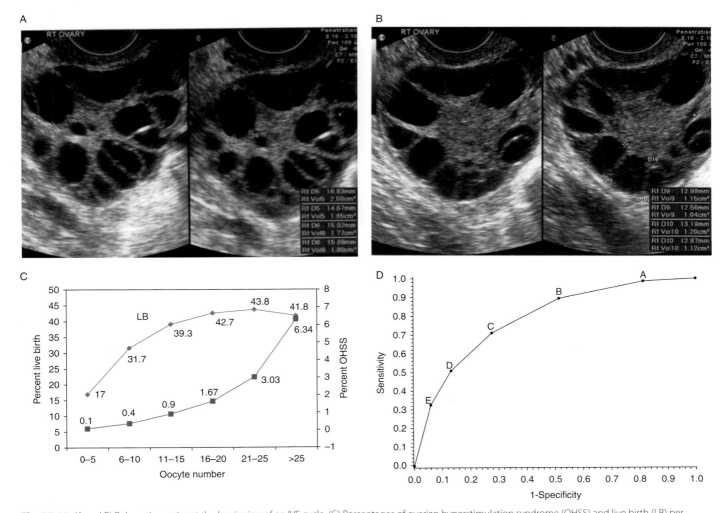

Fig. 37.11 (A and B) Polycystic ovaries at the beginning of an IVF cycle. (C) Percentages of ovarian hyperstimulation syndrome (OHSS) and live birth (LB) per retrieved oocyte numbers per IVF cycle among SART members from 2008 to 2010. (D) Receiver operating characteristic curve for retrieved oocyte number as a predictor of ovarian hyperstimulation syndrome. Oocyte number thresholds: A: 5; B:10; C: 15; D: 20; E: 25. Parts C and D reproduced with permission from Steward RG et al., *Fertil Steril* 2014; **101**(4):967–973.

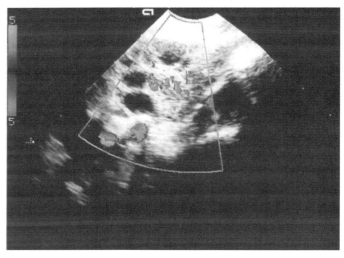

Fig. 37.12 Color Doppler ultrasound image of a polycystic ovary indicating active blood flow. Reproduced with permission from Zaidi et al, *Hum Reprod* 1995; 10: 1992–1996.

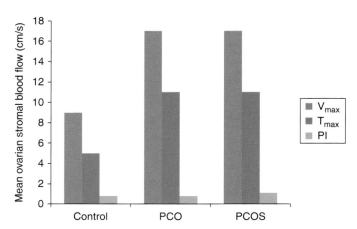

Fig. 37.13 Increased ovarian stromal blood flow in PCOS. Reproduced with permission from Jacobs HS, *Atlas of Clinical Gynecology,* Volume III *Reproductive Endocrinology,* Philadelphia, 1999; Chapter 5, Figure 5.4.

A
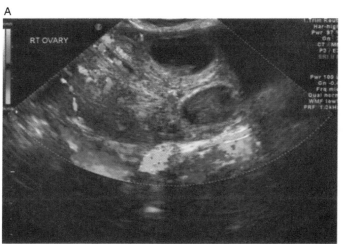

B
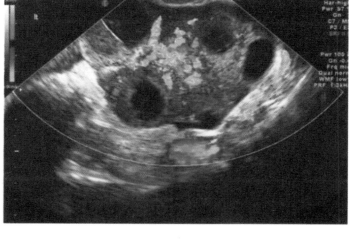

Fig. 37.14 (A and B) Increased ovarian blood flow by Doppler in severe OHSS.

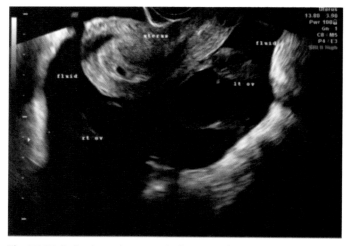

Fig. 37.15 Ascites in moderate ovarian hyperstimulation syndrome in early pregnancy.

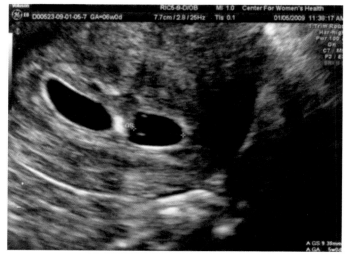

Fig. 37.16 Twins associated with OHSS.

Table 37.2 Technical recommendations for ultrasound assessment of PCO from the 2003 Rotterdam PCOS consensus

- **State-of-the-art equipment operated by appropriately trained personnel.**
- Whenever possible, the transvaginal approach should be used.
- Regularly menstruating women should be scanned in the early follicular phase (cycle days 3–5). Oligo-/amenorrheic women should be scanned either at random or between days 3 and 5 after a progestin-induced withdrawal.
- Calculation of ovarian volume is performed using the simplified formula for a prolate ellipsoid (0.5 × length × width × thickness).
- Follicle number should be estimated both in longitudinal and anteroposterior cross-sections of the ovaries. The size of follicles <10 mm should be expressed as the mean of the diameters measured on the two sections.

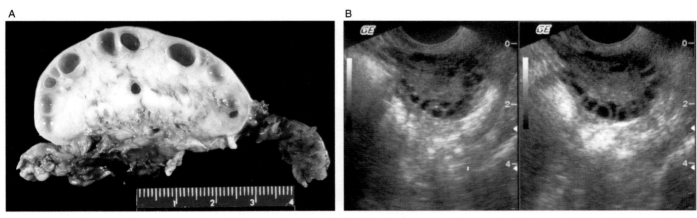

Fig. 37.17 (A) Cut surface of a typical PCO and antral follicles arranged peripherally around a dense core of stroma, which is increased. (B) Sagittal ultrasound images of the ovaries in a patient with PCOS obtained with a 6.5-MHz transvaginal transducer. Small follicles less than 9 mm are arranged around increased ovarian stroma.

the administration of hCG and measurement of serum estradiol, with ultrasound visualization of both small and intermediate follicles used as the basis to measure the likelihood of OHSS.

Prevention of OHSS

Rizk proposed the use of the "Ten Commandments" for preventing OHSS [29]. This list has now been enlarged and separated into two lists of "Ten Commandments" [30]. One list deals with the primary prevention of OHSS, including alternatives prior to stimulation (e.g. ovarian diathermy) and during stimulation (e.g. using low-dosage gonadotropins) [30] (Table 37.4). The other list deals with the secondary prevention of OHSS, including withholding or delaying hCG administration, using luteinizing hormone (LH) or a GnRH agonist instead of hCG to trigger ovulation, and using progesterone for support during the luteal phase (Fig. 37.19; Table 37.5).

Rizk suggested that among the existing alternatives for preventing OHSS, the coasting or delaying of hCG administration (until the estradiol levels decrease to under 3000 pg/mL) is the most widespread technique [23]. With rapidly increasing estradiol levels in women who are undergoing COH because of the simultaneous administration of gonadotropins and GnRH-a, should gonadotropins be withheld and not GnRH-a (because no endogenous gonadotropin secretion is present to maintain follicular growth), a quick decrease in estradiol levels will occur (Fig. 37.19). Whereas healthy developing follicles can bear a short episode of gonadotropin deprivation, smaller follicles'

granulosa cells have decreased tolerance for withheld stimulation from gonadotropins [31–33].

Additionally, further evidence that has the potential to explain coasting physiology relates to expression of VEGF, and secretion is considerably diminished in patients who have been coasted [31]. This explanation for coasting is meant to reduce the risk and severity of OHSS in patients who are at high risk for OHSS [31–33].

For patients who do develop OHSS, the expression of VEGF is excessive. VEGF is made by granulosa-lutein cells and is released into the follicular fluid. The release of VEGF occurs in response to hCG, which induces increased permeability of capillaries. In cultured granulosa-lutein cells of patients who are developing OHSS, hCG induces VEGF expression. Likewise, hCG induces VEGF release in human endothelial cells, which as a result act in an autocrine manner increasing vascular permeability (VP). Therefore, both granulosa cells and endothelial cells could be implicated in VEGF production and release in patients who develop OHSS [31–33].

However, another proposed explanation is that granulosa-lutein cells act as actual endothelial cells [31–33]. VEGF has the capability to reverse hCG's effect on VP by targeting the VEGFR-2 that employs SU5416, which supports the importance of VEGF in OHSS [34]. It additionally provides new insight into the expansion of the strategies used to prevent and treat OHSS based on OHSS's pathophysiological mechanism [34], as opposed to using empirical approaches as we often do today (Figs 37.20–37.22).

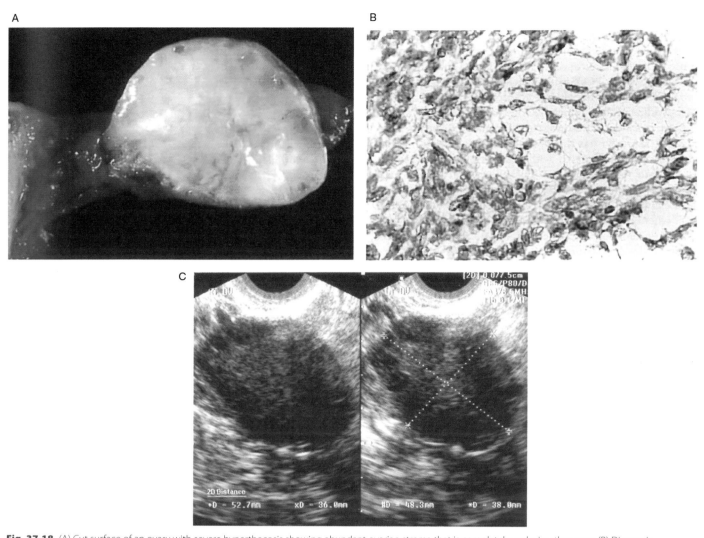

Fig. 37.18 (A) Cut surface of an ovary with severe hyperthecosis showing abundant ovarian stroma that is completely replacing the ovary. (B) Diagnosis confirmed by histological examination – large nests of luteinized thecal cells in the ovarian stroma. (C) Sagittal ultrasound images of hyperthecotic ovaries. Note the complete lack of antral follicles and stroma replacing the ovary.

Table 37.3 Antral follicle count (AFC) and prediction of ovarian hyperstimulation syndrome

Total AFC	Sensitivity	Specificity	PPV	Accuracy
<10	0.94	0.71	0.36	0.76
<12	0.88	0.80	0.44	0.81
<14	0.82	0.89	0.58	0.88
<16	0.47	0.96	0.67	0.88
<18	0.29	0.98	0.71	0.87

PPV, positive predictive value.
Reproduced with permission from Kwee, J. et al. *Reproductive Biology and Endocrinology*, 2007; 5(9): 8.

In animal cancer models, dopamine receptor 2 agonists (when administered at high doses) inhibit not only VEGFR-2 dependent VP, but also angiogenesis. A well-established OHSS rat model that was supplemented with prolactin was used to check whether angiogenesis could be separated from VEGFR-2 dependent VP in a dose-dependent method with cabergoline [35]. A low dose of cabergoline (100 μg/kg) reversed VEGFR-2-dependent VP with no effect on luteal angiogenesis with partial inhibition of ovarian VEGFR-2 phosphorylation levels. There was no observed effect on serum progesterone levels, luteal apoptosis, or other luteolytic effects. Administration of cabergoline also had no effect on VEGF/VEGFR-2 ovarian mRNA levels (Figs 37.20–37.22) [35,36].

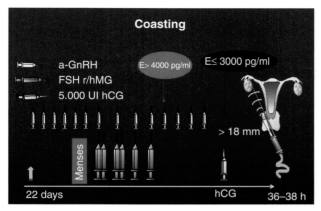

Fig. 37.19 Coasting for prevention of ovarian hyperstimulation syndrome.

Table 37.4 Primary prevention of ovarian hyperstimulation syndrome (OHSS)

The Ten Commandments
1. Prediction of OHSS from history, exam, and ultrasound
2. Laparoscopic ovarian drilling in PCOS patients
3. Metformin in PCOS patients
4. Octreotide in PCOS patients
5. Low-dose gonadotropins in PCOS patients
6. GnRH antagonist protocol
7. Recombinant LH to trigger ovulation
8. GnRH agonist to trigger ovulation
9. In vitro maturation of oocytes
10. Replacement of only one embryo

Reproduced with permission from Rizk B. *Ovarian Hyperstimulation Syndrome: Epidemiology, Prevention and Management.* Cambridge, UK, and New York. (2006) Cambridge University Press.

Table 37.5 Secondary prevention of ovarian hyperstimulation syndrome (OHSS)

The Ten Commandments
1. Withholdings hCG ± continuation of GnRH-a/GnRH antagonist
2. Coasting or delaying hCG: currently most popular method
3. Use of GnRH-a to trigger ovulation
4. Follicular aspiration
5. Progesterone for luteal phase
6. Cryopreservation and replacement of frozen–thawed embryos at a subsequent cycle
7. Dopamine agonist
8. Albumin administration at time of retrieval
9. Glucocorticoid administration
10. Aromatase inhibitors

Reproduced with permission from Rizk B. *Ovarian Hyperstimulation Syndrome: Epidemiology, Prevention and Management.* Cambridge, UK, New York (2006) Cambridge University Press.

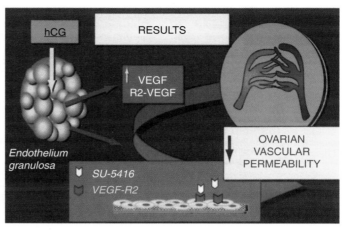

Fig. 37.20 VEGF receptor blockade in prevention of ovarian hyperstimulation syndrome.

In a recent prospective, randomized, controlled trial, Carizza et al. found that, in humans, cabergoline was beneficial in the prevention of early-onset, but not late-onset OHSS [37]. The authors examined 166 patients who had estradiol concentrations of more than 4000 pg/mL on the day of their hCG administration. On the day of oocyte retrieval, all of the patients were given 20 g of intravenous human albumin. These patients were then randomized into two groups. Group A ($n = 83$) were given 0.5 mg of cabergoline orally per day for 3 weeks, beginning the day after oocyte retrieval. Group B ($n = 83$) were not given any medication. In group A, none of the patients developed early OHSS while 9 patients developed late OHSS. In group B, 12 patients developed early OHSS while 3 patients developed late OHSS. The authors proposed that administration of cabergoline significantly diminished the risk of early OHSS ($P < 0.001$), but did not diminish the risk of late-onset OHSS.

Treatment of OHSS

Managing OHSS relies on the appropriate consideration of its severity as well as the presence or absence of complications [38]. The majority of patients who have mild or moderate OHSS are usually treated on an outpatient basis. The physician's comfort and the patient's reliability are essential determinants. Women with mild to moderate OHSS (grades A and B) can be treated in the IVF unit or hospital, as determined by the presence or absence of complications. Women who have severe OHSS (grade C) are often treated in hospital. Table 37.6 lists the indications for hospitalization.

Medical treatment for OHSS that a hospital can provide includes correction of circulatory volume as well as electrolyte imbalance (Fig. 37.23). For women who have developed thromboembolism or are at risk of developing thromboembolism, anticoagulation therapy is given. Currently, a more liberal manner of providing anticoagulation is available and diuretics should not be given to women with severe OHSS, except for women with pulmonary edema. Navot et al. have managed many cases of severe OHSS with albumin and Lasix and their experience should be reviewed for managing these critical patients [4].

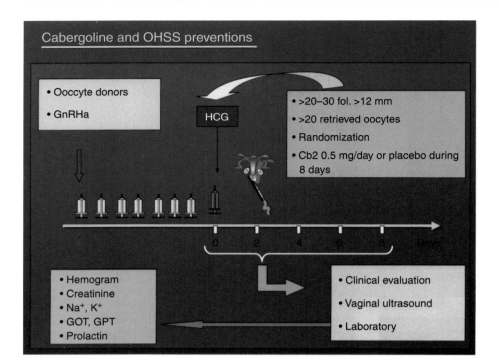

Fig. 37.21 Cabergoline and prevention of ovarian hyperstimulation syndrome.

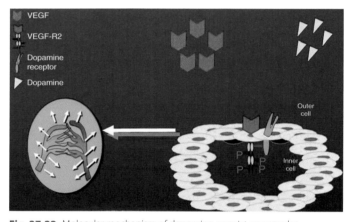

Fig. 37.22 Molecular mechanism of dopamine agonist on vascular permeability.

Table 37.6 Indications for hospitalization of patients with severe OHSS

1. Severe abdominal pain or peritoneal signs

2. Intractable nausea and vomiting that prevents ingestion of food and adequate fluids

3. Severe oliguria or anuria

4. Tense ascites

5. Dyspnea or tachypnea

6. Hypotension (relative to baseline), dizziness, or syncope

7. Severe electrolyte imbalance (hypernatremia, hyperkalemia)

Reproduced with permission from Rizk B. *Ovarian Hyperstimulation Syndrome: Epidemiology, Prevention and Management.* Cambridge, UK, New York (2006) Cambridge University Press.

To manage severe OHSS, the use of ultrasonography is also critical. In 1991, Rizk and Aboulghar proposed the use of ultrasound-guided ascitic fluid aspiration, performed either transvaginally or transabdominally, for tense ascites [38]. Aboulghar et al. observed that transvaginal aspiration improved patients' OHSS symptoms and renal function [39]. Increased intra-abdominal pressure can jeopardize venous return. Therefore, compromised cardiac output, renal edema, and possibly thrombosis may also result. With tense ascites and oliguria, the increased levels of creatinine, or hemoconcentration, that are non-responsive to medical therapy require the use of ultrasound-guided aspiration of ascitic fluid. There is a striking improvement in clinical symptoms (i.e. increase in urine output and creatinine clearance, decline in hematocrit, easing of dyspnea, and alleviation of abdominal discomfort), which supports this treatment approach as safe and particularly

beneficial [40]. Additionally, repeated transabdominal aspiration can be safely performed [41].

To examine the impact of repeated paracentesis on the pregnancy outcome of women with severe OHSS, Chen-Der et al. used color Doppler ultrasonography to study the effects of paracentesis on uterine hemodynamics and intraovarian hemodynamics [41]. In their study, seven pregnant women with tense ascites underwent 41 abdominal paracenteses while three pregnant women with pleural effusion had thoracocenteses performed. The authors measured PI and the maximum peak systolic velocity of both uterine and intraovarian arteries prior to and following each intervention. The mean PI of the uterine arteries declined significantly after paracentesis, although not after thoracocentesis. Additionally, the authors saw a decline in the uterine PI in 13 out of 14 (93%) paracenteses with fewer than 2500 mL of ascites drained as compared with 8 out of 13 (62%) who had more than 2500 mL of ascites drained.

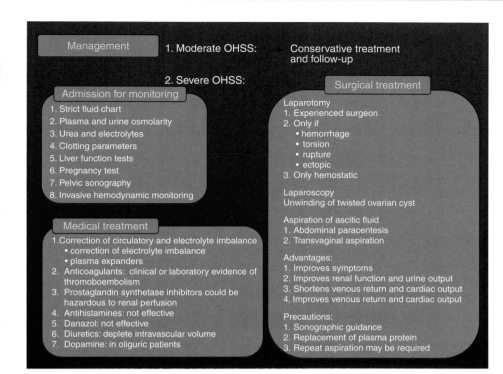

Fig. 37.23 Management of ovarian hyperstimulation syndrome.

Following paracentesis, no noteworthy changes in the intraovarian PI and mean peak systolic velocity in either group were present. Chen-Der et al. [41] noted that there was no difference in miscarriage rates between the two groups. On that basis, they proposed that repeated abdominal paracentesis in patients with severe OHSS increases uterine perfusion with no adverse effects on pregnancy outcome [39].

To decrease the need for paracentesis, Al-Ramahi et al. described three cases where the use of an indwelling peritoneal catheter was employed [42]. With ultrasound guidance, a closed-system Dawson–Mueller catheter with "simp-loc" locking design was inserted in the patient in order to allow non-stop drainage of the ascitic fluid. The authors proposed that, to manage severe OHSS, the nonstop drainage of ascitic fluid is better than repeated abdominal paracenteses.

Abuzeid et al. examined the effectiveness and safety of percutaneous pigtail catheter drainage to manage ascites that complicates severe OHSS [43]. A pigtail catheter inserted with ultrasound guidance and retained until drainage stopped was used. For most patients with OHSS, surgery should be refrained from, except in patients with ovarian torsion or hemorrhage.

Conclusion

In conclusion, ultrasonography is the cornerstone for prediction of OHSS, which is necessary for its prevention. The number of follicles during ovarian stimulation and the number of oocytes retrieved are both associated with increased risk of OHSS. Management of OHSS can also be made safer by the use of ultrasonography for treatment and follow-up.

References

1. Rabau E, Serr DM, David A, et al. Human menopausal gonadotropin for anovulation and sterility. *Am J Obstet Gynecol* 1967; **98**: 92–98.

2. Schenker JG, Weinstein D. Ovarian hyperstimulation syndrome: a current survey. *Fertil Steril* 1978; **30**: 255–268.

3. Golan A, Ron-El R, Herman A, et al. Ovarian hyperstimulation syndrome: an update review. *Obstet Gynecol Surv* 1989; **44**: 430–340.

4. Navot D, Bergh PA, Laufer N. Ovarian hyperstimulation syndrome in novel reproductive technologies: prevention and treatment. *Fertil Steril* 1992; **58**: 249–261.

5. Mozes M, Bogowsky H, Anteby E, et al. Thrombo-embolic phenomena after ovarian stimulation with human menopausal gonadotrophins. *Lancet* 1965; **2**: 1213–1215.

6. Rizk B. Classification of ovarian hyperstimulation syndrome. In: Rizk B (Ed.) *Ovarian Hyperstimulation Syndrome: Epidemiology, Pathophysiology, Prevention and Management.* Cambridge University Press; 2006: 1–9.

7. Serour G. Ovarian hyperstimulation syndrome In: Gerris J, Olivennes F, Delvigne A (Eds.) *Ovarian Hyperstimulation Syndrome.* London: Taylor and Francis; 2006.

8. Schenker JG. Ovarian hyperstimulation syndrome. In: Wallach EE, Zacur H (Eds.) *Reproductive Medicine and Surgery.* St. Louis: Mosby; 1996: 654.

9. Rizk B, Meagher S, Fisher AM. Ovarian hyperstimulation syndrome and cerebrovascular accidents. *Hum Reprod* 1990; **5**: 697–698.

10. Rizk B. Ovarian hyperstimulation syndrome. In: Studd J (Ed.) *Progress in Obstetrics and Gynecology,* Vol **11**. Edinburgh: Churchill Livingstone; 1993: 311–349.

11. Dahl-Lyons CA, Wheeler CA, Frishman GN, et al. Early and late presentation of the ovarian hyperstimulation syndrome: two distinct entities with different risk factors. *Hum Reprod* 1994; **9**: 792–799.

12. Mathur RS, Akande AV, Keay SD, et al. Distinction between early and late ovarian hyperstimulation syndrome. *Fertil Steril* 2000; **73**(5): 901–907.

13. Rizk B. Genetics of ovarian hyperstimulation syndrome. *Reprod Biomed Online* 2009; **19**(1): 14–27.

14. Rizk B, Aboulghar MA, Smitz J, Ron-El R. The role of vascular endothelial growth factor and interleukins in the pathogenesis of severe ovarian hyperstimulation syndrome. *Hum Reprod Update* 1997; **3**: 255–266.

15. Pellicer A, Albert C, Mercader A, et al. The pathogenensis of ovarian hyperstimulation syndrome: in vivo studies investigating the role of interleukin 1-β, interleukin-6 and vascular endothelial growth factor. *Fertil Steril* 1999; **71**: 482–489.

16. Rizk B, Smitz J. Ovarian hyperstimulation syndrome after superovulation for IVF and related procedures. *Hum Reprod* 1992; **7**: 320–327.

17. Delvigne A, Dubois M, Batteu B, et al. The ovarian hyperstimulation syndrome in in-vitro fertilization: a Belgian multicenter study. II. Multiple discriminant analytes for risk prediction. *Hum Reprod* 1993; **8**: 1361–1366.

18. Nagamani M, Chilvers R. Ultrasonography and diagnosis in polycystic ovary syndrome. In: Rizk B (Ed.) *Ultrasonography in Reproductive Medicine and Infertility*. Cambridge University Press; 2010: 75–80.

19. Fox R, Corrigan E, Thomas PA, Hull MG. The diagnosis of polycystic ovaries in women with oligo-amenorrhoea: predictive power of endocrine tests. *Clin Endocrinol* 1991; **34**: 127–131.

20. Danninger B, Brunner M, Obruca A, et al. Prediction of ovarian hyperstimulation syndrome of baseline ovarian volume prior to stimulation. *Hum Reprod* 1996; **11**: 1597–1599.

21. Lass A, Vassiliev A, Decosterd G, et al. Relationship of baseline ovarian volume to ovarian response in World Health Organization Group II anovulatory patients who underwent ovulation induction with gonadotropins. *Fertil Steril* 2002; **78**: 265–269.

22. Rizk B, Nawar MG. Ovarian hyperstimulation syndrome. In: Serhal P, Overton C (Eds.) *Good Clinical Practice in Assisted Reproduction*. Cambridge University Press; 2004: 146–166.

23. Rizk B. Complications of ovulation induction II. Ovarian hyperstimulation syndrome, ovarian torsion. In: Dickey RP, Brinsden PR, Pyrzak R (Eds.) *Manual of Intrauterine Insemination and Ovulation Induction*. Cambridge University Press; 2010: 152–160.

24. Tal J, Faz B, Samberg I, et al. Ultrasonographic and clinical correlates of menotrophin versus sequential clomiphene citrate: menotrophin therapy for induction of ovulation. *Fertil Steril* 1985; **4**: 342–349.

25. Blankstein J, Shalev J, Saadon T, et al. Ovarian hyperstimulation syndrome prediction by number and size of preovulatory ovarian follicles. *Fertil Steril* 1987; **47**: 597–602.

26. Kwee J, Elting M, Schats R, et al. Ovarian volume and antral follicle count for the prediction of low and hyper responders with in vitro fertilization. *Reprod Biol Endocrinol* 2007; **5**: 9.

27. Steward RG, Lan L, Shah AA, et al. Oocyte number as a predictor for ovarian hyperstimulation syndrome and live birth: an analysis of 256,381 in vitro fertilization cycles. *Fertil Steril* 2014 Apr; **101**(4): 967–973.

28. Moohan JM, Curcio K, Leoni M, et al. Low intraovarian vascular resistance: a marker for severe ovarian hyperstimulation syndrome. *Fertil Steril* 1997; **57**: 728–732.

29. Rizk B. Prevention of ovarian hyperstimulation syndrome: The Ten Commandments. Presented at the European Society of Human Reproduction and Embryology symposium, 1993, Tel Aviv, Israel, 1–2.

30. Rizk B. Prevention of ovarian hyperstimulation syndrome In: Rizk B (Ed.) *Ovarian Hyperstimulation Syndrome*. Cambridge University Press; 2006: 130–199.

31. Busso CE, Garcia-Velasco JA, Gomez R, et al. Ovarian hyperstimulation syndrome. In: Rizk B, Garcia-Velasco JA, Sallam H, Madrigiannakis A (Eds.) *Infertility and Assisted Reproduction*. Cambridge University Press; 2008: 243–257.

32. Garcia-Velasco JA, Zuniga A, Pacheco A, et al. Coasting acts through downregulation of VEGF gene expression and protein secretion. *Hum Reprod* 2004; **19**: 1530–1538.

33. Garcia-Velasco JA, Isaza B, Quea G, et al. Coasting for the prevention of ovarian hyperstimulation syndrome: much to do about nothing? *Fertil Steril* 2006; **85**: 547–554.

34. Gomez R, Simon C, Remohi J, et al. Vascular endothelial growth factor receptor-2 activation induces vascular permeability in hyperstimulated rate, and this effect is prevented by receptor blockade. *Endocrinology* 2002; **143**(11): 4339–4348.

35. Gomez R, Gonzalez-Izquierdo M, Zimmermann RC, et al. Low dose dopamine agonist administration blocks vascular endothelial growth factor (VEGF)-mediated vascular hyperpermeability without altering VEGF receptor 2-dependent luteal angiogenesis in a rat ovarian hyperstimulation model. *Endocrinology* 2006; **147**: 5400–5411.

36. Garcia-Velasco JA. How to avoid ovarian hyperstimulation syndrome: a new indication for dopamine agonists. *Reprod Bio Med Online* 2009; **18**(2): 71–75.

37. Carizza C, Abdelmassih VG, Abdelmassih S, et al. Cabergoline reduces the early onset of ovarian hyperstimulation syndrome: a prospective randomized study. *Reprod Bio Med Online* 2008; **17**(6): 751–755.

38. Rizk B, Aboulghar MA. Modern management of ovarian hyperstimulation syndrome. *Hum Reprod* 1991; **6**: 1082–1087.

39. Aboulghar MA, Mansour RT, Serour GI, et al. Ultrasonically guided vaginal aspiration of ascites in the treatment of ovarian hyperstimulation syndrome. *Fertil Steril* 1990; **53**: 933–935.

40. Rizk B, Aboulghar MA. Ovarian hyperstimulation syndrome. In: Aboulghar MA, Rizk, B (Eds.) *Ovarian Stimulation*. Cambridge University Press; 2011: 103–129.

41. Chen-Der C, Yang J, Chao K, et al. Effects of repeated abdominal paracentesis on uterine and intraovarian haemodynamics and pregnancy outcome in severe ovarian hyperstimulation syndrome. *Hum Reprod* 1998; **13**(8): 2077–2081.

42. Al-Ramahi M, Leader A, Claman P, et al. A novel approach to the treatment of ascites associated with ovarian hyperstimulation syndrome. *Hum Reprod* 1997; **12**: 2614–2616.

43. Abuzeid MI, Nassar Z, Massaad Z, et al. Pigtail catheter for the treatment of ascites associated with ovarian hyperstimulation syndrome. *Hum Reprod* 2003; **18**: 370–373.

Chapter

38

Self-operated endovaginal telemonitoring: using internet-based home monitoring of follicular growth in assisted reproduction technology

Jan Gerris

Summary

The need for serial vaginal sonographies to monitor ovarian stimulation for artificial reproductive technology (ART) treatments remains a major practical and organizational drawback for both patients and health care providers. This hampers access to treatment for many couples seeking treatment using IVF or renders it strenuous or expensive from an organizational point of view. It creates a high hidden cost when people have to travel frequently to have their sonograms made or have to plan a prolonged hotel stay near the center where oocyte retrieval and IVF embryology work takes place. We are currently introducing a method allowing patients and/or their partners or, if appropriate, midwives and nurses independent from highly specialized services to make vaginal sonographies at home or near the place where patients live. Specific software has been developed that can be installed on any portable PC or tablet PC. Current experience has shown that after initial teaching, many patients are prepared and competent to make and send video recordings to the center or the physician following them up. They can do this where and when it suits them best. Receipt of images is acknowledged by direct email. After analysis of the growing follicles and uterine lining, a structured response is sent to the patient, comprising dosing advice and next-step instructions. This simplification of the uncontested need to perform these follow-up sonographies, even if applicable to just a selected proportion of IVF patients, could fit in with the general tendency to make IVF more patient-centered and patient-friendly, to implement telemedicine and increase patient empowerment by supervised active participation to their treatment [1]. It opens up access to treatment for patients who live far from IVF centers.

The challenge: bringing new technology to the patient instead of bringing the patient to old technology

Initial attempts by the pioneers of IVF to obtain a pregnancy by in vitro fertilization and embryo transfer (IVF-ET) were conducted in a natural cycle. However, it was soon recognized that ovarian stimulation using injectable hormones was needed in order to obtain more oocytes and increase the chance for success by morphology-based embryo selection. This stimulation needs to be monitored in order to avoid under- or overstimulation as well as for optimal timing of egg retrieval. Since the mid-1980s, this has been done by making vaginal sonograms, whereby a probe is inserted into the vagina. This makes it possible to see the bladder, the uterus and ovaries (especially when stimulated), and the larger vessels of the pelvis. These sonograms are currently made by various care providers: gynecologists, reproductive nurses, radiologists, sonographers. Sonograms are often combined with serial measurements of serum estradiol. Traditionally, for monitoring of ovarian stimulation, women have to come to the center although nowadays, efforts are increasingly being made to bring patient-friendly IVF to the patient instead [1]. The Cochrane Library contains a review indicating that following up the follicular phase of an IVF/ICSI attempt by ultrasound alone does not yield results any different from attempts followed up by both ultrasound and hormone determinations [2], neither in terms of number of oocytes retrieved, nor pregnancies obtained, nor even the incidence of ovarian hyperstimulation syndrome (OHSS). This is not to say that in a case of threatening OHSS, hormone measurements may not be useful nor that measurements of serum progesterone may not be useful in deciding on the cryopreservation of all embryos and replacing them in subsequent natural or artificial cycles [3]. Self-operated endovaginal telemonitoring (SOET) can be combined with salivary determinations of estradiol, which are possible but have gone out of use because of the wide availability of serum estradiol determinations [4]. The goal of SOET is to facilitate the general implementation of ART, which does not exclude that hormone measurements can be performed if indicated.

We have explored the possibility for patients to perform these sonograms themselves and described some aspects of this approach in two early explorative papers [5,6]. It has become clear that many women and/or their partners are perfectly able to do this, if given appropriate teaching. In parallel, we have developed the software that makes it possible to record and send in a very simple way the sonogram video sequences.

Ultrasonography in Gynecology, ed. Botros R. M. B. Rizk and Elizabeth E. Puscheck. Published by Cambridge University Press. © Cambridge University Press 2015.

The need for women to visit the IVF clinic, their treating gynecologist, or another care provider near to the place where they live, in order to perform serial vaginal sonograms, thus falls away. No hard data exist regarding the average number of pre-oocyte-retrieval sonogram visits. It may vary substantially between centers and patients but ranges between two and seven or more. The total annual number of IVF/ICSI attempts amounts to around one million and is still rising. It is not exaggerating to add another one million of non-IVF/ICSI stimulations. This implies between eight and ten million annual sonograms for pre-ovulatory ART monitoring only or, for ~300 working days per year, a daily trek to the IVF clinic for 90 000 women! SOET starts from the principle that recording images using a vaginal probe is in itself an easy procedure, entailing no risks or health hazards. It has become pure routine and is a simple gesture that does not need to be performed by a highly specialized reproductive physician. In fact, these sonograms are already now often performed by other personnel, under the final supervision of reproductive specialists, who are remain responsible for the organization and for the interpretation of the measurements. Aiming at the same quality and personalized follow-up as "live sonograms," SOET thereby also reduces the heavy stress of busy consultations for intrinsically easy procedures. But SOET has more to it than just reducing the number of sonograms performed at a center. It can significantly increase access to treatment itself. Huge distances in large countries, whether they belong to the first, the second, or the third world, where sonography is not available within a reasonable distance from homes, decreases access to IVF/ICSI treatment for many couples who could benefit from it. This is the case in large developed societies, e.g. the USA, Australia, Canada, and other giant countries, but also in many countries in the developing world where assisted reproductive services are scarce though on the rise. The two major impediments to wide access to ART overtly identified are cost of treatment and legal limitations. Recent attention has been given to so-called "IVF in low-resource settings" to be implemented in third-world countries with poor access to treatment because of financial constraints. It is a noble intention of making subfertility a global issue because of its severe social consequences which can devastate a woman's life in some societies. High costs and legal obstacles indeed may hamper treatment. But we must recognize that limited access to ART treatment exists almost everywhere. This follows from the wide variation in the number of ART cycles per number of inhabitants between different countries [7], ranging from >2000 cycles/million inhabitants to just a few hundred cycles/million inhabitants as in the USA or a mere 20/million inhabitants in India. High access rates are usually observed in small countries, e.g. Denmark, Israel, and Belgium. Low access is observed in larger countries, where sheer distance, and/or the time needed to cover it, severely limit treatment utilization, even in high-resource settings. Whether it be the Australian outback, the American Midwest, the Russian steppes, the deep interior of rural India or China, or the more remote areas of many other countries, distance and/or the time needed to reach an expert sonographer plays a preponderant role in making ART a feasible option for many patients who need it.

A solution to the problem

To solve this problem, we have explored the idea to have patients perform their sonograms themselves (Fig. 38.1), after instruction by a midwife, a nurse-practitioner or an experienced sonography technician, using a small, reusable, safe, cheap, and easy-to-use customized device, allowing registration of real-time images under direct visual inspection of the patient or her partner. The instrument consists of a small portable PC or a tablet PC, to which a vaginal probe is connected using USB technology. Images can be sent with proper identification over the internet to the center where a care provider receives, stores, analyses, and interprets the images followed by a report, containing advice regarding the dose of gonadotropins to be self-injected during the following day(s), the timing for a subsequent sonogram, the precise timing of hCG injection and of oocyte retrieval. If extended to intrauterine insemination or freeze/thaw cycles after IVF, even in a natural cycle or after oral ovulation induction, planning of insemination or embryo replacement can be communicated. If needed, these self-operated endovaginal sonograms can be backed up by "live" sonograms in the center. The idea could work for IVF/ICSI cycles but it could be extended to non-IVF ovarian stimulation protocols using oral or intramuscular drugs.

It is *not* the idea to replace *all* vaginal sonography in the context of IVF, let alone *all* gynecological sonograms, by SOET. "Real-time" sonograms will always remain a very important tool in IVF. During a transitional phase of acceptance of SOET, and even if accepted, SOET will not replace "classical" sonograms made by a professional care provider in complicated cases, when abnormal images (cysts, hydrosalpinges, unexpected tumors, endometriosis, etc.) are observed, or on request from anxious patients. It is conceived in the first place to *alleviate* an abnormal amount of time-consuming, routine work and to allow patients living far from the center to make less demanding sacrifices. It may add to the clinical tools at our disposal to conduct judicious treatments in ART.

Potential advantages of self-operated endovaginal telemonitoring (SOET)

A comparison between the disadvantages of the present way of monitoring ovarian stimulation for ART and the advantages of self-operated home sonography is provided in Figs 38.2 and 38.3. The possibility for patients to perform vaginal sonograms themselves at home, or have sonograms made by a "flying nurse" or "flying midwife" or anyone who can operate the system, includes the following advantages. Patients need not come as often to the center to have sonograms performed. They will save time and money spent on petrol, car usage, train, or bus. They and their partners will avoid loss of income

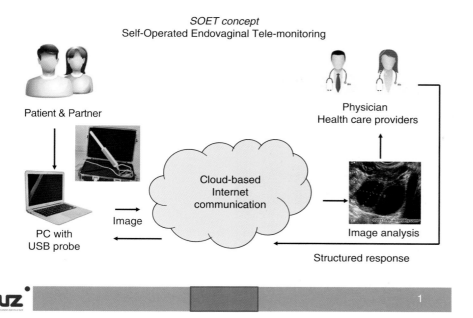

Fig. 38.1 The theoretical concept of self-operated endovaginal telemonitoring (SOET).

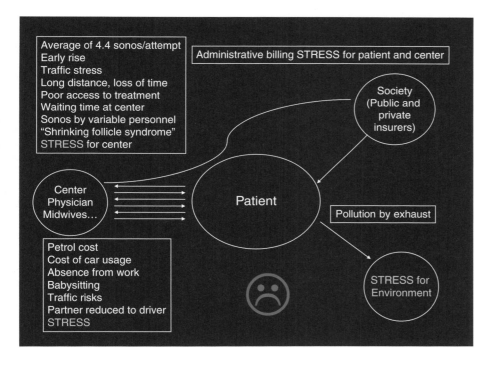

Fig. 38.2 Disadvantages of the traditional way of monitoring ovarian stimulations.

during working hours. Weekends and their important social and household functions will not be interrupted by half- or full-day trips to the center. Patients living far from centers and staying one or two weeks at a hotel near the center will avoid time-consuming and expensive stays. Centers performing IVF will be less crowded by patients only needing a sonogram, mainly during morning hours. Much of this work is at present poorly standardized, relies on authority-based algorithms and decision models, and could for that reason also benefit from improved quality. Indeed, measurements will be more standardized and reproducible and can be performed at ease, allowing

decreased inter-observer variation. Communication with the patient will be smoother, more complete, and more personalized and contain all information needed in print. Images sent can be accompanied by questions that can be answered properly and not in a hurry by a stressed doctor, midwife, or nurse. More time will thus be available for truly necessary interactions between doctors/nurses and patients who still need or prefer to interact in person with the staff at the center, reducing excessively long waiting lists for consultations of new patients. Treatments will become possible for patients who live far from the center, allowing them to show up just before egg retrieval

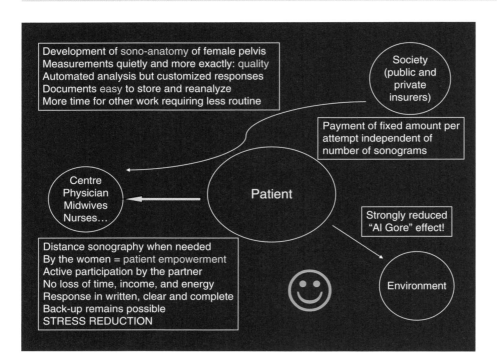

Fig. 38.3 Advantages of monitoring ovarian stimulations using self-operated endovaginal telemonitoring (SOET).

from theoretically anywhere in the world. SOET makes follow-up of ovarian stimulation easier not only for the patient, but for the physician as well, because images can be retrieved and analyzed at any time and in any place where wifi is available. It is a development that fits in a flat world where telemedicine has already found a firm place in other fields of medicine such as radiology, cardiology, and antenatal home cardio-tocography. Structured email communication regarding treatment instructions is undoubtedly in use in many centers. When combined with tele-sonography, it allows patients to be treated in the center of their choice and not necessarily in the center that happens to be closest to their home. It increases patient autonomy. It is conceivable that SOET could have an important place in large countries such as the BRIC countries, where women in rural areas could have sonograms made by a local trained care provider, using one single instrument for several patients, the data being sent with proper identification of patients to the nearest center where egg retrieval and laboratory phase will be conducted. In many of these large countries, patients nowadays simply have no access to treatment due to lack of services [8], although efforts are made to bring simple technology in an affordable way to the third world [9,10]. From the point of view of the center, there will be budgetary advantages: less high-end sonographic instruments have to be invested in; billing stress is reduced by using a fixed price per cycle instead of per sonography. The gain comes from avoiding loss of direct income and transportation cost, apart from more convenience and discretion for the patient and a stronger involvement of the partner, now often reduced to the role of driver.

There may be other, indirect but nevertheless equally important, advantages to SOET. One is the ecological effect. In our quickly changing climate, frequent traveling adds imperceptibly but substantially to using up limited energy resources and creating exhaust. The other is the sheer feeling of empowerment women and their partners may feel when participating actively in their treatment. The often exaggerated personalized contact with the treating physician, already diluted by the team aspect of ART, may be better served by using webcam-mediated personal contacts with the coordinating physician, once he or she is duly known and trusted by the patient. Sonograms can also be made or assisted by the partner who is in 50% of cases at the origin of the subfertility and in many cases will be more than happy to be able to participate in an active way in a treatment that involves his partner more than it does himself.

Clinical experience with SOET

To start with, we questioned 25 couples regarding their attitude towards SOET. Patients' and their partners' positive attitude towards a self-operated vaginal echography technology was highly enthusiastic. Perceived advantages were avoidance of frequent hospital visits, time loss, petrol cost and organizational stress, and the ease of treatment. There were no objections to introducing a device into the vagina. Most partners seemed to be willing to "help" in this regard, potentially replacing a strenuous patient–sonographer encounter by an intimate couple contact. All couples found no problem with basic computer use.

Second, we sought proof of concept using an experimental set-up within our own center. Twenty patients completed their attempt and all performed all sonograms themselves as requested. Images were sent over the hospital intranet as a proxy for the worldwide internet, stored at the receiving end and could be endlessly replayed for quiet measurement and analysis.

All agreed on a very positive experience, as did the midwives involved in this early phase of the study. We therefore conclude that patients' acceptance of self-echography and performance were high. The readiness and reliability of women to visualize their own internal genital organs, recognize the structures, in particular the thickening endometrium and the growing follicles, elicited great interest and cooperation and was highly successful. Relevant images were easily recognized as soon as early follicular development became visible. The need for a didactic reference document exhibiting the most relevant images (bladder, endometrium, follicles) was noted and opens a line for midwife research to standardize and optimize such a teaching tool as an adjunct to "sono-anatomy" of the female pelvis. Illustrations of typical images during treatment are offered to patients and a short movie illustrating the personalized teaching session given by a specialized midwife to each patient is presented.

At present, a prospective randomized trial is being conducted which compares clinical and laboratory outcomes between home sonography and in situ sonogram treatment cycles. This study includes an analysis of the alleged health–economic advantages of SOET, addressing all direct and indirect costs, including ecological, economic, and psychological aspects. Inclusion criteria are: age <41 years, ICSI, no poor response, two ovaries. We used a PC with vaginal probe and a specific web application. Study participants were given sonography training sessions at the center. Fifty-eight randomized patients completed their study cycle with SOET ($n = 29$; 1 drop-out) or non-SOET ($n = 29$); 19/78 (20%) eligible patients declined participation for different reasons. Patient characteristics (age, partner age, body mass index, smoking, treatment rank, anti-müllerian hormone) in SOET and non-SOET are comparable. Similar conception rates were obtained as well as a similar number of follicles >15 mm. The number of ova at ovum pick-up, the number of metaphase II oocytes, $\log_2$ of the number of metaphase II oocytes, the number of transferable embryos available at ET, the number of morphologically excellent embryos, and the number of embryos frozen were all comparable. With respect to patient-reported outcome, the SOET group showed a significantly higher feeling of empowerment and more partner participation than the non-SOET group; comparing SOET patients with their own historic controls in non-SOET attempts showed higher empowerment, partner participation, feeling of discretion, less stress, and a trend towards more contentedness. The health-economic analysis showed SOET cycles to have eight times less productivity loss, four to five times lower transportation cost, more than ten times lower sonogram and consultation costs, but higher personnel cost, probably linked to the extra time needed to follow the strict study protocol.

The preliminary results are thus in line with the non-inferiority hypothesis.

Conclusion

ICT applications are being used increasingly in medicine, creating a wholly new field of tele-medicine. Most of the time, tele-medicine is used to monitor chronic conditions, e.g. hypertension or diabetes, often reducing the need for patients to make frequent visits to the physician. It is also used to improve safety of treatments [11]. In ART, applications so far have been limited to gadgets without real impact on the way treatment is conducted. Of course, we all communicate with patients by phone or email [12]. Recently, there have been a number of developments at the high end of sonography in gynecology, e.g. methods for automatic volume calculation of follicles [13–15], the use of 3D measurement of follicles to determine the timing of hCG administration [16], and the introduction of algorithms to determine the risk of malignancy based on sonographic characteristics of a gynecologic tumor [17,18].

SOET is a low-end development that may fundamentally change the way we organize ovarian hyperstimulation. In selected patients, SOET works, offering practical advantages by empowering patients in urban Western settings, increasing and facilitating access to treatment in large countries, and allowing a disconnection between monitoring and laboratory facilities.

We recorded almost unanimous enthusiasm in all patients and their partners who performed sonograms at home for a further development of SOET as a tool to ease the burden and stress of monitoring follicular growth, due in part to the obstructed traffic in our megalopolitan societies.

We recommend, however, that like all innovative reproductive technologies, SOET should be subjected to thorough evaluation, including randomized clinical trials, in order to be able to assess its possibilities and risks, taking our full responsibility towards our patients [19].

References

1. Pennings G, Ombelet W. Coming soon to your clinic: patient-friendly ART. *Hum Reprod* 2007; **22**: 2075–2079.

2. Kwan I, Bhattacharya S, McNeil A. Monitoring of follicular phase using sonography alone versus sonography and serum determinations of estradiol. Cochrane Menstrual Disorders and Subfertility Group. Published online January 21, 2009. DOI:10.1002/1465 1858.CD005289.pub2.

3. Bosch E, Labarta E, Crespo J, et al. Circulating progesterone levels and ongoing pregnancy rates in controlled ovarian stimulation cycles for *in vitro* fertilization: analysis of over 4000 cycles. *Hum Reprod* 2010; **25**, 2092–2100.

4. Lu Y, Bentley GR, Gann PH, Hodges KR, Chatterton RT. Salivary estradiol and progesterone levels in conception and nonconception cycles in women: evaluation of a new assay for salivary estradiol. *Fertil Steril* 1998; **71**: 863–868.

5. Gerris J, Geril A, De Sutter P. Patient acceptance of self-operated endovaginal telemonitoring (SOET): a step towards more patient friendly ART? *Facts, Views and Vision in Ob/Gyn* 2009; **1**: 161–170.

6. Gerris J, de Sutter P. Self-operated endovaginal telemonitoring (SOET): a step towards more patient-centered ART? *Hum Reprod* 2010; **25**: 562–568.

7. Collins J. An international survey of the health economics of IVF and ICSI. *Hum Reprod. Update* 2002; **8**: 265–277.

8. Makuch MY, Bahamondes L. Barriers to access to infertility care and assisted reproductive technology within the public health sector in Brazil. *Facts, Views and Vision in Ob Gyn* 2012; **4**: 221–226.

9. Cooke I, Gianaroli L, Hovatta O, Trounson AO. On behalf of the Low Cost IVF Foundation. Affordable ART and the Third World: difficulties to overcome. *Hum Reprod* 2008; doi:10.1093/humrep/den145.

10. Ombelet W, Campo R, Frydman R, et al. The Arusha project: accessible infertility care in developing countries – a reasonable option? *Facts, Views and Vision in Ob Gyn* 2010; Monograph, 107–115.

11. Bates DW. Gawande AA. Improving safety with information technology. *N Engl J Med* 2003; **348**: 2526–2534.

12. Mimoni T, Margalioth EJ, Goldberg G, Weiss G, Geva-Eldar T, Tsafrir A. IVF treatment instructions transmitted via the internet: a preliminary experience. Annual Meeting of the ASRM, *Fertil Steril* 2003; **92**(Suppl): S62 (O-211).

13. Raine-Fenning NL, Jayaprakasan K, Clewes JS, Joergner I, Bonaki SD, Chamberlain S. SonoAVC: a novel method of automated volume calculation. *Ultrasound Obstet Gynecol* 2008; **31**: 691–696.

14. Raine-Fenning N, Jayaprakasan K, Chamberlain S, Devlin L, Priddle H, Johnson I. Automated measurements of follicular diameter: a chance to standardize? *Fertil Steril* 2009; **91**: 1469–1472.

15. Ata B, Seyhan A, Reinblatt L, Shalom-Paz E, Krishnamurty S, Tan SL. Comparison of automated and manual follicle monitoring in an unrestricted population of 100 women undergoing controlled ovarian stimulation for IVF. *Hum Reprod* 2011; **26**: 127–133.

16. Vandekerckhove F, Vansteelandt S, Gerris J, De Sutter P. Follicle measurements using sonography-based automated volume count accurately predict the yield of mature oocytes in in vitro fertilization/intracytoplasmic sperm injection cycles. *Gynecol Obstet Invest* 2013; **76**: 107–112.

17. Timmerman D, Testa AC, Bourne T, et al. Logistic regression model to distinguish between the benign and malignant adnexal mass before surgery: a multicenter study by the International Ovarian Tumor Analysis Group. *J Clin Oncol* 2005, **23**: 8794–8801.

18. Timmerman D, Testa AC, Bourne T, et al. Simple ultrasound-based rules for the diagnosis of ovarian cancer. *Ultrasound Obstet Gynecol* 2008; **31**: 681–690.

19. Dondorp W, de Wert G. Innovative reproductive technologies: risks and responsibilities. *Hum Reprod* 2011; **26**: 1604–1608.

Index

Note: page numbers in *italics* refer to figures and tables